Chest Physical Therapy and Pulmonary Rehabilitation

An Interdisciplinary Approach

Second Edition

CHEST PHYSICAL THERAPY AND PULMONARY REHABILITATION
An Interdisciplinary Approach
SECOND EDITION

Donna L. Frownfelter, P.T., R.R.T.

Masters Candidate in Community and Organizational Development
Loyola University of Chicago
Assistant Director, Respiratory Care Services
Rush-Presbyterian-St. Luke's Medical Center
Instructor, Internal Medicine
Rush Medical College
Instructor, Programs in Physical Therapy
Northwestern University Medical School
Chicago, Illinois

Illustrations by
Cheryl Haugh
Kurt Peterson

Photography by
Joseph A. Ficner, Jr.
Mike Horvath
Robert Walker

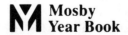

**Mosby
Year Book**

St. Louis   Baltimore   Boston   Chicago   London   Philadelphia   Sydney   Toronto

A Year Book Medical Publishers imprint of Mosby-Year Book, Inc.

Mosby-Year Book, Inc., 11830 Westline Industrial Drive, St. Louis, MO 63146.

4 5 6 7 8 9 0 C M 91

Library of Congress Cataloging-in-Publication Data

Chest physical therapy and pulmonary rehabilitation.

Includes bibliographies and index.
1. Chest—Diseases—Treatment. 2. Physical therapy. 3. Lungs—Diseases—Patients—Rehabilitation. 4. Respiratory therapy. I. Frownfelter, Donna L. [DNLM: 1. Lung Diseases—rehabilitation. 2. Lung Diseases—therapy. 3. Physical Therapy. 4. Respiratory Therapy. 5. Thorax. WF 145 C525]
RC941.C575   1987   617'.54062   86-28153
ISBN 0-8151-3333-2

Sponsoring Editor: Stephany S. Scott
Manager, Copyediting Services: Frances M. Perveiler
Copyeditor: Francis A. Byrne
Production Project Manager: Max Perez
Proofroom Supervisor: Shirley E. Taylor

With Love
to
David, Lauren, Daniel, and Kristin

Contributors

ROBERT BERRY, R.N.
Staff Nurse, Surgical Intensive
Care Unit, Loyola University
Medical Center, Maywood,
Illinois

**LINDA D. CRANE,
M.M.Sc., P.T.**
Associate Professor, Division of
Physical Therapy, University of
New England, Biddeford, Maine,
Board Certified
Cardiopulmonary Specialist

**ELIZABETH DEAN, Ph.D.,
M.C.P.A.**
Associate Professor, School of
Rehabilitation Medicine,
University of British Columbia,
Vancouver, British Columbia,
Canada

**CAROL DICKMAN, P.T.,
R.R.T.**
Consultant, Home Care, Chicago,
Illinois

**DONNA L.
FROWNFELTER, P.T.,
R.R.T.**
Masters Candidate in Community
and Organizational Development,
Loyola University of Chicago;
Assistant Director, Respiratory
Care Services, Rush-Presbyterian-
St. Luke's Medical Center;
Instructor, Internal Medicine,
Rush Medical College; Instructor,
Programs in Physical Therapy,
Northwestern University Medical
School, Chicago, Illinois

WILLY E. HAMMON, P.T.
Chief, Rehabilitative Services,
Oklahoma Memorial Hospital,
Oklahoma City, Oklahoma

**LYN HOBSON, P.T.,
R.R.T.**
Clinical Coordinator, Respiratory
Care Services, Rush-Presbyterian-
St. Luke's Medical Center,
Chicago, Illinois

LUDI ISAAC, B.S.N., R.N.
Medical Chest P.T. Coordinator,
Respiratory Care Services, Rush-
Presbyterian-St. Luke's Medical
Center, Chicago, Illinois

THOMAS JOHNSON, M.D.
Associate Professor in
Radiological Sciences, University
of Oklahoma Health Sciences
Center, Oklahoma City,
Oklahoma

**KIM LITWACK, N.D.,
Ph.D., R.N.**
Unit Leader, Post Anesthesia
Recovery, Rush-Presbyterian-St.
Luke's Medical Center, Chicago,
Illinois

MARY MASSERY, P.T.
Consultant and Lecturer,
Chicago, Illinois

**MARY MATHEWS, B.S.,
R.N., C.C.R.N., R.R.T.**
Neonatal and Pediatrics Chest
P.T., Coordinator, Respiratory
Care Services, Rush-Presbyterian-
St. Luke's Medical Center,
Chicago, Illinois

**LISA SIGG MENDELSON,
M.S.N., R.N.**
Teacher/Practitioner, Post
Anesthesia Recovery, Instructor,
Rush-Presbyterian-St. Luke's
Medical Center, Chicago, Illinois

**ELS MINNIGH, M.Ed.,
P.T.**
Consultant and Lecturer,
Chicago, Illinois

**CASSANDRA JAHNTZ
PECARO, R.R.T.**
Former Director, Respiratory
Rehabilitation, Illinois Masonic
Hospital, Chicago, Illinois

**MAUREEN FOGEL
PERLSTEIN, M.P.H., P.T.,
C.R.T.T.**
Certified ASPO Lamaze
Instructor (ACCE), Florida
Hospital, Orlando, Florida;
Healthsouth Rehabilitation, Inc.,
Winter Park, Florida

**ARTHUR PRANCAN,
Ph.D.**
Associate Professor, Department
of Pharmacology, Rush
University, Rush-Presbyterian-St.
Luke's Medical Center, Chicago,
Illinois

**ANNE R. SMITH, P.T.,
R.R.T.**
Consultant, Home Care, Physical
Therapy, Oak Park, Illinois

**MAUREEN SHEKLETON,
D.N.Sc., R.N.**
Assistant Professor of Nursing,
College of Nursing of Rush
University, Practitioner/Teacher,
Department of OR and Surgical
Nursing, Rush-Presbyterian-St.
Luke's Medical Center, Chicago,
Illinois

CYNTHIA WEBSTER, B.S.R.
Ph.D. Candidate in Educational Psychology, Rehab Consultant to Delta School District, Instructor in Human Development to the Faculty of Education, Vancouver University of British Columbia, British Columbia, Canada

JUDY AMEEN WILCHYNSKI, M.S., P.T.
Formerly Beth Israel Hospital, Physical Therapy Department, Boston, Massachusetts

Forewords

Chest physical therapy and pulmonary rehabilitation are essential forms of therapy for a large segment of our medical population. Donna Frownfelter published the first edition of this excellent text on chest physical therapy and pulmonary rehabilitation in 1978. Since then, many significant changes have occurred in our care of pulmonary patients. Simultaneously, there have been dramatic changes in the economics of health care. This second edition of *Chest Physical Therapy and Pulmonary Rehabilitation* follows the excellent tradition established by the first edition.

This edition has undergone major revision. Every chapter is reorganized with new information, and updated bibliographies are provided. There are major revisions in the chapters on chest assessment, pulmonary rehabilitation, cardiopulmonary pharmacology, review of respiratory anatomy and physiology, cardiac anatomy, and physiology.

Three new chapters are included that deal with the physical therapy approach to respiratory rehabilitation of the patient with neurologic deficits. These are especially important chapters that present important information on patients with spinal cord injuries and neuromuscular weakness. New chapters on inspiratory muscle fatigue and physical therapy and monitoring systems in the ICU are also included, as is an important chapter on patient education.

Physical therapists, respiratory therapists, and nurses who work with respiratory dysfunction patients will find this book useful when working with neonatal, geriatric, critically ill, and pulmonary rehabilitation patients.

In summary, this is an extensively revised book that deals with the advances that have taken place in the last decade and their effect on the patient who requires chest physical therapy and pulmonary rehabilitation. This is certainly a welcome addition to our knowledge on this subject.

ROGER C. BONE, M.D.
THE RALPH C. BROWN PROFESSOR
AND CHAIRMAN OF MEDICINE
CHIEF, SECTION OF PULMONARY
AND CRITICAL CARE MEDICINE
RUSH-PRESBYTERIAN-ST. LUKE'S MEDICAL CENTER
CHICAGO, ILLINOIS

The tremendous growth in the area of cardiopulmonary medicine has presented new horizons and challenges for the physical therapist and allied health professional. The areas of critical care therapy, home care therapy, and pulmonary rehabilitation have necessitated the development of new techniques, procedures, and even equipment.

The revised version of *Chest Physical Therapy and Pulmonary Rehabilitation* provides the practitioner with the content and focus taken by the profession. Each revised chapter includes new treatment approaches and updated bibliographies with current research to support the inclusions, as well as illustrations that add an exciting dimension to the book.

Several contributing authors representing a wide spectrum of skills have given the text a sophisticated approach to problem-solving and clinical management. The chapters on critical care management, written by our Canadian colleague, Elizabeth Dean, enhances the team approach while giving exposure to international methodologies. The new chapters on neuromuscular respiratory rehabilitation address the current problems of patients with multiple diagnoses and the difficulty in establishing treatment goals.

This book once again provides a quality teaching tool for the physical therapist and allied health professionals. The editor and contributing authors should be proud of the role they have taken in shaping the future of pulmonary care.

CATHERINE M. E. CERTO, PH.D., P.T.
ASSISTANT PROFESSOR, PHYSICAL THERAPY
NORTHEASTERN UNIVERSITY
BOSTON, MASSACHUSETTS
CHAIRMAN, CARDIOPULMONARY SECTION
AMERICAN PHYSICAL THERAPY ASSOCIATION

Preface to the First Edition

This book is intended to be used as an instructional and practical guide for physical therapists, respiratory therapists, and nurses. It is meant as a comprehensive clinical means of approaching the respiratory patient. We have included various additional information (from disease entities to a review of respiratory therapy for nurses and physical therapists) in order to have a more comprehensive approach to total patient care. Our approach to this topic is that all therapists and nurses working with the respiratory patient can and should utilize the basic techniques of chest physical therapy with the respiratory patient for optimum care. We are sharing information and ideas with that end in mind.

The physical therapist should be an instructor and consultant in the application of chest physical therapy as well as a participant in patient treatment. Nurses and respiratory therapists desire proper instruction and guidance and form the backbone of the care team. It is only through coordinated and total effort that optimal respiratory care can be achieved.

The preparation of this manuscript is due to the efforts of numerous individuals. The list of thank-yous is extensive. Special notice must be paid to Rush-Presbyterian-St. Luke's Medical Center, a progressive and dynamic institution which encourages and allows such endeavors as this book to take place. The administrative staff is to be highly commended. Mrs. Alla Mae Davis and Mr. Roy White have been extremely helpful and supportive in their administration of our chest physical therapy departmental affairs. Their support has enabled our department to expand and flourish over the last four years. Our past medical director, Dr. Richard Hughes, and present director, Dr. Robert Carton, have given us the ability to grow both professionally and personally. Drs. Ben Carasso and Peter Werner, as well as Doctor Carton, have added much input and constructive criticism as they reviewed the manuscript. Dr. Richard Hughes reviewed and made several suggestions for the chapter on pulmonary rehabilitation. The experience of working with Dr. Hughes in rehabilitation was among the highlights of my professional career. I learned more about sensitivity to patients and individual treatment planning during this time than at any other point in my career. I thank the patients with whom we worked under a grant from the Scholl Foundation. Group studies as well as individual programs proved to be a tremendous learning experience and a great opportunity.

I am grateful for the fine work from the contributors. All contributors either work with or have been employed by our department (with the exception of Dr. Thomas Johnson). They are all well experienced in their own rights and continue to grow and expand their professional careers, either at Rush or at other institutions. It has been a pleasure working with and knowing each one.

Mr. Willy Hammon, R.P.T., wishes to include special acknowledgments: I am very grateful to Thomas H. Johnson, M.D., Associate Professor in Radiological Sciences of the University Hospital and Clinics, for the chest roentgenograms, and to Jacqueline J. Coalson, Ph.D., Professor of Pathology of the University of Oklahoma Health Sciences Center, for the photograph used in the chapter on pathophysiology of chronic pulmonary disease. I wish to thank David C. Levin, M.D., Assistant Professor of Medicine, the Oklahoma University Health Sciences Center, for his critical review of that material, and to express my deep appreciation to Suzanne M. Brown, R.P.T., Director of Rehabilitative Services, and Suzanne Hankinson for their understanding and invaluable help in the preparation of that chapter.

We have had the privilege of working with an outstanding medical illustrator, Cheryl Haugh, whose creative ideas and direct illustrations have brought the text to life. She has been patient and cooperative above and beyond the call of duty; for this we are extremely grateful.

The illustrations in the pediatric chapter were nicely prepared by John E. McClusky.

The photography was done by Robert Walker. We appreciate his work and cooperation.

Thanks to Dr. Anthony J. Schmidt, Professor and Chairman of the Department of Anatomy, Rush University, College of Health Sciences, for assistance in our questions on anatomy.

Special thanks go to the members of our department who have shown great tolerance as well as help and constructive criticism during the time of this manuscript preparation. They often took on additional work and helped in numerous ways. Thanks especially to our three "models," Pat Adney, R.P.T., Tom Lee, R.R.T., and Tim Olsen, C.R.T.T., R.R.T., for posing for several drawings. A special thanks to Debi Swantz, R.P.T., for help in research and midnight typing. Steve Ray, R.R.T., R.N., helped in research for the chapter on clinical assessment.

The manuscript preparation was the work of three fine secretaries, Rose Harris, Jeanne Andrews, and Lola Turner.

Carol Speck made a great contribution in the final preparation. She did a fine job as well as being a great neighbor and friend who offered much encouragement and help during this project.

Penny Randel has efficiently proofread and constructively criticized all aspects of the manuscript. She was most helpful and considerate in her comments.

One of the biggest thanks goes to Pat Wilson, who cares for our daughter, Lauren. She has provided loving care to give me time to prepare this manuscript. She's one in a million!

Thanks to all our families and friends who have followed this through for two years. I am sure they are as happy as we are to have completed "The Book."

Above all, I thank God for the strength and peace of mind to finish this undertaking. He is truly "a Friend that sticketh closer than a brother."

I am most grateful to my husband, David, who has been my greatest supporter all through physical therapy school and respiratory therapy training. He is a truly liberated husband who is able to help in any way necessary. Without him this project would have never succeeded. Thanks also to my dear daughter, Lauren, who has opened up a whole new world of love and happiness. She has helped me rediscover the joys of playing under tables, crawling in boxes, pulling out pans, and walking barefoot through the grass. She also posed for the pictures in the pediatric chapter.

DONNA L. FROWNFELTER, P.T., R.R.T.

Preface to the Second Edition

There have been many changes professionally and personally since the first edition was released. Health care seemed to flourish until about 1984, when many economic changes and realities became apparent in hospitals. Nationwide costs for hospital care increased 617% from 1965 to 1980. The gross national product for hospital care rose from 2% to 3.8%. Medicare expenditures were $4.5 billion in 1970 and $22.8 billion in 1980. The government began to intervene to prevent the continued escalation of costs. In 1983, Medicare introduced a system of prospective payment (PPS) for hospitals. This system is based on diagnostic related groupings (DRGs). In a PPS, payment is determined before services are rendered by DRG classification. It is obvious that the fewer services the patient receives, the less cost to the patient's bill. If the hospital costs are less than the PPS funds allocated, a profit will be realized. On the other hand, if the hospital costs are more than the allotment, there will be a loss to the hospital.

Many significant changes have ensued in hospital staffing. There have been layoffs and decreased patient care. Nurses often have more patients than before, and allied health fields may be cut back to save the salary expenses. Interestingly, some physical therapy colleagues have increased positions and increased treatment of cardiopulmonary patients that are acutely ill. P.T. helps postoperative patients to be discharged more quickly from the hospital and helps to prevent postoperative pneumonia and atelectasis, which could add days to the patient's bill.

Other institutions such as ours have tried to have nurses do the routine chest P.T., with a core group of chest P.T. consultants teaching the nurses, evaluating and setting up treatment plans, and coordinating patient care with the patient's primary care nurse.

The roles of the health care team are in a state of change. As responsibilities for chest P.T. may vary from each facility, these techniques need to be learned by all working with patients with respiratory dysfunction.

Many thanks go to all the contributors and their families and friends for support. We have been excited about the new chapters and the opportunity to work with Canadian physiotherapy colleagues, Elizabeth Dean and Cynthia Webster. It has broadened the perspective of the book tremendously.

I am also especially excited about the information from Mary Massery on the treatment of secondary pulmonary dysfunction. I have never seen such good material used in such a practical clinical manner. Practitioners have been waiting for this information for a long time!

The new photography was well done by Mike Horvath and Joseph Ficner, Jr. Willy Hammon and Mary Massery provided the photography for their chapters. The new artwork is by Kurt Peterson. All were great to work with and are very talented in their respective fields.

Special thanks to Maxine Higgins and Alicia Griffey for their excellent preparation of the manuscript and attention to the details.

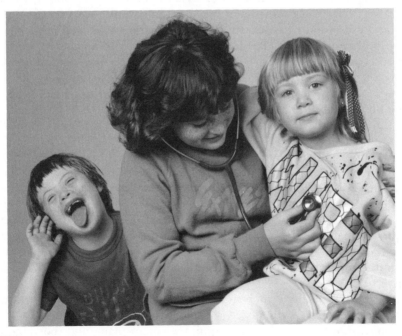

FIG 1.
Now there are three!

Thanks to my sister, Jan, for helping with my child care needs. Now there are three! (See Fig 1.) Their pictures may be spotted in the chest assessment, pediatric, and postural drainage chapters. Yes, they *are* characters!

My family has continued to be a wonderful support source. My husband, David, has always encouraged me and helps me know when I've taken on too much—which seems frequent lately. He has strong shoulders to lean on during book-writing times as well as during the usual chaos of life.

Lauren, Daniel, and Kristin keep me in perspective of life and full of hugs. I can't imagine my life without them. Dull is not in my vocabulary. Thanks kids!

Above all, thank you, Lord, for the strength to complete this task. As the poem "Footsteps in the Sand" states, "During the times of deepest pain and sorrow, You carried me."

DONNA L. FROWNFELTER, P.T., R.R.T.

Introduction

It is interesting to trace the historical beginnings of chest physical therapy and point to several important people and events. Winifred Linton, from England, a nurse who served in many overseas campaigns in World War I, became very much aware of respiratory problems and complications. Following the war, she entered physical therapy training, which she finished in 1921. The 1930s found Miss Linton working a great deal with thoracic surgeons and postoperative patients. In 1934 she went to the famous Brompton Hospital and developed techniques for localized breathing exercises. During World War II, she taught the techniques to both physical therapists and young surgeons. Retiring in 1946, she continued to be clinically active until her death in 1953. In an excerpt from her personal letters, she summarizes the roles of chest physical therapy and of the practitioner:

> To prevent these deformities from occurring, preoperative treatment is all-important. The patient's confidence must be gained and his willing cooperation assured. Treatment should be given at least two weeks before an operation. Success in major surgical disciplines is the product of integrated teamwork, and in considering the role of the physiotherapist in a thoracic team, it is of some historical interest to determine at what stage she became an integral part of the team.

By 1948, chest physical therapy was well recognized (at least in England and the Commonwealth). T. Holmes Sellar included the following in a lecture that year:

> The accepted position of chest surgery as a specialty has been largely due to the cooperation and establishment of well-balanced chest teams or units. Among the integral parts of the team, the part of the physiotherapist is an important member, being largely responsible for restoration of lung function after illness in an operation.

In 1949, Mr. Sellar suggested the "thoracic physiotherapist" should be considered a specialist in his own right.

Postural drainage seemed to begin in a crude form in the 1930s. H. P. Nelson did much to make it a more specialized technique. In 1946, *The Anatomy of the Bronchial Tree* by R. C. Brock was published. This allowed therapists to learn to drain *specific* lung segments in various postural drainage positions.

Several specific major contributors have been cited for work in these early periods; among them are Miss Winnifred Thacker, Miss Reed, Miss Storey, Miss Evans, and Miss MacDowell. The latter two published a paper, one of the first, on *Physiotherapy and Cardiovascular Surgery*. It is an excellent description of the art in cardiac surgery and therapy at the time.

In the United States, chest physical therapy was not practiced as a specialty for many years. A few therapists aware of the techniques used at the Brompton Hospital (or instructed by foreign-trained physical therapists) began to perform modified chest physical therapy treatments in the 1940s during the polio epidemics. Such treatments were still not widely used and techniques were inhibited due to the negative pressure tank ventilators. The development of positive pressure ventilators helped make the patient more accessible for chest therapy treatment.

The basic practice and techniques of chest physical therapy did not greatly change through the 1960s. In the 1960s the development of inhalation therapy was on the rise. With the development of the use of artificial airways, positive pressure ventilators and new surgical procedures, a more aggressive form of therapy for postoperative care of the critically ill patient was necessary. In the late 1960s and 1970s, interest in chest physical therapy increased. Many schools of physical therapy began to include and expand their courses dealing with chest physical therapy.

A sad commentary must be made that at this time many American physical therapy schools have paid little attention to chest physical therapy. During the polio epidemics, attention had been paid to acute care which included respiratory physical therapy. Since then (approximately the late 1950s), physical therapy has not responded to the needs of the critically ill patient. Many graduate physical therapists feel inadequate or fearful and prefer not to treat respiratory patients. Of course, it is much easier to say, "Let respiratory therapy do it!" There are tremendous problems in that type of thinking! Many respiratory therapists lack the background and level of expertise in evaluation and muscle reeducation, chest mobilization, and therapeutic exercise to completely take over the respiratory patient, nor do they wish to take on *more work and responsibility*. Most respiratory therapists desire the chest physical therapist's skill and expertise in teaching, and in many cases also actual treatment of the critically ill or more involved patients. Physical therapists specializing in chest disorders should be available and working with nurses and respiratory therapists at least as consultants and teachers for therapy programs.

There are many short courses now available to update the physical therapist's skills in dealing with respiratory patients, or therapists can spend time working with other chest physical therapy centers. The physical therapist's approach and background may be easily adapted to treat the respiratory patient. Respiratory therapists have tremendous responsibilites in dealing with the critically ill patients. They are able in most cases to perform the basics of chest physical therapy quite well. However, due to the difference in training between the two fields and time constraints, the physical therapist may concentrate on patient evaluation, muscle retraining, and exercise. The respiratory therapist also does much that the physical therapist cannot perform. This should enable us to see our mutual needs and areas for cooperation and overlapping skills.

The physical therapist has now become an important member of the respiratory care team. The scope of practice moved from treating pre- and postoperative patients to include patients with pneumonia, ventilatory failure, after myocardial infarction, trauma, neurologic and spinal cord disorders, and the critically ill. In the late 1960s, the concept of pulmonary rehabilitation was stressed.

Pulmonary rehabilitation programs developed a team approach in the 1970s with the involvement of respiratory therapists (no longer called "inhalation therapists") and nurses as well as physical therapists. There is also an important supportive team including occupational therapy, social service, vocational rehabilitation, consulting physicians and psychologists as well as family and friends. There seems to be a trend toward increasing outpatient care, especially for rehabilitation programs. Ideally, a hospital-based program with the transition to continued home care and outpatient facilities is necessary. Patients are being trained to care for themselves at home, checking and consulting with physicians and therapists on a regular basis.

The future seems unlimited for expanding chest physical therapy services. Neonatal centers are opening and flourishing. Therapists can handle the most critically ill patients with skill and expertise. Teaching and training respiratory care practitioners and nurses provide a total and coordinated program. Physical therapy training must be in more depth. Patient education is being expanded. The therapist needs to be a consultant to national organizations dealing with patients with respiratory ailments as well as to the community at large. Research needs to be done to determine how and why the techniques work as well as to find new ways to accomplish goals of bronchial hygiene, breathing exercise, and rehabilitation. New areas must be explored: the use of biofeedback, transcutaneous nerve stimulators (TNS) to relieve pain, increased coordination of chest physical therapy with respiratory care, and patient education. We should be aware of preventive lung care and determine the role we may play. The possibilities are unlimited.

In 1976, the American Physical Therapy Association (APTA) formed a cardiopulmonary section. It is considering the topic of and criteria for specialization in cardiopulmonary physical therapy. This organization will no doubt greatly improve the quality of and interest in the field as well as patient care. The coordination of medical services needs to be optimal in order for the patient to receive the best respiratory care. Nurses, therapists, physicians, and patients need to learn how to work together effectively as a unit for this to be accomplished. Nurses are utilizing the general chest therapy techniques as a part of their patients' total care plans. Respiratory care practitioners are becoming well versed in techniques and their applications. Several studies have questioned the use of intermittent positive pressure breathing (IPPB) and have caused many respiratory therapy departments to look to chest physical therapy as a replacement for IPPB. Whatever the reason, chest physical therapy in a coordinated fashion is becoming more popular and will undoubtedly be seen as a turning point to better total respiratory care.

In 1985, the Cardiopulmonary Section, now over 700 members strong in the United States, became the first section of the American Physical Therapy Association to develop and administer the first Board Speciality Examination in Cardiopulmonary Physical Therapy. This exam recognizes those physical therapists with advanced competency in cardiopulmonary physical therapy. It has been exciting to be an active member in the section as program chairman for four years and now as vice chairman of the section. It is wonderful to work with such high-quality, dedicated colleagues. I sincerely invite all physical therapists with interest in cardiopulmonary physical therapy to become active in the section.

Where will the future go with DRGs, PPOs, MBOs and all the other new abbreviations we've learned over the last 2 years? It is anyone's guess! However, our goal must always be to strive for the highest quality care in light of the need for cost-efficient management. Let's go for it!

DONNA L. FROWNFELTER, P.T., R.R.T.

Contents

PART ONE

Lung Function in Health and Disease

1

Review of Respiratory Anatomy

Lyn Hobson, P.T., R.R.T.

Elizabeth Dean, Ph.D., M.C.P.A.

This chapter represents the anatomy of the respiratory system including the skeletal features of the thoracic cavity, the muscles of respiration, and the anatomy of the tracheobronchial tree and the lung parenchyma. An understanding of the respiratory system is fundamental to the assessment and treatment of the chest in physical therapy.

THORAX

The bony thorax covers and protects the principal organs of respiration and circulation, as well as the liver and the stomach (Figs 1–1 and 1–2). The posterior surface is formed by the 12 thoracic vertebrae and the posterior part of the 12 ribs. The anterior surface is formed by the sternum and the costal cartilage. The lateral surfaces are formed by the ribs. At birth, the thorax is nearly circular, but during childhood and adolescence it becomes more elliptical, until in adulthood it is wider from side to side than from front to back.

Sternum

The sternum, or breast bone, is a flat bone with three parts—the manubrium, the body and the xiphoid process. The manubrium is the widest and thickest bone of the sternum. Its upper border is scalloped by a

3

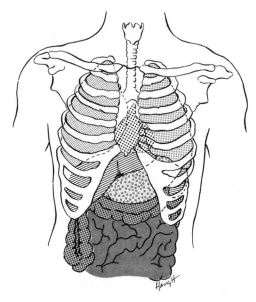

FIG 1–1.
The relationship of the bony thorax and lungs to the abdominal contents (anterior view).

central jugular notch, which can be palpated, and two clavicular notches, which house the clavicles. Its lower border articulates with the upper border of the body at a slight angle, the sternal angle or angle of Louis. This angle can be easily palpated and is a landmark located between thoracic vertebrae T4 and T5 and on a level with the second costal cartilages. The bifurcation of the trachea into the right and left main-stem bronchi also occurs at the sternal angle. The manubrium and body are joined by fibrocartilage which may ossify in later life.

The body of the sternum is twice as long as the manubrium. It is a relatively thin bone, easily pierced by needles for bone marrow aspirations. The heart is located beneath and to the left of the lower third of the body of the sternum. Though attached by cartilage to the ribs, this portion of the sternum is flexible and can be depressed without breaking. This maneuver is used, with care, in closed cardiac massage to artificially circulate blood to the brain and extremities. The lower margin of the body is attached to the xiphoid process by fibrocartilage. This bone is the smallest of the three parts of the sternum and usually fuses with the body of the sternum in later life.

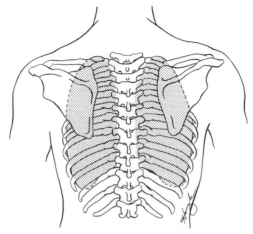

FIG 1–2.
The relationship of the lungs to the bony thorax (posterior view).

Ribs

A large portion of the bony thoracic cage is formed by 12 ribs located on either side of the sternum. The first seven ribs connect posteriorly with the vertebral column and anteriorly through costal cartilages with the sternum. These are known as the *true* ribs. The remaining five ribs are known as the *false* ribs. The first three have their cartilage attached to the cartilage of the rib above. The last two are free or floating ribs. The ribs increase in length from the first to the seventh rib, and then decrease to the 12th rib. They also increase in obliquity until the ninth rib and then decrease in obliquity to the 12th rib.

Each rib has a small head and a short neck that articulate with two thoracic vertebrae. The shaft of the rib curves gently from the neck to a sudden sharp bend, the angle of the rib. Fractures frequently occur at this site. A costal groove is located on the lower border of the shaft of the ribs. This groove houses the intercostal nerves and vessels. Chest tubes and needles are inserted above the ribs and to avoid these vessels and nerves. Each rib is separated from the ribs by the intercostal spaces which contain the intercostal muscles.

MOVEMENTS OF THE THORAX

The frequency of movement of the bony thorax joints is greater than that of almost any other combination of joints in the body. Two types

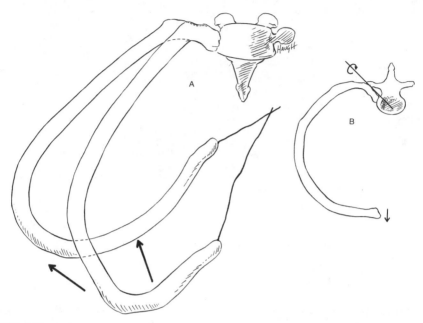

FIG 1–3.
The movements of the ribs. **A,** "bucket handle," lower rib. **B,** "pump handle," first rib.

of movements have been described—the pump-handle movement and the bucket-handle movement (Fig 1–3). The upper ribs are limited in their ability to move. Each pair swings like a pump handle, with elevation thrusting the sternum forward. This forward movement increases the anterior-posterior diameter and the depth of the thorax and is called the *pump-handle movement.* In the lower ribs, there is very little anterior-posterior movement. During inspiration, the ribs swing outward and upward, each pushing against the rib above during elevation. This *bucket-handle movement* increases the transverse diameter of the thoracic cage. Thus, during inspiration, the thorax increases its volume by increasing its anterior-posterior and transverse diameters.

MUSCLES OF RESPIRATION

Inspiration

Diaphragm
The diaphragm is the principal muscle of respiration. During quiet breathing, the diaphragm contributes approximately two thirds of the

tidal volume in the sitting or standing positions, and approximately three fourths of the tidal volume in the supine position. It is also estimated that two thirds of the vital capacity in all positions is contributed by the diaphragm.

The diaphragm is a large, dome-shaped muscle that separates the thoracic and abdominal cavities. Its upper surface supports the pericardium (with which it is partially blended), heart, pleura and lungs. Its lower surface is almost completely covered by the peritoneum and overlies the liver, kidneys, suprarenal glands, stomach and spleen (see Fig 1–4). This large muscle can be divided into right and left halves. Each half is made up of three parts—sternal, lumbar and costal. These three parts are inserted into the central tendon, which lies just below the heart. The sternal part arises from the back of the xiphoid process and descends to the central tendon. On each side is a small gap, the sternocostal triangle, which is located between the sternal and costal parts. It transmits the superior epigastric vessels and is frequently the site of diaphragmatic hernias. The costal parts form the right and left domes. They arise from the inner surfaces of the lower four ribs and the lower six costal cartilages. They interdigitate and transverse the abdomen to insert into the anterolateral part of the central tendon. The lumbar part arises from the bodies of the upper lumbar vertebrae and extends upward to the central tendon. The central tendon is a thin, strong aponeurosis situated near the center of the muscle, somewhat closer to the front of the body. It resembles a trefoil leaf with three divisions or leaflets. The right leaflet is the largest, the middle is the next largest and the left leaflet is the smallest.

Major vessels traverse the diaphragm through one of three openings (Fig 1–4). The vena caval opening is located to the right of the midline in the central tendon and contains branches of the right phrenic nerve and the inferior vena cava. The esophageal opening is located to the left of the midline and contains the esophagus, the vagal nerve trunks and branches of the gastric vessels. The aortic opening is located in the midline and contains the aorta, thoracic duct and sometimes the azygos vein. The diaphragm is also pierced by branches of the left phrenic nerve, small veins and lymph vessels.

The position of the diaphragm and its range of movement vary with posture, the degree of distention of the stomach, size of the intestines, size of the liver and obesity. The average movement of the diaphragm in quiet respiration is 12.5 mm on the right and 12 mm on the left. This can increase to a maximum of 30 mm on the right and 28 mm on the left during increased ventilation. The posture of the individual determines the position of the diaphragm. In the supine posi-

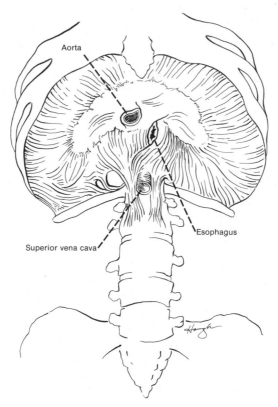

FIG 1–4.
The diaphragm from below.

tion, the resting level of the diaphragm rises. The greatest respiratory excursions during normal breathing occur in this position. However, the lung volumes are decreased due to the elevated position of the abdominal organs. In a sitting or upright position, the dome of the diaphragm is pulled down by the abdominal organs, allowing a larger lung volume. For this reason, individuals who are short of breath are more comfortable sitting than reclining. In a side-lying position, the dome of the diaphragm on the lower side rises farther into the thorax than the dome on the upper side (Fig 1–5). The abdominal organs have a tendency to fall forward out of the way, allowing greater excursion of the dome on the lower side. In contrast, the upper side moves little with respiration in this position. On x-ray, the position of the diaphragm can indicate whether the film was taken during inspiration or

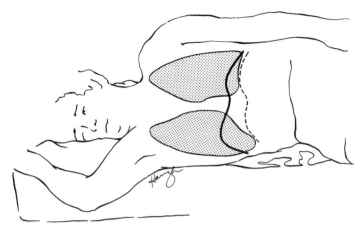

FIG 1–5.
When the patient is lying on his side, the dome of the diaphragm on the lower side rises further in the thorax than the dome on the upper side.

expiration, and may also indicate pathology in the lungs, pleura or abdomen.

Each half of the diaphragm is innervated by a separate nerve, the phrenic nerve on that side. Although the halves contract simultaneously, it is possible for half of the muscle to be paralyzed without affecting the other half. Generally, the paralyzed half remains at the normal level during rest. However, with deep inspiration, the paralyzed half is pulled up by the negative pressure in the thorax. A special x-ray, moving fluoroscopy, is used to determine paralysis of the diaphragm.

Contraction of the diaphragm increases the thoracic volume vertically and transversely. The central tendon is drawn down by the diaphragm as it contracts. As the dome descends, abdominal organs are pushed forward as far as the abdominal walls will allow. When the dome can descend no farther, the costal fibers of the diaphragm contract to increase the thoracic diameter of the thorax. This occurs because the fibers of the costal part of the diaphragm run vertically from their attachment at the costal margin. Thus, contraction of these fibers elevates and everts the ribs (Fig 1–6). If the diaphragm is low in position, it will change the angle of pull of the muscle's costal fibers. Contraction of these fibers will create a horizontal pull, which causes the lateral diameter to become smaller as the ribs are pulled in toward the central tendon.

As the diaphragm descends, it compresses the abdominal organs,

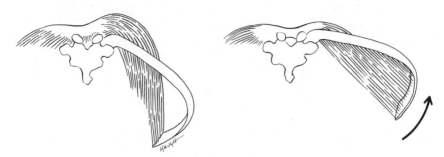

FIG 1–6.
Contraction of the costal fibers of the diaphragm causes rib eversion and elevation.

increasing intra-abdominal pressure. At the same time, the intrathoracic pressure decreases as the lung volume is increased by the descending diaphragm. Inspiratory airflow occurs as a result of this decrease in intrathoracic pressure (see Chapter 2). The pressure gradient between the abdominal and thoracic cavities also facilitates the return of blood to the right side of the heart.

Movement of the diaphragm can be controlled to some extent voluntarily. Vocalists spend years learning to manipulate their diaphragms in order to produce the best sound during singing. The diaphragm ceases to move momentarily when we hold our breaths. The diaphragm is involuntarily involved in parturition, bearing down in bowel movements, laughing, crying and vomiting. Hiccups are spasmodic, sharp contractions of the diaphragm that may indicate disease (such as a subphrenic abscess) if they persist.

Intercostals

The external intercostals extend from the tubercles of the ribs, above, down and forward to the costochondral junction of the ribs below, where they become continuous with the anterior intercostal membrane (Fig 1–7). This membrane extends the muscle forward to the sternum. There are 11 external intercostal muscles on each side of the sternum. They are thicker posteriorly than anteriorly, and thicker than the internal intercostal muscles. They are innervated by the intercostal nerves, and contraction draws the lower rib up and out toward the upper rib. This action increases the volume of the thoracic cavity.

The internal intercostals also number 11 to a side and are considered primarily expiratory in function; they will be discussed in great depth in the context of the expiratory muscles. Recent studies have shown, however, that the intercartilaginous or parasternal portion of the internal intercostals contracts with the external intercostals during inspiration to help elevate the ribs. Besides their respiratory functions, the intercostal muscles contract to prevent the intercostal spaces from being drawn in or bulged out during respiratory activity.

Sternocleidomastoid

The sternocleidomastoid (SCM) is a strong neck muscle arising from two heads, one from the manubrium and one from the medial part of the clavicle (see Fig 1–7). These two heads fuse into one muscle mass that is inserted behind the ear into the mastoid process. It is innervated by the accessory nerve and the second cervical nerve. There

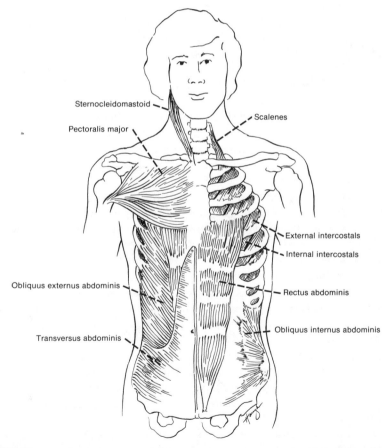

FIG 1–7.
Respiratory muscles (anterior view).

are two of these muscles, one on each side of the neck. When one SCM contracts, it tilts the head toward the shoulder of the same side and rotates the face toward the opposite shoulder. If the two SCM muscles contract together, they pull the head forward into flexion. When the head is fixed, they assist in elevating the sternum, increasing the anteroposterior (AP) diameter of the thorax.

The SCMs are the most important accessory muscles of inspiration. Their contraction can be observed in all patients during forced inspiration and in all patients who are dyspneic. These muscles become visually predominant in patients who are chronically dyspneic (see Chapter 6 on Chest assessment).

The Scalenes

The anterior, medial and posterior scalenes are three separate muscles which we will consider as a functional unit. They are attached superiorly to the transverse processes of the lower five cervical vertebrae and inferiorly to the upper surface of the first two ribs (see Fig 1–7). They are innervated by related cervical spinal nerves. These muscles are primarily supportive neck muscles, but they can assume respiratory responsibilities through reverse action. When their superior attachment is fixed, the scalenes act as accessory respiratory muscles and elevate the first two ribs during inspiration.

Serratus Anterior

The serratus anterior arises from the outer surfaces of the first eight or nine ribs. It curves backward, forming a sheet of muscle that inserts into the medial border of the scapula. It is innervated by the long thoracic nerve (cervical nerves C5, C6, and C7). There are two of these muscles, one on each side of the body. Normally they assist in forward pushing of the arm (as in boxing or punching). When the scapulae are fixed, they act as accessory respiratory muscles and elevate the ribs to which they are attached.

Pectoralis Major

The pectoralis major is a large muscle arising from the clavicle, the sternum and the cartilages of all the true ribs (see Fig 1–7). This muscle sweeps across the anterior chest to insert into the intertubercular sulcus of the humerus. It is innervated by the lateral and medial pectoral nerves and cervical nerves C5, C6, C7, C8, and T1. There are two of these muscles, one on each side of the body. This muscle acts to rotate the humerus medially and to draw the arm across the chest. In climbing and pull-ups, it draws the trunk toward the arms. In forced inspiration when the arms are fixed, it draws the ribs toward the arms, thereby increasing thoracic diameter.

Pectoralis Minor

The pectoralis minor is a thin muscle originating from the outer surfaces of the third, fourth and fifth ribs near their cartilages. It inserts into the coracoid process of the scapula. It is innervated by the pectoral nerves (cervical nerves C6, C7, and C8). There are two of these muscles, one on each side of the body. They contract with the serratus anterior to draw the scapulae toward the chest. During deep inspiration, they contract to elevate the ribs to which they are attached.

Trapezius

The trapezius is two muscles that form a huge diamond-shaped sheet extending from the head down the back and out to both shoulders (Fig 1–8). Its upper belly originates from the external occipital protuberance and curves around the side of the neck to insert into the posterior border of the clavicle. The middle part of the muscle arises from a thin diamond-shaped tendinous sheet, the supraspinous ligaments and the spines of the upper thoracic region, and runs horizontally to insert into the spine of the scapula. Its lower belly arises from the supraspinous ligaments and the spines of the lower thoracic region, and runs upward to be inserted into the lower border of the spine of the scapula. This huge muscle is innervated by the external or spinal part of the accessory nerve and cervical nerves C3 and C4. Its main function is to rotate the scapulae in elevating the arms and to control their gravitational descent.It also braces the scapulae and raises them, as in shrugging the shoulders. Its ability to stabilize the scapulae makes it an important accessory muscle in respiration. This stabilization enables the serratus anterior and pectoralis minor to elevate the ribs.

Erector Spinae

The erector spinae is a large muscle extending from the sacrum to the skull (see Fig 1–8). It originates from the sacrum, iliac crest and the spines of the lower thoracic and lumbar vertebrae. It separates into a lateral iliocostalis, an intermediate longissimus and a medial spinalis column. This muscle mass inserts into various ribs and vertebral processes all the way up to the skull. It is innervated by the related spinal nerves. These muscles extend, laterally flex and rotate the vertebral column. They are considered accessory respiratory muscles through their extension of the vertebral column. In deep inspiration, these muscles extend the vertebral column, allowing further elevation of the ribs.

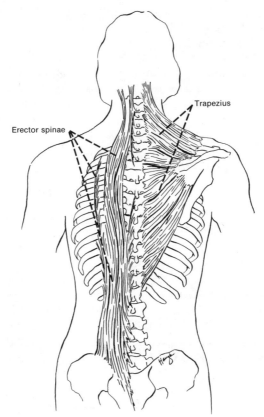

FIG 1–8.
Respiratory muscles (posterior view).

Expiration

Expiration is a passive process, occurring when the intercostals and diaphragm relax. Their relaxation allows the ribs to drop to their preinspiratory position and the diaphragm to rise. These activities compress the lungs, raising intrathoracic pressure above atmospheric pressure, thereby contributing to air flow out of the lungs.

Rectus Abdominis

The rectus abdominis rises from the pubic crest and extends up to insert into the xiphoid process and the costal margin of the fifth, sixth, and seventh costal cartilages (see Fig 1–7). It is innervated by related spinal nerves. Its action will be considered within the context of the other abdominal muscles.

Obliquus Externus Abdominis

This muscle arises in an oblique line from the fifth costal cartilage to the 12th rib (see Fig 1–7). Its posterior fibers attach in an almost vertical line with the iliac crest. The other fibers extend down and forward to attach to the front of the xiphoid process, the linea alba, and below with the pubic symphysis. It is innervated by the lower six thoracic spinal nerves.

Obliquus Internus Abdominis

This muscle originates from the lumbar fascia, the anterior two thirds of the iliac crest and the lateral two thirds of the inguinal ligament (see Fig 1–7). Its posterior fibers run almost vertically upward to insert into the lower borders of the last three ribs. The other fibers join an aponeurosis attached to the costal margin above, the linea alba in the midline and the pubic crest below. It is innervated by the lower six thoracic nerves and the first lumbar spinal nerves.

Transversus Abdominis

The transversus abdominis arises from the inner surface of the lower six costal cartilages, the lumbar fascia, the anterior two thirds of the iliac crest and the lateral third of the inguinal ligament (see Fig 1–7). It runs across the abdomen horizontally to insert into the aponeurosis extending to the linea alba. It is innervated by the lower six thoracic nerves and the first lumbar spinal nerves.

Action of the Abdominal Muscles

These four muscles work together to provide a firm but flexible wall to keep the abdominal viscera in position. The abdominal muscles exert a compressing force on the abdomen when the thorax and pelvis are fixed. This force can be utilized in defecation, urination, parturition and vomiting. In forced expiration, the abdominal muscles help force the diaphragm back to its resting position and thus force air from the lungs. If the pelvis and vertebral column are fixed, the obliquus externus abdominis will aid expiration further by depressing and compressing the lower part of the thorax. Patients with chronic obstructive lung disease have difficulty in exhalation, which causes them to trap air in their lungs. The continued contraction of the abdominal muscles throughout exhalation helps them force this air from the lungs. The abdominal muscles also play an important role in coughing. First, a large volume of air is inhaled and the glottis is closed. Then the abdominal muscles contract, raising intrathoracic pressure. When the glottis opens, the large difference in intrathoracic and atmospheric pressure causes the air to be expelled forcefully at tremendous flow rates (tussive blast). Patients with weak abdominal muscles (from neuromuscular diseases, paraplegia, quadriplegia or extensive abdominal surgery) will frequently have ineffective coughs (see Chapters 11, 12).

The four abdominal muscles have many other nonrespiratory functions both individually and as a group; these will not be discussed here.

Internal Intercostals

There are 11 internal intercostal muscles on each side of the thorax. Each muscle arises from the floor of the costal groove and cartilage and passes inferiorly and posteriorly to insert on the upper border of the rib below. These internal intercostals extend from the sternum anteriorly, around the thorax to the posterior costal angle. They are generally divided into two parts—the interosseous portion located between the sloping parts of the ribs, and the intercartilaginous portions located between costal cartilages. As discussed previously, the intercartilaginous portions are considered inspiratory in function. Contraction of the interosseous portions of the intercostals depresses the ribs and may aid in forceful exhalation. This muscle is innervated by the adjacent intercostal nerves.

SUMMARY OF RESPIRATORY MOVEMENTS

In quiet inspiration, the diaphragm, the external intercostals and the intercartilaginous portions of the internal intercostals are the only muscles that contract. The diaphragm contracts first and then descends, enlarging the thoracic cage vertically. When abdominal contents prevent its further descent, the costal fibers of the diaphragm contract, causing the lower ribs to swing up and out to the side (bucket-handle movement). This lateral rib movement is assisted by the external intercostals and the intercartilaginous portion of the internal intercostals. The transverse diameter of the thorax is increased by this bucket-handle movement. Finally, the upper ribs move forward and upward (pump-handle movement), also through contraction of their external intercostals and the intercartilaginous portions of the internal intercostals. This increases the anterior-posterior diameter of the thorax. In summary, during quiet inspiration, one should first see the epigastric area protrude, then the ribs swing up and out laterally, and finally the upper ribs move forward and upward.

Quiet expiration is passive and involves no muscular contraction. The inspiratory muscles relax, causing intrathoracic pressure to be raised as the ribs and diaphragm compress the lungs by returning to their preinspiratory positions. This increased pressure allows air flow from the lungs.

In forced inspiration, a large number of accessory muscles may contract in addition to the normal inspiratory muscles mentioned. The erector spinae contract to extend the vertebral column. This extension permits greater elevation of the ribs during inspiration. Various back muscles (erector spinae, trapezius and rhomboids) contract to stabilize the vertebral column, head, neck and scapula. This enables accessory respiratory muscles to assist inspiration through reverse action. The sternocleidomastoid raises the sternum. The scalenes elevate the first two ribs. The serratus anterior, pectoralis major and pectoralis minor assist in elevating the ribs. All these accessory muscles tend to elevate the ribs, thus increasing the AP diameter but not the transverse diameter of the thorax. (In fact, the transverse diameter does increase slightly as a result of the increased strength of the contraction of the normal inspiratory muscles.) The marked increase in AP diameter in relation to transverse diameter creates an impression of "en bloc" breathing in the patient using accessory muscles.

In forced expiration, the interosseous portion of the internal inter-costals and the abdominal muscles contract to force air out of the lungs. Forced expiration can be slow and prolonged (as in patients with ob-structive lung disease) or rapid and expulsive (as in a cough). If the abdominal contractions are strong enough, the trunk will flex during exhalation. This flexion further compresses the lungs, forcing more air from them.

UPPER AIRWAYS

Nose

Noses vary in size and shape with individuals and nationalities. Its framework is comprised of bony and cartilaginous parts. Its upper third is primarily bony and contains the nasal bones, the frontal pro-cesses of the maxillae and the nasal part of the frontal bone. Its lower two thirds are cartilaginous (containing the septal, lateral, and major and minor alar nasal cartilages). The nasal cavity is divided into right and left halves by the nasal septum. This cavity extends from the nos-trils to the posterior apertures of the nose in the nasopharynx. The lateral walls of the cavity are irregular due to projecting superior, middle and inferior nasal chonchae. There is a meatus located beneath or lateral to each choncha through which the sinuses drain. The chonchae serve to increase the surface area of the nose for maximum contact with inspired air. The superior chonchae and adjacent septal wall are referred to as the *olfactory region*. They are covered with a thin, yellow olfactory mucous membrane which consists of bipolar nerve cells that are olfactory in function. Only a portion of inspired air reaches the olfactory region to give us our sense of smell. When we wish to smell something specific, we "sniff." This action lifts the inspired air so that more of it comes in contact with the olfactory region.

The anterior portion (vestibule) of the nasal cavity (Fig 1–9) is lined with skin and coarse hairs (vibrissae) that entrap inhaled particles. The

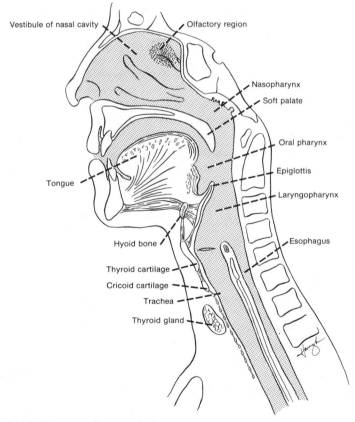

FIG 1–9.
Sagittal section of the head and neck.

rest of the cavity and sinuses (with the exception of the olfactory region) are lined with respiratory mucous membrane. This membrane is composed of pseudostratified columnar ciliated epithelium (Fig 1–10). It contains goblet cells, mucous and serous glands, which secrete mucus and serous secretions. These secretions entrap foreign particles and bacteria. This mucus is then swept to the nasopharynx by the cilia at a rate of 5–15 mm/min, where it is swallowed or expectorated. The mucous membrane is very vascular, with arterial blood supplied by branches of the internal and external carotid arteries. Venous drainage occurs via the anterior facial veins. The mucous membrane is thickest over the chonchae. As air is inhaled it passes around and over the chonchae, whose vascular moist surfaces heat, humidify and filter the inspired air. The mucous membrane may become swollen and irritated in upper respiratory infections and may secrete copious amounts of mucus. Because this membrane is continuous with sinuses, auditory tubes and lacrimal canaliculi, people suffering from colds frequently complain of sinus headaches, watery eyes, earaches and other symptoms. Secretions are frequently so copious that the nasal passages become completely blocked.

Pharynx

The pharynx is an oval fibromuscular sac located behind the nasal cavity, mouth, and larynx. It is approximately 12–14 cm long and extends from the base of the skull to the esophagus below, at the level of the cricoid cartilage opposite the sixth cervical vertebra. Anteriorly it opens

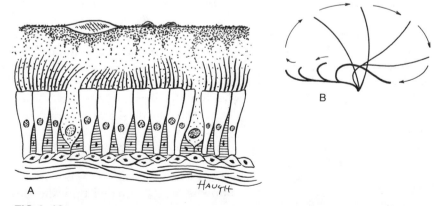

FIG 1–10.
A, pseudostratified columnar ciliated epithelium. **B,** normal movements of cilia.

into the nasal cavity (nasopharynx), mouth (oral pharynx) and larynx (laryngopharynx). The pharyngeal walls are lined with ciliated respiratory mucous membrane in the nasal portion, but stratified squamous in the oral and laryngeal parts.

The nasopharynx is a continuation of the nasal cavities (see Fig 1–9). It lies behind the nose, above the soft palate. With the exception of the soft palate, its walls are immovable, so its cavity is never obliterated, as is the oral and laryngeal pharynx. The nasopharynx communicates with the nasal cavity anteriorly through the posterior apertures of the nose. It communicates with the laryngeal and oral pharynx through an opening, the pharyngeal isthmus. This opening is closed by elevations of the soft palate during swallowing.

The oral pharynx extends from the soft palate to the epiglottis (see Fig 1–9). It opens into the mouth anteriorly through the oropharyngeal isthmus. Its posterior walls lie upon the bodies of the second and third cervical vertebrae. Laterally, two masses of lymphoid tissue, the palatine tonsils, may be seen. These tonsils form part of a circular band of lymphoid tissue surrounding the opening into the digestive and respiratory tracts.

The laryngopharynx lies behind the larynx and extends from the epiglottis above to the inlet of the esophagus below (see Fig 1–9). The fourth to sixth vertebral bodies lie behind the laryngeal pharynx. In front of the laryngopharynx are the epiglottis, the inlet of the larynx and the posterior surfaces of the arytenoid and cricoid cartilages.

Larynx

The larynx is a complex structure composed of cartilages and cords moved by sensitive muscles (Fig 1–11), and is located between the trachea and laryngopharynx whose anterior wall it forms. It acts as a sphincteric valve, with its rapid closure preventing food, liquids and foreign objects from entering the airway. It controls airflow, and at times closes to that thoracic pressure may be raised and the upper airways cleared by a propulsive cough when the larynx opens. Expiratory airflow vibrates as it passes over the contracting vocal cords, producing the sounds we use for speech. (The larynx is not essential for speech. Humans can speak by learning to dilate the upper part of the esophagus so that air vibrates as it passes over; this is called *esophageal speech*.)

The larynx is located between the trachea and the laryngopharynx, whose anterior wall it forms. In adult men it is situated opposite the third, fourth and fifth cervical vertebrae. (It is situated somewhat higher in women and children.) In children the larynx is essentially the

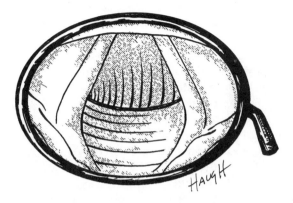

FIG 1–11.
Visualization of the larynx via a laryngoscope.

same in girls as in boys. At puberty the male larynx increases in size considerably until its AP diameter is almost doubled. All the cartilages enlarge, with the thyroid cartilage becoming prominent anteriorly.

The laryngeal skeleton contains the hyoid bone and the cartilages of the larynx (the thyroid, cricoid, epiglottic, right and left arytenoids, corniculates and cuneiforms). The thyroid cartilage is the largest. It has a V-shaped notch in its upper third, which projects forward, forming the "Adam's apple." The entire cartilage is pulled up in swallowing, with the upper part of the cartilage passing beneath the hyoid bone. The cricoid cartilage is shaped like a signet ring, with the signet part facing the posterior. The anterior part of the cartilage is easily palpated just below the thyroid cartilage. It is thicker and more prominent than the tracheal rings which lie below. It is the only cartilage that completely circles the airway. The cricoid cartilage is connected to the thyroid cartilage by the cricothyroid membrane. (This membrane is frequently punctured to establish an airway in an emergency when the upper airway is obstructed.) The epiglottic cartilage is the elastic skeleton of the epiglottis. It is a leaflike structure attached by ligaments to the hyoid bone anteriorly and the thyroid cartilage below. It is considered a vestigial structure, and its removal causes little effect. The last cartilages we will discuss are the arytenoid cartilages. Therapists needing further information on these structures should refer to one of the anatomy books in the reference section. The arytenoid cartilages are two small pyramid-shaped cartilages that articulate with the posterior part of the cricoid cartilage. The vocal cords attach from these cartilages to the thyroid cartilage.

The true vocal cords (or vocal folds) are two pearly white folds of mucous membrane that stretch from the arytenoid cartilage to the thyroid cartilage. The space between the true vocal cords is called the *rima glottidis*. It changes shape with movement of the cords but is generally triangular when the cords are open. The rima glottidis and the true vocal cords are grouped together under the term *glottis*. The glottis is the narrowest part of the adult airway.

Just above the true vocal cords are two shallow grooves in the mucous membrane lining of the larynx. These grooves (ventricles of the larynx) contain numerous glands that secrete the mucus that covers the larynx. The false vocal cords (vestibular or ventricular folds) lie just above the ventricles of the larynx. They are two soft, pink masses of mucous membrane raised slightly from the laryngeal wall. They extend from the thyroid cartilage to the arytenoids. The false cords are not as well developed as the true cords and do not approximate completely during phonation. However, their closure can help protect the airway from aspiration of foreign material.

There are two main groups of muscles that control the opening and closing of the glottis—the abductors and adductors. The posterior cricoarytenoid muscle is the most important muscle in the larynx as it is the only abductor of the vocal folds. It is vital for respiration. Contraction of this muscle separates the vocal folds and widens the lumen of the glottis. There are eight adductors of the vocal folds (aryepiglottic, thyroepiglottic, thyroarytenoid, vocalis, cricothyroid, lateral cricoarytenoid, transverse arytenoid and oblique arytenoid muscles). Contraction of these muscles results in approximation of the vocal cords and narrowing of the glottis. The adductors of the cords are very important in protecting the lower airways. Their contraction prevents fluids, food and other substances from being aspirated. All the intrinsic laryngeal muscles are innervated by the recurrent laryngeal nerve (a branch of the vagus nerve) with the exception of the cricothyroid muscle, which is supplied by the external branch of the superior laryngeal nerve (also a branch of the vagus nerve).

The mucous membrane of the larynx is continuous with that of the laryngopharynx above and the trachea below. It lines the cavity of the larynx and the structures found within. On the anterior surface and upper half of the posterior surface of the epiglottis, the upper part of the aryepiglottis folds and the vocal folds, the mucous membrane is stratified squamous epithelium. The rest of the laryngeal mucosa is ciliated columnar epithelium. The mucous membrane of the larynx has many mucous glands. They are especially numerous in the epiglottis, in front of the arytenoid cartilages and in the ventricles of the larynx. There are also some taste buds located on the epiglottis and irregularly throughout the rest of the larynx.

LOWER AIRWAYS

Trachea

The trachea is a flexible, cartilaginous tube approximately 10–11 cm long and 2.5 cm wide. It lies in front of the esophagus, descending with a slight inclination to the right from the level of the cricoid cartilage (Figs 1–11 and 1–12). It travels behind the sternum into the thorax to the sternal angle (opposite the fifth thoracic vertebra), where it divides to form the right and left main-stem bronchi. The tracheal wall is strengthened by 16–20 horseshoe-shaped cartilaginous rings. The open parts of the tracheal rings are completed by fibrous and elastic

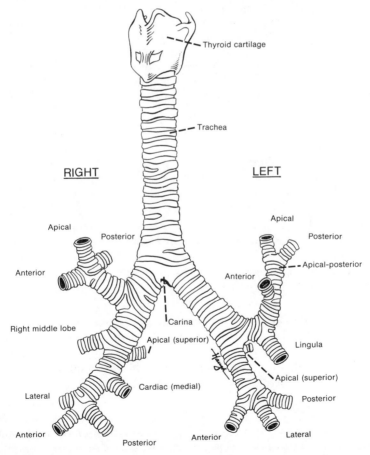

FIG 1–12.
Tracheobronchial tree (a three-quarters view, rotated toward the right side).

tissue and unstriated transverse muscle. This part of the ring faces the posterior and is very flexible. It indents or curves inward during coughing (which serves to increase the velocity of expelled air). These cartilages lie horizontally one above the other, separated by narrow bands of connective tissue. The trachea is lengthened during hyperextension of the head, swallowing (which raises the trachea) and inspiration when the lungs expand and pull the trachea downward. Its cross-sectional area becomes smaller with contraction of the unstriated transverse muscle fibers that complete the tracheal rings.

The mucous membrane of the trachea also contains columnar ciliated epithelium and goblet cells. Each ciliated epithelial cell contains approximately 275 cilia. These structures beat rapidly in a coordinated and unidirectional manner, propelling a sheet of mucus cephalad from the lower respiratory tract to the pharynx, where it is swallowed or expectorated. The cilia beat in this layer of mucus with a strong, forceful forward stroke, followed by a slow ineffective backward stroke which returns the cilia to their starting position. This propelling of mucus by the cilia (mucociliary escalator) is essential. When cilia are paralyzed (by smoke, alcohol, dehydration, anesthesia, starvation or hypoxia), mucus begins to accumulate in distal, gravity-dependent airways, causing infiltrates and eventually localized areas of collapse referred to as atelectasis.

The number of mucus-containing goblet cells is approximately equal to the number of ciliated epithelial cells. Reserve cells lie beneath the ciliated and goblet cells. These reserve cells can differentiate into either goblet cells or ciliated cells. Beneath the reserve cells lie the gland cells. There are approximately 40 times more gland cells than goblet cells. Mucus is composed of 95% water, 2% glycoprotein, 1% carbohydrate, trace amounts of lipid, deoxyribonucleic acid (DNA), dead tissue cells, phagocytes, leukocytes, erythrocytes and entrapped foreign particles. Mucus lines the airways from the trachea to the alveoli. Two separate layers have been observed—the sol layer, which lies on the mucosal surface and contains high concentrations of water, and the gel layer, which is more superficial and more viscous due to its lower concentration of water.

The trachea divides into a right and a left main-stem bronchus (see Fig 1–12). The right main-stem bronchus appears to be an extension of the trachea, being wider, shorter and more vertical than the left main-stem bronchus. Its greater width and more vertical course cause a majority of aspirated foreign material to pass through the right main-stem bronchus. The azygos vein arches over the right main-stem bronchus while the right pulmonary artery lies beneath. The right main-stem bronchus divides to form the right upper lobe bronchus, the right middle lobe bronchus and the right lower lobe bronchus. The right upper lobe divides into three segmental bronchi—apical, posterior and anterior. The apical bronchus runs almost vertically toward the apex of the lung. The posterior bronchus is directed posteriorly in a horizontal direction, while the anterior bronchus runs almost horizontally, anteriorly. The right middle lobe bronchus divides about 10 mm below the right upper lobe bronchus and descends downward anterolaterally. The right lower lobe bronchus divides into five segmental bronchi. The apical or superior bronchus runs almost horizontally, posteriorly. The medial or cardiac bronchus descends downward medially toward the heart. The anterior basal bronchus descends anteriorly. The lateral basal bronchus descends laterally and the posterior bronchus descends posteriorly. Note that each segment describes its position.

The left main-stem bronchus is narrower and runs more horizontally than the right main-stem bronchus. The aortic arch passes over it, while the esophagus, descending aorta and thoracic duct lie behind it. The left pulmonary artery lies anteriorly and above the left main-stem bronchus. The left main-stem bronchus has two major divisions—the left upper lobe bronchus and the left lower lobe bronchus. The left upper lobe bronchus has three major segmental bronchi. The anterior bronchus ascends at approximately a 45-degree angle. The apical-posterior bronchus has two branches; one runs vertically and the other posteriorly toward the apex of the left lung. The lingular bronchus descends anterolaterally, much like the right middle lobe bronchus of the right lung. The right lower lobe bronchus divides into four segmental bronchi. The superior or apical bronchus runs posteriorly in a horizontal direction. The anterior bronchus descends anteriorly. The lateral bronchus descends laterally, while the posterior bronchus descends posteriorly. Again the segments describe their anatomical position.

The bronchi of the airways continue to divide until there are approximately 23 generations (Table 1–1). The main, lobar and segmental bronchi are made up of the first four generations. The walls contain U-shaped cartilage in the main bronchi. This cartilage becomes less well defined and more irregularly shaped as the bronchi continue to divide. In the segmental bronchi the walls are formed by irregularly shaped helical plates with bands of bronchial muscle. The mucous membrane of these airways is essentially the same as in the trachea, but the cells become more cuboidal in the lower divisions.

The subsegmental bronchi extend from the fifth to the seventh generation. The diameter of these airways becomes progressively

TABLE 1–1.
Structural Characteristics of the Air Passages*

	GENERATION (MEAN)	NUMBER	MEAN DIAMETER (MM)	AREA SUPPLIED	CARTILAGE	MUSCLE	NUTRITION	EMPLACEMENT	EPITHELIUM
Trachea	0	1	18	Both lungs	U shaped	Links open end of cartilage		Within connective tissue sheath alongside arterial vessels	Columnar ciliated
Main bronchi	1	2	13	Individual lungs			From the bronchial circulation		
Lobar bronchi	2 → 3	4 → 8	7 → 5	Lobes	Irregular shaped and helical plates	Helical bands			
Segmental bronchi	4	16	4	Segments					
Small bronchi	5 → 11	32 → 2,000	3 → 1	Secondary lobules					
Bronchioles and terminal bronchioles	12 → 16	4,000 → 65,000	1 → 0.5		Absent	Strong helical muscle bands		Embedded directly in the lung parenchyma	Cuboidal
Respiratory bronchioles	17 → 19	130,000 → 500,000	0.5	Primary lobules		Muscle band between alveoli	From the pulmonary circulation		Cuboidal to flat between the alveoli
Alveolar ducts	20 → 22	1,000,000 → 4,000,000	0.3	Alveoli		Thin bands in alveolar septa		Forms the lung parenchyma	Alveolar epithelium
Alveolar sacs	23	8,000,000	0.3						

*From Weibel ER: *Morphometry of the Human Lung.* New York, Springer-Verlag New York, 1963. Used by permission.

smaller, although the total cross-sectional area increases (due to the increased number of divisions of the airways). The mucous membrane is essentially the same, with helical cartilaginous plates and cilia becoming more sparse. These changes continue throughout the eighth to eleventh generations, which are referred to as *bronchioles*.

The terminal bronchioles extend from the 12th to the 16th generation. The diameter of these airways is approximately 1 mm. Cartilage is no longer present to provide structural rigidity. The airways are embedded directly in the lung parenchyma, and it is the elastic properties of this parenchyma that keep these lower airways open. Strong helical muscle bands are present, and their contraction forms longitudinal folds in the mucosa that sharply decrease the diameter of these airways. The epithelium of the terminal bronchioles is cuboidal and no longer ciliated. The cross-sectional area of the airways increases sharply at this level, as the diameter of the terminal bronchioles ceases to decrease as markedly with each generation. All the airways to this level (1–16 generations) are considered conducting because their purpose is to transport gas to the respiratory bronchioles and alveoli where gas exchange will occur. The conducting airways receive their arterial blood from the bronchial circulation (branches of the descending aorta). Airways from below this point receive their arterial blood from the pulmonary arteries.

The respiratory bronchioles extend from the 17th to the 19th generation. They are considered a transitional zone between bronchioles and alveoli. Their walls contain cuboidal epithelium interspersed with some alveoli. The number of alveoli increases with each generation. The walls of the bronchioles are also buried in the lung parenchyma. The airways depend on traction of this parenchyma to maintain their lumen. Muscle bands are also present between alveoli.

Alveolar ducts extend from the 20th to the 22nd generation. Their walls are composed entirely of alveoli, which are separated from one another by their septae, which contain smooth muscle, elastic and collagen fibers, nerves and capillaries. Contraction of the muscle narrows the lumen of the duct. J. F. Nunn in his book, *Applied Respiratory Physiology*, says "About half of the total number of alveoli arise from ducts and some 35% of the alveolar gas resides in the alveolar ducts and the alveoli which arise directly from them."

The 23rd generation of air passages is called *alveolar sacs*. They are essentially the same as alveolar ducts, except that they end as blind pouches. (Actually there is communication between "blind pouches" in the form of the pores of Kohn, which are channels in alveolar walls, and Lambert's canals, which are communications between bronchioles and alveoli. These communications are thought to be responsible for the rapid spread of lung infection. They also provide collateral ventilation to alveoli whose bronchi are obstructed. Although this ventilation does little to arterialize blood, it does help prevent collapse of these alveoli.) Each alveolar sac contains approximately 17 alveoli. There are about 300 million alveoli in an adult man, 85%–95% of which are covered with pulmonary capillaries. Alveolar epithelium is composed of two cell types. Type I cells, squamous pneumocytes, have broad thin extensions which cover about 95% of the alveolar surface. Type II cells, the granular pneumocytes, are more numerous than type I cells but occupy less than 5% of the alveolar surface. This is due to their small, cuboidal shape. These cells are probably responsible for production of surfactant, a phospholipid that lines the alveoli. Surfactant helps keep alveoli expanded by lowering their surface tension. Type II cells have recently been shown to be the primary cells involved in repair of the alveolar epithelium. (This has been shown in experiments where O_2 toxicity was induced in monkeys and in numerous other conditions where type I cells were destroyed.) Type III cells, alveolar brush cells, are very rare and are found only occasionally in humans.

A further type of cell, the alveolar macrophage, is found within the alveolus. These cells are thought to originate from stem cell precursors in the bone marrow and reach the lung through the blood stream. They are large, mononuclear, ameboid cells that roam in the alveoli, alveolar ducts and alveolar sacs. They contain lysosomes which are capable of killing engulfed bacteria. (Recent studies show them to be most effective in neutralizing inhaled gram-positive organisms.) They also engulf foreign matter and are either transported to the lymphatic system or migrate to the terminal bronchioles where they attach themselves to the mucus. They are then carried by the mucus to larger airways and eventually to the pharynx. Since cilia are not present below the 11th generation of air passages, clearance of matter and bacteria from these areas is largely dependent on the macrophages.

Other cells located in the distal airways which are important in the defense of the lung are the lymphocytes and polymorphonuclear leukocytes. Immunoglobulins (IgA, IgG, and IgM) in the blood serum appear to enhance the engulfing activity of the macrophages. There are two types of lymphocytes found in the lung—the B-lymphocyte and the T-lymphocyte. The B-lymphocytes produce gamma globulin antibodies to fight lung infections, while the T-lymphocytes release a substance that attracts macrophages to the site of the infection. The polymorphonuclear leukocytes are important in engulfing and killing blood-borne gram-negative organisms.

LUGS

Two lungs, each covered with its pleura, are in the thoracic cavity. Each lung is attached to the heart and the trachea by its root and the pulmonary ligament. It is otherwise free in the thoracic cavity. The lungs are light, soft spongy organs, whose color darkens with age as they become impregnated with inhaled dust. They are covered with visceral pleurae, thin, glistening serous membranes that cover all surfaces of the lung. The pleurae reflect and continue on the mediastinum and inner thoracic wall where they become known as the *parietal pleurae*. The space between the two pleurae is minuscule and contains a negative pressure at all times, which serves to help keep the lungs inflated. A small amount of pleural fluid lubricates the two pleurae as they slide over each other during breathing. In disease, fluid, tumor cells or air may invade the pleural space and collapse the underlying lung. Each lung presents with an apex, base and three surfaces (costal, medial, and diaphragmatic). There are also three borders (anterior, inferior and posterior). Each lung is divided by fissures into separate lobes. In the right lung the oblique fissure separates the lower lobe from the middle, while the horizontal fissure separates the upper lobe from the middle. The right lung is heavier and wider than the left lung. It is also shorter due to the location of the right lobe of the liver. The left lung is divided into upper and lower lobes by the oblique fissure. It is longer and thinner than the right lung because the heart and pericardium are located in the left thorax. Numerous structures enter the lung at the hilus, or root of the lung (including the main-stem bronchus, the pulmonary artery, pulmonary veins, bronchial arteries and veins, nerves and lymph vessels). The root, or hilus, of the lungs lies opposite the bodies of the fifth, sixth, and seventh thoracic vertebrae. The lungs are connected to the upper airways by the trachea and main-stem bronchi.

Surface Markings

Surface markings of the lungs can be outlined over the chest with a basic knowledge of bony landmarks and gross anatomy of each lung (Table 1–2, Figs 1–13 to 1–15). The apices of both lungs extend one inch above the clavicles at the medial ends. The anterior medial border of the right lung runs from the sternoclavicular joint, to the sternal angle downward to the xiphisternum. The inferior border runs from the xiphisternum laterally to the 6th rib in the midclavicular line, the 8th rib in the midaxillary line, and the 10th rib in the midscapular line. The midscapular line runs downward from the inferior angle of the

TABLE 1–2.

Anatomical Arrangement of the Bronchopulmonary Segments

LOBE	RIGHT LUNG: BRONCHOPULMONARY SEGMENTS	LOBE	LEFT LUNG: BRONCHOPULMONARY SEGMENTS
Upper	Apical—extends above the clavicle anteriorly; smaller area posteriorly.	Upper	Apical posterior—extends above the clavicle anteriorly; occupies comparable area as the apical and posterior segments of the right lung.
	Anterior—occupies area between the clavicle and horizontal fissure.		Anterior—occupies area between the clavicle and the border of the lingula (comparable line to the horizontal fissure of the right lung).
	Posterior—remainder of upper lobe on the posterior aspect down to the oblique fissure.		
Middle	Lateral—extends medially from junction of the two fissures at the 3rd intercostal space to occupy one-third the anterior surface of the lobe.	Lingula‡	Superior—occupies upper half of lingula.
			Inferior—occupies lower half of the lingula.
	Medial—occupies the remaining anterior surface of the lobe.		
Lower (Base)	Anterior—occupies basal area beneath the oblique fissure anteriorly.	Lower (Base)	Anterior—occupies area inferior to the oblique fissure anteriorly.
	Superior*—occupies half the area from the oblique fissure downward on the posterior aspect.		Superior*—occupies one-third of the basal area posteriorly from the oblique fissure downward.
	Lateral—extends from the junction of the middle lobe over the midaxillary area to occupy one third the area inferior to the superior segment on the posterior aspect.		Lateral—occupies the lateral half of the remaining two thirds of the left lower lobe beneath the superior segment on the posterior aspect.
	Posterior—occupies two thirds of the area posteriorly beneath the superior segment.		Posterior—occupies the medial portion of the remaining two thirds of the left lower lobe beneath the superior segment on the posterior aspect.
	Medial†—occupies a space on the inner aspect of the right base.		

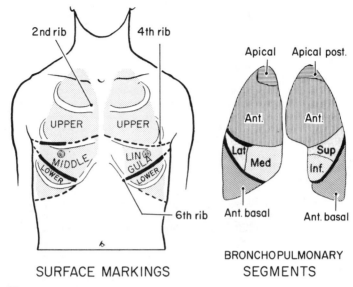

SURFACE MARKINGS

BRONCHOPULMONARY
SEGMENTS

FIG 1–13.
Surface markings of the lungs (anterior aspect). The underlying bronchopulmonary segments are also shown. (From Cherniack RM, et al: *Respiration in Health and Disease*. Philadelphia, WB Saunders Co, 1972. Used by permission.)

scapula with the arm at rest. The inferior border joins the posterior medial border of the lung 2 cm lateral to the 10th thoracic vertebra. The posterior medial border runs 2 cm lateral to the vertebral column from the 7th cervical vertebra to the 10th thoracic vertebra.

The left lung is generally smaller than the right, and accommodates the position of the heart. The medial border on the anterior aspect runs from the sternoclavicular joint to the middle of the sternal angle, down the midline of the sternum to the 4th costal cartilage. A lateral indentation of about an inch and a half forms the cardiac notch at the level of the 5th and 6th costal cartilages. The courses of the inferior and medial borders on the posterior aspect are similar in the

---

←

*This segment can be drained preferentially when the patient lies prone. Superior segments also called apical.

†Medial basal segment has no direct exposure to the chest wall, therefore cannot be directly auscultated. This segment preferentially drains when the patient is positioned for the left lateral basal segment because of the comparable angle of its bronchus.

‡Lingula is not an anatomically distinct area compared with the right middle lobe; rather, it is anatomically part of the left upper lobe.

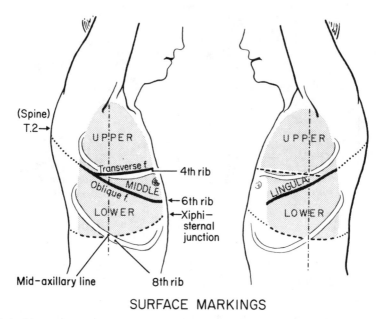

SURFACE MARKINGS

FIG 1–14.
Surface markings of the lungs (lateral aspect). (From Cherniack RM, et al: *Respiration in Health and Disease*. Philadelphia, WB Saunders Co, 1972. Used by permission.)

left and right lungs. In the left lung, however, the inferior border crosses at the level of the 10th thoracic vertebra rather than the 12th observed in the right lung.

The position of the fissures of the lungs can be outlined over the chest wall. In both lungs, the oblique fissure begins between the 2nd to 4th thoracic vertebrae. This can be roughly estimated by following a line continuous with the medial border of the abducted scapula, around the midaxillary line at the 5th rib, and terminating at the 6th costal cartilage anteriorly. The horizontal fissure of the right lung originates from the oblique fissure at the level of about the 4th intercostal space in the midaxillary line, courses medially and slightly upward over the 4th rib anteriorly. The left lung has no horizontal fissure.

Bronchopulmonary Segments
The bronchopulmonary segments lie within the three lobes of the right lung and the two lobes of the left lung. There are ten bronchopulmonary segments on the right and eight on the left. Brief anatomic descriptions of the position of each lobe are provided in Table 1–1. Figure 1–13 illustrates the surface markings on the anterior view of the lungs and the position of the various bronchopulmonary segments

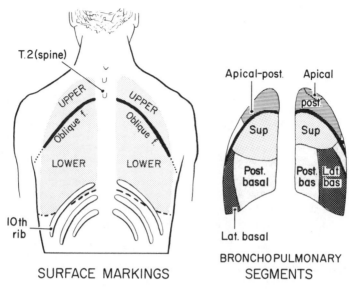

FIG 1–15.
Surface markings of the lungs (posterior aspect). The underlying bronchopulmonary segments are also shown. (From Cherniack RM, et al: *Respiration in Health and Disease*. Philadelphia, WB Saunders Co, 1972. Used by permission.)

within the major anatomic divisions provided by the fissures. Figure 1–14 shows some of these features from the lateral views. Figure 1–15 illustrates the surface markings and bronchopulmonary segments of the posterior aspect of the lungs. Students should be very familiar with the anatomical arrangement of the fissures and bronchopulmonary segments, and be able to precisely outline them using a marking pencil on a partner.

SUMMARY

This chapter has reviewed the anatomy of the respiratory system. The features of the respiratory pump were described with respect to the structure of the bony thorax, the muscles of respiration associated with the chest wall and of the diaphragm. The upper and lower respiratory tracts were described, as well as the relationship of the tracheobronchial tree to the lung/parenchyma. The lung/parenchyma is defined anatomically in terms of discrete bronchopulmonary segments contained within three major divisions of each lung. The specific surface markings defined by the lung fissures and the bronchopulmonary segments are emphasized. A thorough understanding of respiratory anatomy is fundamental to the knowledge base underlying the assessment and management of pulmonary dysfunction by physical therapists.

REFERENCES

Periodicals

Dowell AR, Freeman ER: Lung defense mechanisms: Their importance in respiratory care. *Respir Care* 1970; 22:54.

Green GM: Pulmonary clearance of infectious agents. *Annu Rev Med* 1968; 19:315.

Sorokin SP: Properties of alveolar cells and tissues that strengthen alveolar defenses. *Arch Intern Med* 1970; 126:450.

Wood RE, et al: Tracheal mucociliary transport in patients with cystic fibrosis and its stimulation by Terbutaline. *Am Rev Respir Dis* 1975; 111:733.

Books

Applebaum EL, Bruce DL: *Tracheal Intubation.* Philadelphia, WB Saunders Co, 1976.

Campbell EJ, Agostoni E, Davis JN (eds): *The Respiratory Muscles—Mechanics and Neural Control.* London, Lloyd-Luke Medical Books Ltd, 1970.

Cherniack RM, Cherniack L: *Respiration in Health and Disease,* ed 3. Philadelphia, WB Saunders Co, 1983.

Comroe JH, Jr, et al: *Physiology of Respiration,* ed 2. Chicago, Year Book Medical Publishers, 1974.

Egan DF: *Fundamentals of Respiratory Therapy,* ed 2. St. Louis, CV Mosby Co, 1973.

Gardner E, Gray DJ, O'Rahilly R: *Anatomy: A Regional Study of Human Structure,* ed 4. Philadelphia, WB Saunders Co, 1975.

Gray H: *Anatomy of the Human Body,* ed 29. Philadelphia, Lea & Febiger, 1973.

Haas A, Pinedo H, Haas F, et al: *Pulmonary Therapy and Rehabilitation: Principles and Practice.* Baltimore, Williams & Wilkins Co, 1979.

Hollinshead HW: *The Thorax, Abdomen, and Pelvis.* New York, Harper & Row, 1971.

Lockhart RD, et al: *Anatomy of the Human Body.* London, Faber & Faber, 1981.

Murray JF: *The Normal Lung.* Philadelphia, WB Saunders Co, 1976.

Nunn JF: *Applied Respiratory Physiology,* ed 2. London, Butterworths, 1977.

Quiring DP, Warfel JH: *The Head, Neck and Trunk,* ed 3. Philadelphia, Lea & Febiger, 1967.

Warren R: *Surgery.* Philadelphia, WB Saunders Co, 1963.

Warwick R, Williams PL: *Gray's Anatomy,* ed 36. Philadelphia, WB Saunders Co, 1980.

West JB: *Respiratory Physiology—The Essentials,* ed 2. Williams & Wilkins Co, 1979.

2

Review of Respiratory Physiology

Lyn Hobson, P.T., R.R.T.

Elizabeth Dean, Ph.D., M.C.P.A.

The purpose of this chapter is to review the basics of respiratory physiology. The intent is to enable the therapist and nurse to have a working, clinical understanding of the physiologic mechanisms of their patients. Unless one understands normal physiology, it is difficult to comprehend abnormal processes that occur in disease states. The authors are well aware that a practical, general approach to the subject is difficult since there are always exceptions to general rules. This chapter is not intended to be an exhaustive review of respiratory physiology. For a more in-depth discussion of the subject, the therapist should refer to one of the excellent respiratory physiology texts available (see the references at the end of the chapter).

CONTROL OF BREATHING

The act of breathing is a natural process to which most of us give little thought. Unconsciously, it adjusts to various degrees of activity, maintaining optimum arterial levels of PO_2 and PCO_2, whether we are resting or physically active. Sighing, yawning, hiccuping, laughing and vomiting are all involuntary acts utilizing respiratory muscles. Breathing is also under our voluntary control. We can stop it temporarily by holding our breath or increase it by rapidly panting until we faint (from cerebral vascular constriction due to a decrease in arterial PCO_2).

Exhalation is used in singing, speaking, coughing and blowing, whereas inspiration is used for sniffing and sucking. Parturition, defecation and the Valsalva maneuver are all performed while voluntarily holding our breath. These activities are directed by control centers located in the brain. The centers integrate a multitude of chemical, reflex and physical stimuli before transmitting impulses to the respiratory muscles. The cerebral hemispheres control voluntary respiratory activity, while involuntary respiratory activity is controlled by centers located in the pons and medulla (Fig 2–1).

Medullary and Pontine Respiratory Centers

The respiratory center in the medulla is in the reticular formation. It contains the minimum number of neurons necessary for the basic sequence of inspiration and expiration. Although this center is capable of maintaining some degree of respiratory activity, these respirations are not normal in character.

The apneustic center is in the middle and lower pons. If uncon-

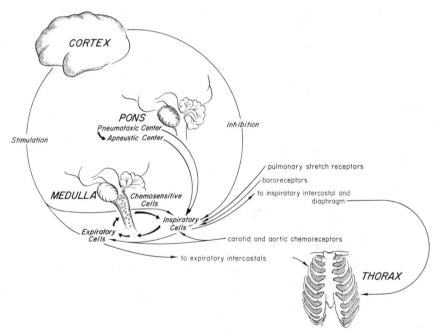

FIG 2–1.
Control of breathing.

trolled by the pneumotaxic center, prolonged inspiratory gasps (apneustic breathing) occur.

The pneumotaxic center is in the upper third of the pons. It maintains the normal pattern of respiration, balancing inspiration and expiration by inhibiting either the apneustic center or the inspiratory component of the medullary center.

Central Chemoreceptors

These receptors are located on the ventral lateral surfaces of the upper medulla. They are bathed in the cerebrospinal fluid (CSF), which is separated from blood by the blood-brain barrier. Although this barrier is relatively impermeable to hydrogen (H^+) and bicarbonate (HCO_3^-) ions. Carbon dioxide (CO_2) diffuses through the barrier easily. Increased stimulation of central chemoreceptors by a rising arterial PCO_2 results in increased rate and depth of ventilation.

Peripheral Chemoreceptors

These receptors are located in the carotid bodies, which lie in the bifurcations of the common carotid artery and in the aortic bodies located above and below the aortic arch. These bodies receive blood from small branches of the vessels on which they are located. The receptors respond to an increase in arterial PCO_2 by increasing ventilation, but are much less important in their response to PCO_2 than are the central chemoreceptors.

The main role of the peripheral chemoreceptors is to respond to hypoxemia by increasing ventilation. If arterial PCO_2 is normal, the PO_2 must drop to 50 mm Hg before ventilation increases. A rising PCO_2 will cause the peripheral chemoreceptors to respond more quickly to a decreasing PO_2. In some patients with severe lung disease, this response to hypoxemia (the hypoxic drive) becomes very important. These patients frequently have a permanently elevated PCO_2 (CO_2 retention). The CSF in these patients compensates for a chronically elevated arterial PCO_2, by returning the pH of the CSF to near normal values. When these patients have lost their ability to stimulate ventilation in response to an elevated PCO_2, arterial hypoxemia becomes their major stimulus to ventilation (hypoxic drive).

REFLEXES

Hering-Breuer Reflex

Hering and Breuer noted in 1868 that distention of anesthetized animal lungs caused a decrease in the frequency of inspiration and an increase in expiratory time. Receptors for this reflex are thought to lie in the smooth muscle of airways from the trachea to the bronchioles. In humans, it takes a lung inflation of more than 800 ml above functional residual capacity to activate the reflex and delay the next breath.

Cough Reflex

Mechanical or chemical stimuli to the larynx, trachea, carina and lower bronchi result in a reflex cough and bronchoconstriction. The high velocity created by the cough sweeps mucus and other irritants up toward the pharynx.

Stretch Reflex

The intercostal muscles and the diaphragm contain sensory muscle spindles that respond to elongation. A signal is sent to the spinal cord and anterior horn motor neurons. These neurons signal more muscle fibers to contract (recruitment) and thus increase the strength of the contraction. Theoretically, such a stretch reflex may be useful when there is an increase in airway resistance or a decrease in lung compliance. Stretching the ribs and the diaphragm may activate the stretch reflex and help the patient to take a deep breath. The fundamental pathways of the stretch reflex are shown in Figure 2–2. Research is needed, however, to establish the therapeutic role of proprioceptive neurofacilitation techniques based upon stretch reflex theory in altering pulmonary function.

Joint and Muscle Receptors

Peripheral joints and muscles of the limbs are believed to have receptors that respond to movement and enhance ventilation in preparation for activity. Ventilation has also been shown to be stimulated by a similar reflex in man and anesthetized animals in response to passive movement of the limbs. The precise pathways for these reflexes have not been well established.

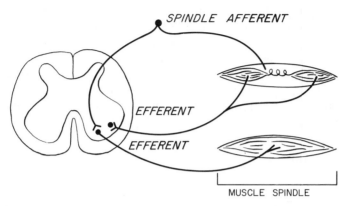

FIG 2–2.
Stretch reflex.

Mechanoreceptors

Changes in systemic blood pressure cause corresponding changes in pressure receptors in the carotid and aortic sinuses. Increase in blood pressure causes mechanical distortion of the receptors in these sinuses, producing reflex hypoventilation. Conversely, a reduction in blood pressure can result in hyperventilation.

MECHANICAL FACTORS IN BREATHING

The flow of air into the lungs is a result of pressure differences between the lungs and the atmosphere. In normal breathing, for inspiration to occur, alveolar pressure must be less than atmospheric pressure. Muscular contraction of the respiratory muscles lowers alveolar pressure and enlarges the thorax. The decreased pressure causes air to flow from the atmosphere into the lungs. Patients who are unable to create adequate negative pressure may have to be mechanically ventilated. The ventilators create a positive pressure (greater than atmospheric pressure) that forces air into the lungs where there is atmospheric pressure. Again, airflow occurs as a result of pressure differences between the atmosphere and the lungs (see Chapter 29). The iron lung used during the polio epidemic of the 1950s assisted ventilation using similar principles. Positive and negative pressures were applied alternately to the chest wall to deflate and inflate the chest, respectively.

Exhalation occurs when alveolar pressure is greater than atmospheric pressure. At the cessation of inspiration, the respiratory muscles return to their resting positions. The diaphragm rises, compressing the lungs and increasing alveolar pressure. As the intercostals relax, the ribs drop back to their preinspiratory position, further compressing the lungs and increasing alveolar pressure. The increased alveolar pressure contributes to air flowing from the lungs. Normally, expiration is a passive process.

Resistance to Breathing

Compliance

The inner walls of the thorax, lined with parietal pleura, and the parenchyma of the lung, lined with visceral pleura, lie in close proximity to one another. They are separated by a small amount of pleural fluid. Muscular contraction of the intercostals and the diaphragm mechanically englarges the thorax. The lungs are enlarged at this time due to their close proximity to the thorax. The healthy lung resists this enlargement and tries to pull away from the chest wall. The ease with which the lungs are inflated during inspiration is known as *compliance* and is defined as the volume change per unit of pressure change. The normal lung is very distensible or compliant. It can become more rigid and less compliant in diseases that cause alveolar, interstitial or pleural fibrosis, and alveolar edema. Compliance increases with age and in emphysema.

The elastic recoil or compliance of the lung is also dependent on a special surface fluid, surfactant, which lines the alveoli. This fluid increases compliance by lowering the surface tension of the alveoli, thereby reducing the muscular effort necessary to ventilate the lungs and keep them expanded. It is a complex lipoprotein that is thought to be produced in the type II alveolar cells (see Chapter 1). A decrease in surfactant causes the alveoli to collapse. Reexpanding these alveoli requires a tremendous amount of work on the part of the patient. The patient may become fatigued and need mechanical ventilation. This occurs in respiratory distress syndrome of the premature infant (previously called hyaline membrane disease) and in adult respiratory distress syndrome (ARDS, also known as shock lung and acute lung injury). In another disease, alveolar proteinosis, there is excessive accumulation of protein in the alveolar spaces. This may be due to excessive production of surfactant or deficient removal of surfactant by alveolar macrophages.

The elastic properties of the lung tend to collapse the lung if not acted on by external forces. The tissues of the thoracic wall also have elastic recoil which cause it to expand considerably if unopposed. These two forces oppose each other, keeping the lungs expanded and the thoracic cage in a neutral position. If these forces are interrupted (as in pneumothorax), the lung collapses and the thoracic wall expands (Fig 2–3). Similarly, the overinflated, barrel-shaped chest of the patient with chronic obstructive disease is explained in part by the elastic ten-

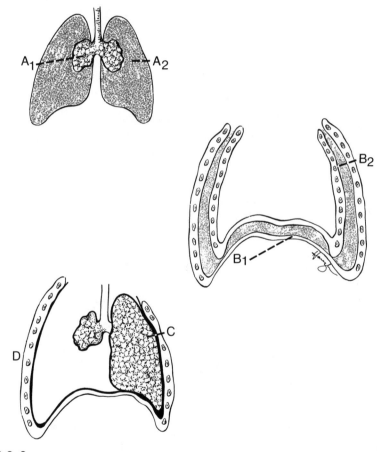

FIG 2–3.
Various relationships between the lungs and the thorax. **A,** 1—the size the lungs would assume if they were not acted on by the elastic recoil of the thoracic wall. 2—normal size of lungs within the thorax. **B,** 1—the size the thorax would assume if it were not acted on by elastic recoil of the lungs. 2—normal position of the chest wall when acted on by elastic recoil of the lungs. **C,** the normal relationship of lung to thorax. **D,** the positions assumed by the lung and thorax in a tension pneumothorax.

sion of the chest wall being unopposed by the usual elastic forces of the lungs which have been damaged by disease.

Pressure Volume Relationships

Pressure volume curves help to define the elastic properties of the chest wall and lungs. The elasticity of the respiratory system as a whole is the sum of its two major components, the lungs, and the chest wall. The so-called relaxation pressure curve is shown in Figure 2–4. The curve illustrates the static pressure of the lungs, chest wall, and the combination of the two measured at given lung volumes. Functional residual capacity reflects the balance of elastic forces exerted by the chest wall and the lungs. This is an important point with significant implications for the clinical presentation and management of patients with chronic lung disease.

The relaxation-pressure curve represents static pressure measurements. This means that the respiratory muscles are inactive, and the volume in the lungs at a given point in the respiratory cycle is determined by the balance of forces between the chest wall and the lungs. The chest wall and lungs exert elastic forces that oppose each other. The chest wall attempts to pull the lung out and the lungs attempt to recoil and pull the chest wall in. The curves labeled lung and chest wall are theoretical and illustrate the elastic force exerted by each when permitted to act unopposed by the other. Normally, these two forces are

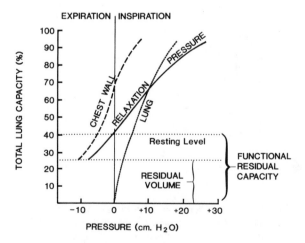

FIG 2–4.
The relaxation pressure curve. The pressure in the lung at any volume reflects elastic forces of the lung and chest wall.

exerted together and give the pressure volume relaxation curve. It can be seen that at functional residual capacity (FRC), these forces are in equilibrium, and therefore functional residual capacity is the resting volume of the respiratory system. Active muscular work is required to effect inspiration. Expiration is normally a passive process. The pressure volume curve also shows the range of lung volumes, specifically tidal volume, over which the energy expenditure for breathing is most economical. In other words, large volume changes result from relatively small changes in pressure as noted from the slope of the curve over tidal volume.

In lung disease, this balance of forces is disrupted. More work and more energy are required to sustain the respiratory effort. The patient is less able to rely on normal elastic recoil of either the chest wall, lungs, or both. Therefore, the patient must put more energy into the system to produce the same respiratory function. The limits of respiratory excursion are determined by both elastic and muscular forces. At total lung capacity, the elastic forces of the respiratory system are balanced by the inspiratory muscle force. At residual volume, the elastic forces of the chest wall are balanced by the maximum expiratory muscle force. This volume excursion from total lung capacity to residual volume reflects vital capacity.

Although the curves representing the elastic forces of the lungs and chest wall are theoretical, they are helpful in understanding the effect of lung dysfunction on pulmonary function and on the clinical presentation of the patient. For example, in chronic obstructive lung disease, the characteristic barrel chest reflects the unopposed elastic forces of the chest wall, succeeding in increasing the excursion of the chest as a result of reduced elastic recoil of the lungs. At the other extreme is the effect of a puncture wound to the chest wall which disrupts the intrapleural pressure gradient that normally keeps the lung expanded and the chest wall contained. The result of such a puncture is to produce a pneumothorax where the lung collapses down to the hilum and the chest wall springs outward (see Fig 2–3).

Airway Resistance

The flow of air into the lungs depends on pressure differences and on the resistance to flow by the airways. *Resistance* is defined as the pressure difference required for one unit flow change. The air passages in humans are divided into upper and lower airways (see Chapter 1). The upper airways are responsible for 45% of airway resistance. The resistance to airflow by the lower airways depends on many factors and is therefore difficult to predict. The branching of the lower airways is irregular, and the diameter of the lumen may vary due to external pressures and contraction or relaxation of bronchial or bronchiolar smooth muscle. The lumen diameter may also decrease due to mucosal congestion, edema or mucus. Any of these changes in the airway diameter may cause an increase in airway resistance. Flow of air through these airways can be either laminar or turbulent (Fig 2–5). *Laminar flow* is a streamlined flow where resistance occurs mainly between the sides of the tubes and the air molecules. It tends to be cone chaped, with the molecules in contact with the walls of the tubes moving more slowly than the molecules in the middle of the tube. *Turbulent flow* occurs when there are frequent molecular collisions in addition to the resistance of the sides of the tubes seen in laminar flow. This type of flow occurs at high flow rates and in airways where there are irregularities caused by mucus, exudate, tumor and other obstructions. In normal lungs, airflow is a combination of laminar and turbulent flow and is known as *tracheobronchial flow.*

The airways are distensible and compressible, and thus are susceptible to outside pressures. As these pressures compress the airways, they alter the airway resistance. *Transmural pressure* is the difference between the pressures in the airways and the pressures surrounding the airways. In erect humans, there is a higher transmural pressure at

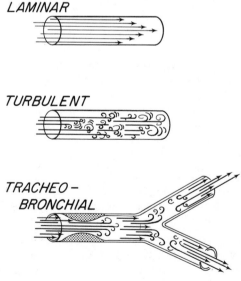

FIG 2–5.
The different types of airflow seen within the tracheobronchial tree.

the apices of the lungs than at the bases. This widens the airways at the apices relative to those at the bases. Although the airways in the apices contain more air at end expiration, the airways in the bases ventilate more. This is because alveoli operating at lower transmural pressures receive more volume than those at higher pressures.

Airway resistance decreases during inspiration as a result of the widening airways. During expiration, airways narrow, thus increasing resistance. The positive alveolar pressure that occurs during expiration partially compresses the airways. If these airways have lost their structural support as a result of disease, they may collapse and trap air distally (as in emphysema).

VENTILATION

Ventilation is the process by which air moves into the lungs. The volume of air inhaled can be measured with a spirometer. The various lung capacities and volumes are defined later in the chapter.

Regional differences in ventilation exist throughout the lung. Studies using radioactive inert gas have shown that when the gas is inhaled and measurements are taken with a radiation counter over the chest wall, radiation counts are greatest in the lower lung fields, intermediate in the midlung fields, and lowest in the upper lung fields. This effect is position or gravity dependent. If supine the apices and bases are ventilated comparably, and the lowermost lung fields are better ventilated than the uppermost lung fields. Similarly, in the lateral or side-lying position, the lower lung fields are preferentially ventilated compared with the upper lung fields.

The causes of regional differences in ventilation can be explained in terms of the anatomy of the lung and mechanics of breathing. An intrapleural pressure gradient exists down the lung. In the upright position, the intrapleural pressure tends to be more negative at the top of the lung, and becomes progressively less negative toward the bottom of the lung. This pressure gradient is thought to reflect the weight of the suspended lung. The more negative intrapleural pressure at the top of the lung results in relatively greater expansion of that area and a larger resting volume. The expanding pressure in the bottom of the lung, however, is relatively small, and hence has a smaller resting volume. This distinction between the upper and lower lung fields is fundamental to understanding the effect on differences in regional ventilation. The regional differences in resting volume should not be confused with regional differences in ventilation volume. Ventilation refers to volume change as a function of resting volume. The relatively higher resting volume in the upper lung fields renders it stiffer or less compliant compared with the low lung volumes and greater compliance in the lower lung fields. The lower lung fields therefore exhibit a greater volume change in relation to resting volume which effects greater overall ventilation compared with the upper lung fields. In summary, ventilation is favored in the lowermost lung fields regardless of the position of the body.

DIFFUSION

Once air has reached the alveoli, it must cross the alveolar-capillary (A-C) membrane (Fig 2–6). The gases must cross through the surfactant lining, the alveolar epithelial membrane and the capillary endothelial membrane. Oxygen has to travel further through a layer of plasma, the erythrocyte membrane and intracellular fluid in the erythrocyte, until it encounters a hemoglobin molecule. This distance is actually very small in normal lungs, but in disease states it may increase. Frequently, the alveolar wall or the capillary membrane become thickened. Fluid, edema, or exudate may separate the two membranes. These con-

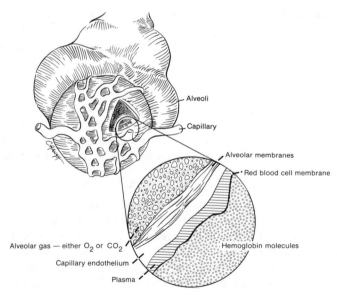

FIG 2–6.
The components of the alveolar-capillary membrane.

ditions are frequently first detected when arterial PO_2 becomes chronically lower than normal. Oxygen diffuses very slowly through the A-C membrane in comparison to CO_2 diffusion. As a result, patients with diffusion problems frequently have hypoxemia with a normal PCO_2. Sarcoidosis, berylliosis, asbestosis, scleroderma and pulmonary edema are some diseases that decrease the diffusing capacity of the gases. The capacity may also decrease in emphysema because of a decrease in surface area for gas exchange.

PERFUSION

Perfusion of the lung refers to the blood flow of the pulmonary circulation available for gas exchange. The pulmonary circulation operates at relatively low pressures compared with the systemic circulation. For this reason, the walls of the blood vessels in the pulmonary circulation are significantly thinner than comparable vessels in the systemic circulation. Pulmonary arterial pressure is low because perfusion of the top of the lung is the most distal area. Compared with the systemic circulation, there is little requirement for significant regional differences in perfusion.

Hydrostatic pressure has a significant effect on perfusion of the lower lobes. The hydrostatic pressure reflects the effect of gravity on the blood, tending to favor perfusion of the lower lung fields. This fact has been substantiated using radioactive tracers in the pulmonary circulation and measuring radiation counts over the lung fields. The nonuniformity of perfusion is believed to reflect the interaction of alveolar, arterial, and venous pressures down the lung. Normally, blood flow is determined by the arterial venous pressure gradient. In the lungs, there are regional differences in alveolar pressure that can exert an effect on the arterial venous pressure gradient. For example, in the upper lung fields, alveolar pressure approximates atmospheric pressure which overrides the arterial pressure and effectively closes the pulmonary capillaries. In the lower lung fields, the opposite occurs. The relatively low volume of air in the alveoli is overridden by the greater capillary hydrostatic pressure. Thus, the capillary pressure effectively overcomes the alveolar pressure.

Pulmonary blood vessels constrict in response to low arterial pressures of oxygen. This is termed hypoxic vasoconstriction. Hypoxic vasoconstriction in the lung is believed to serve as an adaptive mechanism for diverting blood away from underventilated or poorly oxygenated lung areas. Although hypoxic vasoconstriction may have an important role to improve the efficiency of the lungs as a gas exchanger, this mechanism may be potentially deleterious to a patient who has reduced arterial oxygen pressure secondary to pulmonary pathology.

The acid base balance of the blood also affects pulmonary blood flow. A low blood pH or acidemia, for example, potentiates pulmonary vasoconstriction. Thus, impaired ventilatory function can disturb blood gas composition and in turn acid base balance. This effect can be amplified because of the cyclic reaction of pH on pulmonary vasoconstriction. Consideration of these basic physiologic mechanisms are tantamount to optimizing physical therapy intervention.

Ventilation and Perfusion Matching

It is essential that ventilated areas of the lung are in contact with perfused areas of the lung to effect normal gas exchange. Conditions that alter the ventilation or perfusion of part of the lung will also affect the gas exchange in that portion of the lung. Uneven ventilation occurs where there is uneven compliance or uneven airway resistance in different parts of the lung. The lung is more compliant, i.e., easier to inflate at low lung volumes. The apices have a higher resting volume because of a more negative intrapleural pressure than the bases, which renders the apices less compliant than the bases with relatively low resting volumes. Ventilation as previously described is favored in the lower lung regions rather than the apices. Uneven airway resistance may be due to airway narrowing (bronchoconstriction in asthma, mucous plugs, edema, tumor) or collapse due to external pressures as with tumors or emphysema). The lungs may also expand unevenly as a result of the effects of gravity. Uneven compliance may be due to fibrosis, emphysema, pleural thickening, effusions or pulmonary edema.

Nonuniform perfusion or blood flow can be due to gravity, regional differences in intrapleural pressure, regional changes in alveolar pressure, and obstruction or blockage of part of the pulmonay circulation. Gravity increases blood flow in the dependent portions of the lung and decreases it in the nondependent portions of the lung. Regional differences in intrapleural pressure change the transmural pressure of blood vessels and thereby the amount of blood flowing through those vessels. Changes in alveolar pressure also affect the amount of blood flowing through the vessels. Overexpanded alveoli can compress blood vessels, while underexpanded alveoli may allow more blood to flow through those vessels. Blood clots, fat, parasites or tumor cells may constrict or block part of the pulmonary circulation.

As discussed previously, gravity tends to pull blood into the dependent positions of the lung (Fig 2–7). In erect humans, therefore, there is greater blood flow at the bases of the lung. In places, the arterial blood pressure will exceed the alveolar pressure and cause compression or collapse of the airways (Fig 2–8). Blood flow to the apices is decreased due to gravity. Airways in this region are more fully expanded due to high transmural pressures and may further decrease blood flow by compressing blood vessels. It follows that the areas of the best gas exchange will occur where there is the greatest amount of perfusion and ventilation. This occurs toward the base of the lungs in erect humans. Changes in posture cause changes in perfusion and ventilation. Generally, greater air exchange occurs toward the gravity-dependent areas. A person lying on his side will therefore have greater gas exchange in the bottom lung (Fig 2–9).

In normal lungs, there is an optimum ratio or matching of gas and blood. This ratio of ventilation to perfusion is 0.8 to maintain normal blood gas values of P_{O_2} and P_{CO_2}. Therefore, the lungs must be able to supply four parts ventilation to about five parts perfusion. When the ratio is not uniform throughout the lung, the arterial blood cannot contain normal blood gas values. Regions with low ratios (perfusion in ex-

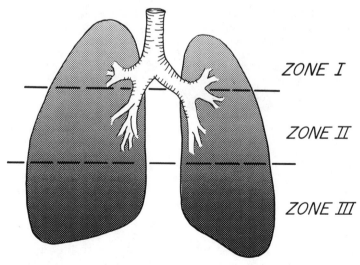

FIG 2–7.
The perfusion of the lung is dependent on posture. In the upright position three areas can be seen. Zone III has perfusion in excess of ventilation, in Zone II perfusion and ventilation are fairly equal and in Zone I ventilation occurs in excess of perfusion.

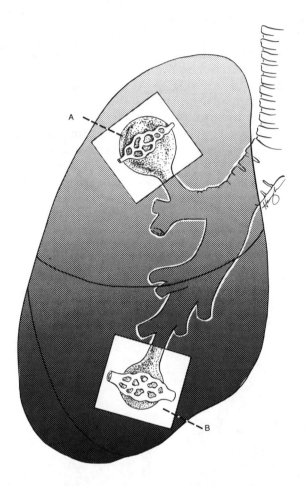

FIG 2–8.
Relationship between the size of the airways and the amount of perfusion in the area in the upright position. **A,** perfusion is decreased in the apices due to gravity. This enables the alveoli to fully expand. This expansion may compress blood vessels and thereby further decrease blood flow. **B,** perfusion is increased in the bases of the lungs due to gravity. The enlarged vessels prevent full expansion of alveoli and may in fact compress them to a smaller size.

cess of ventilation) act as a shunt, while regions with high ratios (ventilation in excess of perfusion) act as dead space (Fig 2–10). Hypoxemia may result if regions of $\dot{V}/\dot{Q}$ ratio predominate. An elevation in arterial P_{CO_2} may also occur unless the patient increases his ventilation. Therapists who are positioning patients with lung pathology may find that

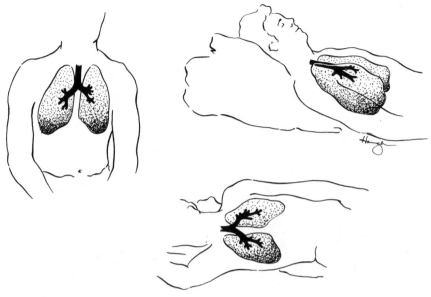

FIG 2–9.
The effect of positioning on perfusion of the lung. Note that gravity-dependent segments have the greatest amount of perfusion.

their patients become very agitated and even cyanotic in certain positions. This restlessness can probably be attributed to ventilation-perfusion inequalities causing poor gas exchange in the dependent lung.

The relationship of ventilation and perfusion in the lung is summarized in the following figures. Figure 2–11 shows increases in ventilation and perfusion down the upright lung. Optimal ventilation and perfusion matching, $\dot{V}/\dot{Q}$, occurs in the mid lung zones. In the upright position, ventilation is in excess of perfusion in the apices, and perfusion is in excess of ventilation in the bases. Figures 2–12 and 2–13 illustrate the effects of shunt and physiologic dead space on $\dot{V}/\dot{Q}$ matching in the upright lung, and their effect on alveolar gas. Specifically, Figure 2–12 shows a schematic representation of regional differences in ventilation and perfusion in the upper, middle, and lower zones of the lungs. These gradients are reflected in the alveolar Po_2 and Pco_2 levels associated with alveolar dead space of the apices, appropriate ventilation-perfusion matching in the mid lung and shunt in the bases. Figure 2–13 shows a graph illustrating the relationship of Po_2 and Pco_2 down the various zones of the upright lung.

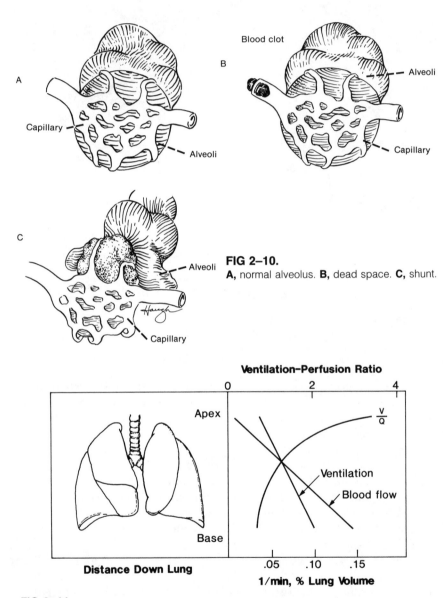

FIG 2–10.
A, normal alveolus. **B,** dead space. **C,** shunt.

FIG 2–11.
The effect of gravity on ventilation, perfusion and ventilation-perfusion matching (V/Q ratio).

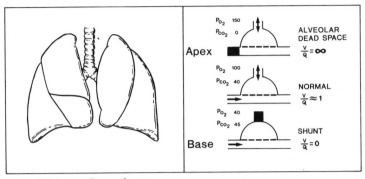

Distance Down Lung

FIG 2–12.
Schemata showing the effect of gravity on ventilation and perfusion down the upright lung.

Clinical Implications

The relationship of ventilation and perfusion have important implications for physical therapists with respect to regulation of blood gases, patient positioning, and optimizing response to chest care and exercise.

The supine position is of particular interest considering most hospitalized patients spend a considerable amount of time in this position. Ventilation and perfusion, hence gas exchange, can theoretically be augmented in the supine position, probably reflecting increased cardiac output. The supine position, however, has a direct effect on lung dynamics which potentiates airway closure and may counter the effect on $\dot{V}/\dot{Q}$ matching. Airway closure is described in a later section. In design-

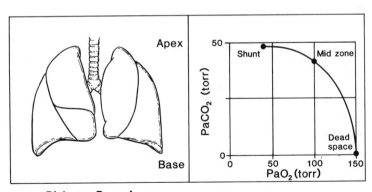

Distance Down Lung

FIG 2–13.
The effect of shunt and physiologic dead space on the P_{O_2} and P_{CO_2} of lung zones.

ing positioning regimen for patients, physical therapists are cautioned to examine the effect of a given position on *all* aspects of lung function. If the position of the patient is supine, lung function is likely to be suboptimal. This may have profound effects on any therapeutic benefit from chest physical therapy or bed exercises.

The beneficial effects of the prone position have been documented in the management of the patient in respiratory failure. Lying prone has been shown to have a more beneficial effect on arterial blood gases than lying supine in some patients. This effect has been shown to be more marked in the prone position with the abdomen free to protrude downward than lying prone with the abdomen restricted. This may reflect in part the favorable effect of this position on lung dynamics by maximizing functional residual capacity and decreasing closing volume. Reports of postponing mechanical ventilation and reducing inspired oxygen concentrations (FIO_2) when incorporating the prone position into the turning regimen are provocative and suggest that the prone position should be considered more often in the routine management and prevention of pulmonary dysfunction.

Traditional chest physical therapy has focused on removing secretions, thereby improving ventilation. Optimizing gas exchange and maintaining or improving blood gases are also treatment priorities. Optimal gas exchange reflects adequate ventilation and perfusion matching throughout the lungs. This is effected by reducing undue shunt and physiologic dead space. Thus, the therapist or nurse needs to consider the gas exchange and the variables that affect it, e.g., lung disease, age, position, smoking history, or treatment and exercise prescription. With greater understanding of these factors, physical therapy interventions are likely to be more beneficial and to reduce untoward adverse effects.

Transport of Oxygen by the Blood

Once oxygen reaches the blood, it rapidly combines with hemoglobin to form oxyhemoglobin. A small proportion of oxygen is dissolved in the plasma. The use of the hemoglobin molecule as an oxygen carrier allows for greater availability and efficiency of oxygen delivery to the tissues in response to changes in metabolism. Saturation of the oxygen-carrying sites on the hemoglobin molecule is curvilinearly related to the partial pressure of oxygen in the tissues. This relationship is called the oxyhemoglobin dissociation curve and is a sigmoid or S-shaped curve (Fig 2–14). The hemoglobin of arterial blood is 98% or almost completely saturated with oxygen. Under normal circumstances, arterial

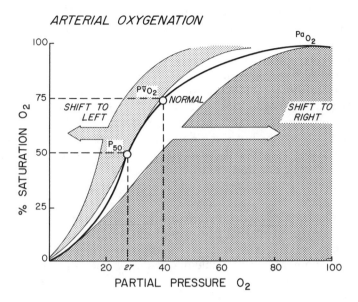

FIG 2–14.
The oxyhemoglobin dissociation curve.

blood is mixed with a small proportion of venous blood from the coronary and pulmonary circulation, resulting in arterial saturation of less than 100%. The graph shows a range of partial pressures of oxygen that may exist in the tissues. At relatively high arterial oxygen pressures, the oxygen saturation is high. This reflects high association or low dissociation between oxygen and hemoglobin. Saturation does not fall significantly until the partial pressure of oxygen falls below 80 mm Hg. Even at PO_2 levels of 40 to 50 mm Hg, arterial saturation is still 75%. This suggests an enormous capacity of the oxyhemoglobin dissociation system to meet the varying needs of different tissues without severely compromising arterial saturation. A PO_2 of less than 50%, for example, has a profound effect on arterial saturation. This demonstrates an adaptive response of hemoglobin dissociation to respond to low oxygen tissue pressures by greater dissociation of oxygen from hemoglobin as the need arises. As the PO_2 improves as a result of increased supply of oxygen or decreased demand, the affinity between oxygen and hemoglobin increases, and arterial saturation increases. Thus, oxygen is not released unless there is a need for greater oxygen delivery in the tissues.

Different conditions can increase or decrease hemoglobin affinity for oxygen and thereby cause a shift in the oxyhemoglobin dissociation curve (see Fig 2–14). A shift to the right results in decreased oxygen affinity and greater dissociation of oxygen and hemoglobin. In this instance, for any given partial pressure of oxygen, there is a lower saturation than normal. This means that there is more oxygen available to the tissues. Shifts in the curve to the right occur with increasing concentration of hydrogen ions (i.e., decreasing pH), increasing P_{CO_2}, increasing temperatures, and increasing levels of 2,3-DPG (diphosphoglycerate), a byproduct of red blood cell metabolism. West suggests, "A simple way to remember these shifts is that an exercising muscle (increased metabolic demand), is acid, hypercarbic, (hypercapnic) and hot, and it benefits from increased unloading of oxygen from its capillaries."

A shift of the curve to the left results in increased oxygen affinity. Thus, for any given partial pressure of oxygen, there is a higher saturation than normal. This means that there is less oxygen available to the tissues. This occurs in alkalemia, hypothermia, and decreased 2,3-DPG.

Anemia (reduced red blood cell count and hemoglobin) and polycythemia (excess red blood cells and hemoglobin) produce changes in oxygen content of the blood as well as saturation. Anemia shifts the curve to the right and lowers the maximal saturation achievable. Polycythemia has the opposite effect. The curve is shifted to the left and maximal saturation approaches 100%.

TRANSPORT OF CARBON DIOXIDE

Carbon dioxide is an acid produced by cells as a result of cell metabolism. It is carried in various forms by venous blood to the lungs, where it is eliminated. Most of the CO_2 added to plasma diffuses into the red blood cells, where it is buffered and returned to the plasma to be carried to the lungs. The buffering mechanism is so effective that large changes in dissolved carbon dioxide can occur with small changes in blood pH.

The transport of CO_2 has an important role in the acid-base status of the blood. The lung excretes 10,000 mEq of carbonic acid per day. (Carbonic acid is broken down into water and carbon dioxide. The carbon dioxide is buffered and eliminated through the lungs.) The kidney can excrete only 100 mEq per day of acids. Therefore, alterations in alveolar ventilation can have profound effects on the body's acid-base status. A decrease in the lung's ability to ventilate causes a sharp rise in

PCO_2 and a drop in pH. This causes an *acute respiratory acidosis*. If this change occurs gradually, the pH will remain within normal limits while the PCO_2 is elevated. This is known as a *compensated respiratory acidosis*. Hyperventilation or excessive ventilation will cause rapid elimination of carbon dioxide from the blood. This results in a decreased PCO_2 and an increased pH and is known as an *acute respiratory alkalosis*. Again, if the change occurs gradually, the pH will remain within normal limits even though the PCO_2 is decreased. This is a *compensated respiratory alkalosis*.

PULMONARY FUNCTION TESTS

A series of studies, pulmonary function tests (PFT), are helpful in evaluating the mechanical function of the lungs. These studies can determine if the lungs are functioning normally or if there is a problem of which even the patient is unaware. Such tests are being used more frequently in hospitals and medical centers to localize and monitor lung disease, and as presurgical studies to predict postoperative respiratory complications. In dealing with patients with respiratory problems, the pulmonary function tests will help the therapist understand the nature of the patient's problem and the type of therapy that is most appropriate for that problem. The most common pulmonary function tests are discussed below, as well as the significance of deviations from normal. Normal values are not given because they vary with height, weight, and age.

Dead Space

The most important function of the lungs is to supply the body with sufficient oxygen (O_2) to meet its metabolic needs and to remove the excess carbon dioxide (CO_2) that is produced. As this gas exchange occurs continuously at the alveolar level, air must move in and out of the lungs frequently enough to keep alveolar O_2 levels high and alveolar CO_2 levels low. Fresh air does not go directly to the alveoli but moves first through the conducting airways where no gas exchange occurs.

As air passes through the conducting airways (the nose or mouth, pharynx, larynx, trachea, bronchi and bronchioles), it is filtered, heated and humidified (see Chapter 1). The volume of these conducting airways is known as the *anatomic dead space* and is approximately equal in milliliters to an adult's ideal weight in pounds (about 150 ml). A normal breath, the *tidal volume* (TV), must be large enough to reach the alveoli beyond the anatomic dead space. In a normal adult, the TV is 450–600 ml, 150 ml of which ventilates dead space. The other 300–450 ml reaches alveoli and is referred to as *alveolar ventilation.*

There are many diseases or conditions that can alter the volume of dead space that must be ventilated. In some cases, dead space decreases, as in a pneumonectomy where it is physically removed or in asthma where bronchospasm may narrow the airways. In other conditions, such as pulmonary embolus, dead space increases when ventilated areas of lung cease to be perfused. The alveoli continue to receive fresh gas but there is no blood available for gas exchange. This type of dead space is known as *physiologic dead space.*

In cases of increased dead space, a larger percentage of the tidal volume is ventilating the dead space, leaving a smaller percentage for alveolar ventilation. The patient must work harder to get enough air to the functioning alveoli. This causes increased work of breathing and frequently results in patient fatigue. In other cases, a patient may be unable to take his normal tidal volume because of respiratory muscle weakness secondary to disease (Guillain-Barré, myasthenia gravis or quadriplegia) or because he is in a compromised state from a disease (cancer) or surgery. If his tidal volume drops, for example, from 450 ml to 300 ml, then only 150 ml will be available for alveolar ventilation. Again, a larger percentage of each breath is ventilating dead space, which results in increased work of breathing for the patient.

Lung Volumes

The lung contains four volumes, tidal volume (which we have already discussed), inspiratory reserve volume (IRV), expiratory reserve volume (ERV) and residual volume (RV) (Fig 2–15). *Inspiratory reserve volume* is the maximum amount of air that can be inhaled from the end of a normal inspiration. The *expiratory reserve volume* is the maximum amount of air that can be expired after a normal exhalation. The *residual volume* is the volume of gas that remains in the lungs at the end of a maximum expiration.

Changes in the residual volume can help diagnose certain conditions. An increase in RV means that even with maximum effort, the patient cannot exhale excess air from his lungs. This results in hyperinflated lungs and indicates that certain changes have occurred in the pulmonary tissue, which in time may cause mechanical changes in the chest wall (i.e., increased AP diameter, flattened diaphragm, etc., see Chapter 4). These changes may be reversible in patients with partial

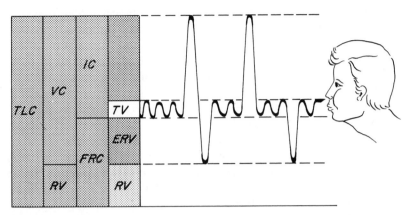

FIG 2–15.
A spirogram (pulmonary function testing).

bronchial obstruction (as in young asthmatics) or irreversible as in patients with emphysema. A decrease in residual volume can occur in diffuse restrictive pulmonary diseases (see Chapter 4) and in diseases in which alveoli are occluded in many portions of the lung (cancer, diffuse microatelectasis).

Capacities

The lung contains four capacities, each of which contain two or more volumes (see Fig 2–15). They are total lung capacity (TLC), vital capacity (VC), inspiratory capacity (IC) and functional residual capacity (FRC). *Total lung capacity* is the amount of gas the lung contains at the end of a maximum inspiration. It contains all four lung volumes (see Fig 2–15). A decrease in TLC can indicate extensive pulmonary disease or the presence of certain conditions (restrictive disease—see Chapter 3, edema, exudate, atelectasis, neoplasms). A decrease in TLC can also occur when pulmonary tissue is compressed (pleural effusions, pneumothorax, hemothorax) or if there is a nonpulmonary limitation to full expansion (kyphoscoliosis, obesity, pregnancy, ascites, and other conditions). TLC may be increased in emphysema.

Vital capacity is defined as the maximum amount of gas that can be expelled from the lungs by forceful effort following a maximum inspiration. It contains the inspiratory reserve volume, tidal volume and expiratory reserve volume (see Fig 2–15). A decrease in VC can occur as a result of absolute reduction in distensible lung tissue. Examples of this are pneumonia, atelectasis, pulmonary congestion, occlusion of a major bronchus by a tumor, bronchiolar obstruction, pulmonary edema, restrictive diseases and surgical excision of pulmonary tissue.

Decrease in vital capacity can also occur where there is no disease of lung tissue or airways. There may be decreased respiratory movements secondary to depression of the respiratory centers or due to neuromuscular diseases (myasthenia gravis, Guillain-Barré, and others). Limitation of thoracic expansion (as in scleroderma, kyphoscoliosis, or pain from surgery or fractured ribs) may also cause a decrease in VC. Pregnancy, ascites, and abdominal tumor may limit the descent of the diaphragm and therefore decrease the amount of air in the lungs. If the lungs cannot fully expand (as with pleural effusion, pneumothorax, diaphragmatic hernia, or marked cardiac enlargement), there will also be a decrease in vital capacity.

Inspiratory capacity is the maximum amount of air that can be inspired from the resting expiratory level. it contains the inspiratory reserve volumes and the tidal volume. The *functional residual capacity* is the volume of air remaining in the lungs at the resting expiratory level. It contains the expiratory reserve volume and the residual volume. The FRC prevents large fluctuations in alveolar PO_2 with each breath. An increase in FRC represents hyperinflation of the lungs. It causes the thorax to be larger than normal, resulting in muscular inefficiency and some mechanical disadvantage. In some conditions (as in shock lung), patients who are hypoxemic mechanically have their FRC increased through positive end-expiratory pressure (PEEP) or continuous positive airway pressure (CPAP) to help keep their alveoli open and maintain a high alveolar PO_2 with each breath.

SUMMARY OF PATHOPHYSIOLOGIC PULMONARY FUNCTION

Figure 2–16 shows the relative differences in lung volumes and capacities in obstructive and restrictive lung disease compared with the healthy individual. Although disease has a profound impact on pulmonary function, tidal volume usually constituting 10% of total lung capacity may remain remarkably constant until disease is relatively severe. Physiologic pulmonary reserves in obstructive and restrictive lung diseases, however, are likely to be compromised and limit the patient's exercise tolerance. In obstructive lung disease, TLC, FRC, and RV are markedly increased. If severe, the increased FRC compromises VC. Considerably more energy may need to be expended to breathe (up to a tenfold increase) compared with the healthy individual. This effect

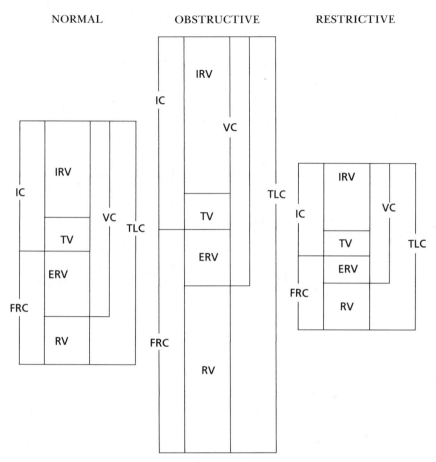

FIG 2–16.
Examples of proportional changes of lung volumes and capacities characteristic of obstructive and restrictive lung diseases.

may be disproportionately increased with minimal amounts of activity.

In restrictive lung disease, restriction of the chest wall or lung tissue can produce a decrease in TLC. A VC of 80% predicted for a patient (based on age and weight) is considered a diagnostic feature. A residual decline in FRC potentiates airway closure.

The phenomenon of closing volume in the lungs has particular significance for physical therapists who prescribe breathing exercises and body positioning, and thereby alter pulmonary mechanics and gas exchange. These treatment interventions may have a pronounced effect on lung volumes and airway closure. At low lung volumes, e.g., breathing at FRC, head-down position, and in lung disease, intrapleural pressures are generally less negative and the pressure of dependent lung regions may equal or exceed atmospheric pressure. Intrapleural pressure is less negative because the lung is less expanded and elastic recoil less pronounced. As a result, airway closure is potentiated. In young individuals, closure is evident at RV; however, in older individuals, closure is observed at higher lung volumes, e.g., at FRC. Premature closure of the small airways results in uneven ventilation and impaired gas exchange with a given lung unit. Airway closure occurs more readily in chronic smokers and in patients with lung disease.

Aging has a significant effect on airway closure. With aging is a loss of pulmonary elastic recoil resulting in a loss of intrapleural negative pressure. In older individuals, therefore, airway closure occurs at higher lung volumes. For example, closure has been reported to occur at the age of 65 in the upright lung during normal breathing. In the supine position where FRC is reduced, closure occurs at a significantly younger age (about 44). In addition to the often compounding effect of age, the lung volume at which airway closure occurs increases with chronic smoking and lung disease, and is changed with alterations in body position.

FORCED EXPIRATION

One of the most useful tests in the measurement of a single expiration after a maximum inspiration; this is known as a *forced vital capacity* (FVC). It should be the same as the vital capacity. In chronic obstructive lung disease, the FVC is frequently decreased while the vital capacity is normal. The forceful expiration causes higher transpulmonary pressures so that bronchiolar collapse, obstructive lesions and air trapping are all exaggerated. Measurements can be taken at different time intervals throughout the FVC. These are known as the forced expiratory volumes (FEV) and are marked by seconds. FEV_1 is the forced expiratory volume at one second and should be at least 80% of the vital capacity. In obstructive diseases (see Chapter 4), the FEV_1 is reduced much more than the vital capacity, giving a low FEV/VC%. In restrictive diseases, both the FEV_1 and the VC are decreased, giving a normal FEV/VC%.

Another useful way of looking at forced expiration is with a flow volume curve. This curve (Fig 2–17) shows that flow rises rapidly to a high value, and then declines over most of expiration. The expiratory

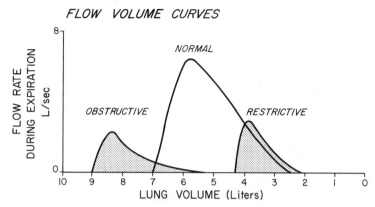

FIG 2–17.
Comparison of flow volume curves in the normal patient and in the patient with obstructive or restrictive lung disease.

flow curve is independent of effort and therefore very useful in diagnosing disease. In restrictive diseases, the maximum flow rate is reduced, as is the total volume exhaled (see Fig 2–17). In obstructive diseases, the flow rate is very low in relation to lung volume and a scooped-out appearance is often seen (see Fig 2–17).

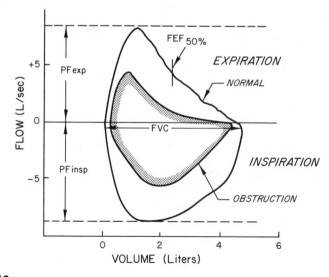

FIG 2–18.
Comparison of flow volume loops in the normal patient and in the patient with obstructive lung disease.

Another diagnostic test that utilizes forced expirations is the flow volume loop. It is a graphic analysis of the flow generated during a forced expiratory volume maneuver followed by a forced inspiratory volume maneuver (Fig 2–18). This graph offers a pictorial representation of data from many individual tests (peak inspiratory and expiratory flow rates, FVC, FEV, etc.). The shape of the graph may also be helpful in diagnosing disease (see Fig 2–17).

CLOSING VOLUME AND AIRWAY CLOSURE

The assessment of closing volume is used to help diagnose small airway disease. A test called the single breath nitrogen (N_2) washout is used for assessing closing volume and closing capacity of the small airways. In this test, the subject takes a single VC breath of 100% oxygen. During complete exhalation, the N_2 concentration can be measured. The characteristic tracing of N_2 concentration versus lung volume reflects sequential emptying of differentially ventilated lung units, hence different and expiratory N_2 concentrations. Four phases can be identified (Fig 2–19). Phase I contains pure dead space and virtually none of the potential N_2 from the RV. Phase II is associated with an increasing N_2 concentration of a mixture of gas from the dead space and alveoli. The plateau in N_2 concentration observed in Phase III reflects pure alveolar gas emanating from the bases and middle lung zones. Phase IV occurs toward the end of expiration and is characterized by an abrupt increase

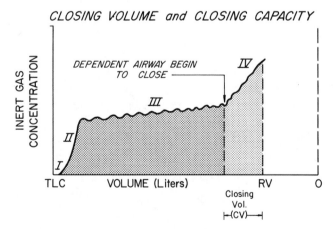

FIG 2–19.
The single breath nitrogen washout test to assess airway closure.

in N_2 concentration. This high N_2 concentration reflects closure of airways at the base of the lungs and gas being expired from the upper lung zones because in the single breath of 100% oxygen, less oxygen was initially directed to this area.

Closing volume is the lung volume at which the inflection of Phase IV, the marked increase in N_2 concentration after the plateau, is observed. Closing capacity refers to closing volume and RV. The same characteristic tracing of the single breath nitrogen washout test can be obtained with an inhalation of a bolus of tracer gas, e.g., argon, helium, xenon-133.

The closing volume is 10% of the vital capacity in young, healthy individuals. It increases with age and is 40% of the vital capacity at 65 years of age. Closing volume is used as an aid to the diagnosis of small airway disease and as a means of evaluating treatment or drug response.

SUMMARY

This chapter presented an overview of both central and peripheral mechanisms, e.g., muscle, joint, and lung and chest wall stretch receptors involved with the regulation of respiration. Mechanical factors of breathing, lung compliance, and airway resistance are described. The elastic properties of the respiratory system, i.e., chest wall and lungs, are reflected in the pressure volume relaxation curve. This curve has important implications for the clinical presentation of the patient with lung dysfunction, and in particular, the efficiency and energy requirement of the respiratory system.

Ventilation and perfusion matching is the basis of gas exchange and the adequacy of lung function. Many factors in addition to disease, however, can affect ventilation and perfusion matching, including age, position, and smoking history. The relationship of such factors are discussed.

Arterial PO_2 and PCO_2 are normally maintained within certain prescribed limits. Oxyhemoglobin dissociation helps to ensure adequate oxygen delivery to the tissues once oxygen has diffused through the alveolar capillary membrane into the circulation.

Assessment of pulmonary function can be clinically performed simply and noninvasively. Physical therapists need a thorough understanding of the implications of altered lung function on the tolerance of the patient to treatment and exercise and on response to these. Airway closure is one factor interfering with ventilation and perfusion matching. Care must be observed in avoiding premature airway closure and deterioration in ventilation and perfusion matching during physical therapy, in patients who are likely to have higher than normal closing volumes.

REFERENCES

Periodicals

Clauss RH, Scalabrini BY, Ray JF, et al: Effects of changing body position upon improved ventilation perfusion relationships. *Circulation* 1968; 37(Suppl 2):214.

Dean E: The effect of body position on pulmonary function. *Phys Ther* (in press).

Douglas WW, Rehder K, Froukje BM: Improved oxygenation in patients with acute respiratory failure: The prone position. *Am Rev Respir Dis* 1977; 115:559.

Ferris, BG, Pollard DS: Effect of deep and quiet breathing on pulmonary compliance. *J Clin Invest* 1959; 39:143.

Goldman M: Mechanical interaction between diaphragm and rib cage. *Am Rev Respir Dis* 1979; 119(Part 2):23.

Konno K, Mead J: Measurement of separate volume changes of rib cage and abdomen during breathing. *J Appl Physiol* 1967; 22:407.

Leblanc P, Ruff F, Milic-Emili J: Effects of age and body position on airway closure in man. *J Appl Physiol* 1970; 28:448.

Mead J: Respiration: Pulmonary mechanics. *Ann Rev Physiol* 1973; 35:169.

Perutz FM: Hemoglobin structure and respiratory transport. *Sci Am* 1978; 239:92.

Rahn H, Otis AB, Chadwick LE, et al: The pressure-volume diagram of the thorax and lung. *Am J Physiol* 1946; 146:161.

Ray J F, et al: Immobility, hypoxemia, and pulmonary arteriovenous shunting. *Arch Surg* 1974; 109:537.

Riley RL, Cournand A: "Ideal" alveolar air and the analysis of ventilation-perfusion relationships in the lungs. *J Appl Physiol* 1949; 6:825.

Sears TA: Breathing a sensorimotor act. *Sci Basis Med* 1971; 7:129.

West JB: Blood-flow, ventilation, and gas exchange in the lung. *Lancet* 1963; 2:1055.

Books

Bates DV, Macklem PT, Christie RV: *Respiratory Function in Disease.* Philadelphia, WB Saunders Co, 1971.

Brobeck JR (ed): *Best and Taylor's Physiological Basis of Medical Practice,* ed 10. Baltimore, Williams & Wilkins Co, 1979.

Burrows B, Knudson RJ, Quan SF, et al: *Respiratory Disorders: A Pathophysiologic Approach,* ed 2. Chicago, Year Book Medical Publishers, 1983.

Cherniack RM, Cherniack L: *Respiration in Health and Disease,* ed 3. Philadelphia, WB Saunders Co, 1983.

Comroe JH, Jr, et al: *The Lung,* ed 2. Chicago, Year Book Medical Publishers, 1973.

Comroe JH, Jr: *Physiology of Respiration,* ed 2. Chicago, Year Book Medical Publishers, 1974.

Egan DF: *Fundamentals of Respiratory Therapy,* ed 2. St. Louis, CV Mosby Co, 1973.

Murray JF: *The Normal Lung.* Philadelphia, WB Saunders Co, 1976.

Nunn JF: *Applied Respiratory Physiology,* ed 2. London, Butterworths, 1977.

West JB: *Respiratory Physiology—The Essentials,* ed 2. Baltimore, Williams & Wilkins Co, 1979.

West JB: *Pulmonary Pathophysiology: The Essentials,* ed 2. Baltimore, Williams & Wilkins Co, 1981.

3

Review of Cardiac Anatomy and Physiology

Lyn Hobson, P.T., R.R.T.

Elizabeth Dean, Ph.D., M.C.P.A.

The heart lies in series with the lungs. Virtually all the blood returned to the right side of the heart passes through the lungs and is delivered to the left side of the heart for ejection to the systemic, coronary, and pulmonary circulations. Because of this interrelationship, changes in either lung or heart function can exert changes in the function of the other organ. The therapist or nurse must therefore have a thorough understanding of both heart and lung mechanics and how they perform synergistically when treating cardiorespiratory dysfunction. This chapter presents the anatomy of the heart and its physiology in terms of its electrical and mechanical activity. An introduction to basic electrocardiography is also presented. Special attention is given to the coordination of the electrical and mechanical behavior of the heart needed to effect adequate pulmonary and systemic circulation as efficiently as possible. An understanding of these interactions is essential to health care personnel involved with cardiopulmonary patients as well as with other patient groups who will undergo the physical stress of therapeutic exercise and other interventions.

THE HEART

The heart is a conical, hollow muscular pump enclosed in a fibroserous sac, the pericardium. Its size is closely related to body size and corresponds remarkably to the size of an individual's clenched fist. It is positioned in the center of the chest behind the lower half of the sternum. The largest portion of the heart lies to the left of the midsternal line; the apex is found approximately 9 cm to the left in the fifth intercostal space.

The heart as a whole is freely movable within the pericardial cavity, changing position during both contraction and respiration. During contraction, the apex moves forward, strikes the chest and imparts the chest and apex beat, which may be felt and seen. *Abnormal position of the apex beat can indicate cardiac enlargement or displacement.* During breathing the movements of the diaphragm determine the position of the heart. This is due to the attachment of the central tendon of the diaphragm to the pericardium. Changes in position during quiet breathing are hardly noticeable, but with deep inspirations, the downward excursion of the diaphragm causes the heart to descend and rotate to the right. The opposite occurs during expiration. Pathology of the lungs can also change the position of the heart. Atelectasis shifts the heart to the same side. In tension pneumothorax where air enters the chest usually through an opening in the chest wall and cannot escape, the positive pressure shifts the heart away from the side of the pathology.

The heart is enclosed by the pericardium, whose two surfaces can be visualized by considering the heart as a fist which is plunged into a large balloon. The outer surface, a tough fibrous membrane, is called the visceral pericardium. It encases the heart and the organs and terminations of the great vessels. This membrane is so unyielding that when fluid accumulates rapidly in the pericardial cavity it can compress the heart and impede venous return. When this occurs frequently, a window is cut in the pericardium, allowing the fluid to escape. The inner surface, the parietal pericardium, is a serous membrane that lines the visceral pericardium. This inner surface is reflected onto the heart, where it becomes the epicardium. Ten to 20 ml of clear pericardial fluid separates and moistens the two pericardial surfaces. The pericardium with its fluid lubricates the moving parts of the heart, minimizing friction during contraction. It also holds the heart in position and prevents dilation.

The heart is divided into right and left halves by an obliquely placed longitudinal septum (Fig 3–1). Each half has two chambers—the atrium, which receives blood from veins, and the ventricles, which eject blood into the arteries. The superior vena cava, inferior vena cava and intrinsic veins of the heart deposit venous blood into the right atrium. Blood then passes through the tricuspid valve to the right ventricle. The right ventricle projects the blood through the pulmonary valve

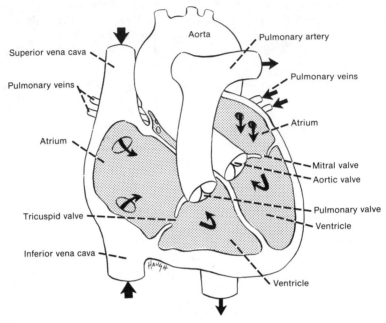

FIG 3–1.
Blood flow of the heart.

into the pulmonary arteries, which are the only arteries in the body containing unoxygenated blood. Pulmonary veins return the blood to the left atrium and from there it passes through the mitral valve to the left ventricle. From the left ventricle it is ejected through the aortic valve into the main artery of the body, the aorta.

The heart is divided into three layers–the epicardium, myocardium, and endocardium. The outermost layer, the epicardium, is visceral pericardium and is frequently infiltrated with fat. The coronary blood vessels that nourish the heart run in this layer before entering the myocardium. The myocardium consists of cardiac muscle fibers. The thickness of the layers of cardiac muscle fibers is directly proportional to the amount of work they perform. The ventricles do more work than the atria, and their walls are thicker. The pressure in the aorta is higher than that in the pulmonary trunk. This requires greater work from the left ventricle, so its walls are twice as thick as those of the right ventricle. The innermost layer, the endocardium, is the smooth endothelial lining of the interior of the heart.

The arterial supply of the heart muscle is derived from the right and left coronary arteries which arise from the aortic sinuses (Fig 3–2). The left coronary artery (LCA) divides into the anterior descending artery and the left circumflex artery. These arteries supply most of the left ventricle, the left atrium, most of the ventricular septum and, in 45% of people, the sinoatrial (SA) node. The right coronary artery (RCA) supplies most of the right ventricle, the atrioventricular (AV) node and, in 55% of people, the SA node. Infarction of these arteries or their branches can thus cause interruption or cessation of the conduction system and death of the myocardial muscle in the area supplied by the artery. The severity of the infarction is dependent on the size of the artery and the importance of the area it supplies.

The heart is drained by a number of veins. Most of the veins of the heart enter the coronary sinus, which then empties into the right atrium. A small portion of veins, the thebesian veins, empty directly into the right and left ventricles.

Innervation of the heart involves a complex balance between its intrinsic automaticity and extrinsic nerves (Fig 3–3). The SA and AV nodes provide the heart with an inherent ability for spontaneous rhythmic initiation of the cardiac impulse. The rate of this impulse formation is regulated by the automatic nervous system, which also influ-

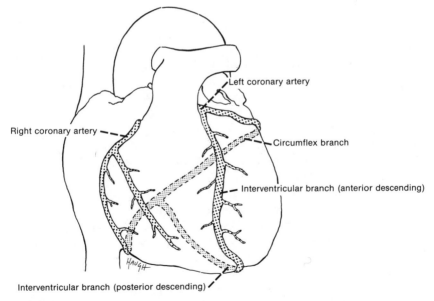

FIG 3–2.
Blood supply of the heart.

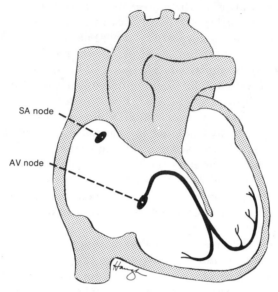

FIG 3–3.
Electrical conduction of the heart.

ences other phases of the cardiac cycle. It controls the rate of spread of the excitation impulse and the contractility of both atria and ventricles.

The automatic nervous system extends its influence to the heart via the vagus nerve (parasympathetic) and upper thoracic nerves (sympathetic). These nerves mingle together around the root and arch of the aorta near the tracheal bifurcation, forming the cardiac plexus. Extensions from the cardiac plexus richly supply the SA and AV nodes. They are so well mingled that scientists are unable to determine which nerves supply which parts of the heart. Stimulation of the sympathetic nervous system causes acceleration of the discharge rate in the SA node, increase in AV nodal conduction, and increase in the contractile force of both atrial and ventricular muscles. Stimulation of the vagus nerve causes cardiac slowing and decreased AV nodal conduction. Thus, the parasympathetic system seems to operate as a brake on the heart, while the sympathetic system operates in emergencies to accelerate cardiac activity.

Intrinsic innervation of the heart centers around the SA node, which lies near the junction of the superior vena cava and the right atrium. It is the normal pacemaker of the heart, sending concentric waves of excitation throughout the atrium. Without neural influence, impulse formation from this node would be greater than 100 beats per minute. However, vagal influence decreases the impulse formation to 60–90 beats per minute. The SA node retains its position as pacer of the heart as long as it generates impulses at a faster rate than any other part of the myocardium and as long as these impulses are rapidly conducted from atria to the ventricles. Normal impulse formation may be interrupted by vascular lesions (occlusion of the coronary arteries) or by cardiac disease (pericarditis). The SA node is especially susceptible to pericarditis and all other surface cardiac diseases due to its superficial position immediately beneath the epicardium.

The concentric waves of excitation sent out by the SA node must travel through the AV node in order to reach the ventricles. This node is located in the floor of the right atrium, just above the insertion of the tricuspid valve. Its main function is to cause a 0.04 second delay in the atrioventricular transmissions. This has two advantages. It postpones ventricular excitation until the atria have had time to eject their contents into the ventricles. It also limits the number of signals that can be transmitted by the AV node. The AV node also has its own inherent rhythmicity, firing at a much slower rate than the SA node (40–60 beats per minute). Its main pathology is due to occlusion of the right coronary artery which supplies the AV node in 90% of the cases. From the AV node arises a triangular group of fibers known as the AV bundle or bundle of His. This bundle divides in the ventricular septum into two branches—the left bundle branch and the right bundle branch. Each of these bundles continues to divide into many fine strands which spread across the ventricles. At the end of the bundle's ramifications are Purkinje's fibers which are continuous with the cardiac muscle. The waves of excitation pass through the bundle of His, down the bundle branches, through Purkinje's fibers to the cardiac muscle, which then contracts.

The four valves of the heart, although delicate in appearance, are designed to withstand repetitive closures against high pressures (see Fig 3–1). They frequently operate for more than 80 years without need of repair or replacement. The tricuspid and mitral valves function differently from the other valves of the heart. Being located between the atria and ventricles, they must effect a precise closure within a contracting cavity.

During diastole, the two leaflets or cusps of the mitral valve and the three cusps of the tricuspid valve relax into the cavities of the ventricles, allowing blood to flow between the two chambers. As the ventricular chambers fill with blood, the cusps of the valves are forced up into a closed position. Fibrous cords, the chordae tendinae, are located on the ventricular surfaces of these cusps. These cords connect the cusps of the valve with the papillary muscles of the ventricular walls. As pressure builds in the ventricular chambers, contraction of these muscles prevents the cusps from being forced up into the atria. Dysfunction or rupture of the chordae tendinae or the papillary muscles may undermine the support of one or more valve cusps, producing regurgitation from the ventricles to the atria.

The pulmonic and aortic valves are similar in appearance but the aortic cusps are slightly thicker than the pulmonic cusps. Each valve has three fibrous cusps, the bases of which are firmly attached to the root of the aorta or the pulmonary artery. The free edges of these valves project into the lumen of the vessels. At the end of systole, blood in the aorta and pulmonary artery forces the cusps of the valves shut. These valves are attached in such a manner that they cannot be everted into the ventricles by increased pressure in the vessels. During diastole the cusps support the column of blood filling the ventricles. Contraction of the ventricles during systole increases pressure within the ventricular chambers, forcing the cusps to open and allow blood flow into the vessels.

The vascular system is a complex series of tubes throughout the entire body. It conveys nutrition and oxygen to all tissues of the body and carries away their waste products. The driving force for this system is the heart. The vascular system can be considered to have two major components—systemic and pulmonary circulation.

Systemic circulation begins with the aorta, the largest artery in the body. Branches from this artery carry blood to the head, viscera and limbs. As the arteries branch they become smaller and smaller until they form arterioles. The arterioles regulate the flow of blood to the capillaries through contraction or relaxation of smooth muscle in their walls. Contraction of the vessels raises blood pressure by limiting the blood volume to a smaller area. The reverse occurs with muscle relaxation. Many factors (nervous impulses, hormonal stimulation, drugs, oxygen and carbon dioxide concentrations) determine the degree of contraction of vascular smooth muscle and whether contraction occurs locally or throughout the entire body.

Arterioles branch to form the smallest vessels, the capillaries, which consist of a single layer of endothelial cells forming lumen just large enough for the red blood cells to roll along. The capillary bed is enormous, its capacity far exceeding 10 pints. Its network is finer and denser in active tissue like muscle and brain, and less dense in less active tissue such as tendon. Gas exchange occurs in the capillary bed, where the red blood cells give up their oxygen, and blood plasma transudes capillary walls, carrying nutrition to tissue.

Capillaries form venules, which are the smallest veins. These veins branch and become increasingly larger. Blood flow through the veins is largely dependent on muscular or visceral action or pressures. These pressures are intermittent and, were it not for double-cusped valves located within the veins, blood would flow backward when the pressure ceases. In the extremities, muscular contractions move blood into the trunk. In the pelvic and abdominal region blood flow is dependent on intra-abdominal pressure exceeding intrathoracic pressure. Blood flows through the trunk in veins which become increasingly larger until they finally enter the superior and inferior venae cavae. These empty directly into the right atrium. Blood flow through the right side of the heart and lungs is known as *pulmonary circulation.*

The quantity of blood flowing through the pulmonary circulation is approximately equal to that flowing through systemic circulation. Blood flows from the right ventricle into the pulmonary artery, which divides into right and left branches 4 cm from the ventricle. These branches then separate, one going to each lung, where they continue to divide into smaller arteries. The pulmonary arteries and arterioles are much shorter, have thinner walls and larger diameters and are more distensible than their systemic counterparts. This gives the pulmonary system a compliance as great as that of the systemic arterial system, thereby allowing the pulmonary arteries to accommodate the stroke volume output of the right ventricle. Pulmonary vascular resistance and arterial pressure are one-sixth that of the systemic system (pulmonary arterial pressure is 20/10 mm Hg as compared to 120/80 mm Hg systemically).

Pulmonary capillaries are very short and arise abruptly from much larger arterioles. They form a dense network over the walls of the alveoli, making a minimum distance over which gas exchange occurs. The pulmonary veins are also very short but have distensibility characteristics similar to those of the systemic system. Unlike systemic veins, these veins have no valves. Pulmonary veins act as a capacitance vessel or a blood reservoir for the left atrium. Contraction of smooth muscle in the veins makes the reservoir constrict. This increases blood volume in relation to the internal volume of the vessels. The pulmonary veins become larger and larger until they converge into two veins from each lung, which then carry oxygenated blood to the left atrium.

The surface markings of the heart can be traced by joining four points over the anterior chest wall. On the right, the heart extends from the third to the sixth costal cartilages at a distance of about 10 to

15 mm from the sternum. On the left, the heart extends from the second costal cartilage to the fifth intercostal space 12 to 15 mm and 9 cm from the left sternal border, respectively.

Joining the two points on the left side outlines the left atrium and ventricle. The heart is rotated to the left in the chest, resulting in the right side of the heart being foremost. Thus, joining the two uppermost points outlines the level of the atria and joining the two lower points represents the margin of the right ventricle.

BASIC ELECTROCARDIOGRAPHY

The electrocardiogram (ECG) is used to monitor the electrical activity in the heart. It graphically traces the depolarization and repolarization of the heart from different angles, depending on the leads being used. The typical ECG represents a cardiac cycle, with the P wave, QRS complex, S-T segment and T wave (Fig 3–4). This sequence triggers the release of calcium into and from within the cardiac cells to effect interaction of the myofilaments and contraction of the cardiac muscle.

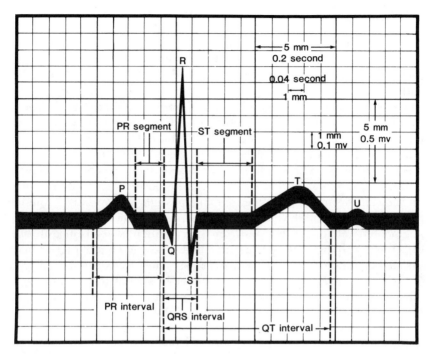

FIG 3–4.
A normal electrocardiogram showing characteristic waves, intervals, and segments, and some of the features of the tracing paper.

Polarization

Resting cardiac muscle maintains a negative charge on the inside of the cell membrane and a positive charge on the outside of the cell membrane. During depolarization, an influx of sodium to the inside of the cell renders the inside of the cell positive and the outside negative. An electric field is generated between the depolarized parts of the myocardium and the polarized or resting cardiac muscle. It is this current that is recorded on the ECG. The P wave represents atrial depolarization and corresponds to atrial contraction. The QRS complex represents ventricular depolarization and contraction. During repolarization, the cardiac muscle regains its negative charge within each cell and the cardiac muscle is physically inactive. The repolarization of the atria is buried within the QRS complex. The T wave represents ventricular repolarization.

Standard Leads

The electrodes used to record the ECG are placed equidistant from the heart. They form a triangle (Einthoven's triangle) with the heart located in the center. Electrodes are placed on the right arm, left arm and left leg. A ground is placed on the right leg. The sides of the triangle are labeled I, II, and III, and represent leads. Each lead is formed by two electrodes, one positive and one negative. For example, in lead II the right arm is negative and the left leg is positive. Three more leads, the augmented leads, use the same standard limb leads mentioned above. The negative electrode is formed by combining leads I, II and III. Their algebraic sum is 0. The positive electrode is placed on the right arm (AV_R-augmented voltage right arm positive), the left arm (AV_L-augmented voltage left arm positive) or the left leg (AV_F-augmented voltage left leg positive). The augmented leads measure the difference in potential between the limb and the center of the heart (located at 0 potential). There are also six chest leads numbered from V_1 to V_6. An electrode is placed on the right side of the sternum (V_1). This electrode is a suction cup that is moved to different positions on the chest from the right side to the left to obtain the six chest leads. All 12 leads enable one to view the electrical activity of the heart from many different angles. Certain pathologies may be concealed in one lead but become evident when viewed from another lead.

The therapist working with acutely ill patients should be familiar with the normal ECG pattern and be able to recognize the major arrhythmias. Being familiar with all 12 leads is impractical and unnecessary for our purposes. Most hospitals use limb leads I, II or III on their monitors. The therapist should be familiar with normal strips on the lead that the hospital uses most frequently. When working with a monitored patient, one should take time to familiarize oneself with that patient's pattern, and check with the nurse to see if the patient has had any arrhythmias and, if so, the nature of those arrhythmias. During treatment, the therapist should check the monitor periodically to determine if changes in the heart rhythm or rate have occurred. Percussion and vibration cause artifacts on the ECG monitor and may activate monitor alarms. In some circumstances monitor alarms may have to be turned off. This should be done only after discussion with the patient's nurse. The alarms should be reactivated after treatment. With experience, the therapist will quickly notice subtle changes on the monitor. If significant changes and/or arrhythmias do occur, the treatment should be stopped and the nurse and physician notified.

The rhythms discussed below are basic and are intended to be a review. Pediatric electrocardiography is very different and is not covered in depth. Therapists working in those areas should familiarize themselves with the specific variations found in this specialty area. Therapists unfamiliar with ECGs should take the responsibility to independently pursue increased knowledge in this area. There are many excellent references and self-program texts available. The resources of specially trained therapists, nurses and physicians in the field, as well as educational programs, should be tapped.

The Normal ECG Complex

Figure 3–4 illustrates the normal ECG. ECG paper is marked in 1 mm horizontal and vertical units in boxes of 5 mm at a paper speed of 25 mm per second, that is 1 mm every 0.04 seconds. The therapist or nurse can calculate the heart rate from the frequency of QRS complexes per unit time. Changes in shape, amplitude, and duration of the P, QRS, T and possibly U waves may suggest the presence of specific conduction abnormalities, pathology, or both. At normal resting heart rates, the time required for each upstroke or QRS wave, the intervals and segments of the ECG are proportional. For example, at a rate of 75 beats per minute, the cardiac cycle lasts 0.8 seconds, the QRS takes 0.08 seconds, the ST segment is twice as long as the PR segment, the QT interval is almost three times as long as the PR interval. As the heart rate increases, the cardiac intervals and segments decrease correspondingly. At extremely high heart rates, i.e., during exercise, ventricular filling may be reduced as a result of reduced ventricular filling time. This results in reduced cardiac output; hence, decreased performance.

SUPRAVENTRICULAR RHYTHMS

Normal Sinus Rhythm

This is the normal ECG pattern originating in the sinus node and producing a rate of 60–100 beats per minute (Fig 3–5).

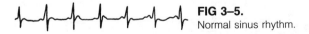

FIG 3–5.
Normal sinus rhythm.

Sinus Arrhythmia

This is a normal pattern where the heart rate varies with respiration, increasing with inspiration and decreasing with expiration. It is frequently seen in healthy children and athletic adults (Fig 3–6).

FIG 3–6.
Sinus arrhythmia.

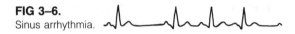

Sinus Bradycardia

This rhythm has the same pattern as the normal sinus rhythm but the rate is less than 60 per minute. It can occur during suctioning as a combined result of hypoxemia and vagal stimulation. It is also seen in patients who are hypoxemic or have increased intracranial pressure (Fig 3–7). This is a serious sign and if it occurs, the chest physical therapy treatment should be stopped immediately and the nurse notified. Neonates and infants are considered bradycardic when their heart rate drops to less than 100. When this occurs in neonates, the therapist should immediately oxygenate and stimulate the neonate while calling the nurse.

FIG 3–7.
Sinus bradycardia.

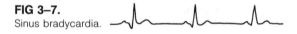

Sinus Tachycardia

This arrhythmia has a normal sinus pattern, but the rate has increased up to 160 beats per minutes. The increased rate causes increased myocardial work and may be due to pulmonary embolus, congestive heart failure, or fever (Fig 3–8).

FIG 3–8.
Sinus tachycardia.

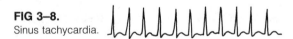

Paroxysmal Atrial Tachycardia (PAT)

PAT is a sudden onset of a rapid, regular atrial tachycardia that usually ends as it began. The rate varies between 150 and 240 beats per minute. Possible causes of PAT include emotional stress, fatigue, and digestive and electrolyte disturbances. It is treated by having the patient perform the Valsalva maneuver, carotid sinus massage, or digitalis or quinidine treatment (Fig 3–9).

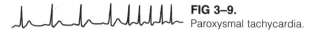

FIG 3–9.
Paroxysmal tachycardia.

Premature Atrial Contractions (PAC)

PAC is a transient arrhythmia that occurs when an ectopic site in the atria causes premature contraction of the atria. It causes an irregular rhythm and is frequently seen after an excess of coffee, alcohol or tobacco (Fig 3–10).

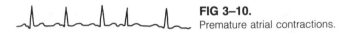

FIG 3–10.
Premature atrial contractions.

Atrial Flutter

Atrial flutter originates from one ectopic focus in the atria, which causes the atria to contract several times before there is a ventricular response. This is a form of heart block, and the ventricular response will usually be 2:1, 3:1, or 4:1 depending on the amount of heart block present. On the ECG strip, a series of P waves appear in a sawtoothed pattern between each QRS complex. This arrhythmia is seen in patients with heart and lung disease and is treated with digitalis (Fig 3–11).

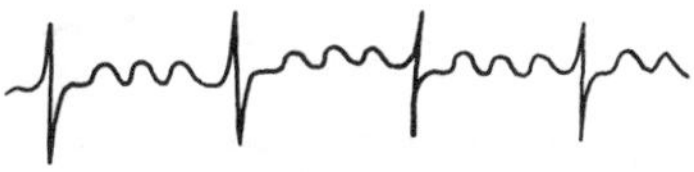

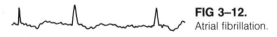

FIG 3–11.
Atrial flutter.

Atrial Fibrillation

Atrial fibrillation presents with totally irregular, indistinguishable baseline undulations between QRS complexes. The rhythm is irregular, with a heart rate varying between 100 and 160 beats per minute. This rhythm is seen in patients with mitral stenosis, acute myocardial infarctions and acute infections. It is treated with quinidine and digitalis (Fig 3–12).

FIG 3–12.
Atrial fibrillation.

Junctional Rhythm

This rhythm originates in the region of the atrioventricular junction and is characterized by a slow heart rate (40–60 beats per minute). It is differentiated from sinus bradycardia by inverted P waves and occurs only if the SA node fails to fire (Fig 3–13).

FIG 3–13.
Junctional rhythm.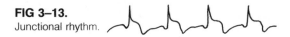

Ventricular Rhythms

Premature Ventricular Contraction (PVC)

A PVC occurs when the ventricles contract before the next expected sinus node stimulated contraction. On the ECG, PVCs appear bizarre, taller and wider than the normal ventricular contractions (Fig 3–14). They occur when an ectopic focus in the ventricular muscle discharges. PVCs occurring from one ectopic focus are identical in appearance and are referred to as *unifocal PVCs*. PVCs that are different in appearance are referred to as *multifocal PVCs,* since they are caused by more than one ectopic focus in the ventricles. PVCs indicate increased irritability of the myocardium and may be caused by drugs, surgery, electrolyte imbalance, acute and chronic heart disease, and hypoxemia. They are treated with several drugs including lidocaine, atropine and propanolol. Chest physical therapy treatments should be stopped immediately and the nurse notified when more than six PVCs occur per minute or if the PVCs are multifocal.

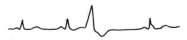

Premature ventricular contraction

FIG 3–14.
Premature ventricular contractions.

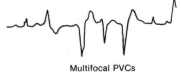

Multifocal PVCs

Unifocal PVCs

Trigeminy.   This arrhythmia is characterized by two normal beats followed by a PVC (Fig 3–15).

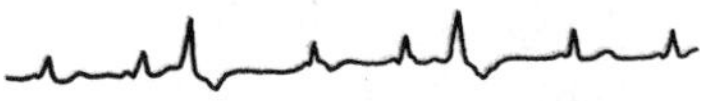

FIG 3–15.
Trigeminy.

Bigeminy.   This arrhythmia is characterized by a PVC occurring after every normal beat (in other words, every other beat is a PVC) (Fig 3–16).

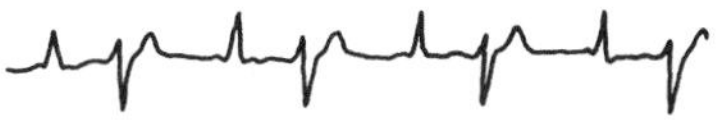

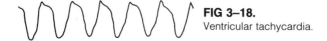

FIG 3–16.
Bigeminy.

Coupling. PVCs occurring together are known as *coupled* PVCs. The nurse or physician should be notified as they may indicate impending ventricular tachycardia (Fig 3–17).

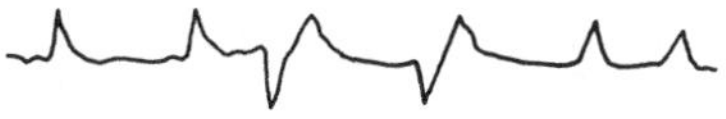

FIG 3–17.
Coupling.

Ventricular Tachycardia. Three or more PVCs together are known as ventricular tachycardia. It is a dangerous arrhythmia that is frequently a precursor to ventricular fibrillation and death. It produces an ECG pattern of widely bizarre premature ventricular contractions (PVCs) and is usually treated with medical therapy and direct current (DC) cardioversion. Cardiac output drops markedly during this arrhythmia, necessitating external cardiac massage until a more normal rhythm occurs (Fig 3–18).

FIG 3–18.
Ventricular tachycardia.

Ventricular Fibrillation. Ventricular fibrillation appears as disorganized ventricular flutters on the ECG. The ventricles have ceased to contract and are merely quivering. There is no cardiac output and death will ensue unless normal rhythm is restored within three minutes. This arrhythmia is treated with immediate DC cardioversion (Fig 3–19).

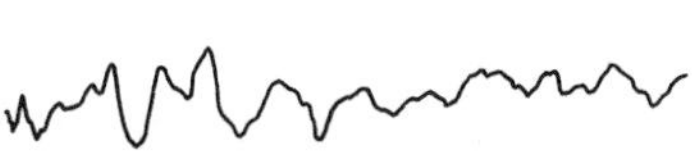

FIG 3–19.
Ventricular fibrillation.

PACEMAKERS

A pacemaker is an electronic device that delivers electric impulses to the heart muscle which cause the ventricles (or atria) to contract. Pacemakers are used when there is a block in the conduction system or when the sinus node is not functioning well. There are two types of pacemakers—temporary and permanent. The temporary pacemakers are used for transient problems and in emergencies. They can be used for up to one month.

Both types of pacemakers are inserted either transvenously or trans-thoracically. They are operated by a battery implanted under the skin. Wires from this battery are passed through the venous system (transvenous) into the right ventricle, or sewn directly into the ventricular wall (epicardial). This battery emits an electric impulse seen on the ECG strip as a vertical spike which is immediately followed by an atrial beat (atrial pacing) or a ventricular beat that resembles a PVC (ventricular pacing). The pacemaker can be set to pace at a fixed rate or on demand (fires when it does not sense a QRS wave).

On bedside monitors, pacemaker spikes are frequently difficult to visualize and may be read as PVCs by the therapist. Therapists are advised to be conservative and to check with the nurse or physician when in doubt of the rhythm (Fig 3–20).

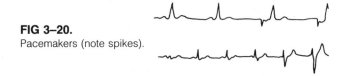

FIG 3–20.
Pacemakers (note spikes).

IMPLICATIONS FOR THE PHYSICAL THERAPIST

Therapists working with patients on ECG monitors should discuss the patient's condition and the nature of the arrhythmias with the nurse caring for the patient. Therapists uncomfortable with watching the patient's monitor should ask the nurse to stay throughout the treatment. Therapists who work frequently with these patients, however, should be familiar with ECG interpretation.

With the greater emphasis on optimization of treatment effects and reducing any potential risk to the patient, ECG interpretation is fast becoming an integral part of the skills of the therapist. The advent of ECG telemetry systems is permitting the therapist to monitor patients more stringently during activity, rather than disconnecting ECG leads during treatments that could potentially be detrimental either by over- or under-treating the patient. Working routinely with ECG monitors where these are indicated will undoubtedly help to improve treatment effectiveness.

COORDINATION OF CARDIAC EVENTS

The electrical and mechanical events of the cardiac cycle are summarized in Figure 3–21. These events include the spread of the wave of electrical excitation throughout the myocardium, the resulting sequence of contraction of the atria and ventricles followed by dynamic changes in pressure and blood volume in the heart chambers, the heart sounds and the timing of these events. The cardiac cycle takes 0.8 second in a heart beating at 75 beats per minute. Ventricular systole or ejection takes about one-third of this time. Its onset and termination are marked respectively by closure and opening of the atrioventricular valves (mitral and tricuspid). Diastole, or the period between successive

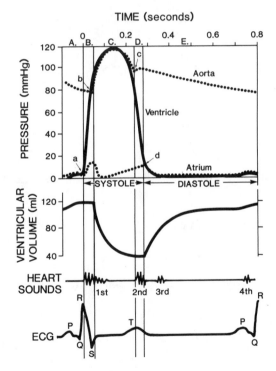

FIG 3–21.
Summary of electrical and mechanical events of the heart. **A,** atrial systole. **B,** isovolumetric contraction. **C,** ejection. **D,** isovolumetric relaxation. **E,** rapid inflow, diastasis, and active rapid filling. Note relationship of ventricular pressure and volume. *(a)* closure of the atrioventricular valves; *(b)* opening of the semilunar valves; *(c)* closure of the semilunar valves; *(d)* opening of the atrioventricular valves.

ventricular systoles in which the ventricles fill with blood, takes two-thirds of the 0.8 second of each cardiac cycle.

Phases of Systole and Diastole

Ventricular systole normally has three phases: isovolumetric contraction period, rapid ejection period, and a slower ejection period.

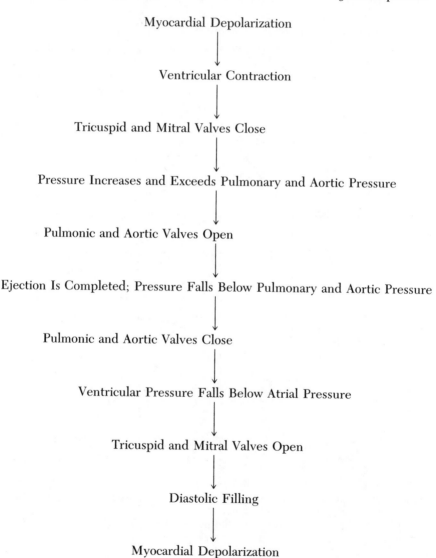

FIG 3–22.
The sequence of pressure changes in the heart during the cardiac cycle.

Ventricular diastole also has three phases: passive rapid-filling phase, diastasis (a slower filling phase), and active rapid-filling phase.

Heart Sounds

The heart sounds are described as a low-pitched long duration sound (S_1) followed by a higher pitched slower duration sound (S_2) that resembles the phonic sounds of LUB-dub. S_1 is associated with closure of the atrioventricular valves. S_2 is associated with closure of the semilunar valves. In inspiration, the aortic valve closes several milliseconds before the pulmonic valve, resulting in a splitting of the second heart sound, S_2. During inspiration, intrathoracic pressure becomes more negative, venous return and right heart volume increase, hence pulmonary ejection is prolonged in this situation, and closure of the pulmonary valve is delayed. Other variations in splitting of S_2 occur with pathology. The presence of a third (S_3) or fourth (S_4) heart sound is usually considered abnormal. S_3 is usually associated with the passive rapid-filling phase, and S_4 with the active rapid-filling phase.

Volume and Pressure Changes

Changes in the ventricular volume curve and aortic pressure wave reflect changes in atrial and ventricular pressure during systole and diastole. The sequence of events appears in a flow chart in Figure 3–22. Pressure gradients within the heart are responsible for the opening and closing of the valves. Coordinated valve opening and closure are important in promoting the forward movement of blood and preventing mechanical inefficiency of the heart pump due to valvular regurgitation of blood during ventricular contraction. Regurgitation of blood in the retrograde direction gives rise to heart murmurs audible on auscultation of the heart.

SUMMARY

This chapter covered the anatomy and physiology of the heart. The electrical conduction system and the mechanical action of the heart are emphasized because the coordination of these events is essential for maintaining cardiopulmonary status and is paramount to good physical performance. The heart and lungs work synergistically as a unit. Dysfunction of either the heart or the lungs can therefore produce dysfunction in the other organ because the heart and lungs are aligned in series with one another.

An introduction to basic electrocardiography is presented. Physical therapists working in areas using routine ECG monitoring need to become familiar with ECG interpretation. Greater familiarity with the singularly important, nonivasive ECG monitoring system can help therapists enhance treatment effectiveness and reduce potential risk to the patient in any setting.

Optimization of heart and lung function helps to promote better treatment outcomes related to both exercise and other therapeutic modalities. A thorough understanding of this complex subject is essential to the optimization of therapeutic response in any patient.

REFERENCES

Andreoli KG, Hunn VK, Zipes DP, et al: *Comprehensive Cardiac Care,* ed 5. St Louis, CV Mosby Co, 1983.

Berne RM, Levy MN: *Cardiovascular Physiology,* ed 4. St Louis, CV Mosby Co, 1981.

Brobeck JR (ed): *Best and Taylor's Physiological Basis of Medical Practice,* ed 10. Baltimore, Williams & Wilkins Co, 1979.

Cherniack RM, Cherniack L: *Respiration in Health and Disease,* ed 3. Philadelphia, WB Saunders Co, 1983.

Criley JM, Ross RS: *Cardiovascular Physiology.* Tarpon Springs, Florida, Tampa Tracings, 1971.

Dubin D: *Rapid Interpretation of EKGs,* ed 3. Tampa, Florida, Cover Publishing Co, 1974.

French WG, Criley JM: *Practical Cardiology: Ischemic and Valvular Heart Disease.* New York, John Wiley & Sons, 1983.

Ganong WF: *Review of Medical Physiology,* ed 11. Los Altos, Lange Medical Publications, 1983.

Gardner E, Gray DJ, O'Rahilly R: *Anatomy: A Regional Study of Human Structure,* ed 4. Philadelphia, WB Saunders Co, 1975.

Gould SE: *Pathology of the Heart and Blood Vessels.* Springfield, Illinois, Charles C Thomas, Publisher, 1968.

Gray H: *Anatomy of the Human Body,* ed 29. Philadelphia, Lea & Febiger, 1973.

Hurst JW, Logue RB, Schlant RC, et al: *The Heart, Arteries and Veins,* ed 3. New York, McGraw-Hill Book Co, 1974.

Katz AM: *Physiology of the Heart.* New York, Raven Press, 1977.

Marriott HJL: *Practical Electrocardiography,* ed 7. Baltimore, Williams & Wilkins Co, 1983.

Marriott HJ, Conover MH: *Advanced Concepts in Arrhythmias.* St Louis, CV Mosby Co, 1983.

Murray JF: *The Normal Lung.* Philadelphia, WB Saunders Co, 1976.

Nunn JF: *Applied Respiratory Physiology.* London, Butterworths, 1971.

Oram S: *Clinical Heart Disease,* ed 2. London, William Heinemann Medical Books Ltd, 1981.

Rushmer RF: *Cardiovascular Dynamics,* ed 4. Philadelphia, WB Saunders Co, 1976.

Rushmer RF: *Structure and Function of the Cardiovascular System,* ed 2. Philadelphia, WB Saunders Co, 1976.

Warren R: *Surgery.* Philadelphia, WB Saunders Co, 1963.

Warwick R, Williams PL: *Gray's Anatomy,* ed 35. Philadelphia, WB Saunders Co, 1973.

West JB: *Respiratory Physiology—The Essentials,* ed 2. Baltimore, Williams & Wilkins Co, 1979.

4

Pathophysiology of Chronic Pulmonary Disease

Willy E. Hammon, P.T.

This chapter describes the pathophysiology of chronic pulmonary disease. Chronic pulmonary disease can be categorized broadly into obstructive and restrictive disorders. Overlap between the two categories does exist. For example, chronic obstructive lung disease over the long term is associated with decreased lung and chest wall compliance, which are common features of the restrictive lung diseases. Similarly reduced airway compliance seen in some restrictive diseases may increase resistance by effectively obstructing airflow.

An understanding of the pathophysiology of lung disease is important in relating the signs and symptoms to treatment goals and prioritizing, selecting, and applying the appropriate treatment interventions.

OBSTRUCTIVE LUNG DISEASES

Several abbreviations can be found in the literature for a pulmonary disorder characterized by increased airway resistance, particularly noticeable by a prolonged forced expiration. Some of these are COPD (chronic obstructive pulmonary disease), COAD (chronic obstructive airway disease), CAO (chronic airways obstruction), and COLD (chronic obstructive lung disease).

The first part of this chapter considers chronic bronchitis, emphysema, asthma, and bronchiectasis individually. With the possible exception of bronchiectasis, however, it is unusual in the clinical setting to find a patient with only one of these conditions. Most patients have some combination of chronic bronchitis, emphysema and asthma, and in this chapter we have chosen to refer to these individuals as having COPD. These patients have intermittent episodes of wheezing, along with a variable degree of chronic bronchitis and emphysema. Radiologically, they may have hyperinflated lungs, flattened diaphragms, and an enlarged right ventricle due to increased pulmonary artery pressure. Other findings vary from patient to patient, depending on the predominant disease process contributing to their COPD.

COPD is becoming more and more common. Estimates by the American Lung Association place the number of new patients with COPD seen in 1985 at 144,000, with the total number of U.S. patients with COPD perhaps as high as 18.5 million. Deaths from COPD have increased consistently and numbered 70,000 in 1985. It is the sixth ranked cause of major disability and the fifth leading cause of death.

CHRONIC BRONCHITIS

Chronic bronchitis is a disease characterized by a cough producing sputum for at least three months and for two consecutive years.

Pathologically, one finds an increase in the size of the tracheobronchial mucous glands (increased Reid index) and goblet cell hyperplasia. Mucous cell metaplasia of bronchial epithelium results in a decreased number of cilia. Ciliary dysfunction and disruption of the continuity of the mucous blanket are common. In the peripheral airways, we observe bronchiolitis, bronchiolar narrowing and increased amounts of mucus.

The etiology of chronic bronchitis is believed to be related to long-term irritation of the tracheobronchial tree. The most common cause of irritation is cigarette smoking. Inhaled smoke stimulates the goblet cells and mucous glands to secrete more mucus. This smoke also inhibits ciliary action. The hypersecretion of mucus and impaired cilia lead to a chronic productive cough. The fact that smokers secrete an abnormal amount of mucus makes them prone to develop respiratory infections and it takes them longer to recover from these infections. In addition, the smoke irritation of the tracheobronchial tree causes bronchoconstriction. Although smoking is the most common cause of chronic bronchitis, other agents that have been implicated are air pollution, certain occupations, and bronchial infections.

These patients are referred to as "blue bloaters" because they usually have stocky body build and are "blue" due to hypoxemia. Although many of these patients have a high P_{CO_2}, the pH is normalized by renal retention of bicarbonate (HCO_3^-). The chronic bronchitic's bone marrow tries to compensate for chronic hypoxemia by increased production of red blood cells, leading to polycythemia. Polycythemia, in turn, makes the blood more viscous, forcing the heart to work even harder to pump it. Long-term hypoxemia leads to increased pulmonary artery pressure and right ventricular hypertrophy.

Bronchitics have tenacious, purulent sputum that is difficult to expectorate. In an exacerbation, usually due to infection, they have an even greater amount of sputum and retained secretions. Retained secretions lead to ventilation-perfusion abnormalities, which increase hypoxemia and CO_2 retention because perfused areas of the lung cannot be ventilated effectively. The respiratory rate increases, as does the use of respiratory accessory muscles. The resultant increased work of breathing requires greater oxygen consumption by these inefficient muscles, with a greater production of carbon dioxide than the respiratory system can adequately meet. This contributes to a further drop in PO_2 and a rise in PCO_2. The hypoxemia and acidemia increase pulmonary vessel constriction, which raises pulmonary artery pressure and ultimately leads to right heart failure (cor pulmonale).

So the patient admitted to the hospital with an exacerbation of chronic bronchitis presents the following picture: He usually is of stocky body build, his color is dusky, and he breathes with moderate to marked use of the respiratory accessory muscles, depending on the degree of respiratory distress. Wheezing may be audible or noted by auscultation. Intercostal (or sternal) retractions may be present, again depending on the degree of respiratory distress. Edema in the extremities (especially in the ankle area) and neck vein distention reflect decompensated cor pulmonale. The patient may report that this breathing difficulty began with increased amounts of secretions (with a change in their normal color) or decreased amounts of sputum (reflecting increased retention of secretions). Arterial blood gases show the bronchitic to have a lowered PO_2, a raised PCO_2 and a lowered pH.

Pulmonary function tests indicate a reduced vital capacity, FEV_1, maximum voluntary ventilation and diffusing capacity, as well as an increased functional residual capacity and residual volume.

During an exacerbation, these patients are usually treated with intravenous fluids, antibiotics, bronchodilators and low-flow oxygen. Diuretics and digitalis are often given to treat cor pulmonale. Postural drainage may be requested to help the patient expectorate secretions. Breathing retraining and, during recovery, exercise with supplemental oxygen may also benefit the patient. It is important for these patients to stay away from bronchial irritants (cigarette smoke, air pollution, and others) and to drink large volumes of water to keep their secretions thin enough to be easily expectorated.

Emphysema

There are two main types of emphysema—centrilobular and panlobular. It has been suggested that centrilobular emphysema is 20 times more common than panlobular emphysema, although both types are often found in the same pair of lungs.

As its name implies, centrilobular emphysema is characterized by destruction of the respiratory bronchiole (Fig 4–1) as well as edema, inflammation, and thickened bronchiolar walls. These changes are more common and more marked in the upper portions of the lungs. This form of emphysema is found more often in men than in women, is rare among nonsmokers, and is common among patients with chronic bronchitis.

Panlobular emphysema, on the other hand, is characterized by destructive enlargement of the alveoli, distal to the terminal bronchiole

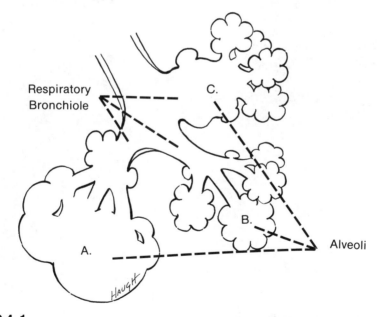

FIG 4–1.
A, panlobular emphysema is characterized by a destructive enlargement of the alveoli. **B,** a normal respiratory bronchiole and alveoli. **C,** centrilobular emphysema is characterized by a selective enlargement and destruction of the respiratory bronchiole.

(see Fig 4–1). This type of emphysema is also found in subjects that have α-antitrypsin deficiency. Airway obstruction in these individuals is caused by loss of lung elastic recoil or radial traction on the bronchioles. When individuals with normal lungs inhale, the airways are stretched open by the enlarging elastic lung, and during exhalation the airways are narrowed due to the decreasing stretch of the lung. However, the lungs of patients with panlobular emphysema have decreased elasticity due to disruption and destruction of surrounding alveolar walls. This in turn leaves the bronchiole unsupported and vulnerable to collapse during exhalation.

Bullae, emphysematous spaces larger than 1 cm in diameter, may be found in patients with emphysema (Fig 4–2). It is thought that they develop from an obstruction of the conducting airways that permits the flow of air into the alveoli during inspiration but does not allow air to flow out again during expiration. This causes the alveoli to become hyperinflated and eventually leads to destruction of the alveolar walls

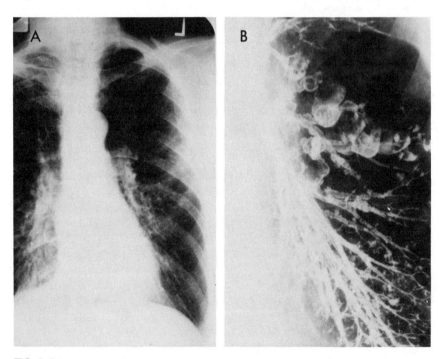

FIG 4–2.
A, AP chest film reveals bullous emphysema with multiple, thin, rounded fibrotic lucencies. **B,** the spot film bronchogram of the left midlung field shows intact bronchi and distal emphysematous blebs. (Courtesy of T.H. Johnson, M.D.)

with a resultant enlarged air space in the lung parenchyma. These bullae can be more than 10 cm in diameter, and by compression, can compromise the function of the remaining lung tissue (Fig 4–3). If this happens, surgical intervention to remove the bulla is often necessary. Pneumothorax, a serious complication, can result from the rupture of one of these bullae.

The emphysema patient's most common complaint is dyspnea. Physically, these patients appear thin and have an increased anterior-posterior chest diameter. Typically, they breathe using the accessory muscles of inspiration. These patients are often seen leaning forward, resting their forearms on their knees, or sitting with their arms extended at their sides, pushing down against the bed or chair in order to elevate their shoulders and improve the effectiveness of the accessory muscles of inspiration. They may breathe through pursed lips during the expiratory phase of breathing. These patients have been

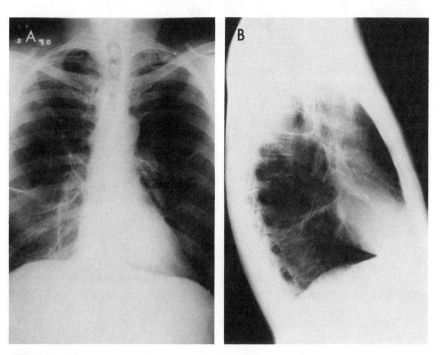

FIG 4–3.
A, AP and lateral **B** views of the chest of a patient with advanced bullous emphysematous changes. Note the bullae in the upper lung fields. The lateral film reveals an increased A-P diameter of the thorax, flattening of the diaphragms and an increased anterior clear space. (Courtesy of T.H. Johnson, M.D.)

referred to as "pink puffers" due to the increased respiratory work they must do in order to maintain relatively normal blood gases. On auscultation, decreased breath sounds can be noted throughout most or all of the lung fields. Radiologically, we find that the emphysema patient has overinflated lungs, a flattened diaphragm and a small, elongated heart (Fig 4–4). Pulmonary function tests show a decreased vital capacity, FEV_1, maximum voluntary ventilation and a greatly reduced diffusing capacity. The total lung capacity is increased, while the residual volume and functional residual capacity are even more increased. Arterial blood gases reflect a mildly or moderately lowered PO_2, a normal or slightly raised PCO_2 and a normal pH. These patients, unlike chronic bronchitics, normally will develop heart failure in the end stage of their disease (Fig 4–5).

Treatment of progressive emphysema that requires hospitalization

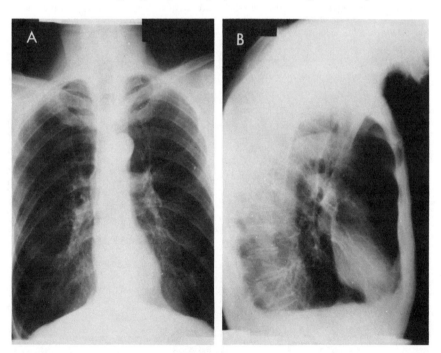

FIG 4–4.
A, AP chest film reveals the increased lucency of lung fields and flattening of the diaphragm of emphysema. The vascular structures are crowded medially. **B,** lateral chest film reveals an increased AP diameter and flattening of the diaphragms. There is an increase in the anterior clear space. These are all findings of emphysema. (Courtesy of T.H. Johnson, M.D.)

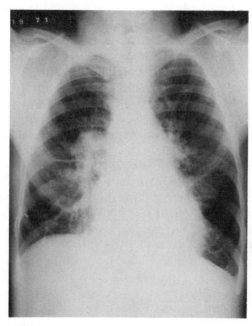

FIG 4–5.
The chest film reveals peripheral emphysematous lucency. The hilar areas are tremendously enlarged by the pulmonary arteries in a typical cor pulmonale configuration. Cardiomegaly is also present. (Courtesy of T.H. Johnson, M.D.)

often includes intravenous fluids, antibiotics and low-flow oxygen. Some of these patients also receive bronchodilators, diuretics and digitalis. Postural drainage may be requested to aid the patients in mobilizing and expectorating secretions if the patients have pneumonia (pure emphysema patients are "dry"). Breathing retraining can be very helpful to relieve dyspnea in these individuals. As these patients recover, they often can benefit from pulmonary rehabilitation.

The etiology of emphysema is uncertain. It is known that the incidence of emphysema increases with age. It is most often found in chronic bronchitics, and there is no question that emphysema is much more prevalent in cigarette smokers than in nonsmokers. There seems to be an hereditary factor too, as evidenced by the severe panlobular emphysema that patients with an α_1-antitrypsin deficiency develop relatively early in life, even though they may never have smoked. Repeated lower respiratory tract infections may also play a role. However, the interrelationship of these and other factors in producing emphysema is still not well understood.

Prognosis of Chronic Bronchitis and Emphysema

Chronic bronchitis and emphysema are marked by a progressive loss of lung function. At the end of five years, patients with COPD have a death rate four to five times greater than the normal expected value. Death rates reported by various studies depend on the method of selection of patients, types of diagnostic tests and other criteria. In general, the death rates five years after diagnosis are 20%–55%. Burrows and Earle reported an overall mortality of 47% at the end of five years. They felt five-year survival rates could be estimated as follows: 80% in patients with an FEV_1 greater than 1.2 L; 60% for those with an FEV_1 close to 1.0 L; and 40% for patients with an FEV_1 less than 0.75 L. However, if the above flow rates are found in patients with complications of resting tachycardia, chronic hypercapnia and a severely impaired diffusing capacity, the survival rates should be reduced by 25%. Other factors that have been associated with a poor prognosis are cor pulmonale, weight loss, radiologic evidence of emphysema, a dyspneic onset, polycythemia and Hoover's sign (an inward movement of the ribs on inspiration).

The most frequent causes of death in patients with COPD (in descending order of frequency) are congestive heart failure (secondary to cor pulmonale), respiratory failure, pneumonia, bronchiolitis and pulmonary embolism.

ASTHMA

Asthma is a disease characterized by an increased responsiveness of the trachea and bronchi to various stimuli, and is manifested by widespread narrowing of the airways that changes in severity either spontaneously or as a result of treatment. During an asthma attack, the lumen of the airways is narrowed or occluded by a combination of bronchial smooth muscle spasm, inflammation of the mucosa and an overproduction of a viscous, tenacious mucus.

Asthma is certainly a widespread disease in the world today. Its incidence is about 10 persons per 1,000, or 1%. It is found more often in children under 15 years old, where estimates of prevalence vary from 5% to 15%. It is noteworthy that about 80% of asthmatic children do not have asthma after the age of 10.

Asthma that begins in patients under the age of 35 is usually allergic or extrinsic. These asthma attacks are precipitated when an individual comes in contact with a specific substance to which he is sensitive, such as pollens or household dust (Table 4–1). Often asthmatics are allergic to a number of substances, rather than just one or two.

If a patient's first asthma attack occurs after the age of 35, often there is evidence of chronic airway obstruction with intermittent episodes of acute bronchospasm. These individuals, whose attacks are not triggered by specific substances, are referred to as having nonallergic or intrinsic asthma (see Table 4–1). Chronic bronchitis is commonly found in this group and this is the type of asthmatic usually seen in the hospital setting.

The asthmatic patient presents the following picture during an attack. He has a rapid rate of breathing and is using his accessory respiratory muscles (Fig 4–6). The expiratory phase of breathing is prolonged with audible wheezing and rhonchi. The patient may cough frequently, though unproductively, and may complain of tightness in his chest. Radiologically, the lungs may appear hyperinflated or show small atelectatic areas from retained secretions. Early in the attack, ar-

TABLE 4–1.

Factors That May Precipitate
an Asthma Attack

I. Allergic or extrinsic asthma
    A. Pollen—especially
        ragweed
    B. Animals
    C. Feathers
    D. Molds
    E. Household dust
    F. Food
II. Nonallergic or intrinsic asthma
    A. Inhaled irritants
        1. Cigarette smoke
        2. Dust
        3. Pollution
        4. Chemicals
    B. Weather
        1. High humidity
        2. Cold air
    C. Respiratory infections
        1. Common cold
        2. Bacterial bronchitis
    D. Drugs
        1. Aspirin
    E. Emotions
        1. Stress
    F. Exercise

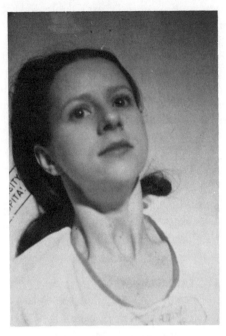

FIG 4–6.
A patient in respiratory distress during an acute asthma attack. Note the marked use of the sternocleidomastoids and other accessory muscles during inspiration.

terial blood gases reflect slight hypoxemia and a low P_{CO_2} (from hyperventilation). If the attack progresses, the P_{O_2} continues to fall as the P_{CO_2} climbs above the normal range. As obstruction becomes severe, deterioration of the patient is evidenced by a high CO_2, a low P_{O_2}, and a pH of less than 7.30 (see Chapter 26).

It is not unusual to see hospitalized asthmatics treated with intravenous fluids, bronchodilators, supplemental oxygen and corticosteroids. Breathing retraining in the acute attack may be helpful. It is most beneficial in teaching patients to relax and try to "prevent" further attacks, or to deal with them more effectively. Postural drainage during the acute phase is felt to be ineffective but is indicated when the patient improves and his cough becomes productive. It is important that these patients avoid bronchial irritants and substances that might precipitate an asthma attack.

An asthma attack that persists for hours and is unresponsive to medical management is referred to as *status asthmaticus*. The patient may appear dehydrated, cyanotic and near exhaustion from labored breathing. In contrast to the audible wheezing and rhonchi heard early in the attack, the chest now has greatly diminished or absent breath sounds. Status asthmaticus results in a significant death rate and is regarded as a medical emergency. Patients in respiratory failure may require mechanical ventilation.

If we examine the lungs of a patient who has died from status asthmaticus, we find the lungs are very much hyperinflated. Examination of the airways reveals a mucosa that is edematous and inflamed. Characteristic of asthma, the basement membrane is thickened. The mucous glands are enlarged and there is an increase in the number of goblet cells. Evidence of bronchospasm is seen by the hypertrophied and thickened smooth muscle. The lumens of most bronchioles, down to the terminal bronchioles, are filled with viscous, sticky mucus (Fig 4–7). It is evident that the occluded bronchioles have caused death by asphyxiation. Secretions in the tracheobronchial tree of the asthmatic are a combination of mucus (secreted by the mucous glands) and an exudate from the dilated capillaries just below the basement membrane. It has been shown that cilia do not sweep the mucoserous fluid nearly as effectively as pure mucus. Additionally, sheets of ciliated epithelium have been shed into the bronchial lumen, further contributing to the stasis of secretions. Although the alveoli are overinflated, the permanent destructive changes found in emphysema are not present.

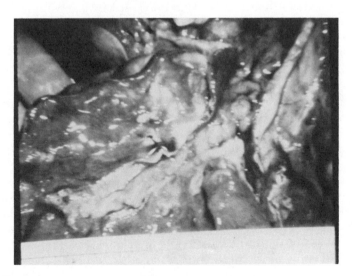

FIG 4–7.
Gross specimen of lung showing large mucus plug within the bronchial tree of a patient who died from status asthmaticus. (Courtesy of J.J. Coalson, Ph.D.)

Prognosis of Asthma

Most studies following children with asthma for a number of years report a death rate of about 1%. One large study of 1,000 asthmatics of all ages in England reported a mortality of 7% due to asthma or its complications. This study reported that 2% of the patients with intermittent asthma died, compared with 9% of those with continuous asthma. During the 1960s, there was a sharp increase in the number of asthmatic deaths reported by countries around the world. At the peak of this increase, England and Wales reported that 7% of the deaths in children between 10 and 14 years of age were attributable to asthma. This reflected a sevenfold increase in only seven years. Some medical authorities feel this increase in deaths was related to widespread use or abuse of certain pressurized aerosol nebulizers containing isoproterenol, but this has been disputed.

BRONCHIECTASIS

Bronchiectasis is defined as an abnormal dilation of medium-sized bronchi and bronchioles (about the fourth to ninth generations), generally associated with a previous, chronic necrotizing infection within these passages. Ordinarily, there is sufficient cartilage within the walls of the larger bronchi to protect them from dilation.

The airway deformities can be classified into three types. *Cylindrical* (or longitudinal) bronchiectasis is the most common type, with a uniform dilation of the airways. *Varicose* bronchiectasis refers to a greater dilation than in cylindrical bronchiectasis, causing the walls of the bronchi to resemble varicose veins (Fig 4–8). *Saccular* (or cystic) bronchiectasis refers to airways that have intermittent spherical ballooning (Fig 4–9).

Bronchiectasis is usually localized in a few segments or in an entire lobe of the lung. Most commonly it is unilateral (although 40%–50% of the cases are bilateral) and affects the basal segments of the lower lobes, in particular those of the left lung, more often than the upper lobes. When the left lower lobe is involved, it is not unusual to find bronchiectasis in the lingula of the left upper lobe as well. Interestingly, bronchiectasis of the right middle lobe is relatively common in elderly people and can contribute to both hemoptysis and repeated infections of this lobe.

Pathologically, the mucosa appears edematous and ulcerated. Destruction of the elastic and muscular structures of the airway walls is

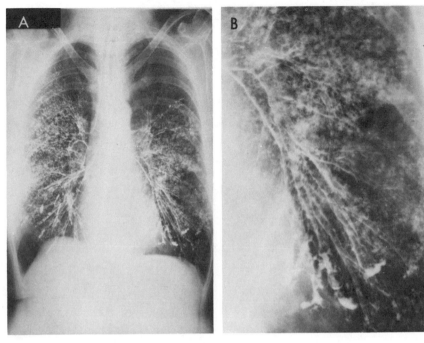

FIG 4–8.
A, AP chest film of a bronchogram with cylindrical and varicose bronchiectasis in the lower lung fields. **B,** close-up view of cylindrical and varicose bronchiectatic changes in the left lower lobe. (Courtesy of T.H. Johnson, M.D.)

evident with resultant dilation and fibrosis. The walls are lined with hyperplastic nonciliated mucus-secreting cells that have replaced the normal ciliated epithelium. This change is significant because it interrupts the mucociliary blanket and causes pooling of infected secretions which further damage and irritate the bronchial walls.

The etiology of bronchiectasis is related to obstruction of the airways and respiratory infections. Some 60% of the cases of bronchiectasis are preceded by an acute respiratory infection. The infection stimulates an increased production of mucus. The mucus is, in turn, infected and the infection advances to involve the bronchial walls. Portions of the mucosa are destroyed and are replaced by fibrous tissue. The radial traction of the lung parenchyma on the damaged bronchi causes the involved airways to become permanently dilated and distorted. These areas, devoid of normal ciliated cells, contain secretions that eventually become chronically infected.

Obstruction can cause bronchiectasis by collapsing lung tissue distal

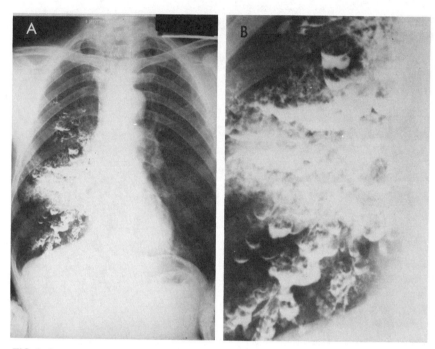

FIG 4–9.
A, AP chest film of a bronchogram shows saccular bronchiectasis. **B,** close-up view of bronchiectatic areas with grapelike saccular bronchiectasis. (Courtesy of T.H. Johnson, M.D.)

to the obstruction. The increased negative pressure in the chest (from the collapsed lung) exerts a greater traction on the airways, causing them to expand and become distorted. Secretions are retained, and if the obstruction is prolonged, there is an infection that begins to destroy the walls of the bronchi as described above. There has been a significant reduction in the number of patients with bronchiectasis since the introduction of antibiotics to treat respiratory infections.

Patients that have severe, diffuse, long-standing bronchiectasis are rarely seen today. Physically, they are emaciated, and as many as 25% of them may have clubbed fingers. A chronic cough, with expectoration of unpleasant tasting, purulent sputum, is typical in these patients. When their sputum is collected and allowed to stand, it may separate into three distinct layers: the uppermost layer is frothy, the middle layer is serous or mucopurulent, and the lowest layer is purulent and may contain small grayish or yellowish plugs. Changes of body position, while sleeping or on arising, often stimulate coughing as the pooled secretions are spilled onto the mucosa of normal, larger airways. These individuals may have cor pulmonale from fibrosis that has extended to involve the pulmonary capillary bed. Patients with widespread bronchiectasis appear dyspneic and have increased work of breathing due to hypoxemia and hypercapnia from ventilation-perfusion mismatching. Anastomosis of the bronchial and pulmonary vascular systems causes shunting of the systemic blood from the hypertrophied bronchial arteries and may contribute to a decreased ability to take oxygen into the involved segments of the lung.

Most patients complain of relatively few symptoms, except during a respiratory infection when they have an increased cough and sputum production. The amount of sputum expectorated and the severity of the cough vary from patient to patient, according to the amount of involvement. Hemoptysis does occur in about half of the elderly patients, evidently due to erosion of enlarged bronchial arteries that accompany the dilated bronchi.

Effective postural drainage is an important part of the management of bronchiectasis. It should be done at least twice daily in patients with a productive cough. Postural drainage should be done an hour before retiring at night in order to facilitate the expectoration of secretions that would interfere with rest by stimulating violent coughing when the patient changes positions. It should also be done on arising in the morning to clear the lungs of secretions that have accumulated overnight. Therapists teaching the patient postural drainage positions devised to drain the involved segments should keep in mind that this disease causes distortion and dilation of the bronchi; hence, the traditional positions found in books may be of limited value in determining the precise segment of the lung that is the source of the secretions. If the involvement is in the lower lobes, we suggest that the patient be in the Trendelenburg position and be gradually rotated from lying on one side, to supine, to lying on the opposite side, and prone, if tolerated, with percussion and vibration 5–10 minutes per segment over all surfaces of the lower lobe being treated. A similar procedure may be followed while sitting if the upper lobes require drainage, but these segments rarely require drainage as they usually drain during the course of the day while the individual is in a more or less erect position. Positions that are especially productive should be emphasized and drained longer. The patient should be instructed to do the postural drainage even if the treatment seems unproductive. Secretions may be mobilized during treatment and it can take several minutes for the remaining cilia to sweep the mucus far enough up the tracheobronchial tree to be expectorated or swallowed.

Pulmonary function tests of patients with localized bronchiectasis show few or no abnormalities. However, in more widespread disease, there is a reduction in the FEV_1, maximum midexpiratory flow rate and maximal voluntary ventilation (MVV), and an increase in the residual volume (see Chapter 2).

Hospitalized patients with bronchiectasis may be treated with postural drainage, intravenous fluids, antibiotics, supplemental oxygen and other medications. Long-term medical management may include a broad-spectrum antibiotic taken orally 10–14 days per month, low-flow oxygen for hypoxemia, postural drainage, avoidance of bronchial irritants (e.g., cigarette smoke and air pollution) and other measures. Some patients may have surgical resection if their area of involvement is quite limited. It is most important that these patients drink large volumes of water each day (2–3 quarts) to keep their secretions thin so they can be expectorated more easily (unless their fluid intake is limited for cardiac reasons). These individuals may benefit greatly from pulmonary rehabilitation. Clinical experience has shown that patients with bronchiectasis may have dramatic increases in exercise tolerance (tenfold) following pulmonary rehabilitation.

Prognosis of Bronchiectasis

Before the antibiotic era, the prognosis for individuals with bronchiectasis was poor. As might be expected, infection was usually the precipitating cause of death. However, at the present time, the prognosis of patients with proper medical management is much improved. Most studies show that about 75% of the patients have an improved symptom complex since diagnosis and lead relatively normal lives. Cor pulmonale, a complication of diffuse, long-standing bronchiectasis, accounts for about 50% of the deaths. Pneumonia and hemorrhage are less frequent causes of death. With modern therapy, only a few patients succumb to respiratory infections or their complications. Few children who develop bronchiectasis live beyond their forties. Repeated bronchopulmonary infections can contribute to worsening pulmonary function and an earlier death. Before the antimicrobial era, most patients with untreated, widespread, severe bronchiectasis died within 15 years. Today, prognosis for each individual depends on the extent of the disease process at the time of diagnosis and on proper medical management. Patients with moderate, localized disease, treated properly, may have a relatively normal life expectancy.

BREATHING PATTERNS

The COPD patient deviates from the normal breathing pattern for several reasons. First, the emphysematous lung is hyperinflated, causing a flattened diaphragm, which is particularly disadvantaged during expiration, when it must try to rise against gravity and the hyperinflated lung. In an effort to maintain adequate pulmonary ventilation, the COPD patient tries to compensate for this disadvantaged diaphragm by using his accessory respiratory muscles. However, this not only results in a labored breathing pattern, but also significantly increases his work of breathing. Over a period of time, we find these patients' breathing patterns are only 30% diaphragmatic and 70% accessory respiratory rate and relieving dyspnea in emphysematous patients. Pursed-lips breathing may decrease air trapping by reducing bronchiolar collapse during expiration. Care must be exercised not to teach the The sensation of air hunger makes the COPD patient's pattern even more abnormal as he reacts by initiating inspiration before expiration has been completed. The result is a dyspneic patient with a very inefficient and uncoordinated pattern of breathing.

How can the breathing pattern be improved? The ideal breathing pattern is one that supplies a maximum amount of alveolar ventilation with a minimum amount of effort. The patient must learn to relax his accessory breathing muscles and retrain the diaphragm to be the main respiratory muscle. Some therapists teach COPD patients to relax accessory breathing muscles using Jacobson's techniques or other relaxation measures. The retraining of the diaphragm has been described by Rusk in his book, *Rehabilitation Medicine.* More recently, feedback devices have been used to relax accessory breathing muscles and teach diaphragmatic breathing. Leaning forward 30–40 degrees from the erect position is effective in relaxing the accessory respiratory muscles and stimulating diaphragmatic breathing. This evidently enhances the descent of the diaphragm during inspiration due to the decreased tension of the abdominal muscles and the reduced pressure exerted by the viscera attached to the diaphragm. The dyspneic patient can be taught these techniques while sitting and later they may be incorporated during standing and walking.

Exhaling through pursed lips is also effective in reducing the respiratory rate and relieving dyspnea in emphysematous patients. Pursed-lips breathing may decrease air trapping by reducing bronchiolar collapse during expiration. Care must be exercised not to teach the patient to forcefully exhale since this increases bronchiolar collapse. Breathing retraining results in an improved ventilation at a slower respiratory rate (which decreases the work of breathing).

The COPD patient must be taught that it is important to use his diaphragm as the main respiratory muscle and relax his accessory breathing muscles during everyday life. This pattern of breathing is essential during periods of dyspnea.

PHYSICAL CONDITION

The COPD patient becomes inactive due to a distressing cycle of events (see Chapter 14). Let us analyze physiologically what happens when the pulmonary disabled patient tries to exercise. A small amount of physical exertion requires increased oxygen consumption and carbon dioxide production in the muscles. This, in turn, causes an increased respiratory rate (which increases work of breathing) and cardiac output. The inability of the lungs to meet the increased oxygen demand and carbon dioxide production adequately, due to ventilation-perfusion abnormalities, will cause a further decrease in the P_{O_2} and a greater increase in P_{CO_2}. Patients who have increased pulmonary artery pressure at rest (due to hypoxemia and acidemia) can be expected to have an additional increase in pulmonary artery pressure during exercise, with resultant increased work for the right ventricle. It is not unusual for chronically hypoxic patients to have premature ventricular contractions while exercising, evidently due to a combination of increased pulmonary artery pressure, increased work of the right heart and a hypoxic myocardium.

Subjectively, the patient finds that minimum physical activity causes him to become short of breath and fatigued. To avoid this discomfort, he simply greatly restricts his physical activity. Lack of physical exercise leads to decreased muscle tone and less efficient muscles. This, in turn, causes the muscles to become more easily fatigued, and the pulmonary cripple has therefore even greater dyspnea on exertion. The result is atrophied muscles that demand more oxygen than normal muscles from a severely handicapped respiratory system, just to do a small amount of work.

POSTURAL DRAINAGE

Postural drainage must be performed properly on these patients. First, many COPD patients have an increased amount of secretions and this in itself predisposes them to respiratory tract infections. Second, they have a disrupted mucociliary blanket, which is further inhibited if they smoke. Third, these patients have a cough that is seriously impaired. The effectiveness of a cough depends upon the high velocity of air passing out from the airways during the cough. The COPD patient has a reduced expiratory velocity due to increased airway resistance and loss of elastic recoil. In fact, if he has an FEV_1 less than 700 cc, his cough is very ineffective. In the normal lung, the airways are compressed during a cough, which increases the velocity of air leaving the lungs. However, some evidence suggests that in these patients the already decreased velocity of air leaving the lungs is further reduced because compression may take place only in lobar and larger airways. If this is the case, then these patients can effectively clear secretions only down to the lobar bronchi. Retained secretions lead to further ventilation-perfusion imbalances, which increase respiratory rate, myocardial work and work of breathing. Rusk has reported on the effectiveness of postural drainage in removing secretions from emphysematous lungs. In view of the impaired mechanisms for removing secretions and the effectiveness of postural drainage, we feel the importance of postural drainage to COPD patients is evident, with emphasis to the middle and lower lobes. However, in draining the superior and posterior segments of the lower lobes, many COPD patients find it very difficult to breathe while lying prone. Evidently this restricts the normal rise of the abdomen (as the diaphragm descends) during inspiration. As a result, many of these patients must be positioned on their sides or three-quarters toward prone in order to individually drain the superior or posterior basal segment of the uppermost lung, rather than bilaterally draining these segments while the patient is lying prone (see Chapter 12).

PERSONALITY CHARACTERISTICS

Most COPD patients seen in the hospital setting are unable to work because of their pulmonary condition. As has already been discussed, their physical activity may have become very limited due to the dyspnea that accompanies or follows physical exertion. They are no longer able to do many of the enjoyable things that they could do only a few months or years before. Many have become restricted to the boundaries of their home or perhaps their yard. It may be that their physician, too, has become discouraged at the progression of the disease despite all efforts at treatment and has advised the COPD patient to "take it easy." In view of the progression of the disease and the physical limitations it brings, it is not surprising that depression is one of the most consistent personality characteristics of the COPD patient. Typically, they are unwilling to accept the irreversibility of their disease. If these patients have been to a number of physicians and hospitals with no appreciable improvement, they are distrustful, frustrated and perhaps even hostile. COPD patients are pessimistic, their morale is low, and the inability to work has caused their self-image to be undermined. Additional personality characteristics of COPD patients include withdrawal and insecurity. With these emotions in mind, it is important for the therapist to maintain a positive attitude and a cheerful outlook when dealing with these individuals, emphasizing their rehabilitation potential (or progress while in a program) rather than dwelling on their disability.

RESTRICTIVE LUNG DISEASES

A restrictive disease is characterized by lungs that are prevented from expanding fully. Normally during inspiration the diaphragm descends, the chest wall moves upward and outward, and the lung tissue expands as it fills with air. Hence, an abnormality in any of these areas can produce a restrictive pattern. For example, a decrease in compliance or elasticity of the lung parenchyma (i.e., interstitial fibrosis, sarcoidosis, pneumoconiosis, scleroderma) can produce this defect. Pleural abnormalities, such as pleural effusion (by direct compression), can prevent the lungs from expanding fully. Thoracic changes, such as kyphoscoliosis and ankylosing spondylitis, can cause lung restriction. Obesity and ascites, by limiting diaphragmatic movement, can also produce a restrictive defect. Atelectasis, the adult respiratory distress syndrome (ARDS), neuromuscular disorders of the thorax, abdominal and thoracic surgery and central nervous system depression (by disease or drugs) have been referred to as *acute restrictive diseases.*

Pulmonary functions generally show a decreased vital capacity, inspiratory capacity and total lung capacity, while the residual volume can be normal or reduced. If the restriction is pulmonary in origin, there is a reduction in the lung compliance and the diffusing capacity.

In the rehabilitation of pulmonary patients, it is important to recognize that the restrictive lung disease patient has an ideal breathing pattern which is different from the individual with COPD. An increased respiratory rate in the COPD patient results in a markedly increased work of breathing. Therefore, it is important for him to breathe at a slow rate. However, the patient with a restrictive defect *must* breathe at an increased respiratory rate. Therefore, modification of such a patient's breathing pattern, by breathing retraining, is usually not indicated.

Many of these restrictive disorders are discussed elsewhere in this book. Since obstructive lung diseases are encountered much more often than restrictive disorders in the hospital setting, they have been discussed in greater detail. We will briefly consider some of the restrictive lung diseases here.

The Adult Respiratory Distress Syndrome (Acute Lung Injury)

The adult respiratory distress syndrome is an acute pulmonary restrictive condition that can result from a variety of insults and has been referred to in the past by a number of different names (Table 4–2). This syndrome is characterized by respiratory distress (evidenced by dyspnea and tachypnea), severe hypoxia that does not respond to high concentrations of oxygen (due to intrapulmonary right-to-left shunting from areas of the lungs that are perfused but not ventilated), decreased lung compliance (reflected by ventilator pressures of 80 cm H_2O or higher to inflate the lung to a normal volume) and a roentgenogram of the chest showing diffuse infiltrates (similar to pulmonary edema, but in ARDS the heart and pulmonary vessels are usually normal in size) (Fig 4–10).

ARDS can follow gram-negative sepsis, diffuse aspiration or viral pneumonia, pulmonary or nonpulmonary trauma, multiple fat embolisms, drug overdose, inhalation of toxic chemicals, shock of any etiology, pancreatitis, cardiopulmonary bypass or other causes. Following the pulmonary insult is a latent period of several hours before the onset of respiratory distress and other features of this syndrome.

Regardless of the specific insult that causes ARDS, diffuse pulmonary capillary bed injury is the common feature of this condition. The capillary bed becomes more permeable, with edema and red blood cells

TABLE 4–2.
Other Names in the Medical Literature for the Adult Respiratory Distress Syndrome

Acute respiratory distress syndrome
Adult hyaline membrane disease
Congestive atelectasis
Da Nang lung
Noncardiac pulmonary edema
Post pump lung
Posttraumatic pulmonary insufficiency
Posttraumatic wet-lung syndrome
Shock lung
Wet lung
Acute lung injury

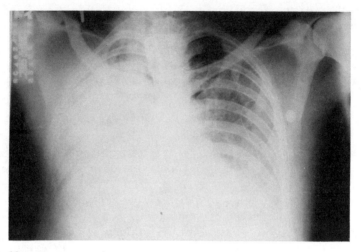

FIG 4–10.
The portable AP chest film reveals confluent and patchy consolidations throughout both lung fields of the adult respiratory distress syndrome (ARDS), which in this case was caused by gram-negative shock. ARDS is characterized by a white-out of the lungs. (Courtesy of T.H. Johnson, M.D.)

entering the interstitial spaces and subsequently the alveoli, where surfactant or its production is impaired. This, in turn causes a decrease in lung compliance and areas of atelectasis. Ventilation-perfusion mismatching causes right-to-left shunting and hypoxemia. In the acute phase, this hypoxemia is often the cause of death.

Many ARDS patients require mechanical ventilation. If the inspired oxygen fraction needed to maintain adequate oxygenation exceeds 50%, PEEP is usually used. Important in the reduction of atelectasis are mechanical ventilation with large tidal volumes (15 ml/kg body weight), periodic hyperinflations, chest physical therapy for mobilization and control of secretions, careful suctioning techniques and turning the patient frequently to reduce the accumulation of secretions in one area. Careful fluid regulation (to avoid fluid overloading) and diuresis of overhydrated patients are indicated. Antibiotics are given to treat sepsis or superimposed infections. Large doses of corticosteroids may be used if fat embolism or aspiration pneumonia has precipitated the ARDS. The use of extracorporeal membrane oxygenators (ECMO) in treating ARDS patients is currently being evaluated in several institutions. However, even with such aggressive treatment, only 20%–50% of these patients survive.

Atelectasis

The term *atelectasis* is derived from the Greek words "ateles" (imperfect) and "ektasis" (expansion) and refers to a condition in which one or more segments or lobes of the lung are collapsed. Atelectasis can be caused by compression of the lung tissue (from increased pleural fluid, pneumothorax, etc.) or more often from an obstructed airway (by secretions or tumor) with subsequent absorption of the "trapped" air by the pulmonary capillary bed and resulting in a collapse of the lung tissue distal to the obstruction.

On examination, the patient with atelectasis is noted to have diminished chest movement and absent breath sounds over the involved area. A roentgenogram of the chest shows an increased density over the involved area, with a shift of the trachea and mediastinum toward the collapsed lung tissue. The patient is often tachypneic and cyanotic (due to shunting) and has a spiked temperature.

The ventilator patient is predisposed to developing atelectasis due to an increased production of mucus in the tracheobronchial tree (from tracheostomy, endotracheal tube, etc.), decreased ciliary activity (especially when high concentrations of oxygen are required), loss of an effective cough due to an artificial airway, limited physical activity (causing pooling of secretions in gravity-dependent areas of the lung) and pooling of secretions (which occlude airways and lead to atelectasis and pneumonia).

Atelectasis is a particularly common complication after thoracic or upper abdominal surgery. Following surgery, these patients have a reduced total lung capacity, functional residual capacity and residual volume. General anesthesia, narcotics, and postoperative pain contribute to an abnormally shallow breathing pattern following surgery, with an absence of spontaneous hyperinflations which are normally done every 5 or 10 minutes.

It has recently been shown that patients who have undergone intra-abdominal vascular surgery have markedly ineffective ciliary activity with subsequent pooling of secretions and a high incidence of postoperative pulmonary complications. Neurologic patients, especially those with increased tracheobronchial secretions, are also predisposed to developing atelectasis.

It has been reported that chest physical therapy is very effective in reducing the incidence of postoperative pulmonary complications in patients undergoing upper abdominal procedures. Roentgenographically, we have seen dramatic clearing of extensive atelectasis following effective postural drainage, percussion and vibration to the involved areas (Fig 4–11). Postural drainage and other chest physical therapy techniques are very effective in preventing and treating atelectasis caused by retained secretions.

Sarcoidosis

Sarcoidosis is a granulomatous disorder of unknown etiology which can effect multiple body systems. Typically, initial findings can include bilateral hilar adenopathy, pulmonary infiltration and skin or eye lesions. The lungs are the organs most often involved and some 20%–50% of these patients first seek medical attention because of respiratory symptoms. It affects blacks 10–12 times more frequently than whites, females twice as often as males. It usually occurs in the third or fourth decade of life.

The intrathoracic changes can be classified into four stages. In the first stage, the patient is asymptomatic, with the chest x-ray showing bilateral hilar adenopathy and right paratracheal adenopathy (Fig 4–

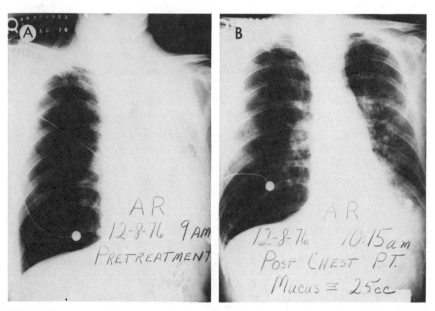

FIG 4–11.
A, portable AP chest film of a COPD patient shows almost complete atelectasis of the left lung. **B,** immediately following a 20-minute treatment of postural drainage, percussion and vibration to all segments of the left lower lobe (during which 25 ml of mucus was expectorated), a chest film reveals almost complete reexpansion of the involved lung.

12,A). In the second stage a diffuse pulmonary infiltration is found along with the bilateral hilar adenopathy. Interstitial infiltration or fibrosis, without hilar adenopathy, characterizes the third stage (Fig 4–12,B). In the fourth stage, emphysematous changes, cysts and bullae are found.

In 60%–90% of these patients with hilar adenopathy, the disease spontaneously regresses over a period of 1 to 2 years. About one-third of the patients with sarcoidosis involving the lungs also have a spontaneous regression, usually leaving some residual fibrosis. The remaining two-thirds that have chronic sarcoidosis have progressive pulmonary impairment, along with a variable degree of involvement of the heart, liver, spleen, lymph nodes, muscles, bones, and central nervous system.

Most patients with sarcoidosis need no treatment. At the present time, corticosteroids are the most effective form of therapy for patients with sarcoidosis that requires treatment.

Diffuse Interstitial Pulmonary Fibrosis

This is a disease characterized by a diffuse inflammatory process distal to the terminal bronchiole with thickening of the alveolar walls and a tendency to fibrosis. Large mononuclear cells are usually present within the alveolar spaces. The most common early symptoms are fatigue, dys-

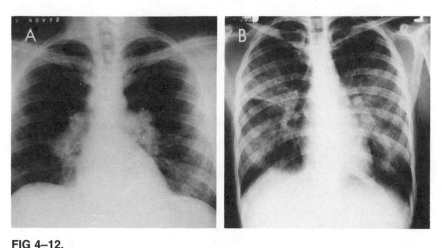

FIG 4–12.
A, sarcoidosis in its first stage is manifested by bilateral hilar adenopathy. Usually there are no significant physical symptoms. **B,** disseminated sarcoidosis (third stage) reveals widespread parenchymal changes with scarring. The hilar adenopathy is usually decreased. (Courtesy of T.H. Johnson, M.D.)

pnea on exertion and a chronic unproductive cough. As the disease progresses, the patient becomes steadily more dyspneic and cyanotic. On auscultation, one notes sharply crackling rales. Chest expansion is reduced and clubbing of the digits is often present.

Pulmonary function tests show a reduced vital capacity and total lung capacity with no impaired flow rates. Compliance is markedly reduced to less than half of the predicted value. A reduced diffusing capacity is the earliest and most consistent change. At first, the arterial P_{O_2} may be normal at rest but drops significantly with exercise. The P_{CO_2} is reduced due to hyperventilation, and the pH is kept normal by renal compensation. Later the P_{O_2} is markedly reduced due to the thickened alveolar membrane and ventilation-perfusion mismatching.

The etiology of this condition is uncertain. Similar conditions can be produced by certain drugs or poisons and are found in patients with rheumatoid arthritis and systemic sclerosis. There appears to be a genetic factor, as twins, siblings and other members of the same family have been reported with diffuse interstitial pulmonary fibrosis. This condition has also been reported in a few individuals with Raynaud's disease, ulcerative colitis and other diseases, but their exact relationship remains unclear. Corticosteroids are the only effective treatment for diffuse interstitial pulmonary fibrosis.

Patients with the subacute form described by Hamman and Rich usually die within six months. Patients with the chronic form, treated with steroids, may survive for as long as 15 years. Untreated, these patients most often succumb within 2–4 years. Cause of death is usually related to respiratory or heart failure, although an unexpected number have died from adenocarcinoma and undifferentiated or alveolar cell carcinoma of the lung.

Progressive Systemic Sclerosis (Scleroderma)

Progressive systemic sclerosis (scleroderma) is a rare disease that causes thickening and fibrosis of the connective tissue of multiple parts of the body with replacement of many elements of the connective tissue by colloidal collagen. The skin is most often involved, although the lungs, heart, kidneys, bones and other parts of the body can also be affected.

Approximately one-half to two-thirds of the patients with progressive systemic sclerosis have pulmonary involvement.

Many of these patients with pulmonary involvement are asymptomatic, although symptoms can include weight loss, progressive dyspnea, low-grade fever and cough (sometimes producing mucoid sputum). Chest x-rays show a characteristic fibrosis of the mid and lower lung fields. Auscultation often reveals bibasilar rales. Pulmonary function tests reveal a restrictive defect with impaired diffusion.

Corticosteroids are the only treatment for pulmonary involvement in patients with progressive systemic sclerosis.

Prognosis of patients with only skin and joint involvement is much better than for those that have involvement of the heart, lungs and kidneys. In the latter group progression results in death after several years. Women seem to have a poorer prognosis than men. The average survival for whites is reported to be about seven years compared with two years for blacks.

Pulmonary Alveolar Proteinosis

Pulmonary alveolar proteinosis is a rare disease of unknown etiology, characterized by alveoli filled with a lipid-rich "proteinaceous" material and no abnormality of the alveolar wall, interstitial spaces, conducting airways or pleural surfaces. Most often it is found in men between the ages of 30 and 50, although it has been reported in patients of all ages and both sexes.

The most common symptoms are progressive dyspnea and weight loss, with cough, hemoptysis and chest pain reported less frequently. Roentgenograms of the chest reveal diffuse bilateral (commonly perihilar) opacities (Fig 4–13). Physical findings may include fine inspira-

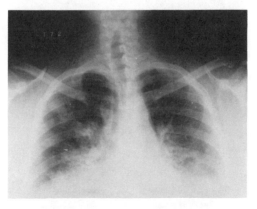

FIG 4–13.
Pulmonary alveolar proteinosis. PA chest film demonstrates an irregular, patchy, poorly defined confluence of acinar shadows which are symmetrical in both lower lung fields. The appearance is very similar to pulmonary edema. (Courtesy of T.H. Johnson, M.D.)

tory rales, dullness to percussion and, in the later stages, cyanosis and clubbing. Pulmonary function studies usually show a decreased vital capacity, functional residual capacity and diffusing capacity. Arterial blood gases indicate a low PO_2, especially during exercise, with normal PCO_2 and pH.

The treatment of choice for patients with moderate to severe dyspnea on exertion from alveolar proteinosis is bronchopulmonary lavage. The patient is taken to the operating room where, after general anesthesia and placement of a Carlen's tube (which isolates each lung), the patient is turned in the lateral decubitus position with the lung to be lavaged downward. The Carlen's tube enables the patient to be ventilated by his uppermost lung while the lower lung is carefully filled with saline to the functional residual capacity. Then an additional 300–500 ml saline are alternately allowed to run into and out of the lung by gravitational flow. As the saline flows out, percussion is done over the lung being lavaged, and this greatly increases the amount of proteinaceous material washed from the lung (Fig 4–14). We (at the University of Oklahoma) have compared the effectiveness of mechanical vibration, manual vibration and manual percussion in removing this

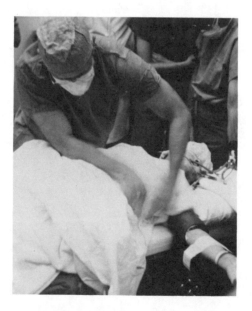

FIG 4–14.
A patient with pulmonary alveolar proteinosis in the operating room undergoing bronchopulmonary lavage of her left lung. Percussion is done over the left lung as the saline runs out, increasing the amount of proteinaceous material removed during this procedure.

material from involved lungs and have found manual percussion to be superior. In this process, patients are usually lavaged with 20–30 L saline, after which they are taken to the recovery room and later back to their own room. After two or three days the procedure is repeated on the opposite lung.

Most patients have significant clinical improvement following bronchopulmonary lavage, and many have an improvement in their chest roentgenograms. After lavage, for reasons that are unclear, the material may reaccumulate slowly or not at all. Some patients do have spontaneous remissions without undergoing lavage.

Before bronchopulmonary lavage was done on these patients, almost all children with alveolar proteinosis died, and 20%–25% of the adults died within five years, usually due to respiratory failure or cor pulmonale. Some 60%–70% improved greatly or recovered. The effect that bronchopulmonary lavage has on the long-term outcome remains to be seen, but present results are encouraging.

THORACIC DEFORMITY

Respiratory insufficiency can result from abnormalities of the chest wall secondary to congential deformity, acquired disease, and trauma. Congenital deformity of the chest wall reduces the mobility of the bony thorax and thereby increases the work of breathing. Shallow, rapid breathing often results. Minute ventilation is increased at the expense of alveolar ventilation. Examples of chronic deformities that impinge on pulmonary function are kyphoscoliosis secondary to poliomyelitis, tuberculous osteomyelitis, and other causes, and ankylosing spondylitis. Other examples of deformity include traumatic injury of the vertebral column, ribs, and sternum. Routine chest assessment should include a musculoskeletal examination of the thoracic spine.

Normal pulmonary function and gas exchange depend on symmetry of pulmonary anatomy, hence physiological function. Asymmetry of the chest wall is therefore likely to interfere with the regional gradients of ventilation and perfusion in the lungs. The effects of physiologic dead space and shunt may be magnified, producing hypoxemia and hypercapnia. With severe chest deformity, a cycle of respiratory acidosis, pulmonary hypertension, and cor pulmonale can result in a life-threatening situation.

Some common chest deformities are reviewed briefly. The severity of these deformities and any underlying disorders determine the effect on pulmonary function.

Kyphoscoliosis

Kyphoscoliosis is characterized by a curvature of the spine laterally and in the anteroposterior direction. Kyphosis refers to the increased curvature of the thoracic spine forward. Scoliosis refers to the lateral curvature of the vertebral column. The bodies of the vertebrae rotate, forcing the ribs opposite the convexity to bulge. The ribs on the concave side of the lateral curvature are sunken and depressed. The opposite occurs anteriorly, with the ribs on the convex side being sunken and the ribs on the concave side being prominent. In kyphoscoliosis or when both deformities coexist, total lung capacity and vital capacity can be reduced if the condition is severe. Airway resistance tends not to be affected.

Kyphosis can be associated with chronic obstructive lung disease and the adaptive increase in anteroposterior diameter of the chest. In this situation, functional residual capacity tends to be increased, and the results of pulmonary function tests tend to be compatible with the picture of chronic obstructive lung disease. Patients with kyphosis in the absence of chronic obstructive lung disease tend to have reduced total lung capacities but otherwise relatively normal pulmonary function.

Ankylosing Spondylitis

Ankylosing spondylitis is characterized by chronic inflammation of the joints of the vertebral column. The natural course of the disease results in ankylosis or loss of mobility of the affected joints. Pulmonary function is not usually severely affected. Compensation by the respiratory system for the progressive rigidity of the vertebral column helps to maintain adequate diaphragmatic excursion. The patient is reliant on diaphragmatic motion for ventilation. Vital capacity is reduced; however, ventilatory capacity is usually adequate.

Rib Fractures

Rib fractures constitute the most common form of chest wall injury. Rib fractures tend to be painful, resulting in splinting and guarding of the chest. Breathing is impaired; thus, tidal volume is reduced. Cough is inhibited. Rib injuries can range from bruising and crack fractures to multiple fractures, flail chest, and lung puncture. If properly diagnosed and managed at the outset, rib fractures do not usually constitute a major long-term problem.

Chest Trauma

Blunt chest trauma is a major cause of serious pulmonary dysfunction. Chest trauma is a leading cause of death in individuals under 45 years. Chest trauma may be due to accidents, i.e., motorcycles, car, falls, or contact sports. These serious cases of chest trauma may also lead to lung contusions as well as other structural lacerations or trauma of the lungs or diaphragm.

The practitioner may be asked to work with patients with rib fractures or flail chest. Flail chest is defined as two or more ribs broken in two or more places. Consequently, there is a "flailing" or paradoxical movement on inspiration. There will be a tendency for atelectasis in the chest area of fractured ribs or flail chest due to poor stability and lack of expansion of the chest wall. Pain from fractured ribs will also be a strong limiting factor to deep breathing even if the chest wall is intact.

Management of rib fractures mainly involves good pain control, frequent positioning to prevent pooling of secretions, and encouragement to deep breathe and move the chest wall. Epidural morphine drip has been a very helpful adjunct to the more traditional methods in these patients.

Flail chest management is accomplished by placing the patient on a mechanical ventilator for "internal stabilization" by positive pressure breathing often with PEEP (positive end expiratory pressure).

Pulmonary contusion has been seen in 30%–70% of patients with chest trauma. Hemorrhage may be present in alveolar structures and also in the interstitial spaces. Chest PT can be a helpful adjunct to the care of patients with pulmonary contusions by maintaining airway clearance.

OTHER SKELETAL VARIATIONS

The following skeletal deformities are often associated with other medical conditions. The degree of impairment of pulmonary function therefore depends on both the deformity and the nature of any underlying conditions.

Cervical Ribs

Cervical ribs are bony growths of the costal processes of the seventh cervical vertebrae that have well-defined heads and necks. As they grow, they may eventually impinge on nerves and vessels, causing various obscure symptoms. If they become too troublesome, they can be removed surgically.

Rickets

In this disease, the ends of the ribs that join the costal cartilages become enlarged, forming visible knots on the anterior chest known as the *ricket rosary*. A groove forms laterally on either side of these enlargements as the softening ribs sink. Harrison's sulcus and pigeon breast may also be present in these patients. (See text below.)

Harrison's Sulcus

A transverse groove may occur just above the costal arch in patients who have soft bones and a chronically distended abdomen. This occurs as a result of the lower ribs being pushed out by abdominal distention. It is frequently seen in patients with rickets.

Pigeon Breast

Pigeon breast is a prominent forward projection of the sternum. It frequently indicates the presence of rickets or spinal curvature.

Funnel Breast

Funnel breast occurs when the lower part of the sternum and the xiphoid process are deeply depressed, producing a hollow in the lower sternal region. This may also be referred to as *pectus excavation.*

Barrel Chest

This abnormality is frequently seen in patients who have emphysema. The chest appears to be in a permanent state of inspiration, with the ribs held in a horizontal position. Upon examination, the side-to-side diameter is almost equal to the front-to-back diameter. The chest frequently appears frozen, moving only up and down vertically as a whole. Occasionally paradoxical movements may be seen, with the ribs flaring up and out during exhalation and down and in during inspiration. This occurs as a result of the permanent flattening of the diaphragm.

SUMMARY

This chapter has described the essential pathophysiological features of obstructive and restrictive lung diseases. Obstructive lung disease is associated with mechanical airway obstruction producing air trapping distal to the site of obstruction, hyperinflation of the chest wall, and flattening of the hemidiaphragms. Increased work of breathing and possible respiratory muscle fatigue can predispose the patient to right ventricular hypertrophy, elevated pulmonary artery pressure, and right heart failure (cor pulmonale).

Restrictive lung disease impairs pulmonary function as a result of reduced lung and chest wall compliance. Reduced lung compliance is commonly associated with prolonged inhalation of inorganic and organic materials, in addition to proteinosis and atelectasis. Reduced chest wall compliance occurs secondary to chest wall deformities, including kyphoscoliosis and congenital deformities.

A knowledge of the pathophysiology of pulmonary dysfunction assists the practitioner in relating the pathophysiology to the clinical signs and symptoms, and the appropriate treatment goals and interventions.

REFERENCES

Periodicals

Aldrich TK, Arora, NS, Rochester DF: The influence of airway obstruction and respiratory muscle strength on maximal voluntary ventilation in lung disease. *Am Rev Resp Dis* 1982; 126:195.

American Thoracic Society (statement by the Committee on Diagnostic Standards for Non-Tuberculous Respiratory Diseases): Definitions and classification of chronic bronchitis, asthma, and pulmonary emphysema, *Am Rev Respir Dis* 1962; 85:762.

Askutosh K, et al: Asynchronous breathing movements in patients with chronic obstructive pulmonary disease. *Chest* 1975; 67:553.

Barach AL: Chronic obstructive lung disease: Postural relief of dyspnea. *Arch Phys Med Rehabil* 1974; 55:494.

Bartlett RH, et al: Mortality prediction in adult respiratory insufficiency. *Chest* 1975; 67:680.

Bartlett RH, Gazzaniga AB, Geraghty TR: Respiratory maneuvers to prevent postoperative pulmonary complications, *JAMA* 1973; 224:1017.

Block JD, et al: A feedback device for teaching diaphragmatic breathing. *Am Rev Respir Dis* 1969; 100:577.

Bousky SF, et al: Factors affecting prognosis in emphysema, *Dis Chest* 1964; 45:402.

Burrows B, Earle R: Predictability of survival in patients with chronic airway obstruction. *Am Rev Respir Dis* 1969; 99:865.

Frownfelter DL: A coordinated approach to the treatment of atelectasis. *Respir Ther* 1977; 7:54.

Gamsu G, et al: Postoperative impairment of mucus transport in the lung. *Am Rev Respir Dis* 1976; 114:673.

Gandevia B: Pressurized sympathomimetic aerosols and their lack of relationship to asthma mortality in Australia. *Med J Aust* 1973; 1:273.

Gibson GJ, Pride NB, Davis JN, et al: Pulmonary mechanics in patients with respiratory muscle weakness. *Am Rev Resp Dis* 1977; 115:389.

Gold WM: Asthma. *Basics Respir Dis* 1976; 4:1.

Hamman L, Rich AR: Acute diffuse interstitial fibrosis of the lungs. *Bull Johns Hopkins Hosp* 1944; 74:177.

Hapke EJ, Meak, JC, Jacobs J: Pulmonary function in progressive muscular dystrophy. *Chest* 1972; 61:41.

Hilding A: Physiology of drainage of nasal mucus: Experimental work on accessory sinuses. *Am J Physiol* 1932; 100:664.

Hodgkin JE, et al: Chronic obstructive airway diseases—current concepts in diagnosis and comprehensive care. *JAMA* 1975; 232:1243.

Hopewell PC, Murray JF: The adult respiratory distress syndrome. *Ann Rev Med* 1976; 27:343.

Hyatt RE: Role of bronchial obstruction in chronic lung disease. *Arch Phys Med Rehabil* 1968; 49:333.

Johnston R, Lee K: Myofeedback: A new method of teaching breathing exercises to emphysematous patients. *Phys Ther* 1976; 56:826.

Konietzko NF, Carton RW, Leroy EP: Causes of death in patients with bronchiectasis, *Am Rev Respir Dis* 1969; 100:852.

Matzen RN: Vocational rehabilitation—the culmination of physical rehabilitation. *Chest (Suppl)* 1971; 60:21.

Mead J, et al: Significance of the relationship between lung recoil and maximum expiratory flow. *J Appl Physiol* 1967; 22:95.

Miller WF: Rehabilitation of patients with chronic obstructive lung disease. *Med Clin North Am* 1967; 51:349.

Mitchell RS, Webb WC, Filley GF: Chronic obstructive bronchopulmonary disease. III. Factors influencing prognosis. *Am Rev Respir Dis* 1964; 89:878.

Muller RE, Petty TL, Filley GF: Ventilation and arterial blood gas changes induced by pursed-lip breathing. *J Appl Physiol* 1970; 28:784.

Ogilvie AG: Asthma: A study on prognosis of 1,000 patients. *Thorax* 1962; 17:183.

Petty TL, Guthrie AG: The effects of augmented breathing maneuvers on ventilation in severe chronic airway obstruction. *Respir Care* 1974; 16:104.

Pierce AK, Paez PN, Miller WE: Exercise training with the aid of a portable oxygen supply in patients with emphysema. *Am Rev Respir Dis* 1965; 91:653.

Public Health Service Publications, Nos. 1529 and 1802: Chronic respiratory disease control program (Arlington, Virginia, National Center for Chronic Disease Control, 1968).

Reid L: Anatomy of the lung and patterns of structural change in disease. *Physiotherapy* 1976; 62:44.

Renzehi AD: Prognosis in chronic obstructive pulmonary disease. *Med Clin North Am* 1967; 51:363.

Rochester DF, Brown NM: Chronic obstructive pulmonary diseases. *Res Staff Phys* 1976; 22:44.

Rogers RM: Shock lung or respiratory distress syndrome of adults. *Cont Educ Fam Phys* 1975; 3:26.

Rogers RM, Graunstein MS, Shuman JF: Role of Bronchopulmonary lavage in the treatment of respiratory failure: A review. *Chest (Suppl 2)* 1972; 62:95.

Rogers RM, Tatum KR: Bronchopulmonary lavage: A new approach to old problems. *Med Clin North Am* 1970; 54:755.

Sharma OD: A clinical picture sarcoidosis: Treatment and prognosis. *Res Staff Phys* 1977; 23:123.

Simon G, Medvei VC: Chronic bronchitis: Radiologic aspects of a five-year follow-up. *Thorax* 1962; 17:5.

Simpson DG: Bronchiectasis. *Hosp Med* 1975; 11:94.

Stoley PD: Asthma mortality. *Am Rev Respir Dis* 1972; 105:883.

Thoman RL, Stoker GL, Ross JC: The efficacy of pursed-lip breathing in patients with chronic obstructive pulmonary disease. *Am Rev Respir Dis* 1966; 93:100.

Thoren L: Postoperative pulmonary complications; observations on their prevention by means of physiotherapy. *Acta Chir Scand* 1954; 107:193.

Thurlbeck WM: Chronic bronchitis and emphysema—the pathophysiology of chronic obstructive lung disease. *Basics Respir Dis* 1974; 3:1.

Treatment of status asthmaticus. *Br Med J* 1972; 4:563.

Webber BA: Current trends in the treatment of asthma. *Physiotherapy* 1973; 59: 388.

Williams H, McNicol RN: Prevalence, natural history, and relationship of wheezy bronchitis and asthma in children: An epidemiological study. *Br Med J* 1969; 4:321.

World Health Organization: World Health Statistics Manual, 1973–1976.

Books

Bates DV, Mackle MPT, Christie RV: *Respiratory Function in Disease,* ed 2. Philadelphia, WB Saunders Co, 1971.

Baum GL (ed): *Textbook of Pulmonary Diseases,* ed 3. Boston, Little, Brown & Co, 1983.

Bergofsky EH: Respiratory insufficiency in mechanical and neuromuscular disorders of the thorax, in Fishman AP (ed): *Pulmonary Diseases and Disorders.* New York, McGraw-Hill Book Co, 1980.

Burrows B, Knudson RJ, Quan SF, et al: *Respiratory Disorders: A Pathophysiologic Approach,* ed 2. Chicago, Year Book Medical Publishers, 1983.

Cherniak RM, et al: *Respiration in Health and Disease,* ed 3. Philadelphia, WB Saunders Co, 1983.

Comroe JH, Jr, et al: *The Lung: Clinical Physiology and Pulmonary Function Tests,* ed 2. Chicago, Year Book Medical Publishers, 1962.

Crofton J, Douglas A: *Respiratory Diseases,* ed 3. Oxford, Blackwell Scientific Publications, 1981.

Dunnill MS: The morphology of the airways in bronchial asthma, in Stein M (ed): *New Directions in Asthma.* Park Ridge, Illinois, American College of Chest Physicians, 1975.

Egan DF: *Fundamentals of Respiratory Therapy,* ed 2. St Louis, CV Mosby Co, 1973.

Hinshaw HC: *Diseases of the Chest,* ed 4. Philadelphia, WB Saunders Co, 1980.

Jacobson E: *Progressive Relaxation,* ed 3. Chicago, University of Chicago Press, 1974.

Joint Committee of the Allergy Foundation of American Thoracic Society: *Asthma—A Practical Guide for Physicians.* National Tuberculosis and Respiratory Disease Association, 1973.

Leigh D, Morley E: *Bronchial Asthma—A Genetic Population, and Psychiatric Study.* Oxford, Pergamon Press, 1967.

Lester DM: The psychological impact of chronic obstructive pulmonary disease, in Johnston RF (ed): *Pulmonary Care.* New York, Grune & Stratton, Inc, 1973.

Millard M: Lung, pleura, and mediastinum, in Anderson WA (ed): *Pathology,* vol 2. St Louis, CV Mosby Co, 1971.

Perry TL (ed): *Intensive and Rehabilitative Respiratory Care: A Practical Approach to the Management of Acute and Chronic Respiratory Failure,* ed 3. Philadelphia, Lea & Febiger, 1982.

Robbins SL, Angell M: *Basic Pathology,* ed 3. Philadelphia, WB Saunders Co, 1980.

Rusk HA: *Rehabilitation Medicine,* ed 3. St Louis, CV Mosby Co, 1971.

Shapiro BA, Harrison RA, Trout CA: *Clinical Application of Respiratory Care,* ed 2. Chicago, Year Book Medical Publishers, 1979.

Pulmonary Disease

Carasso B: Therapeutic options in COPD. *Geriatrics* 1982; 37(5):99–102, 106.

Davis P, di SantAgnese PA: Diagnosis and treatment of cystic fibrosis. An update. *Chest* 1984; 85 (6) 802–809.

Geddes DM: Chronic airflow obstruction. *Postgrad Med J* 1984; 60(701):194–200.

Geddes DM: Chronic airflow obstruction. *Postgrad Med* 1984; 75 (5):241–242, 248.

Hogg JC: the pathology of asthma. *Clin Chest Med* 1984; 5(4)567–571.

Kawakami Y, Terai T, Yamamoto H, et al: Exercise and oxygen inhalation in relation to prognosis of chronic obstructive pulmonary disease. *Chest* 1982; 81(2):182–188.

Lewiston NJ: Bronchiectasis in childhood. *Pediatr Clin North Am* 1984; 31 (4): 865–878.

Make B: Medical management of emphysema. *Clin Chest Med* 1983; 4 (3): 465–482.

Miller WF: Chronic pulmonary disease. *Annu Rev Rehabil* 1980; 1:333–355.

Miller WF: Chronic obstructive pulmonary disease. *Hosp Pract* 1981; 16(2):89–106.

Moller P: Skeletal muscle adaptation to aging and to respiratory and liver failure. *Acta Med Scand (Suppl)* 1982; 654:1–40.

Scano G, VanMeerhaeghe A, Willeput R, et al: Effect of oxygen on breathing during exercise in patients with chronic obstructive lung disease. *Eur J Respir Dis* 1982; 63(1):23–30.

Smith JM: The recent history of the treatment of asthma: A personal view. *Thorax* 1983; 38 (4):244–253.

Stein DA, Bradley BL, Miller WC: Mechanisms of oxygen effects on exercise in patients with chronic obstructive pulmonary disease. *Chest* 1982; 81(1):6–10.

Rees J: ABC of asthma. Definition and diagnosis. *Br Med J (Clin Res)* 1984; 5;288 (6427): 1370–1372.

5

Occupational Lung Disease

Maureen Fogel Perlstein, M.P.H., P.T., C.R.T.T.

INTRODUCTION AND HISTORY

The relationship between occupations and disease has been observed from early history. References to this relationship can be found in Greek and Roman literature. In the late Middle Ages, the topic was more closely studied. The most significant study of occupational disease was conducted by Bernardo Ramizzini in his classical treatise, *De Morbis Artificum Diatriba, Diseases of Workers*, which was written in 1713.

Ramizzini described the plight of workers in the preface of his book: "For we must admit that the workers in certain arts and crafts sometimes derive from them grave injuries, so that where they hoped for a subsistence that would prolong their lives and feed their families, they are too often repaid with the most dangerous diseases, and finally uttering curses on a profession to which they had devoted themselves, they desert their post among the living." Ramizzini studied more than 50 occupational categories, including miners of metals, bakers, millers, sifters of grain and farmers. He proposed that in addition to asking the usual questions about symptoms, a physician should also ask a patient about his occupation.

Concern about occupational health and safety in the United States dates as far back as 1914 with the establishment of the Federal Office of Industrial Hygiene and Sanitation. Federal legislation regarding occupational lung diseases, however, has only recently been promulgated. Coal workers' lung disease was not recognized as a specific disease entity until the early 1940s in Great Britain. Research conducted in the

United States by the Pennsylvania Department of Health (1959–1961) and by the U.S. Public Health Service (1963–1965) demonstrated the serious health problems related to coal mining.

The old saying "An ounce of prevention is worth a pound of cure" is so often ignored. In the early 1900s, working conditions in mines were designed for efficiency of production, to increase profit margins regardless of the danger to employees' health. As is often the case, public attention was finally drawn to the plight of coal miners and their families by disaster. In November 1968, a mine explosion killing 78 men in Farmington, West Virginia, triggered the passage of Public Law 91–173, the Federal Coal Mine Health and Safety Act of 1969. This act was designed to protect the health and safety of miners. It placed responsibility for reducing dust concentrations in mines on the coal industry, subject to federal inspection. The act also provided for a radiologic screening program to identify workers with coal mine worker's pneumoconiosis, known as black lung. This original law, which required evidence of positive radiologic findings, was amended by the Black Lung Benefits Act of 1972. Now an individual working in the mines for more than 15 years who is totally disabled by lung disease is eligible for federal benefits regardless of x-ray findings. Federal benefits paid to disabled miners or to their widows were $144.50 per month in 1970 and were increased to more than $200 per month in 1974. Higher payments are made to miners or their widows when there are qualified dependents.

The government's commitment to provide safe and healthful working conditions, which began with the Federal Coal Mine Act, was expanded to all American industry with passage of the Occupational Safety and Health Act (OSHA) of 1970. Today, the National Institute for Occupational Safety and Health (NIOSH) in the Department of Health, Education and Welfare (HEW), and the U.S. Department of Labor are responsible for the implementation of OSHA. The Department of Labor's responsibilities include setting standards for the workplace, enforcing standards, operating a national record keeping and reporting system, and promoting employer-employee relations. NIOSH directs its efforts toward health and safety research, hazard evaluations, compiling an annual list of toxic substances, conducting industrywide studies, and developing manpower.

The promulgation of government standards regarding occupational safety and health is motivated not only by an altruistic social concern, but also by cost containment. Obviously, controlling the incidence of occupationally acquired diseases at their source is the ultimate goal of both government and industry.

PATHOPHYSIOLOGY OF OCCUPATIONAL LUNG DISEASES

The term *pneumoconiosis* comes from the Greek words "pneumo" (lungs) and "konis" (dust). Simply translated, it means dusty lungs. Pneumoconiosis is now used as a generic term defined as ". . . the presence of inhaled dust in the lungs and their non-neoplasmic reaction to it." These dusts may be inorganic (mineral) in origin or of organic (nonmineral) origin. Reactions to inorganic and organic dusts comprise the first two major categories of occupational diseases. The third category, which will be discussed, includes pulmonary reactions to fumes and gases.

These three categories share in common the pathologic and radiologic characteristic of widespread pulmonary parenchymal involvement, representing a fibrotic reaction. Functional abnormalities that result may reflect restrictive, obstructive or perfusion defects. In some cases, two or all three of these defects occur in combination.

Dust Deposition

The topic of dust deposition is preliminary to any discussion of specific disease entities. Dust particles, like any other form of matter, are under the influence of gravity. The manner in which inhaled particles behave is determined by their aerodynamic particle size. Aerodynamic particle size, a concept used as a common denominator for a means of comparison, reflects particle size, shape, density and surface characteristics. In this way, the behavior of irregularly shaped particles with various compositions can be compared to a particle that is spherical, has a diameter of 1 μ and is of unit density.

Particles that are 10 μ in size or larger are usually filtered out by the hair in the nose. The mucociliary escalator (see Chapter 1) acts as a clearance mechanism for the lungs, removing most particles between 5 and 10 μ in size by raising them up to the throat where they can be coughed up or swallowed. Particles that are not removed in this manner may be deposited in the respiratory tract by one of four mechanisms—sedimentation, inertial impaction, interception and diffusion.

Sedimentation

Sedimentation is a settling of particles due to the force of gravity. The rate at which they settle is a function of particle density and diameter. Deposition in the larger airways occurs mainly by sedimentation of particles with an aerodynamic size of less than 2 μ.

Inertial Impaction

The respiratory tract consists of many branching tubes. Branching causes changes in the direction of airways. Particles in an air stream, however, tend to continue their original path due to inertia, and impinge on bronchial walls. Inertial impaction is a function of particle density and diameter, airway diameter and airflow characteristics. This mechanism affects particles larger than 10 μ and, as mentioned above, is the primary means of deposition in the nose.

Interception

Particles with irregular shapes tend to become wedged in the walls of bronchioles, especially at their bifurcations. This wedged deposition, called *interception,* is a factor of the particle shape rather than of its falling speed or mass. Long, thin fibers such as asbestos, fiberglass and talc act in this manner.

Diffusion

Very small particles, less than 0.1 μ in diameter, are deposited by diffusion. These particles are greatly influenced by their Brownian motion, the random movement of minute particles. Those in close proximity to alveolar walls are able to diffuse across and be deposited within the alveolus. Other particles this size leave the lungs during normal exhalation.

Reaction to Inorganic Dusts

Silicosis

Silicosis is a fibrotic lung disease caused by the inhalation of dust containing silicon dioxide, SiO_2. This mineral can be found in large quantities all over the world, and in fact is one of the most important constituents of the earth's crust, so the risk of exposure is great. Silicon dioxide is in sandstone, granite and slate. The ores of other metals that are found in silica-containing rock include gold, tin, copper, silver, nickel, uranium, mica and graphite. Workers at the greatest risk of exposure are those involved in mining, quarrying and tunneling. Other sources of exposure occur in occupations of stone cutting, masonry, glass manufacture, abrasives manufacture, blasting, foundry work, ceramics and enameling.

Some of the inhaled particles will be removed by the mucociliary escalator (MCE), which may fail to remove small, irregularly shaped silicon dioxide fibers that penetrate into small airways and alveoli.

These particles are deposited chiefly by sedimentation and interception.

Once within the alveoli, the macrophage defense mechanism is triggered. Macrophages, the body's scavenger cells, engulf foreign particles. Both silica and asbestos fibers may injure lysosomal membranes within the macrophages. The lysosomes then release digestive enzymes, initiating autodigestion and causing the entire macrophage to disintegrate. The liberated particles are reingested by other macrophages, and the cycle begins again.

In order to prevent the spread of this destructive process, fibroblasts and collagen fibers proliferate in an attempt to wall in the dust particles. This results in the formation of local fibrous lesions known as *silicotic nodules*. Silicotic nodules, 3–5 mm in diameter, tend to cluster and are distributed primarily in the upper lobes and superior segments of the lower lobes. Nodules increase in both size and number with continued exposure. Alveolar walls become thickened by the deposition of collagenous fibers. The fibrotic process also affects the visceral and parietal pleura, which may become adherent.

The diagnosis of silicosis is made by history of exposure and x-ray findings of nodular shadows. In its simple form, uncomplicated by chronic bronchitis or infection, silicosis may not progress clinically.

The devastating feature of silicosis, as well as other pneumoconioses, is that there may be no overt symptoms until the disease is in an advanced state. Then the worker may experience a dry cough and dyspnea on exertion. Dyspnea is the result of a restrictive lesion caused by the fibrotic process. Pulmonary function tests in uncomplicated silicosis may be within normal limits. When abnormalities occur, the studies reflect a decrease in total lung capacity, vital capacity and functional reserve capacity, as with other restrictive lesions (see Chapter 2). Breath sounds are normal or decreased by pleural thickening. Adventitious breath sounds are not heard in uncomplicated cases.

Silicosis has been found to predispose to the development of pulmonary tuberculosis. Silicosis is frequently complicated by emphysema and chronic bronchitis, due to cigarette smoking, and by superimposed respiratory infections. In this case, the disease assumes an obstructive lesion and diffusion defects as well. Severe progressive dyspnea, a productive cough and wheezing develop, finally resulting in total disability. When silicosis is extensive in both its simple and complicated forms, pulmonary hypertension and cor pulmonale eventually occur.

There is no specific therapy other than removing the individual from the source of exposure. Methods of prevention are discussed at the conclusion of this chapter.

Asbestosis

"Asbestos" is the Greek word for unquenchable. The name is derived from the fact that this group of fibrous minerals is noncombustible. Because of its fireproof qualities, asbestos has thousands of uses, among them building insulation, fireproof textiles, automobile brake linings, floor coverings and ironing board coverings. NIOSH has estimated that up to 500,000 workers may be exposed to the manufacture and handling of asbestos products.

Exposure to asbestos is associated with three lesions—asbestosis, lung cancer and mesothelioma. Asbestosis results from prolonged exposure to asbestos fibers. The elongated shape of asbestos fibers allows them to be deposited deeply into the respiratory tract, primarily by interception. Over many years, massive pulmonary fibrosis and pleural thickening occur. Clinically, progressive dyspnea and cough are usually present. The cough is often dry or productive of a small amount of sputum. Iron-coated asbestos fibers called *ferrugenous bodies* are often found in the sputum. Ferrugenous bodies are dumb-bell shaped and approximately 20–100 μ long.

Pulmonary function tests of people with asbestosis reveal both a restrictive lesion and a diffusion defect. Cor pulmonale is a common end-stage complication of the disease. The radiologic appearance includes diffuse interstitial fibrosis of the lower lobes, pleural thickening and blunting of the costophrenic angles. As with the other pneumoconioses, there is no specific treatment for asbestosis.

Exposure to asbestos may result in neoplasm. Both bronchogenic carcinoma and mesotheliomas of the pleura and peritoneum have been linked to asbestos. The exposure typically occurs 20 years prior to development of bronchogenic carcinoma, and approximately 30–40 years before the appearance of mesothelioma. A possible synergistic effect of asbestos and cigarette smoking has been reported to contribute to the incidence of bronchogenic carcinoma among insulation workers.

Talc

Talc is a hydrated magnesium silicate whose chemical formula is $Mg_3Si_4O_{10}(Oh)_2$. It is used in the manufacture of rubber and is commonly found in cosmetics such as dusting powder. Talc, like silica and asbestos, causes interstitial fibrosis and pleural thickening. The clinical picture of progressive dyspnea and cough has been previously described.

Coal Mine Worker's Pneumoconiosis: Black Lung

The severity of this disease varies primarily with the type of coal mined and its silica content. Anthracite or hard coal is associated with a higher incidence of black lung than is bituminous or soft coal. Workers may also be exposed to varying degrees of coal dust (graphite) depending on their individual task and physical location in the mine. Workers at the coal face, where the actual cutting operation occurs, are at the greatest risk of exposure.

Coal mine worker's pneumoconiosis gets the nickname black lung from black pigmented dust particles, called *macules,* which collect in the lungs. The dust macules, 2–5 mm in diameter, are located predominantly in the upper lobes but may be distributed throughout the lungs.

Nodular lesions containing carbon dust, macrophages, and collagen fibers develop along respiratory bronchioles. These nodules result in dilation of the bronchioles and centrilobular emphysema. Massive lesions called progressive massive fibrosis (PMF) and cavitation are also associated with coal mine worker's pneumoconiosis. Rheumatoid coal pneumoconiosis (Caplan's syndrome) is a modified form of the disease associated with rheumatoid arthritis.

As in the case of the other pneumoconioses, the simple or uncomplicated form is uncommon. Coal mine worker's pneumoconiosis is often associated with chronic bronchitis and infections. This obstructive lesion is associated with progressive symptoms of cough, sputum production, dyspnea on exertion and disability. Radiologic findings of nodules may or may not be present. Decreased breath sounds related to emphysema and expiratory wheezes related to superimposed chronic bronchitis may be heard on auscultation. Pulmonary function tests may reveal decreased FEV_1 and maximum expiratory flow rates with normal vital capacity.

While there is no cure for coal mine worker's pneumoconiosis, the complications of chronic bronchitis and cor pulmonale (in the case of PMF) must be treated.

Beryllium Disease

Workers may be exposed to beryllium fumes and dusts in welding, aircraft manufacture and rocket fuel production. Beryllium may cause a contact dermatitis in addition to respiratory lesions. The respiratory manifestations of beryllium disease occur in both acute and chronic forms.

The acute form occurs after an intensive exposure of several days duration or following limited exposures over a one-year period. This form of the disease is characterized by an acute pneumonitis with intra-alveolar edema. Scattered moist rales may be heard on auscultation. The patient usually has a nonproductive cough in addition to dyspnea, cyanosis and tachycardia. Although acute beryllium disease may be fatal, most patients recover within six months.

Chronic beryllium disease is characterized by interstitial fibrosis with the formation of granulomas which resembles idiopathic sarcoidosis. Progressive dyspnea, weakness and a nonproductive cough are common symptoms. Complications include cor pulmonale and spontaneous pneumothorax.

Siderosis, Stannosis, and Baritosis

Workers in welding, iron ore mining and smelting industries are exposed to dusts containing iron oxide, tin oxide and barium sulfate. These metals may be retained as dust deposits in the lungs, and the conditions are known as siderosis (iron), stannosis (tin) and baritosis (barium). Due to the absence of fibrosis formation, the exposed workers are usually asymptomatic.

Reactions to Organic Dusts

Occupational lung diseases are not restricted to miners, welders and construction workers. Workers exposed to organic material such as fungal spores and plant fibers may develop serious pulmonary reactions. This type of reaction, known as *extrinsic allergic alveolitis*, is defined by Parkes as: ". . . a disorder related to the inhalation of organic material and characterized by the presence of specific precipitating antibodies (precipitins), and by lymphocytic infiltration and sarcoid-like granulomas in the walls of alveoli and small airways." These reactions, also known as *allergic interstitial pneumonias*, are caused by a variety of agents summarized in Table 5–1.

The pulmonary manifestations of these diseases are caused not by hay, maple trees or sugar cane, but rather by the molds and fungi which grow on bales and logs that have been stored unprotected from moisture.

The diagnosis of pneumoconiosis of an organic origin is made by occupational history and clinical manifestations, which commonly include abrupt onset of dyspnea, fever, chills and a nonproductive cough. Both restrictive and diffusion defects may be found on pulmonary function tests. Symptoms may be reversed by removing the worker from the exposure by a change of jobs, by modifying the materials handling process or by using protective clothing and masks. Re-

TABLE 5–1.
Agents That Cause Allergic Interstitial Pneumonitis*

FORM OF HYPERSENSITIVITY	AGENT
Farmer's lung	*Micropolyspora faeni*
Moldy hay disease	*M. faeni* and *Aspergillus fumigatus*
Bagassosis	*Thermoactinomyces vulgaris*
Mushroom worker's disease	*M. faeni* and *T. vulgaris*
Suberosis (oak bark)	*M. faeni* and *T. vulgaris*
Malt worker's lung	*A. fumigatus* and *A. clavatus*
Maple-bark stripper's lung	*Cryptostroma corticale*
Sequoiosis	*Graphium* and *Auerobasidium*
Cheese worker's lung	*Penicillium*
Insect antigen's lung (wheat weevil)	*Sitophilus ghonvirus*
Pituitary-snuff-taker's lung	Pituitary snuff
Pigeon breeder's disease	Pigeons and budgerigars (avian antigen)
Enzyme lung	*Bacillus subtilis*
Sisal worker's disease	Unknown
Coffee worker's disease	Unknown
Wood-dust pneumonitis	Oak and mahogany dust
Humidifiers and air conditioner pneumonitis	Thermophilic actinomycetes
Byssinosis	Cotton fibers, flax and hemp dust

*Adapted from Harrison T: *Principles of Internal Medicine,* ed 7. New York, McGraw-Hill Book Co, 1974.

peated exposure to these organic dusts may result in nonreversible interstitial fibrosis.

Reaction to Fumes and Gases

Ramizzini never treated a patient with polymer fume fever. Surely, he never heard the work *plastic.* In our highly industrialized society, we use products manufactured from man-made compounds such as Teflon pots and pans containing polyfluorines and packaging materials made of polyvinylchlorides. When these polymers are heated at high temperatures, they release fumes that cause symptoms including high fever, chills, malaise, dry cough and headache. This syndrome is known as *polymer fume fever.* Workers in the meat packing industry who use heating elements to seal meat in plastic wrappers are exposed to these fumes, as well as those workers involved in the manufacture of plastics.

Metal workers may develop a similar syndrome known as *metal fume fever.* The most common exposures are in chrome and copper plating, zinc used in brass founding, and iron welding. With brief exposures, the symptoms above are self-limiting, typically disappearing over the weekend only to reappear on Monday afternoon. Over prolonged periods, however, chronic cough and hemoptysis may develop with impairment of diffusing capacity.

Smog, that distinctive combination of smoke and fog, results from the photochemical oxidation of car exhaust fumes containing nitrous oxides and hydrocarbons. Nitrogen dioxide (NO_2) and ozone (O_3) are toxic byproducts of this reaction. Ozone is also produced in the welding process when oxygen is ionized.

Both NO_2 and O_3 are toxic to the respiratory tract. Ozone is especially irritating due to its strong oxidizing properties. In the lungs, ozone damages ciliated endothelial cells lining bronchioles and impairs the mucociliary clearance mechanism. Bronchospasm may also occur in the susceptible individuals, including the very young and old, those with preexisting lung disease and heavy smokers.

Carbon monoxide (CO), another common air pollutant, combines 200 times more quickly with hemoglobin than does oxygen. When carbon monoxide is bound to hemoglobin, its oxygen-carrying capacity is decreased. Carbon monoxide also shifts the oxyhemoglobin dissociation curve to the left so that oxygen is not normally released by blood, resulting in tissue hypoxia. Victims of carbon monoxide poisoning have a characteristic "cherry red" cyanosis due to the bright red color of carboxyhemoglobin.

The Environmental Protection Agency (EPA) has sponsored legislation designed to clean up the air. Unfortunately, air pollution will continue to be a major health problem in this country as long as it is cheaper for industry to pay fines for releasing waste products into the ambient air than to develop safer means of disposal; and as long as car owners disconnect catalytic converters in an effort to get better mileage from their "lead-free" gasoline.

HOW TO TAKE AN OCCUPATIONAL HISTORY

Determining the etiology of any disease is an essential step in selecting an effective therapeutic treatment. In the field of occupationally related diseases, determining the etiology is especially critical for four reasons:

1. Recurrence may be prevented by removing the worker from the hazardous exposure or providing him with protective clothing.

2. Chronic disease occurrence should be prevented. In most cases, occupational lung diseases discovered in the early stages can be treated and arrested. Chronic disease, however, is usually irreversible.

3. Each worker becomes a guinea pig for others.

The following example illustrates the above points. If a foundry worker goes to his private physician complaining of a chronic productive cough, he may be stamped with a diagnosis of COPD. This patient is usually treated symptomatically with expectorants and prophylactic antibiotics. He then returns to work and continues to be exposed to the dust and fumes that caused his disease. Without knowledge of the patient's occupation, the physician would be unable to counsel the patient about further disease prevention. In addition, the patient's fellow workers would continue to be exposed to the same hazards. Some who were asymptomatic would go on to develop disease symptoms over a period of time. Others, with occasional symptoms dismissed as an allergy or the flu, could develop chronic irreversible disease. Determining the specific etiology of an occupationally related disease has implications, therefore, not only for an individual worker, but in fact for *all* those exposed to the hazard.

4. Etiology determination is also in industry's interest. Factories cannot operate efficiently with many workers absent due to illness. Eliminating occupational hazards helps to keep production levels up and insurance rates down in the long run.

The skill of taking a complete medical history will not be presented here. The nature of symptoms, their onset and duration, family history for genetic factors, and past medical history are included in the patient's general medical history. Ascertaining this type of information is generally reserved for the physician or physician's assistant. Because the organized study of occupationally related diseases is in the developing stages, the impact of occupation on workers' health is not widely taught in medical schools, nor is it usually considered by clinicians. Therefore, it is appropriate to present the technique of taking a work history to allied health professionals with direct patient contact who have an opportunity to obtain this information from the patient during the general patient evaluation.

Taking a work history is a process of asking specific questions relating to the workplace:

1. Obtain a detailed chronology of the job history, including job titles, duration of employment and the age at which the patient began each job. Age is a significant factor in disease susceptibility. Also, many occupational lung diseases have very long incubation periods. A worker exposed to asbestos, for example, may develop bronchogenic carcinoma 20 years following the exposure, asbestosis after 25–30 years and mesothelioma 40 years after the initial exposure. When a person is asked his or her occupation, he usually gives the present or most recent occupation. The disease, however, may be the result of an occupational exposure experienced many years before. Typically, workers with debilitating lung diseases have "end jobs" such as clerk or front door guard. These sedentary jobs given as the present occupation have little or no relation to their 20-year stint in a steel mill or foundry which they were forced to leave 10 years ago due to shortness of breath.

2. Determine the exact nature of the job, not just its title. Ask questions such as:

What actual procedures did you do at work?

What materials did you work with? (These often have common trade names.)

Where exactly were you located in the factory or mine? (A coal worker at the cutting face has a much greater exposure to dust than one who drives a lift truck for the company, yet they may both be called miners.)

What machines did you work with?

3. Determine the general sanitary conditions in the workplace by asking such questions as:

How often did you have to wash your hands or change clothes because they were dusty?

What were the ventilation conditions like? Did the air always look or smell dirty? Were there any exhaust hoods to remove dust or fumes, or did fans merely blow it around?

How often did floors have to be swept due to accumulation of dust?

Did workers eat in the same area where they worked, or were separate facilities provided?

Did workers take their contaminated clothing home with them?

Did other workers cough or complain about working conditions, and were others often absent due to illness?

4. Consider the concept of total body burden of a toxic substance. This is the overall effect on the body of:

(*a*) Multiple sources of a single material: a worker who uses a degreasing solvent in an aerosol can to clean a machine at work may also use aerosol-propelled spray paint in his hobby and a spray deodorant.

(*b*) Multiple materials affecting a single target organ: a worker's lungs may be exposed to dust on the job, frequent air pollution in the city, and two packs of cigarettes per day.

(*c*) A single material may affect multiple target organs: Asbestos causes disease of both the lungs and the diaphragm.

5. Synergistic effects must also be considered. This refers to a greater than additive effect of two or more factors.

(*a*) Multiple exposures: People commonly have several jobs during their lives. A migrant farm worker who is exposed to the fungus, thermophilic actinomyces, which produces farmer's lung, may travel to a city where he can get a higher paying job as a steel mill worker. Foundry work involves exposure to silica in the molding process.

(*b*) There is no centralized pharmaceutical data bank for prescription drugs issued to people. Many drugs containing bronchodilators can be bought across the counter. This means that an individual can obtain a variety of medications whose *collective* administration can have harmful side effects although they are safe when taken individually.

(*c*) Cardiopulmonary disease: The heart and lungs are so closely related in their function of maintaining tissue oxygenation that impairments in either organ are reflected in the other. An individual with coronary artery disease who works in a brewery would be at great risk of suffering a myocardial infarction due to his occupational exposures of higher than average levels of CO_2 in the ambient air, heat in the rooms and heavy lifting tasks.

(*d*) Genetic factors: Alpha$_1$-antitrypsin deficiency, a disease carried by an autosomal recessive gene, is associated with emphysema and chronic bronchitis. If an individual with this genetic predisposition to emphysema works as a concrete mixer and is exposed to sand with high silica content, his lungs' reserve capacity may be completely destroyed.

(*e*) Habits: This category includes diet, consumption of alcohol, hobbies, and, most important, *smoking*. There have been numerous studies illustrating the relationship between cigarette smoking, chronic bronchitis, emphysema, and lung cancer. The prevalance of these diseases used to be much higher among men than women. Increasingly, women have adopted men's most dangerous habit:

smoking. It is not surprising, therefore, that the prevalence of these lung diseases, especially bronchogenic carcinoma, is on the rise among women and is rapidly approaching rates among men. Cigarette smoking combined with occupational exposures appears to have a synergistic effect on the lungs.

PREVENTION

As stated previously, there is no specific cure for any of the pneumoconioses. Workers who have acquired any of these diseases must be treated symptomatically. Postural drainage, chest percussion and vibration, and deep breathing exercises are appropriate for maintaining bronchial hygiene in those patients with retained secretions. A comprehensive program of pulmonary rehabilitation is vital to improve not only the debilitated worker's cardiopulmonary exercise tolerance, but also to improve his quality of life.

Unfortunately, most people with occupational lung disease are asymptomatic until the disease is in an advanced state. The key, therefore, to reducing the incidence of new cases and consequently the prevalence of this category of disease, is prevention, which can be achieved by:

1. Prejob screening: In some workplaces, hospitals for example, preemployment physical examinations are required of all prospective workers. Information obtained from the history and physical, in addition to laboratory data, can be used to identify workers with preexisting lung disease and those at high risk of developing lung disease, such as those with extensive smoking histories. These individuals can then be placed in areas where their exposure to dusts and fumes is low. On an industrywide basis, basic prejob screening can be done by specially trained allied health personnel under a physician's supervision.

2. Yearly physical examinations: Health screening as discussed above should be repeated at regular intervals to identify individuals who have early evidence of lung (or other) disease. Pulmonary function tests including spirometry, maximum midexpiratory flow (MMEF) and closing volumes are believed to have high predictive value for early evidence of lung pathology. When such evidence is detected, workers should receive job counseling and assistance in securing another position which will remove them from the hazardous exposure. Statistical information obtained from screening programs should be used in epi-

demiologic studies to identify health hazards so that they can be eliminated from the workplace, rather than exposing other workers to the same risk.

3. Masks and protective clothing: Mining and industrial engineers must strive to design manufacturing processes that keep human exposure to dusts and fumes at a minimum. Masks and protective clothing can also be useful in reducing the volume of inhaled particles and chemicals. Unfortunately, many face masks are left in lockers because workers find them hot and uncomfortable to wear.

4. Ventilation: Maintaining proper ventilation in the workplace is an essential component. Particles and fumes should be removed by filtration and not merely blown about by fans or routed out into the ambient air, exposing the surrounding community to pollution.

5. Strict adherence to threshold limit values (TLV): In order to establish national standards for industry, the American Conference of Governmental Industrial Hygienists has published a list of TLVs: "Threshold limit values refer to airborne concentrations of substances and represent conditions under which it is believed that nearly all workers may be repeatedly exposed day after day *without* adverse effect." Due to the wide variation of biologic adaptability, as well as preexisting disease, some individuals may be affected by levels of substances that are below the TLV. Therefore, these values should be ". . . used as guides in the control of health hazards and should not be used as fine lines between safe and dangerous concentrations."

At the time of this writing, programs for industrywide inspections under OSHA have been inadequately funded. Adherence to TLV standards is consequently at the discretion of the individual employer.

REFERENCES

Periodicals

Epler GR, Saber FA, Gaensler EA: Determination of severe impairment (disability) in interstitial lung disease. *Am Rev Respir Dis* 1980; 121(4):647–659.

Howard J, Mohsenifar Z, Brown HV, et al: Role of exercise testing in assessing functional respiratory impairment due to asbestos exposure. *J Occup Med* 1982; 24(9):685–689.

Kelley MA, Daniele RP: Exercise testing in interstitial lung disease. *Clin Chest Med* 1984; 5(1):145–156.

Pearle J: Exercise performance and functional improvement in asbestos-exposed workers. *Chest* 1981; 80(6):701–705.

Rogan J, et al: Role of dust in the working environment in the development of chronic bronchitis in British coal miners, *Br J Ind Med* 1973; 30:217.

Scano G, Garcia-Herreros P, Stendardi D, et al: Cardiopulmonary adaptation to exercise in coal miners. *Arch Environ Health* 1980; 35(6):360–366.

Selikoff I, Chung J, Hammon E: Asbestos exposure and neoplasia. *JAMA* 1964; 188:22.

Selikoff I, Hammond E, Chung J: Asbestos exposure, smoking and neoplasm. *JAMA* 1968; 204:106.

Walker D, Archibald R, Attfield M: Bronchitis in men employed in the coke industry. *Br J Ind Med* 1971; 28:58.

Weidermann HP, Gee JB, Balmes JR, et al: Exercise testing in occupational lung disease. *Clin Chest Med* 1984; 5(1):157–171.

Books

Clague E: *The Health-Impaired Mines Under Black Lung Legislation.* New York, Praeger Publishers, 1973.

Harrison T: *Principles of Internal Medicine,* vols. 1 and 2, ed 7. New York, McGraw-Hill Book Co, 1974.

Mayers M: *Occupational Health: Hazards of the Work Environment.* Baltimore, Williams & Wilkins Co, 1969.

McAteer J: *Coal Mine Health and Safety: The Case of West Virginia.* New York, Praeger Publishers, 1973.

Morgan W, Seaton A: *Occupational Lung Diseases.* Philadelphia, WB Saunders Co, 1975.

Parkes R: *Occupational Lung Disorders.* London, Butterworths, 1974.

Ramizzini B: *De Morbis Artificum Diatriba; Diseases of Workers* (1713; original volume: Chicago: University of Chicago Press, 1940). Translated from the Latin text by Wilmer Cave Wright. New York, Hafner Publishing Company, 1964.

Slonim N, et al: *Respiratory Physiology,* ed 2. St Louis, CV Mosby Co, 1971.

Miscellaneous

Agnes F, Marcus M, Lorin E: Enemies in the dust: Occupational respiratory diseases. Reprinted from the bulletin of the American Lung Association, September 1974.

Definitions and classifications of noninfectious reactions of the lung, a statement of the Committee on Diagnostic Standards in Respiratory Diseases, American Thoracic Society, Am. Rev. Respir. Dis. 93, no. 6, pp. 1–16, 1966.

Lectures presented at the University of Illinois School of Public Health, Chicago, Illinois: Principles of Occupational Health and Environmental Medicine (course title) by Bertrand Carnow, M.D., 1976.

Lloyd Davis J: *Respiratory Diseases in Foundrymen: Report of a Survey.* London, Department of Employment, 1971.

Papers and proceedings of the National Conference on Medicine and the Federal Coal Mine Health and Safety Act of 1969, Public Law 91–173, June 15–18, 1970, Washington, D.C.

Royal College of Physicians Report: Air Pollution and Health, London, 1970.

The Health Consequences of Smoking: A Report of the Surgeon General, 1972. U.S. Department of HEW, Publication #72–7516.

TLVs: Threshold Limit Values for Chemical Substances and Physical Agents in the Workroom Environment with Intended Changes for 1975, © 1975 by the American Conference of Governmental Industrial Hygienists.

United States Public Health Service Publications, No. 1076: Silicosis in the metal mining industry: A re-evaluation 1958–1961 (Washington D.C.: U.S. Government Printing Office, 1963).

PART TWO

Clinical Techniques and Application of Chest Physical Therapy

6

Chest Assessment

Lyn Hobson, P.T., R.R.T.

Willy E. Hammon, P.T.

The information in this chapter will be approached from a slightly different perspective than in most texts. Chest assessment will be presented from the perspective of the clinician evaluating patients with chronic pulmonary problems as well as the acutely ill hospitalized adult. Numerous references are made to abnormalities and conditions actually encountered during chest evaluations by the authors and their significance. In this way, the majority of our readers can make a more direct application of this information to their own setting.

Chest assessment enables the therapist to determine valuable information for several reasons:

1. It provides a means for the therapist to compare the day-to-day change in the patient's pulmonary status.

2. Abnormalities can be identified in specific lobes of the lung to which the therapist can direct treatment efforts.

3. A basis is established from which to gauge the patient's tolerance to treatment.

4. It provides a pretreatment standard to compare the posttreatment assessment with, in order to determine the effectiveness of the chest physical therapy performed.

147

5. The assessment may reveal a new or previously undiscovered pulmonary complication. If this occurs, the therapist can notify the physicians and facilitate the delivery of appropriate care.

ANATOMIC CONSIDERATIONS

It is useful to have in mind the surface anatomy of the lobes of the lungs in relationship to the chest wall. Common lines of reference are the midclavicular line (a perpendicular line descending from the center of the clavicle), the anterior axillary line (a vertical line descending from the anterior axillary fold), the midaxillary line (a similar line descending from the center of the axilla), and the posterior axillary line (descending from the posterior axillary fold). Posteriorly, additional lines of reference include the scapular line (a vertical line passing through the inferior angle of each scapula) and the vertebral line passing over the spinous processes of the vertebral column).

Although anatomists divide the lungs into upper, middle, and lower lobes, from the actual surface anatomy it would be more descriptive to refer to them as anterior and posterior lobes. The left lung has only two lobes—the upper and lower. These lobes are divided by the horizontal fissure, located posteriorly at the level of the fourth rib, laterally at the fifth rib, and anteriorly at the six rib. The lower margin of the lung is located at approximately the tenth rib posteriorly and tracts superiorly and anteriorly to the sixth rib at the sternum.

The right lung is divided into three lobes—the upper, middle, and lower. Posteriorly, the upper and lower lobes (unlike the left lung) are divided by the major fissure at the level of the fourth rib. However, at the midaxillary line, the lower margin of the upper lobe becomes horizontal and continues anteriorly to the sternum at approximately the fourth rib. The lower margin descends slightly as it progresses anteriorly from the same point in the midaxillary line, terminating at the level of the sixth rib, approximately 5 cm lateral to sternum.

CHART ASSESSMENT

Therapists should peruse the patient's chart (Fig 6–1) to determine the nature of the pulmonary problem. Before reading the history of the patient, look at the admission data on your patient. How old is he? Does he work? Where? Is he married? Is this a planned admission or an emergency admission? Then read the chart. The following ques-

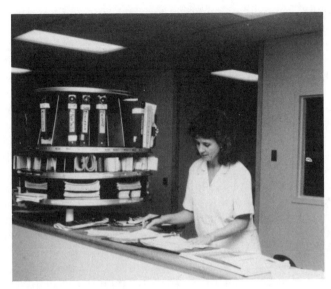

FIG 6–1.
A thorough chart review is an essential part of patient evaluation.

tions should be answered. Is he being admitted for a primary pulmonary problem? What is his admission diagnosis? Does it indicate to you what his pulmonary problem might be? What past pulmonary problems has the patient had? What is his past medical history? (This should help you in determining the condition of the patient, and provide you with a clue to his current pulmonary problem.) Has he ever smoked? What environmental substances has he been exposed to? Do they cause pulmonary problems? Does he have a current pulmonary problem? Is it chronic or acute? If chronic, is it obstructive or restrictive? Does the patient have a musculoskeletal or neuromuscular problem that predisposes him to pulmonary problems? These could include muscular dystrophy, scoliosis, ALS, Guillain-Barré, and so on. Does the patient have an immunity deficit that predisposes him to pulmonary disease? These would include AIDS, leukemia, and other cancers.

Read the admitting physician's notes on the patient's respiratory and cardiovascular status. Does the patient have adventitious sounds? Are there other problems that would cause you to modify your treatment? Heart or renal problems? A hiatal hernia? A tendency to bleed? Flail chest or rib fractures? Rib metastases? A tendency to aspirate?

There is also data that must be collected before treating the patient. What is the platelet count? If the count is extremely low, i.e., below 30,000, the patient could hemorrhage during treatment. Be cautious! If the patient's platelets are fluctuating wildly, it may be better to modify your treatment to breathing exercises and/or vibration. What is the PT/PTT? These should fall within the normal ranges: 21–31 for PTT, 70–130 for PT. At our institution, percussion is done when values fall outside the normal ranges. This is with the approval of our medical director and the Department of Hematology. Based on a study we did in which 500 patients were treated, none of them hemorrhaged, even when PT/PTT were abnormal. Platelet count above 30,000 was significant. Please check with your own medical director and hematology department before instituting this as a policy.

What organisms are being cultured from sputum cultures? What does the pulmonary function test show? What does the admission chest x-ray show? Frequently, chronic changes on CXR are listed on the admission CXR only. At our institution, there was one incident when fractured ribs were only mentioned once. The therapist in charge of the patient should check the CXR herself and have a doctor confirm that there were indeed rib fractures. CXRs frequently reveal areas of problems that cannot be found in the chest assessment, and therefore should be checked on a regular basis.

Once all this information has been evaluated, you are ready to interview the patient. This should occur before you physically examine him. The things he tells you should provide a clue as to where to look for the problem. Find out if the problem is chronic or acute. Is the patient high-strung and anxious? Does he get short of breath as he talks to you? All of these can occur in patients who have advanced pulmonary disease, or who are extremely sick. When this happens, plan on being low keyed and patient. Do not rush the patient or you may miss valuable information.

GENERAL CONSIDERATIONS

As you approach the patient's bedside, take a moment to note his immediate surroundings. Is the oxygen therapy equipment properly attached and functioning? Are his nasal prongs or oxygen mask placed properly? Is there water bubbling in the oxygen or ventilator tubing? If so, this should be drained before continuing the physical assessment as it may distort or mask pulmonary abnormalities. Repositioning the patient for treatment may cause this water to drain into patient's airways, triggering coughing paroxysms. What kind of cough is the patient exhibiting? Is it productive or nonproductive? A dry cough that occurs acutely can be the precursor of a viral infection of the upper

and/or lower respiratory tracts. It may also indicate bronchogenic carcinoma, early stages of left heart failure, or if short and abrupt may
simply be a nervous habit. Time of occurence of cough can also be
informative; when it is worse at night upon reclining, it can indicate
bronchiectasis or sinusitis. A cough spasm that awakens the patient is
frequently seen in patients with bronchial asthma or left heart failure.
A patient who coughs during or following meals may be aspirating.

Has the patient been expectorating sputum? Is the amount, color,
and consistency of sputum normal for this patient? If it is, it indicates
a chronic pulmonary problem; if not it indicates a new problem. Scan
the bedside table for a sample of sputum, often in the emesis basin.
Take note of the color, purulence, odor, and consistency to help determine the type of ongoing pulmonary process (Fig 6–2). Is it thick and

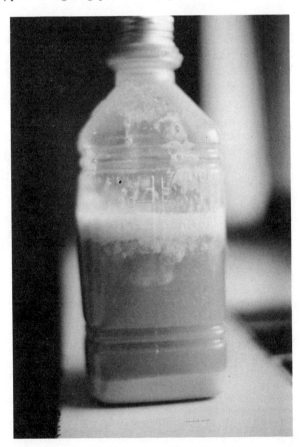

FIG 6–2.
Layering of 24-hour sputum collection in a patient with bronchiectasis.

difficult to expectorate? The patient may need increased hydration or aerosol treatment to thin the secretions so they can be more easily expectorated. Does the patient have hemoptysis? If so, the cause must be known before proceeding. Bloody sputum is common following pulmonary contusions, and generally these patients tolerate chest PT well. However, at least two fatal pulmonary hemorrhages have occurred in patients with lung cancer that were having hemoptysis. These individuals should be carefully evaluated and treated with caution. Common sputum color and characteristics are summarized in Table 6–1.

Posture

What posture does the patient assume? The leaning forward posture (stool position) (Figs 6–3, 6–4, 6–5), sitting erect with elbows extended or reclining with the head of the bed almost at 90 degrees all correlate well with increased respiratory distress as these enhance the effectiveness of the respiratory accessory muscles. Subtle indications of long-term use of the leaning forward posture are discolored skin patches above the knees (target signs). Does he prefer to recline primarily on one side? The patient usually does this to optimize his oxygenation by lying with the best functioning lung in a dependent position (sidelying). Also, this maneuver can diminish pleuritic chest pain secondary to pneumonia or pulmonary embolism.

TABLE 6–1.
Common Causes of Colored Sputum

COLOR DESCRIPTION	CAUSE
Red	Blood (hemoptysis)
Red pigmentation	*Serratia marcescens*
Red-currant jelly	*Klebsiella* pneumonia
Rusty	Lobar pneumonia
Green	Stasis
Green (sweet odor)	*Pseudomonas* infection
Brown (fecal odor)	Anaerobic infection/lung abscess
Yellow	Jaundice
Yellow (purulent)	Infection
Milky (reportedly salty)	Bronchoalveolar carcinoma
Pink frothy	Pulmonary edema
Black	Pulmonary anthrosilicosis

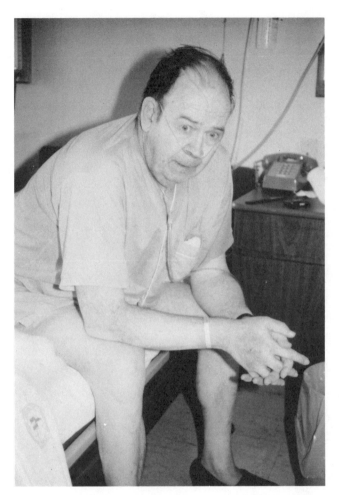

FIG 6–3.
Stool position assumed by a patient with COPD.

Patient History

Does the patient complain of dry or productive cough? Is he expectorating more or less secretions than normal for him? Are they bloody or blood-streaked? Is he short of breath at rest? Upon exertion? At night? Does he have chest pain? Where? When? These are the problems that bring most patients with pulmonary problems to the doctor, and are the types of questions one should ask the patient with pulmonary

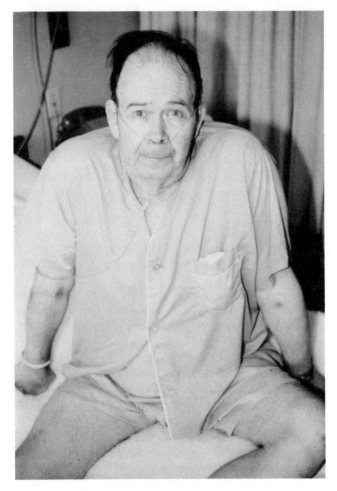

FIG 6–4.
Frog position assumed by a patient with COPD to decrease shortness of breath. Note pursed lip breathing and accessory muscle use.

symptoms. The former questions are dealt with in depth later in the chapter; the latter are covered here.

Shortness of breath (SOB) is one of the primary symptoms that sends patients to pulmonary specialists. Does the patient complain that he cannot get air "down to the bottom of the lung"? Does your patient demonstrate this problem by taking a deep breath? This type of SOB is associated with tension or anxiety and occurs in only a few patients

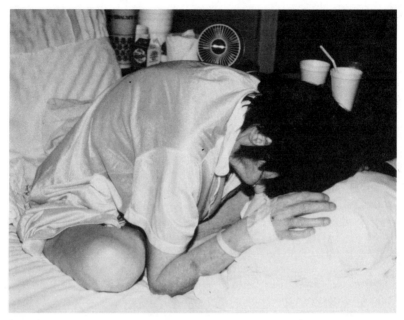

FIG 6–5.
Patient positions herself to decrease dyspnea. This position is frequently seen with cystic fibrosis patients.

who are SOB. Does your patient complain that he can't lie flat without feeling like he is "suffocating"? Does he require four or five pillows for comfort? Patients with these complaints may have mitral stenosis, left ventricular failure, advanced chronic bronchitis, or emphysema. In the latter two pulmonary diseases, these symptoms occur late in the disease. Does the patient complain of SOB, dyspnea during exertion (DOE)? After exercise? It may indicate exercise-induced asthma, bronchitis, desaturation, or some other organic disease. Do these symptoms of DOE occur in a patient with a history of a productive cough or along with another symptom such as a tightness in the chest? In the former it may indicate progression of a chronic pulmonary disorder, while in the latter it may indicate coronary insufficiency.

Does your patient complain of chest pain? Does his chest hurt during a deep inspiration? Does it "catch" at the end of inspiration and then disappear during a breath hold or exhalation? If so, it is probably a pleural pain, especially if the pain cannot be elicited by palpation. Pain that increases with pressure is usually chest wall pain, frequently muscle pain. Does the patient complain of "squeezing" or "pressing" pain through chest, shoulders, neck, jaw, or extending to the left arm or both arms? This is usually angina or an anginal equivalent pain or due to massive pulmonary embolism, acute pericarditis, or some other critical condition. Do not continue treatment in these patients. Did the pain begin during coughing? Does it increase when you apply pressure to the ribs? If so, it may be due to a fractured rib. This occurs frequently in patients who have frequent severe coughing (patients with COPD, chronic bronchitis), especially if they are on long term steroids.

Personal History

The personal habits and life-styles of patients may point the way to pulmonary problems. Does he or has he ever smoked? What? Cigarettes, cigars, marijuana? While smoking cigars rarely causes lung problems, smoking cigarettes can lead to multiple pulmonary problems including chronic bronchitis, emphysema, and bronchiogenic carcinoma as well as heart disease. Make a note of the number of packs of cigarettes smoked times the number of years the patient smoked (pack years). The greater the number of pack years, especially over 60 pack years, the greater the probability of a pulmonary problem such as those mentioned above. Smoking marijuana can cause acute pulmonary problems due to the substances that are mixed with the marijuana, i.e. pulmonary edema.

Does the patient drink excessively? Aspiration pneumonia is common among alcoholics as is pneumococcal and klebsiella pneumonia. Does the patient use nose drops frequently or put vaseline in the nares? This is a common cause of lipoid pneumonias. Does the patient abuse drugs? Heroin? Is he chronically ill with diabetes, cancer, or a blood dyscrasia? These disorders predispose patients to infection by conventional organisms such as pneumococci, staphylococci, gram-negative bacilli, tubercle bacilli as well as infection by an opportunistic organism such as *Nocardia, Candida, Aspergillus, Pneumocystis* or cytomegalovirus. Does the patient worry excessively? Is the patient obese or on a diet? These situations predispose the patient to disease. Has the patient had contact with any animals, domestic or wild? Acute pneumonic lesions are found in patients who have contracted ornithosis from sick birds or tularemia from wild rabbits. Exposure to diseased pigeons can cause interstitial pneumonitis associated with psittacosis. Is there a familial historyof pulmonary disease? Have family members had asthma, TB, cystic fibrosis, or emphysema at an early age? The latter condition occurs when there is an α_1-antitrypsin deficiency, and can cause death at an early age.

Occupational and Residential History

Where has the patient lived throughout his life? Has he lived in an industrial environment? A farming community? Emphysema and chronic bronchitis are frequently seen in patients who live in industrial areas; histoplasmosis is seen in the valleys of great rivers, and in old wood and soil; coccidioidomycosis is more frequently found in the deserts of southern California, Arizona, or New Mexico. Farmers are subject to extrinsic allergic alveolitis (farmer's lung), histoplasmosis (in chicken farmers), and silo-filler's disease.

What kind of job has the patient held? Go back to the patient's first job. Recently cases of asbestosis have been found in patients whose contact with asbestos occurred on a limited basis years ago. Did the patient ever work in a mine? Patients develop silicosis years later (see Chapter 5).

Inspection

What is the color of the patient's face, nose, lips, tongue? Is central cyanosis present? Is the patient exhaling with pursed lips? (See Fig 6–3.) Do you observe nasal flaring? Examine his fingertips for clubbing (Fig 6–6) and peripheral cyanosis. Is his face flushed or are his eyes

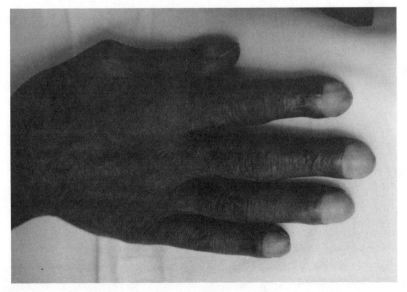

FIG 6–6.
Clubbing in a patient with lung cancer.

bloodshot? Keep in mind the signs and symptoms of hypoxemia and carbon dioxide (CO_2) retention (Tables 6–2 and 6–3).

For example, one of the authors was asked to treat a 60-year-old man with COPD. On approaching the bedside, the patient was noted to be reclining with the head of the bed at almost 90 degrees, very somnolent, and breathing with very small respiratory excursions. The man's face was red. The therapist shook his shoulder and asked if he was all right. The patient then opened his eyes (which were red and bloodshot) and tried to speak. His speech was slurred and unintelligible. Rather than doing the requested treatment, the physicians were called. An arterial blood gas showed the patient had a very high PCO_2 and was significantly acidotic. He was moved to the ICU, intubated, and mechanical ventilation was instituted.

TABLE 6–2.

Signs and Symptoms of Hypoxia

Signs	Cyanosis (central with or without peripheral)
	Sympathetic Response
	Mild hypertension
	Tachycardia
	Peripheral vasoconstriction
	Nonsympathetic Response
	Bradycardia
	Hypotension
Symptoms	Similar to alcohol intoxication
	Loss of judgment
	Paranoia
	Restlessness
	Agitation
	Dizziness
	Confusion

TABLE 6–3.

Signs and Symptoms of CO_2 Narcosis

Signs	Vasodilatation
	Redness of skin, sclera, and conjunctiva (due to increased cutaneous blood flow)
	Sympathetic Response
	Hypertension (both systolic and diastolic)
	Tachycardia
	Diaphoresis
	Metabolic encephalopathy
	Cognitive defects
Symptoms	Headache
	Mild Sedation → Somnolence → Coma

On another occasion, a 45-year-old man was two days status post second intercostal space thoracotomy for an open lung biopsy. On entering the room, the patient was observed reclining with the head of the bed flat. He was noted to have marked central cyanosis, although wearing a nasal cannula. However, on tracing the length of the oxygen tubing, it was found wedged under the head of the bed, and disconnected from the humidifier at the wall. The patient admitted to lowering the head of the bed a few minutes earlier. An arterial blood gas drawn just prior to the reattachment of oxygen showed an extremely low Po_2. The patient responded quickly to the supplemental oxygen. In both of these cases, being familiar with the signs and symptoms of hypoxia and CO_2 retention enabled the therapist to facilitate the delivery of appropriate care, other than chest physical therapy.

Observe the patient's respiratory rate. Normal for adults is 15–17 breaths per minute. An increased rate, equal to or greater than 24 per minute is highly indicative of an acute pulmonary process. Ask him "how do you feel?" Listen as he answers, as it helps determine his degree of respiratory distress. A patient with significant respiratory distress will give short, one- or two-word answers, or will pause to take a breath several times during a single sentence. Is audible congestion present? This congestion may contribute to increased work of breathing and arterial blood gas abnormalities.

Compare the anteroposterior and lateral dimensions of the chest. Is the ratio of dimensions normal (1:2 to 5:7)? An increased anteroposterior diameter (barrel chest) is strongly suggestive of COPD. However, it is important to differentiate between barrel chest and kyphosis. The distance between the bottom of the rib cage and the anterior-superior iliac crest should be at least three finger widths. If this distance is preserved in a barrel-chested individual, suspect COPD. If there is little or no distance between the bottom of the rib cage and the anterior-superior iliac crest, suspect that the problem is in the spine (i.e., osteoporosis) rather than in the chest. Another way to confirm COPD at the bedside is to ask the patient to take a deep inspiration and exhale as rapidly as possible while you observe the length of time it takes to complete this maneuver. If the forced exhalation takes longer than 3–4 seconds, it strongly suggests COPD.

Scoliosis is another type of thoracic cage deformity encountered on occasion. It is an S-shaped deformity of the entire spine with an elevation of one shoulder and pelvis. Kyphoscoliosis is a combination of kyphosis and scoliosis (Fig 6–7). Its etiology may be related to severe unilateral lung disease, old major thoracic surgeries such as thoracoplasty, various musculoskeletal conditions, or even unknown causes. Many pa-

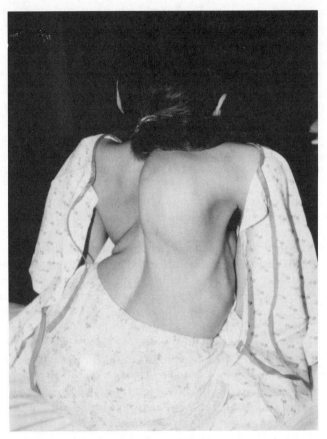

FIG 6–7.
Kyphoscoliosis in a young woman.

tients develop respiratory and cardiac failure secondary to significantly reduced lung volumes. (Table 6–4).

The pigeon breast deformity (pectus carinatum) is an abnormal protuberance of the sternum. The funnel breast (pectus excavatum) is an opposite deformity, with a depressed sternum giving the appearance of a hollow anterior chest (Fig 6–8).

What is the appearance of the skin? Are the chest vessels abnormally prominent, suggesting a superior vena cava syndrome (Fig 6–9)? Is jugular vein distension present, suggesting congestive heart failure? Carefully inspect the chest for scars, bandaids, or needle marks (secondary to thoracentesis, subclavian punctures, etc.). If these diagnostic procedures have been performed in the past few hours, make certain

TABLE 6–4.

Clinical Description of Respiratory Failure and Cough Impairment of Various Conditions*

| CONDITIONS | INCIDENCE | | |
	RESPIRATORY FAILURE	SECRETIONS ATELECTASIS, PNEUMONIA	COUGH IMPAIRMENT
Thoracic Cage			
Scoliosis	Common	Normal	None
Severe scoliosis kyphosis	Common	Increased	+ +
C-cord injury 5	Common	Increased	+ + +
Postpolio	Common	Increased	+ + +
ALS	Common	Increased	+ + +
MD	Common	Increased	+ + +
Miscellaneous			
Advanced COPD	Common	Increased	+ +
Bronchiectasis	Uncommon	Increased	+ +
Comatose	Common	Increased	+ +
Chest trauma/surgery	Common	Increased	+ +

*Key to abbreviations: ALS = amyotrophic lateral sclerosis; MD = muscular dystrophies; COPD = chronic obstructive pulmonary disease; + + = moderately severe; + + + = severe.

the postprocedure chest x-ray does not indicate a pneumothorax. One of the authors had a patient arrest during a postural drainage treatment following an undocumented thoracentesis. The patient had a small iatrogenic pneumothorax following the procedure, which the physicians elected to follow without chest tube placement (but failed to chart). The postresuscitation chest x-rays showed a significantly enlarged pneumothorax.

Analysis of Breathing Pattern

As the patient is reclining, examine the neck and anterior chest. Are the neck accessory muscles contracting with inspiration? Does the trachea descend excessively as the patient inhales?

Is the breathing pattern normal? Is inspiration active, with the abdomen rising, followed by bilateral symmetrical expansion of the lateral ribs? In thoracic trauma patients, do you observe an inward movement of some portion of the ribs with inspiration (flail chest)? Do the lower ribs move inward with inspiration (Hoover's sign) rather than outward? This is indicative of advanced COPD. Are inter

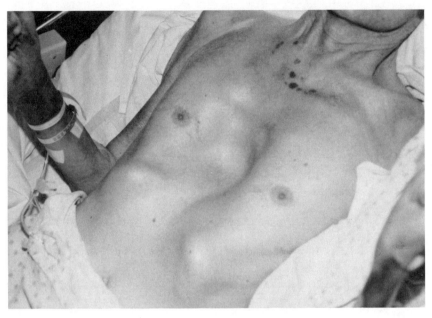

FIG 6–8.
Pectus excavatum or funnel breast is characterized by a depressed sternum; patient's
deformity limited his cough ability.

costal or sternal retractions present? Do the intercostal spaces appear
equal? Decreased unilateral intercostal spaces reflect a unilateral process. Prominent bilateral intercostal spaces suggest an increased work
of breathing.

Expiration is normally passive. Does the patient actively contract
his abdominal muscles during expiration (forced expiration)? This is
indicative of an obstructive airway disease. Does the abdomen "bounce"
following expiration? In COPD patients, this is a sign of fatiguing respiratory muscles. Two additional clinically recognizable signs of inspiratory muscle fatigue are abdominal paradox (an inward displacement
of the abdomen with inspiration) and respiratory alternans (a cyclic alteration between a series of abdominal respirations followed by a series
of respirations using primarily rib cage movements—apparently the
body is alternately tying to rest an overtaxed diaphragm and inspiratory accessory muscles). With these significant findings, the clinician
would avoid placing the patient in Trendelenburg as this would require
increased inspiratory effort (against gravity and the abdominal cavity)
from the already failing inspiratory muscles.

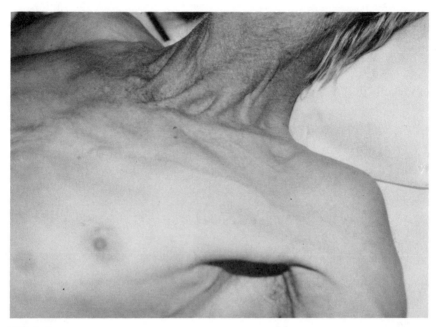

FIG 6–9.
Superior vena cava syndrome. Note blood vessel proliferation over anterior chest and jugular vein distention.

Nonrespiratory Movements of the Chest

Is there a pulsating heartbeat visible in the epigastrum, and just to the left of the epigastrum? During inspection a mediastinal shift may be suggested by observing a displacement in the position of the pulsating heart. For example, one of the authors, while assessing a 19-year-old quadriplegic in acute respiratory distress noted the position of the pulsating heart was shifted laterally into the left anterior and midaxillary lines. Auscultation, percussion, and a chest x-ray demonstrated complete left lung atelectasis with significant left mediastinal shift. A chest PT treatment was performed, with expectoration of several milliliters of sputum. The lung reexpansion was evident by restored breath sounds, resonance to percussion, a near midline position of the pulsating heartbeat, and confirmed by the posttreatment chest x-ray.

Palpation

Abnormalities of the chest identified by inspection should be palpated. These include asymmetries, abnormal contours, lumps or masses, soft tissue swelling, skin discolorations, edematous areas, needle-marks, areas adjoining margins of surgical incisions, and bandages, dilated superficial vessels, etc. Even areas that appear normal to inspection should be briefly palpated before initiating treatment. Abnormalities discovered by the authors while palpating normal appearing areas include subcutaneous air (from a pneumothorax) and unstable rib fracture that "popped" with inspiration and coughing. In both cases, the therapist's approach to the patients' treatment was significantly altered by these findings. Also by palpating the margins of a surgical dressing, intermittently open bronchocutaneous fistula was first identified by feeling the skin move abnormally with deep inspirations.

It is also useful to have the patient say "ninety-nine" while the therapist uses the ulnar or palmar surface of his hands to compare the vibration produced through the same part of the chest wall over each lung by voice (vocal fremitus) (Fig 6–10). Causes of increased vocal fremitus are pneumonia, atelectasis, lung mass, etc. Decreased vocal fremitus is usually caused by conditions that interfere with the transmission of sound through the chest wall. Common causes of decreased fremitus include pleural effusions, pleural thickening, pneumothorax, etc. Abnormalities identified by inspection and palpation should be carefully evaluated by auscultation and percussion.

Evaluate the chest for symmetrical expansion during respiration. Place your hands over the anterior chest wall, as the upper lobes are located anteriorly above the fourth and fifth ribs. The fingers should extend above the clavicles and cover the upper trapezius. Pull the underlying skin taut medially with the thumbs extended, until they are touching at the midsternal line. As the patient inhales and exhales, compare the movements of the right and left hands. In particular, note the separation of the thumb tips. Are they symmetrical? If one side has diminished movement, suspect underlying unilateral pulmonary pathology.

The right middle lobe and the lingular portion of the left upper lobe are beneath the fifth and sixth ribs anteriorly. Again, with the tips of the examiner's thumbs touching at the midsternal line at the xiphoid process, extend the fingers laterally toward the axillae. As the patient inhales and exhales, compare one side with the opposite and the motion noted previously over the upper lobes.

The lower lobes are examined with the patient seated with his back toward the therapist. These lobes underly the seventh to tenth ribs, with thoracic inspiratory expansion taking place almost entirely in a lateral direction. The therapist usually places his hands high in the axilla with the fingers touching the anterior axillary fold. Both hands are

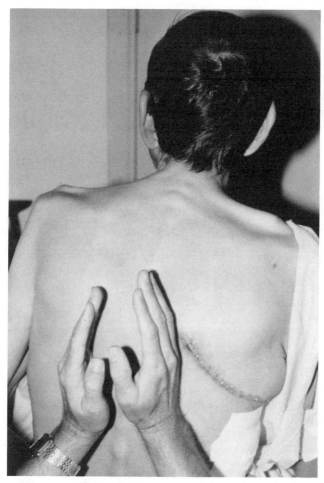

FIG 6–10.
Vocal fremitus evaluation.

approximated toward the vertebral line, pulling the underlying skin taut. The thumb tips should touch over the spinous processes of the vertebra (Fig 6–11). Then, with inspiration, the hands should move with chest expansion, separating the thumb tips.

Movement of the diaphragm should be assessed in patients with impaired inspiratory effort. The patient is placed supine and the therapist lightly rests his thumbs along the costal margins, with the tips almost touching the midsternal line at the xiphoid process. The fingers are extended upward and laterally along the lower ribs. The movement

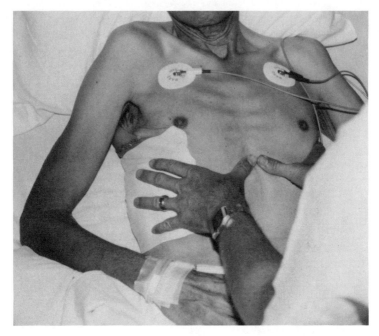

FIG 6–11.
Measuring symmetry of lower chest wall in a patient after a thoracotomy.

of the diaphragm should be easily seen and palpated in normal conditions. Lack of abdominal movement or an inward displacement of the abdomen with prominent chest expansion suggests diaphragm dysfunction or paralysis (Figs 6–12 to 6–14). This assessment can affect the treatment plans of patients as these cases illustrate.

A 26-year-old male was transferred to our hospital following a motor vehicle accident, in which he sustained a complete spinal cord injury at the level of C_5. He required mechanical ventilation for several weeks, and despite several attempts at weaning, remained ventilator dependent. Several of the physicians believed the diaphragm was paralyzed and that he would be unable to be weaned. Using the above technique, the physical therapist was able to demonstrate that the patient's diaphragm was functioning. Using inspiratory muscle exercises as part of a comprehensive respiratory care program, the patient's inspiratory muscle strength improved and he was successfully weaned in an additional two weeks.

A 24-year-old male with a progressive muscular dystrophy was transferred to our hospital because of respiratory failure. He required

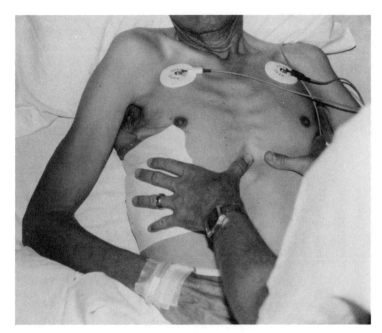

FIG 6–12.
Finishing positioning following full inspiration.

mechanical ventilation and was difficult to wean. Some professionals believed he was uncooperative and this lengthened the weaning process. However, the physical therapist assessed diaphragmatic movement and pointed out the paradoxical abdominal movement with prominent chest expansion that strongly suggested paralysis of the diaphragm. Further studies confirmed a minimally functioning diaphragm. Some improvement was made with inspiratory muscle exercises, but he required a rocking-bed for respiratory assistance before he could be discharged from the ICU.

Percussion

There are two techniques for percussion of the chest: direct percussion and mediate or indirect. Direct percussion refers to directly striking the chest wall with one finger or slapping the chest while listening to the percussion note produced. The preferred technique, mediate or indirect percussion, involves placing the middle finger of one hand (usually the nondominant hand) firmly against the chest wall while rapidly strik-

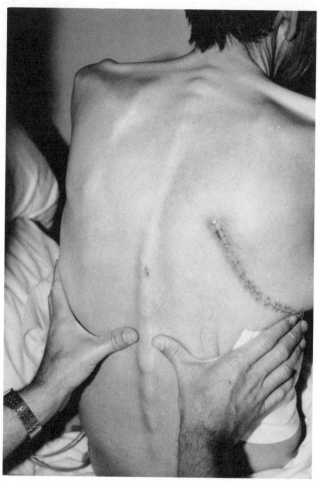

FIG 6–13.
Posterior chest wall exam.

ing it just below the nail by the tip of the middle finger of the other hand (Fig 6–15). The motion for this is entirely at the wrist joint. The sound produced is usually categorized as resonant (over normal lung tissue), hyperresonant (emphysematous lungs, or pneumothorax), tympanic (normally over the stomach bubble), dullness (lung with decreased air), and flat (absolute or extreme dullness).

   This skill is frequently unmastered by therapists, yet the authors have found it useful in the assessment and treatment of pulmonary

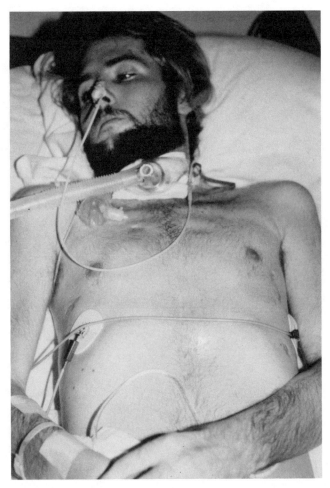

FIG 6–14.
Paradoxical abdominal descent during inspiration in a quadriplegic patient.

patients. Percussion prior to auscultation helps to identify areas of abnormalities. It is also useful to determine the patient's tolerance to percussion with the entire hand during postural drainage. Individuals that are sensitive to this evaluation technique often cannot tolerate that latter type. Dullness over one of the lower posterior and lateral hemithoraces that becomes resonant as the patient reclines on the opposite lung usually indicates a pleural effusion. The percussion note is also useful when treating patients with atelectasis. The pretreatment assessment

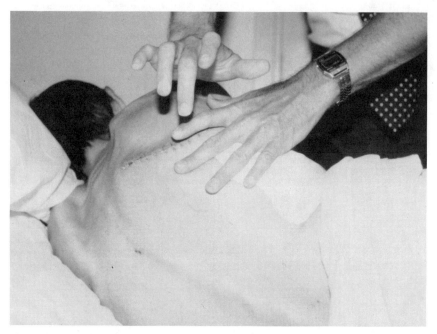

FIG 6–15.
Mediate percussion.

reveals a dull or flat note. As the underlying lung tissues are reexpanded, there is usually a sudden expulsion of mucus, and the percussion note becomes resonant.

The percussion note can be effective in differentiating a patient's cause for respiratory distress. For example, a flat percussion note in the case described under *Nonrespiratory Movements of the Chest* was crucial in ruling out a pneumothorax and allowing the therapist to proceed with vigorous postural drainage, percussion, and vibration. One other case was that of a 24-year-old male following laparotomy for an abdominal gunshot wound. This patient was reported to have atelectasis. However, on assessment there was minimal expansion of the right hemithorax, hyperresonance to percussion, and absent breath sounds. On reading the chest x-ray that was taken shortly before the therapist arrived to see the patient, an almost complete right pneumothorax was discovered. The physicians were notified and placed a chest tube that resolved the pneumothorax. These cases illustrate how mastering percussion can be invaluable to therapists doing chest physical therapy.

Auscultation—Things to Consider

Auscultation should confirm what the therapist has already determined in the chart assessment, patient interview (Fig 6–16), and physical assessment. Is the patient in a good position to accurately assess auscultated sounds? Is he leaning toward one side or the other? Is he slumping? Is he splinting due to pain? Does he have abnormal posture due to muscular, neurological, or skeletal problems? Ideally, the patient should be sitting erect, shoulders and back relaxed, arms loose at his sides. If the patient is in bed, you can raise the head of the bed and have the patient lean forward with you or with his nurse supporting him, or you can have him sit on the side of the bed. If he cannot sit, auscultate the patient as he lies on his side. Have you compared the left lung to the right lung as the patient lies first on one side, then on the other? Comparing the auscultated sounds in both positions will give you a more accurate idea of what is happening in the patient's lungs. The dependent or "down" lung should sound louder due to ventila-

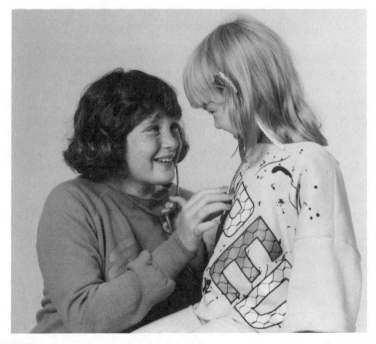

FIG 6–16.
Assessment is a time for rapport building when a relationship is established with your patient.

tion/perfusion changes. Placing the patient on his other side will clarify what is being auscultated. A patient with normal breath sounds who is placed on his right side will seem to have louder breath sounds in that lung and softer or diminished sounds in the left lung. The reverse will occur when the patient is placed on his left side. Comparing the breath sounds in both positions will help you determine more accurately what is being auscultated.

Did you auscultate the patient with the diaphragm or with the bell of the stethoscope? The diaphragm filters out low-pitched sounds (heart sounds) so that high-pitched sounds (breath sounds) are heard more clearly. It is used primarily to auscultate the lung sounds. The bell filters out high-pitched sounds making the low-pitched sounds (heart sounds) clear. It can also be used to auscultate patients who are very young or very thin. Patients with emphysema are frequently very thin, with ribs held permanently in an end-inspiration position. Breath sounds are very distant if audible at all when auscultated with the diaphragm. Using the bell, one can press it against intercostal muscles between the ribs to hear more clearly distant breath sounds. Until you are comfortable with the bell, auscultate these latter patients with both the bell and the diaphragm of your stethoscope.

Have you auscultated the patient with his clothes on or off? It is important to auscultate over bare skin. Auscultating over clothes distorts lung sounds so that they sound like adventitious sounds (Fig 6–17). An extremely hairy chest may also have this effect. Have you auscultated the chest from top to bottom comparing the left lung to the right lung? It is a matter of preference whether you auscultate the anterior or posterior chest first. When you auscultate the patient's back, have you had the patient push his shoulders as far forward as possible? This gives you a greater surface area over which to auscultate as the scapula move away from the spine as the shoulders go forward. Do not auscultate over the scapula as bone does not transmit breath sounds. Have you auscultated all surfaces of the chest comparing the left lung to the right lung? Anteriorly? Posteriorly? Laterally under the arms? When you auscultate, did the patient breathe quietly? Or did he breathe noisily? Did he vocalize? Patients frequently must be coached so that they do not vocalize with each breath. The sounds audibly heard distort what is auscultated. Have you made note of the location of the sounds auscultated? Have you noted when there are differences auscultated between the left and right lung, as well as adventitious sounds. Have you notated the location of the abnormal sounds? The location of abnormal sounds should be described by surface (anterior, posterior, or lateral lung fields) and by position on the surface (upper, mid, or lower lung fields). Although topographic charts are available to

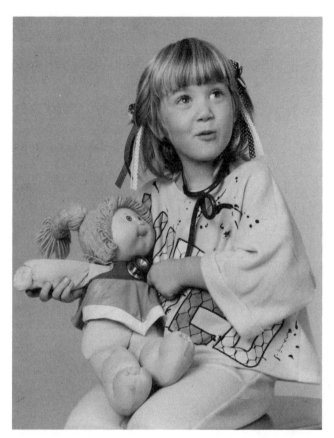

FIG 6–17.
Crackles! I heard crackles!

pinpoint the exact location on the chest of each lung segment, they are used to describe auscultated lung sounds. Topographic charts are based on positions of the lungs in cadavers. In life, the lung segments change position from breath to breath and when there is lung pathology. Describe what you hear and the location of the sound. For example: posterior lower lung fields, anterior mid-lung fields, right lateral mid-lung fields.

Normal Breath Sounds

When you auscultate the patient, what do you hear? Do you hear soft, rustling noises that sound like a gentle breeze? Are these sounds heard continuously through inspiration and early exhalation? Is the inspiratory phase louder, longer, and higher pitched than the expiratory phase? Are these sounds heard throughout all lung fields, except for the anterior upper lung fields next to the sternum? If so, you are hearing vesicular breath sounds also known as "normal" breath sounds. Are the breath sounds diminished or absent? This can occur secondary to neuromuscular disease, or weakness. It may occur when there is diminished air entry as in atelectasis or in obstruction of the bronchus from secretions, tumor, or fluid. A reduction in compliance of the lung as in pulmonary fibrosis can cause decreased breath sounds. There may be destruction of lung tissue as in emphysema. There may be air, fluid, or fat acting as a barrier between the lung and the chest. All of these conditions cause normal breath sounds or vesicular breath sounds to be diminished or absent.

Do you hear very loud, high-pitched, tubular or hollow sounds next to the sternum, especially on the right? Is the expiratory phase loud, clearly audible, and of longer duration than the inspiratory phase? Is there a short pause between the two phases? If so, these are *bronchial or tracheal breath sounds* and are normal when heard next to the sternum, between the scapula, or over the trachea. Heard elsewhere they may indicate consolidation, pneumonia, pleural effusion, tumor, or atelectasis. The bronchial sound is created when consolidated tissue surrounding patient airways allows transmission of that sound without distraction to the periphery. It is like the sound heard over the trachea. In some patients a different type of breath sound is auscultated over the large airways.

Do you hear sounds that are a combination of bronchial and vesicular breath sounds? Are the inspiratory and expiratory phases loud and roughly equal in length and intensity with no gap between the two phases? These are known as *bronchovesicular breath sounds* and can be heard over partially consolidated alveoli, fluid filled alveoli, and in early pneumonia. These sounds are normal when heard anteriorly under the clavicles next to the sternum (especially on the right), and when heard posteriorly between the scapula.

Adventitious Sounds

Do you hear abnormal sounds? Are they prolonged whistling notes or musical in character, changing pitch during the respiratory cycle? Are they high-pitched sounds that start and end at different times during inspiration, expiration, or both? These are *wheezes* and can occur when a tumor blocks an airway, in asthma, where airways are narrowed, and in patients with diffuse interstitial fibrosis such as asbestosis or fibrosing alveolitis. In the latter two diseases, the wheezes are located primarily in the lower lung fields. Wheezes may be single or multiple as in asthma.

Do you hear low-pitched, loud, coarse continous sounds heard primarily during exhalation? Do they have a bubbling or moaning quality? Do the sounds start and end together (unlike wheezes). These are rhonchi and thought to be created by air moving through fluid such as mucus or edema. These sounds are heard primarily in the congested patient who has retained secretions. They have been called *"death rattles"* when heard audibly.

Do you hear brief, explosive, interrupted sounds? Are they fine? These sounds are called *rales* or *crackles* (see Fig 6–17). Fine rales are persistent, multiple, and frequently occur in showers of clicks at the end of inspiration. They are frequently found in patients with heart failure, pulmonary edema, and pneumonia. They are heard in patients with connective tissue diseases such as lupus erythematosus and rheumatoid lung, as well as in patients with interstitial lung disease such as pulmonary fibrosis, silicosis, and asbestosis. In the interstitial fibrosing diseases, rales correlate with the pathological severity of the disease.

Are the rales coarse in nature? Coarse rales are bubbling sounds associated with secretions or fluid in the airways. These sounds are heard earlier in the inspiratory cycle than "fine" rales. Coarse rales are heard in patients with pneumonia, tuberculosis, bronchitis, bronchiectasis, and lung abscesses.

Are the rales low-pitched or high-pitched? Loud or faint? Do they occur singularly or do they sound like showers of clicks? All of these words describe rales. Two descriptive terms that were purposefully omitted are "moist" and "dry." In past years, these terms were the primary descriptive terms used to describe rales. In recent years, their use has been discouraged as the associations of the two terms implies insight into the cause of the sounds. Since one cannot determine the underlying pathology that creates the rales, describing them as moist or dry is at best subjective and as such should be avoided.

Rales can be heard in patients with normal lungs and in patients who have lung pathology. In those who do not have primary or secondary problems such as bedridden or elderly patients, rales usually disappear after the patient coughs or takes several deep breaths. In this patient population, the rales are thought to be atelectatic alveoli opening up. As soon as the alveoli are open, the rales disappear. Patients who are developing lung pathology (for instance, postoperatively) may have rales that disappear with coughing. In their case secretions have been coughed up to a larger airway where they can no longer be heard.

Rales that do not disappear after coughing indicate lung pathology (pneumonia, heart failure, interstitial lung disease, connective tissue damage).

Are the rales "posttussic"? *"Posttussic"* rales is a phrase found often in the charts of patients. It is found in patients who are candidates for developing pulmonary congestion. It is elicited by having the patient deeply inhale, exhale, and cough. As he takes his next breath, fine rales are heard in the initial phase of inspiration. These rales are not heard during normal auscultation of the patient. They appear only after a deep breath and cough. They are probably due to atelectatic bronchial walls suddenly opening with the deep breath and cough.

Do you hear a grating, creaking noise that sounds like a squeaky door or two pieces of leather rubbing together? Is it loudest at the end of inspiration? Does the patient complain of pain at the exact location? This is a *pleural rub* and it occurs when roughened parietal and visceral pleura rub together during respiration. You can create a close version of that sound by placing one hand over your ear and then rubbing the back of it with a finger of your other hand. This sound is frequently heard at the lower anterior and lateral rib cage, where chest movement is the greatest. A pleural rub indicates primary pleural disease due to trauma, neoplasm, inflammation, or an underlying pulmonary neoplasm, infarction, or pneumonia. It disappears when fluid forms and separates the two membranes.

Having the patient speak may confirm suspicion of an area of fluid or of lung consolidation. When the patient says "ninety-nine," do you hear soft, confused, barely audible sounds or do the words sound loud and distinct? In normal lungs, spoken words do not transmit well. At best they are very distant, soft, confused noises. When you have the patient whisper the words, "one, two, three," do you hear the sounds clearly? This is known as "whispering pectoriloquy." In cases where the spoken word is transmitted loudly and clearly to the periphery, you have bronchophany. It indicates lung consolidation. If the patient says "ee," does it transmit as "aa"? If so, the patient has *egophany*. It is associated with pleural effusions and heard at the upper margins of an effusion. It is heard rarely at the border of a consolidation. There are other sounds that you may hear during your professional career.

When auscultating the patient, do you find the breath sounds switching in midcycle to a totally different sound? Say from vesicular to tubular or vesicular to a wheeze. The change in sound occurs when a bronchus suddenly opens or closes as a foreign object or pedunculated tumor changes position in the airways. They are called *metamorphosing breath sounds*. Do you hear a high-pitched, metallic sound?

TABLE 6–5.
Chest Assessment Findings

CONDITION	INSPECTION	PALPATION (TACTILE FREMITUS)	PERCUSSION	BREATH SOUNDS	VOCAL SOUNDS; WHISPERED VOCAL SOUNDS	ADVENTITIOUS SOUNDS	CONDITION
					AUSCULTATION		
Normal	Symmetry in motion	Present	Resonant	Vesicular everywhere but next to sternum, bronchovesicular next to sternum	Muffled, distant, indistinct sounds	None	Normal
Heart failure	Symmetry in motion, increased respiratory rate	Present	Resonant	Vesicular	As in normal lungs	Fine rales or crackles in dependent portions of lung; occasional wheezes	Heart failure
Pleural effusion (moderate to large)	Decreased motion on affected side, tachypnea Trachea deviated away from affected side	Decreased to absent	Dull to flat	Decreased to absent breath sounds over fluid Above fluid, bronchial breath sounds	Decreased Bronchophony, egophony, whispered pectoriloquy above fluid and over lung compressed by fluid	— May have pleural rub	Pleural effusion

(Continued)

TABLE 6–5. (*Continued*)

CONDITION	INSPECTION	PALPATION (TACTILE FREMITUS)	PERCUSSION	AUSCULTATION			
				BREATH SOUNDS	VOCAL SOUNDS; WHISPERED VOCAL SOUNDS	ADVENTITIOUS SOUNDS	CONDITION
Pneumothorax (greater than 15%)	Decreased motion on affected side, tachypnea, trachea deviated to side opposite pneumothorax	Decreased to absent	Hyperresonant	Absent or decreased breath sounds	Decreased or absent	Amphoric or cavernous breath sounds	Pneumothorax
Pneumonia	Decreased motion on affected side, tachypnea	Increased	Dull	Bronchial/tubular breath sounds	Increased whispered pectoriloquy egophony	Coarse rales/ crackles, do not clear with cough, rhonchi, expiratory wheezing, may have pleural rub	Pneumonia
Airway obstruction	Chest held near full inspiration (en bloc movement), heavy use of accessory muscles, decreased to absent	Decreased	Hyperresonant	Decreased breath sounds with prolonged expiratory phase	Decreased or absent	None or rales, ronchi, wheezes	Airway obstruction

Asthma (during moderately severe attack)	motion, prolonged expiratory phase, Hoover's sign Use of accessory muscles, symmetry of motion, tachypnea	Decreased	Resonant or hyperresonant	Decreased breath sounds, bronchial breath sounds, prolonged expiratory phase	Decreased	Inspiratory and expiratory wheezes, ronchi	Asthma
Bronchitis	Decreased motion on affected side, occasional use of accessory muscles, prolonged expiratory phase	Increased ronchal fremitus	Resonant	Normal—may have prolonged expiration	Normal	Coarse rales/crackles, ronchi/wheezes change or clear with cough	Bronchitis
Bronchiectasis	Decreased motion on affected side, clubbing, tachypnea	Increased ronchal fremitus	Normal	Normal	Normal	Rales	Bronchiectasis
Fibrosis	Decreased motion throughout thorax,	Decreased to absent	Dull	Decreased breath sounds	Decreased	Fine rales/crackles, wheezes	Fibrosis

(Continued)

TABLE 6–5. (*Continued*)

CONDITION	INSPECTION	PALPATION (TACTILE FREMITUS)	PERCUSSION	AUSCULTATION			CONDITION
				BREATH SOUNDS	VOCAL SOUNDS; WHISPERED VOCAL SOUNDS	ADVENTITIOUS SOUNDS	
	symmetry of motion, tachypnea, intercostal retractions						
Consolidation, unobstructed bronchus	Decreased motion on affected side	Increased	Dull	Bronchial/ tracheal breath sounds	Bronchophony, egophany, whispering pectoriloquy, absent	Rales	Consolidation, unobstructed bronchus
Obstructed bronchus	Decreased motion on affected side	Decreased	Dull	Absent breath sounds		None	Obstructed bronchus
Atelectasis	Decreased motion on affected side, trachea deviated to affected side, tachypnea	Decreased	Dull to flat	If complete, decreased to absent breath sounds; if incomplete, bronchial or metamorphosing breath sounds	Decreased to absent	Rales	Atelectasis

Does it sound like the noise made by blowing across the mouth of an empty bottle? These are *amphoric* breath sounds and are heard over a pneumothorax or when a bronchus is in opposition to a collapsed or consolidated lobe. Does it have a low-pitched hollow reverberating quality? This is a cavernous sound and occurs over a cavity or pneumothorax. The sounds mentioned in this paragraph are rarely heard but unforgettable when they occur. Table 6–5 summarizes and correlates the patient's respiratory condition with chest assessment findings.

Conclusion

A good assessment of the patient's records, history, personal habits, and chest assessment requires time and effort. The more the therapist studies and practices these skills, the more proficient he becomes. In this chapter, we have presented the information from the perspective of the physical therapist clinician, using clinical examples from our respective practices. We urge clinicians to do daily assessments in order to better monitor changes that are occurring. This is particularly helpful in rapidly changing pulmonary processes such as developing pneumonias or consolidations. The evaluation enables the practitioner to

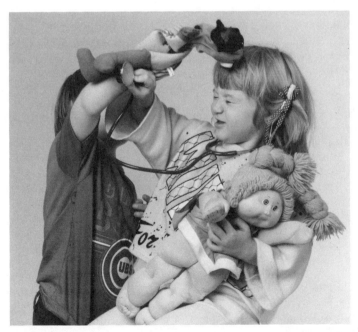

FIG 6–18.
There is not always full agreement regarding chest assessment.

find and treat the areas of the lung that are congested. There is not always full agreement regarding chest assessment (Fig 6–18). Reevaluating the patient will tell the clinician whether or not the therapy has been effective. Treatment plans can then be modified and changed as necessary. This helps to ensure the delivery of appropriate care to the patient.

REFERENCES

Barbee R: The medical history in pulmonary disease, in *Basics of Respiratory Disease,* vol 2. no 3. 1983.

Baum G, Wolinsky E: *Textbook of Pulmonary Diseases,* ed 3. Boston, Little, Brown & Co, 1983.

Burton G, Gee G, Hodgkin J: *Respiratory Care: A Guide to Clinical Practice.* Philadelphia, JB Lippincott Co, 1977.

Cugell DW: Sounds of the lungs. *Chest* 1978; 73:3.

Davies G: *Office Diagnosis and Management of Chronic Obstructive Pulmonary Disease.* Philadelphia, Lea & Febiger, 1981.

Epler C, Carrington C, Gaensler E: Crackles (rales) in the interstitial pulmonary diseases. *Chest* 1978; 73:3; 333–339.

Fishman A: *Pulmonary Diseases and Disorders.* New York, McGraw-Hill Book Co, 1980.

Flenley DC: *Respiratory Medicine.* London, Bailliere Findall-London-Cassell Ltd, 1981.

Forgacs P: Breath sounds (editorial). *Thorax* 1978; 33(6):681–683.

Forgacs P: The functional basis of pulmonary sounds. *Chest* 1978; 73:3:399–405.

Fraser R, Pare JA: *Diagnosis of Diseases of the Chest.* Philadelphia, WB Saunders Co, 1977.

Gracey DR: *Pulmonary Disease in the Adult.* Chicago, Year Book Medical Publishers, 1981.

Listening to the lungs (editorial). *Br Med J* 1978; 2(6151):1515.

Longe R, Taylor T, Calvert JC: The thorax and the lungs. *Drug Intell Clin Pharm* 1981; 15:166–174.

Loudon RG: Auscultation of the lung, in *Clinical Notes on Respiratory Diseases.* Fall pp 3–7, 1982.

Loudon RG: The lung speaks out. *Am Rev Respir Dis* 1982; 126(3):411–412.

MacDonnell K, Segal M: *Current Respiratory Care.* Boston, Little, Brown & Co, 1977.

Murphy R, Holford S: Lung sounds. *Basics of Respiratory Disease.* American Thoracic Society, 1980.

Murphy R: Auscultation of the lung: Past lessons, future possibilities. *Thorax* 1981; 36:99–107.

Ploysongsana V, Yongyudh A, Schonfeld J, et al: Mechanism of production of crackles after atelectasis during low-volume breathing. *Am Rev Respir Dis* 1982; 126:413–415.

Rifas E: How to listen in on breath sounds. *Nursing* 1984; March: 30–33.

Sackner M: *Diagnostic Techniques in Pulmonary Disease,* Part 1. New York, Marcel Dekker, Inc, 1980.

Schare B, Stehlin C: What those breath sounds are telling you to do. *Nursing* 1981; December 48–49.

Sharma O, Balchum O: *Key Facts in Pulmonary Disease,* New York, Churchill Livingstone, Inc, 1983.

Wilkins R, Levinsky N: *Medicine Essentials of Clinical Practice.* Boston, Little, Brown & Co, 1983.

7

Musculoskeletal Evaluation as Related to Breathing Exercise Programs, Posture Analysis and Correction

Els Minnigh, M.Ed., P.T.

The necessity of performing a musculoskeletal evaluation on a routine basis is often overlooked as a source of collecting valuable information. The evaluation is important not only to determine prognosis and progress in all chest physical therapy treatments, but also to assess a quality pulmonary rehabilitation program.

In short, we should be able to determine on a routine evaluation: (1) the necessity for pulmonary rehabilitation and the individualized treatment programs for hospitalized patients, (2) the areas where medical complications might occur, (3) the need for general physical fitness programs and (4) objective data for research and charting.

The musculoskeletal evaluation in chest physical therapy should be performed on a routine basis. The areas of concern are discussed below.

MOBILITY OF THE THORACIC SPINE AND RIB CAGE

The mobility of the thoracic spine and rib cage is directly related to the availability of lung space and secondary lung function (expansion).

In chest physical therapy, the emphasis is most likely concentrated on abnormal lung physiology and secondarily on the limitations of the patient. This is an unfortunate trend because temporary attempts to correct these abnormalities are readily available during hospitalization, but the long-lasting effects, in the form of reeducation, are often forgotten.

The decrease in mobility of the thoracic spine and rib cage is considered a normal process, as a part of aging. Some of the first noticeable signs of aging are found in, at, and around the joint spaces. In the past, these normal signs have been grossly ignored. However, the current literature and information to the public have been focusing on physical fitness by stressing various exercise programs and encouraging deep breathing. In reviewing these various exercise programs, it has become apparent that the majority place the emphasis on mobilization of the spine, shoulders and hip joints. In physical therapy, similar trends are noticeable. Special courses are presently offered on the various mobilization techniques of the joints to alleviate discomfort, stiffness and dysfunction. This form of mobilization, however, requires special skills and can be applied only by therapists trained in these techniques. However, *general mobilization exercises* should be an integral part of therapy for all respiratory patients.

POSTURE

Posture is considered the mirror of the soul. In our everyday life, we reflect our feelings of happiness, tiredness or malaise by our posture. In pantomine, entire stories are performed by body movements alone. Therefore, it is of no surprise that pathologic conditions are often recognized by the posture of the patient. In many instances the observations trigger the suspicion for further careful examination. For example, a patient with chronic obstructive pulmonary disease is often characterized by a kyphotic posture and a forward tilted head-neck position. A postoperative patient often projects or holds the place of incision while walking down the hall and reflects the area of his surgery by his posture.

ESTABLISHING THE NEEDS FOR BREATHING EXERCISE PROGRAMS

The concept of including breathing exercises for all patients receiving chest physical therapy is by no means new. It is a well-known and accepted fact that active range of motion exercises to the shoulders or chest expansion exercises and lateral flexion exercises stimulate deep breathing and often create a spontaneous cough reflex. In short, they enhance the mobilization of secretions.

Breathing exercise programs can be divided into two major categories—*short-term* exercise programs for all patients receiving chest physical therapy to enhance successful bronchial hygiene, and *long-term* exercise programs for the after-hospitalization period (home programs).

These programs are primarily aimed at:

1. Patients with clinical symptoms of retained secretions.

2. Postsurgical patients with thoracic or abdominal or head and neck surgeries.

3. Neurologic patients with myasthenia gravis, myotrophic lateral sclerosis, post-cerebrovascular accidents, multiple sclerosis, Parkinson's disease, debilitation, Guillain-Barré syndrome, neuromuscular weakness and spinal cord injuries.

4. Cancer patients receiving chemotherapy.

5. Chronic lung abnormalities.

Preestablished home instruction programs might be helpful to guarantee a carry-over at home.

GENERAL GUIDELINES FOR EVALUATION

Time of evaluation: First visit. Routine evaluation is done to all patients, including preoperative patients.

Purpose of evaluation: To collect data as a preventive and/or precautionary measure or to establish appropriate treatment if pathology exists. The data will establish baselines to guide the therapist in setting up therapy programs and gauging improvement and progress. For example, limited diaphragmatic breathing with limited costal expansion before surgery may indicate the potential site of atelectasis following surgery. These findings will assist the therapist in planning a program that will include laterocostal and deep breathing as a preventive measure to avoid atelectasis.

Results of evaluation are used to establish short- and long-term goals and to document areas of concern. The main goals in chest physical therapy are to increase lung function and to strive for a more normal pattern of breathing.

Areas of concern in chest physical therapy enhance the establishment of priorities. Areas of concern are:

1. Restricted chest areas as well as potential areas of restriction.

2. Habitual breathing patterns and the need for corrective exercises.

3. Habitual posture and body mechanics and the need for corrective exercises.

4. Muscle strength of the surrounding musculatures of the abdominals, thoracic spine, rib cage and shoulder girdle, and the need for active strengthening exercise programs.

5. Endurance and the need for endurance exercises, including functional activities such as stair climbing, lifting and activities of daily living (ADL).

PROCEDURES FOR EVALUATION

General

The evaluation is divided in four major categories—inspection, palpation of bony and soft tissues (Fig 7–1), active and passive range of motion (Fig 7–2) and muscle test.

Positions

The evaluation is performed in the following positions: standing, sitting and lying down, if the others are impractical.

Areas of Inspection

The inspection is best done from the following views: anterior, lateral and posterior.

Focus

The evaluation is focused on:

1. Inspection and palpation.
> Posture: general (habitual)—specific.
> Symmetry: shoulder lines—clavicles.
> Muscle contour: hypertrophy—atrophy (Fig 7–3).
> Chest contour: various shapes of the chest.

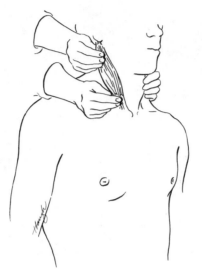

FIG 7–1.
Palpation of the sternocleidomastoid muscle.

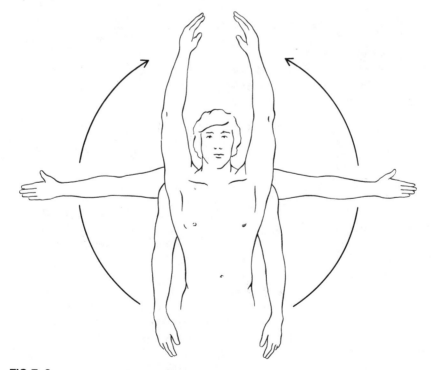

FIG 7–2.
Evaluation of active full range of motion.

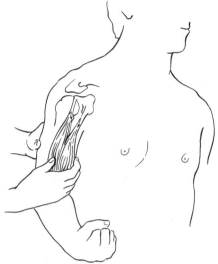

FIG 7–3.
Evaluation of muscle tone (palpation).

2. Active movement.

    Mobility of the thoracic spine, rib cage and shoulder girdle.
    Range of motion: shoulder girdle (Figs 7–4 to 7–6).
    Breathing pattern: various patterns (Fig 7–7).
    Muscle strength: regular 5-point scale (Table 7–1).

Evaluation Form
To collect objective data, it is advisable to use a standard form.

General Guidelines

1. An evaluation is only of value when all personnel in a drop chest physical therapy department follow the same basic routine.

2. A standard form should include basic normal standards to be valid.

3. A good evaluator needs experience.

THE MOST COMMONLY OCCURRING PATHOLOGIC FINDINGS

This listing is compiled to assist the evaluator in developing a routine evaluation technique.

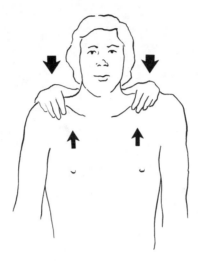

FIG 7–4.
Check shoulders for the patient's level of relaxation, muscle strength of the trapezius, mobility, and posture evaluation.

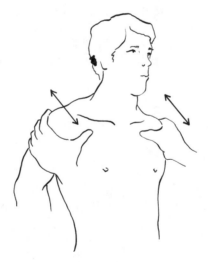

FIG 7–5.
Check shoulders for mobility and potential chest expansion.

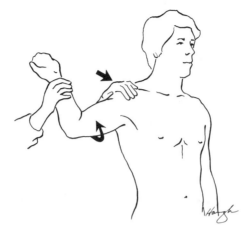

FIG 7–6.
Evaluation of internal and external rotation of the shoulder.

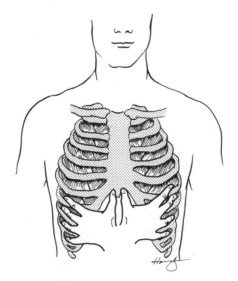

FIG 7–7.
Palpation of the intercostal spaces for evaluation of laterocostal and diaphragmatic excursion.

TABLE 7–1.

Muscle Grading Chart

MUSCLE GRADATIONS	DESCRIPTION
5–Normal	Complete range of motion against gravity with full resistance
4–Good	Complete range of motion against gravity with some resistance
3–Fair	Complete range of motion against gravity
2–Poor	Complete range of motion with gravity eliminated
1–Trace	Evidence of slight contractility with no joint motion
0–Zero	No evidence of contractility

Observation (Inspection)

While the patient is telling his version of his disease, his *posture, movements, breathing patterns, speech patterns,* and *areas of tension* or *lack of movement* should be observed.

Palpation

Palpation always follows the general observation. Palpation is performed with the fingertips. Only the established areas that require further information should be palpated. Information such as *muscle tension, muscle tone* (hypertrophy or atrophy), and movement of the diaphragm and ribs should be noted (see Fig 7–3).

Pathologic Findings

Pathologic findings can be observed in various aspects of body alignment. Once abnormalities are observed, corrective exercise programs are developed. Some program suggestions are made as guidelines for therapists.

ABNORMALITIES IN THE SPINE

Thoracic kyphosis.   Patient appears to have a round back, with his arms hanging loosely from his body, in front of his hips. This disorder is most noticeable in the lateral and posterior views. The patient exhibits difficulty in chest expansion and pulling the shoulder blades together.

Recommendations: (1) deep breathing exercises, (2) relaxation exercises (also instruct the patient to stand and sit up tall), (3) chest expansion exercises, (4) active (range of motion) exercises to the shoulders and (5) extension exercises for the thoracic spine.

Cervical lordosis. The patient appears to have his head shifted forward and the neck curved forward. This disorder is most noticeable in the lateral and posterior views. The patient experiences difficulty in bringing his chin to his chest and looking over his shoulders. Often it is a result of the excessive use of the accessory muscles. Most likely the patient will have a high, superficial breathing pattern.

Recommendations: (1) deep breathing exercises, (2) relaxation exercises of shoulder and neck muscles, (3) posture correction exercises (use of a mirror might be helpful), and (4) extension exercises of the spine.

Scoliosis (Fig 7–8). Lateral curvature of the spine. The patient appears to have one shoulder higher than the other. The scapula on the side of the curvature may be winging. Severe conditions are often corrected by a Milwaukee brace (spinal orthosis) and/or surgery. The disorder is most noticeable in the posterior view. The patient has difficulty standing erect with his shoulders at an even level.

Recommendations: (1) special scoliosis exercise programs provided by physical therapists—these exercise programs place emphasis on postural correction and deep breathing especially for patients in a brace

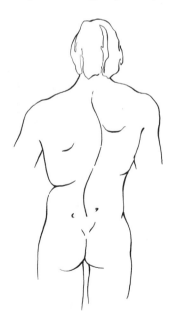

FIG 7–8.
Scoliosis posture.

and/or following surgery, (2) chest expansion exercises, (3) extension exercises for the spine and (4) active range of motion exercises to shoulders.

Kyphoscoliosis.   The patient appears to have a lateral scoliosis and a kyphosis in the thoracic area. This disorder is most noticeable in the lateral and posterior views. The patient exhibits difficulty in chest expansion and pulling the shoulder blades together.

Recommendations are the same as for scoliosis and kyphosis.

Lumbar lordosis (Fig 7–9).   The patient appears to have a hollow, low back, often with a protruding abdomen. This is most often found in combination with thoracic kyphosis. The disorder is most noticeable in the lateral and posterior views. The patient experiences difficulty in flexion (bending over). His cough is most likely weak or superficial.

Recommendations: (1) strengthening of abdominal muscles, (2) extension exercises of the spine and (3) deep breathing exercises.

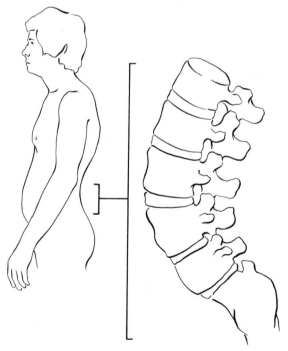

FIG 7–9.
Posture of kypholordosis.

Rigid spine. In this disorder, the entire spine is rigid. The patient has difficulty in bending over, including lateral bending.

The disorder is most noticeable in lateral and posterior views during active movement. The patient experiences difficulty in fully expanding the chest.

Recommendations: (1) mobilization exercises of the spine and (2) deep breathing exercises.

CHEST DEFORMITIES

Barrel chest The sternum is seen to protrude and has a larger circumference in the upper part of the chest than in the lower part. It is not uncommon to also find a cervicothoracic kyphosis of the spine. The disorder is most noticeable in the anterior and lateral views. The patient experiences diffculty in standing erect and breathing deeply. A high superficial breathing pattern is most commonly present. This is often seen in patients with chronic obstruction pulmonary disease.

Recommendations: (1) extension exercises of thoracic and cervical spine, (2) chest mobilization exercises and (3) deep breathing exercises with emphasis on diaphragmatic movement rather than on upper chest movement.

Pectus excavatum.   In this disorder, the sternum is in a "caved-in" position. The lower ribs are winging and the intercostal spaces are often narrowed. The patient primarily uses diaphragmatic breathing and the abdomen protrudes. This disorder is most noticeable in the anterior and lateral views. The patient experiences difficulty in standing up erect and fully expanding the chest. Lateral costal expansion is diminished.

Recommendations: (1) extension exercises of the thoracic spine, (2) active range of motion exercises to the shoulders, (3) chest expansion exercises, (4) segmental breathing exercises and (5) active exercises to abdominal musculature.

Flat chest.   The rib cage appears flat in anterior and posterior views. The intercostal spaces are often narrowed. The thoracic spine appears rigid in active movements. The disorder is most noticeable in anterior and lateral views. The patient experiences difficulty in segmental and deep breathing. He has a tendency toward superficial breathing.

Recommendations: mobilization exercises of the thoracic spine, active range of motion exercises to shoulders, segmental breathing exercises, deep breathing exercises and endurance exercises.

Muscle contour. The muscles that are most commonly visible in patients with a chronic pulmonary disorder are the accessory muscles. These include the sternocleidomastoids, scalenes and upper part of the trapezius (see Chapter 1).

Visible accessory muscles indicate a high superficial breathing pattern. A wheezing sound may be audible. The speech pattern is often marked by a high-pitched voice with frequent inhalations between the words. Accessory muscles are most noticeable in the anterior view.

The patient experiences difficulty in exhalation and deep breathing during activity.

Abdominal muscles frequently show weakness. They should also be tested.

Recommendations for treatment are: (1) relaxation exercises, (2) segmental breathing exercises, (3) deep breathing exercises, (4) endurance exercises and (5) corrective breathing exercises.

Musculoskeletal deformities may develop secondarily to a neurologic disorder. By observation, *asymmetry* of the shoulder lines and clavicles, in addition to hypertrophy or atrophy in the muscle contour, may be noticed.

The most important factor to be closely watched is pulmonary function. The pulmonary functions (especially vital capacity) decrease when muscle weakness is present in the diaphragm, abdominals, long back extensors and the muscles covering the rib cage. In many cases the patient experiences difficulty in deep breathing and coughing and is unable to handle his own bronchial hygiene.

Recommendations for treatment are: (1) bronchial hygiene to prevent pulmonary complications, (2) deep breathing exercises, (3) segmental exercises, (4) endurance exercises, (5) muscle test and (6) muscle strengthening exercises.

CONCLUSION

This chapter outlines the importance of evaluating all patients who are receiving chest physical therapy. The results of the evaluation are primarily used to establish individualized breathing exercise programs. It is common knowledge that bronchial hygiene is of primary importance to overcome pulmonary dysfunctions. However, breathing exercises in addition to bronchial hygiene will assure a carryover and longer-lasting effects. Breathing exercises in general are a valuable measure for preventing pulmonary dysfunction in patients whose physical condition will predispose to pulmonary complications. Guidelines for evaluation precedures are discussed in this chapter in addition to a listing of the most common pathologic musculoskeletal disorders prone to pulmonary dysfunction.

REFERENCES

Books

Blount WP, Moe JH: *The Milwaukee Brace.* Baltimore, Williams & Wilkins, 1973.

Hoppenfeld S: *Physical Examination of the Spine and Extremities.* New York, Appleton-Century-Crofts, 1976.

Hoppenfeld S: *Scoliosis, A Manual of Concept and Treatment.* Philadelphia, JB Lippincott Co, 1967.

Kendall HO, Kendall FP: *Posture and Pain.* Huntington, New York, R.E. Krieger, 1970.

Myers CR, Golding LA, Sinning WE: *The Y's Way to Physical Fitness. A Guide Book for Instructors.* New York, Popular Library, 1973.

Zohn DA, Mennell J: *Musculoskeletal Pain, Diagnosis and Physical Treatment.* Boston, Little, Brown & Co, 1976.

8

Relaxation Principles and Techniques

Donna Frownfelter, P.T., R.R.T.
Maureen Fogel Perlstein, M.P.H., P.T., C.R.T.T.

Relaxation has been defined as a state of lessened tension, a recreative state or diversion and a mitigation of pain. Individuals who are able to achieve relaxation states (or the "relaxation response" advocated by Benson) exhibit better mental and physical health and an improved ability to cope with stress and tension in their lives.

Benson relates the physiology behind the relaxation response as "an integrated hypothalamic response which results in generalized decreased sympathetic nervous system activity, and perhaps also increased parasympathetic activity." These changes seem to be the opposite of the "fight or flight" response first described by Walter B. Cannon. This response will increase blood pressure, heart rate, respiratory rate, body metabolism and blood flow to the extremities. In animals, this response allows them to prepare for a fight or run away. In humans, the reaction virtually is the same but may be elicited for what often seem trivial matters such as running for a bus, figuring out a problem, changing environment or life situation, worrying and stress.

Patients with respiratory disorders tend to be extremely nervous and tense. Often they relate they do not know if their next breath will come. Tension has the added effect of tightening the chest wall and spine, which renders breathing more difficult and further impinges on respiration. "Normal" individuals experience difficulty breathing in stressful situations. One can understand the extreme respiratory problems a patient encounters when his already compromised breathing is further taxed by stress.

Therapists should learn to observe signs of stress and tension in their patients. When these signs are noted, relaxation techniques discussed further in this chapter may be beneficial and should be included in therapy.

SIGNS OF TENSION AND STRAIN

Rathbone, in her excellent book *Relaxation,* discusses several signs often noted in tense individuals. A few clinically applicable to our patients will be noted.

Appearance.   Tense people are generally well groomed, often to an extreme. They are generally not flabby but have hypertonic muscles, firm and well rounded. Their movements are not graceful, but tight and restricted.

Mannerisms.   Tense individuals tend to fidget, twitch, tremble, bite their nails, wring their hands and perform other nervous gestures. They tend to hold their bodies stiff and seem cramped. Their shoulders are often in a hunched position. They may appear to be grimacing or generally uncomfortable.

Restrictions in Joint Flexibility.   Tense people do not move easily or freely. They may exhibit limitations in mobility or the full range of motion at the joints. This is especially true of the spine.

Restriction in Breathing.   Breathing is decreased due to limitations of the chest and spine. Signs of excess tension in the respiratory system are choking attacks, asthma, laryngospasm, spasmodic coughing and irregular breathing.

Poor Circulation.   Tense individuals often complain of increased perspiration and feeling cold (cold, clammy hands). There may be skin flushing. Often muscle tension causes a decrease in circulation leading to tension headaches.

Digestive System.   Dysfunctions of the stomach, colon and liver are often observed in tense individuals. This may take the form of an "acidic" stomach, indigestion, constipation, or diarrhea.

Hyperactivity of Other Organs.   Frequency of urination is a common problem during stress. The uterus may also be affected, causing dysmenorrhea.

Pain.   Pain may be caused by stress (as in tension headaches). There must be close observation to determine whether pain is primary or secondary. For example, did pain cause the stress or vice versa?

Irritability to Environmental Factors.   Tense individuals tend to be "touchy." They may seem to "make mountains out of molehills." Things that under normal circumstances would be irrelevant may seem earth-shaking.

Overactivity.   It has been noted that tense individuals will continue to overwork and continue in hyperactivity.

Insomnia.   Complaints of insomnia in our patients are frequent and may be related to any number of reasons from hypoxemia to stress. The cause of insomnia should be pursued.

Treatment of Tension

When these signs are observed in patients, therapy should be initiated with *goals of relaxation and chest mobilization.* Patient education is also very important at this point. Patients should understand the effects of stress on their condition. They need to learn to control their body's response to stress so it does not further impair their condition. Patient education should include realization of the importance of proper diet, exercise and rest.

Proper diet should include nourishing meals and few stimulating drinks. Moderation should be a keynote. Fluid intake should be monitored. Tense individuals do not drink much water. Especially those that partake in efforts demanding tonic muscle contractions for long periods of time increase their need for water. We have all experienced dry lips and tongue as well as a distressing thirst during times of increased fear and anxiety. Increased perspiration and frequent urination in stress situations also deplete fluid levels.

Exercise to induce relaxation should not be too strenuous. Suggestions in general are for rhythmic, loose, swinging exercise. Often an alteration between stretching a muscle and releasing tension may be done *slowly* through its full range of motion to increase joint mobility.

Proper rest following activity is essential for relaxation to take place. Patients should strive for adequate sleep at night. They need to attempt to "wind down" from the day's activity and stress *before* retiring. Exercise right before going to bed is contraindicated as the patient will be too stimulated to be able to sleep.

There are several relaxation approaches to patients with increased tension. A few of them will be discussed at this time and related on a practical, clinical level that may be modified for patient care.

The most common proven current approaches to relaxation are: Jacobsen's progressive relaxation, biofeedback, yoga, transcendental meditation, hypnosis, Benson's relaxation response and, from a physical therapy standpoint, chest mobilization for relaxation exercise and guided imagery or visualization. Each of these will be briefly discussed.

JACOBSEN'S PROGRESSIVE RELAXATION EXERCISES

Jacobsen was a Chicago physiologist and physician. His progressive relaxation technique seeks to achieve an increase in the patient's discriminative control of his skeletal muscles. Jacobsen states that anxiety and muscular relaxation are opposite physiologic effects and cannot exist simultaneously.

The patient is instructed to contract isolated muscles and muscle groups to recognize tension. Then he is instructed to "go in the negative direction" to achieve relaxation. (This extreme contraction-relaxation may not be stressed strongly if the patient has a less extreme case of tension.)

To achieve progressive relaxation, the patient is positioned supine in a quiet atmosphere. He is asked to maintain a passive attitude. He learns to recognize the feeling of even the slightest muscular contraction so he can avoid it and achieve maximal muscle relaxation. In the first session, the patient may start with the legs and hips or arms and shoulders. Later emphasis is placed on the chest, back, neck, and face. In a typical therapy session, the patient is asked to be comfortable, close his eyes, clench his fist and hold it tightly, then let the arm fall limply. "Relaxing is the negative of doing." When the arm falls, he is not to move it but let it rest and relax further. Repetitions will be included. The relaxation process will include all muscle groups, i.e.: (1) Bend both feet down and let them go limp. (2) Wrinkle your forehead, let it go. (3) Frown, let it go. (4) Pull shoulder blades together, relax. (5) Pull buttocks together, relax. The goal is to let the patient feel the contraction, then experience the relaxation of that muscle group.

In applying these techniques to respiratory patients, attention is specifically focused on the upper chest, neck, shoulder and abdominal muscles. Relaxation in these muscle groups will facilitate improved ventilation (Tables 8–1 to 8–6).

TABLE 8–1.

Relaxation Technique No. 1: Relaxation of Arms (Time: 4–5 minutes)

First	Settle back as comfortably as you can and allow yourself to relax to the best of your ability. Clench your right fist, tighter and tighter, and study the tension as you tighten. Keep it clenched and feel the tension in your fist, hand, and forearm. Relax. Let the fingers become loose. Observe the contrast in your feelings. Let yourself go and try to become more relaxed all over.
Second	Clench your right fist tightly again. Hold it and notice the tension. Relax. Your fingers straightened out and you notice the difference once again.
Third	Repeat the procedure with your left fist. Clench the fist while the rest of your body relaxes. Clench the fist tighter and feel the tension. Relax, then repeat the procedure, enjoying the contrast. After clenching, relax for a minute or two.
Fourth	Clench both fists, tighter and tighter. Both fists and forearms should be tense. Study the sensations. Relax. Straighten your fingers and feel the relaxation. Continue relaxing your hands and forearms more and more.
Fifth	Bend your elbows and tense your biceps. Tense them harder and study the feelings. Straighten your arms, then let them relax. Feel the difference. Let the relaxation develop. Once more, tense your biceps. Hold the tension and observe it carefully. Straighten your arms and relax. *Pay close attention to your feelings each time you tense and relax.*
Sixth	Straighten your arms until you feel most tension in the triceps muscles along the back of your arms. Stretch your arms and feel the tension, then relax. Get your arms back into a comfortable position. Allow the relaxation to proceed on its own. The arms should feel comfortably heavy as you allow them to relax. Straighten the arms once more so that you feel the tension in the triceps muscles. Feel the tension. Then relax.
Seventh	Concentrate on pure relaxation in the arms without any tension. Get your arms into a comfortable position, then let them relax. Continue to relax them even more. Even when your arms seem fully relaxed, try to go that extra bit further; try to achieve deeper and deeper levels of relaxation.

TABLE 8–2.

Relaxation Technique No. 2: Relaxation of Facial Area, Neck, Shoulders, Upper Back (Time: 4–5 minutes)

First	Let all your muscles go loose and heave. Settle back quietly and comfortably. Wrinkle your forehead; wrinkle it tighter. Stop, relax, and smooth it out. Picture the entire forehead and scalp becoming smoother as the relaxation increases.

TABLE 8–2. (*Continued*)

Second	Frown and crease your brows and study the tension. Release the tension. Smooth out the forehead once more. Close your eyes tighter and tighter. Feel the tension. Relax your eyes. Keep your eyes closed (good luck reading this with your eyes closed). They should be closed gently, comfortably. Notice the relaxation.
Third	Clench your jaws, studying the tension throughout your jaws. Relax. Let your lips part slightly. Appreciate the relaxation.
Fourth	Press your tongue hard against the roof of your mouth. Feel the tension. Let your tongue return to a comfortable and relaxed position.
Fifth	Purse your lips, pressing them tighter and tighter together. Relax. Note the contrast between tension and relaxation. Feel the relaxation all over your face, forehead, scalp, eyes, jaws, lips, tongue, and throat. The relaxation progresses further and further.
Sixth	For the neck . . . Press your head back as far as it can go and feel the tension in the neck. Roll your head to the right and feel the tension shift; now roll it to the left. Straighten your head and bring it forward. Press your chin against your chest. Let your head return to a comfortable position and study the relaxation. Let the relaxation develop.

TABLE 8–3.

Relaxation Techniques No. 3: Relaxation of Chest, Stomach, and Lower Back
(Time: 4–5 minutes)

First	Relax your entire body to the best of your ability. Feel the comfortable heaviness that accompanies relaxation. Breathe easily and freely in and out. Notice how the relaxation increases as you exhale. Feel that relaxation as you breathe out.
Second	Breathe in and fill your lungs; inhale deeply and hold your breath. Study the tension. Now exhale; let the walls of your chest grow loose and push the air out automatically. Continue relaxing and breathe freely and gently. Feel and enjoy the relaxation.
Third	With the rest of your body as relaxed as possible, fill your lungs again. Hold your breath. Breathe out and appreciate the relief. Just breathe normally. Continue relaxing your chest and let the relaxation spread to your back, shoulders, neck, and arms. Let go and enjoy the relaxation.
Fourth	Now pay attention to your abdominal muscles. Tighten your muscles to make your abdomen hard. Notice the tension, then relax. Let the muscles loosen and notice the contrast. Once more, press and tighten your stomach muscles. Hold the tension and study it. Relax. Notice the general well-being that comes with relaxing your stomach.
Fifth	Draw your stomach in. Pull the muscles right in and feel the tension this way. Now relax and let your stomach out. Continue breathing normally and easily and feel the gently massaging action all over your chest and stomach. Pull your stomach in again and hold the tension. Now push out and tense. Hold the tension. Once more, pull in and feel the tension.
Sixth	Relax your stomach fully. Let the tension dissolve as the relaxation grows deeper. Each time you breathe out, notice the rhythmic relaxation both in your lungs and in your stomach. Notice how your chest and stomach relax more and more. Try to let go of all contractions anywhere in your body.

TABLE 8–4.

Relaxation Techniques No. 4: Relaxation of Shoulders, Upper and Lower Back

First	Using your imagination, think of yourself on a soft, fluffy white cloud. Your whole body is floating. Let yourself go. Let your muscles go loose and heavy. Feel that comfortable "all is well" feeling as you totally relax. Notice how the relaxation increases as you exhale.
Second	Feel tension in your shoulder muscles as you shrug your shoulders. Pretend you are a turtle pulling its head into its shell. Hold the tension. Now relax and let go. Move your shoulders about until you sense the feeling of relaxation. Try to remember the feeling of tightness and tension as you shrug your shoulders again. Bring your shoulders up and forward. Hold the tension, being aware of the feeling. Now let go. Feel the muscles across your shoulders and the back of your neck grow limp. As you shrug your shoulders this time, bring them up and back. Tense those muscles, hold, then let go. Be aware of the change in feeling.
Third	As you tense your shoulder muscles this time, tighten your neck, throat, jaws, and facial muscles. Bring your shoulders up and forward now as you squeeze muscles in your neck, throat, jaws, and face. Hold it. Relax and note the difference in feeling. Feel the relaxation spread deep in your shoulders, right into the back of your neck, throat, and face. Let go. Let the feeling go deeper and deeper.
Fourth	Now direct your attention to your lower back. Arch your back, making it hollow, and feel the tension along the spine. Recognize that feeling and settle down again, relaxing the lower muscles. Keep the rest of the muscles throughout your body as relaxed as possible as you do that again. Arch your back, tighten the muscles, recognize the feelings as you localize the areas of tension. Now let go, settle down, feel the ease, warmth, and comfort. Notice the changed feeling and how restful it is.
Fifth	With your attention focused on the lower back, bend sideways to the right, feel the tension of the muscles on the left of your lower spine. Straighten your back and notice the relaxed feeling. Bend sideways to your left; bend a little more. Think of the muscles in your lower back. Now straighten and relax.
Sixth	This time, try to flatten your lower back so your spine is as straight as possible. Lying on the floor, flatten your back so you can't put a finger between it and the floor. Feel the tension, then release. Study the difference between the tensed and relaxed states.
Seventh	Relax your entire body as best you can. Move your shoulders and upper back until they are comfortably positioned. Now do the same with your lower back, moving from side to side as necessary to find the most comfortable position. Mentally check your back muscles for looseness. Mentally talk to these muscles, telling them to let go.

TABLE 8–5.
Relaxation Techniques No. 5: Relaxation of Hips and Calves; Complete Body Relaxation

First	Let go of all tensions and relax. Now flex your buttocks and thighs. Flex your thighs by pressing down your heels as hard as you can. Relax and note the difference. Straighten your knees and flex your thigh muscles again. Hold the tension. Relax your hips and thighs. Allow the relaxation to proceed on its own.
Second	Press your feet and toes downward, away from your face, so your calf muscles become tense. Study the tension. Relax your feet and calves.
Third	This time, bend your feet toward your face so you feel tension along your shins. Bring your toes right up. Relax again. Keep relaxing for a while. Let yourself relax further, all over. Relax your feet, ankles, calves, shins, knees, thighs, buttocks, and hips. Feel how heavy and relaxed you have become.
Fourth	Now spread the relaxation to your stomach, waist, lower back. Let go more and more. Feel that relaxation all over. Let it proceed to your upper back, chest, shoulders and arms, and right to the tips of your fingers. Keep relaxing more and more deeply. Make sure that no tension has crept into your throat. Relax your neck, jaws, and all your facial muscles. Keep relaxing your whole body like that for a while.
Fifth	Now you can become twice as relaxed as you are, merely by taking in a real deep breath and slowly exhaling. With your eyes closed to avoid distractions and to keep surface tensions from developing, breathe in deeply and feel yourself becoming heavier. Take in a long, deep breath and let it out very slowly. Feel how heavy and relaxed you have become.
Sixth	In a state of perfect relaxation, you should feel unwilling to move a single muscle in your body. Think about the effort that would be required to raise your right arm. Now you decide not to lift the arm but to continue relaxing. Observe the relief and the disappearance of tension.
Seventh	Continue relaxing like that. When you wish to get up, count backwards from four to one. You should then feel refreshed, wide awake, and calm.

TABLE 8–6.
Relaxation Technique No. 6: Total Body Relaxation

First	Position yourself as comfortably as possible, with a pillow under your head and another one under your knees. Bring the pillow under your head close to your shoulders. Allow your knees to fall apart, supported by the pillow under them.
Second	Beginning with your scalp and ending with your toes, you are going to tense and relax groups of muscles. Be conscious of the feeling of tension and the opposite feeling of release. You may sense feelings of hostility, aggravation, frustration, fear, and similar emotions as you tense your muscles. You may feel peaceful, loving, restful, accepted, forgiven, and similar comfortable feelings as you relax.
Third	Tense your scalp—relax. Wrinkle your forehead, hard—relax. Frown, crease your brows tightly—relax. Study the tension and relaxation feelings. Close

(Continued)

TABLE 8–6. *(Continued)*

	your eyes, squeeze hard—relax. Press your tongue hard against the roof of your mouth—relax, allowing your tongue to go flat and limp. Clench your jaws, bite your teeth together—relax. Purse your lips and press them together hard—relax. Press your head back, study the neck muscles—relax. Press your head forward onto your chest—relax. Roll your head to the left and press—relax. Roll your head to the right—relax.
Fourth	Clench both fists—relax. Stretch your fingers—relax. Flex your biceps with clenched fists—relax. Straighten your arms, bending the backs of your hands upward—relax.
Fifth	Take in a deep breath and hold it—relax as you exhale. Tighten your abdominal muscles, pinch, and squeeze—relax. Push out and tense the muscles that way—relax.
Sixth	Shrug your shoulders up and forward—relax. Shrug your shoulders up and backward—relax. Arch your back—relax. Push back with the small of your back—relax.
Seventh	Flex your buttocks and thighs—relax. Press your feet and toes away from you; feel the pull on the leg calf muscles—relax. Press your feet and toes toward your face so you feel tension along the shins—relax. Curl your toes, squeezing hard—relax. Now bend your toes out and relax.
Eighth	Take in a long, deep breath, and feel how heavy you are. Let your muscles go limp, sort of flow. Listen to your heart beat and notice the slow inhalation and exhalation of your breathing. Mentally check out each area of your body and let it go—head and face, arms, chest and abdomen, back hips, legs, and feet. You are totally relaxed.

BIOFEEDBACK

Biofeedback for relaxation is utilized by teaching the patient to mentally recognize a biologic function and then gain control over that function. For example, if the patient was using neck accessory muscles, surface electrodes would be placed on the accessory muscles. The patient would direct his attention to decreasing the electrical activity observed and heard to a resting state activity level. This has been used both in teaching relaxation and for facilitation of muscle groups desired (muscle reeducation). It seems to be a very helpful technique for relaxation. The author's experience is limited, but there are many current articles that seem to highly recommend the technique. We need to pursue the use of biofeedback for relaxation since it offers another resource to draw upon. The following is a script the therapist could read to the patient to attempt to improve the relaxation state.

Relaxation

Just find a comfortable chair and make whatever minor adjustments you need to make to *allow* yourself to be as comfortable and unrestricted as possible and let your mind just *drift* throughout your body and check that everywhere is loose, relaxed and that there is no restrictive clothing or uncomfortable position to your body. Again, take whatever *minor adjustments* you need to make now to allow yourself to be in a most comfortable position. Then let your attention just drift to the very top of your head, to your scalp and forehead—smoothing out all the muscles in your scalp and forehead. Just let them go, relax them. *Smooth* those muscles out and let your scalp rest very comfortably on top of your head. Let that relaxation just *flow* on over your eyebrows, eyelids, even relaxing the back of your eyes, letting your eyes rest quite comfortably. *Continue* to let the relaxation flow over your cheeks, lips, and chin, letting your whole face become comfortably heavy and relaxed. *Pay special attention* to your jaw, allowing the muscles that hold up your jaw to relax—just let them go. You will notice that your jaw will be tugged down slightly by gravity and as that happens your lips will part slightly.

As you relax your face and jaw, also let go of your tongue, throat and your vocal chords, letting your vocal chords become very quiet with your tongue resting very comfortably on the floor of your mouth.

Let the relaxation continue to flow down the back of your head, letting go of all the muscles along your neck and down your shoulders. Smooth out all the muscles of your neck and shoulders. You might even think of them as tiny knotted rope that you untie and let hang loose and limp. Smooth them out and just let them hang loose, limp, and relaxed. Continue to relax your shoulders and neck and let that relaxation flow down into your arms, relaxing all the muscles of your upper arm down to your elbows and your forearm, smoothing out those muscles and letting them go. Let go of the muscles around your wrists and hands all the way down to your fingertips, letting your arms become comfortably heavy and relaxed. As your arms become more and more relaxed and heavy, let the blood flow more comfortably into your fingertips and realize as you let go of the tension in your arms and shoulders, the blood flows more comfortably and easily into the fingertips.

As you continue to relax your head and face, your neck and shoulders and your arms, let your attention now drift to the upper back and smooth out all the muscles along your shoulders and upper back. Continue to relax all the way along your spine, down your middle back, smoothing out all the muscles and down into your lower back, letting go all the way down into your waist and buttocks.

Let that relaxation come around the sides of your body, letting go of all the muscles around your rib cage, smoothing them out and letting go. With every breath, allow your chest to become more and more comfortably relaxed. Just observe your breathing with every breath. Just notice the inhalation of the air through your nostrils, down, down into your lungs, filling up the lungs and then exhaling back out again and allow your breathing to be just normal, rhythmic, smooth. With every breath, allow yourself just to float down into that chair. Let the relaxation spread down to your abdomen, your waist, smoothing out all the muscles in your stomach to become relaxed. Just observe it.

Let go of all the muscles around your hips, waist, and pelvis, letting your whole pelvic area relax and smooth out. Continue to let that re-laxation flow down to your thighs, knees, down to your shins, calves, letting your legs become heavy, comfortably heavy, and relaxed. Let go of your ankles, heels, feet—even the soles of your feet and toes. As your legs become comfortably heavy, blood flows again more easily to the toes allowing your feet to become comfortably warm.

Your whole body from the very top of your head, all the way down to the ends of your toes is relaxed, peacefully calm, quiet inside. With every breath now, allow your body to let go a little bit more. With every exhale, let your body just float on down through the chair, comfortably heavy and relaxed. As you relax more and more and more deeply, remain *awake and aware* but very relaxed. Relaxation allows the whole system to have a very deep rest while you are awake and aware. Relax-ation is *different from tiredness.* While tiredness is a drain of energy pro-duced by too much tension in the system, relaxation allows you to *con-serve* the *energy* that was formerly used up by tension through deep relaxation, such as you are experiencing now. The body can get a very deep rest and you can feel *refreshed* and *rejuvenated.*

As you practice these techniques of deep progressive relaxation, realize, as with any other *skill,* you become more and *more capable* and effective at *relaxing more quickly* and more *efficiently.* So that soon, rather than going through the entire process, muscle by muscle group, the words "calm," "quite quiet," or "relax" will allow you to achieve the same quality of relaxation that you are experiencing now and, with practice, the depth of relaxation can also be increased. Again, allow yourself to be conscious and awake but relaxed and quite quiet inside, and when you are ready, become aware of the room and the environ-ment around you and let your eyes open, remaining relaxed, feeling good all over and refreshed as if you have had a very deep rest. When you are ready, just let your eyes open and become aware of the room.

YOGA AND TRANSCENDENTAL MEDITATION (TM)

Yoga exercise, or asana, consists generally of slowly stretching and bending into a particular position without strain or pain, holding that position for a length of time (usually 10 seconds to 5 minutes or more) and then releasing the pose as slowly as it was assumed. A brief rest period will follow the exercise. The rest period allows for the maximal relaxation effect of the pose, prevents fatigue and has a soothing, pleasurable feeling. Some purported effects of the asanas are increased flexibility (especially of the spine), improved circulation, stimulation of glands, organs and skeletal muscles, as well as better posture. Breathing exercises (pranayamas) are also included, generally to initiate meditation and relaxation. Complete breaths and cleansing breaths are used to begin exercise. They have a calming effect and are a step to induce mental and physical relaxation.

A patient should receive clearance from his physician before starting yoga due to the exercise involved. Many elderly patients are able to do the techniques; however, it seems especially ideal for younger patients that have more endurance and resiliency.

Transcendental meditation is a form of yoga. It is taught as a very systematic method of repeating a word without attempting to concentrate specifically on the word. Meditation is recommended for 15–20 minutes twice a day in a comfortable position with the eyes closed. (The use of a word to focus on has been found in the literature dating back to Judaism in the second century B.C. It is seen in Eastern religions such as Zen and Yoga, and in the 14th century monks and Christians mention the meditation technique.)

In studies of individuals practicing TM, the following results were observed: decreased oxygen consumption, CO_2 elimination, heart rate, respiratory rate, minute ventilation and arterial blood lactate.

HYPNOSIS

Hypnosis involves making an appropriate suggestion to achieve a desired mental or physical behavior. The results have been varied. The author has no personal experience with this in relation to relaxation, although some sources claim success. Clinically, we have had patients stop smoking after they were hypnotized.

THE RELAXATION RESPONSE

This technique proposed by Herbert Benson induces relaxation by eliciting four elements.

1. *A quiet environment:* there should be decreased stimulation. The
patient's eyes should be closed.

2. *A mental device:* this is a constant stimulus—a word or a phrase
repeated either silently or audibly. This may also be accomplished by
fixed gazing at an object. The purpose of this maneuver is to shift from
logical externally oriented thought to the word or object. A prayer may
be appropriate and elicit the same response.

3. *A passive attitude:* the patient is encouraged to disregard
thoughts, to concentrate on the relaxing technique.

4. *A decrease in muscle tone:* the patient should assume a comfortable
position that requires minimal work to maintain. The patient should
not fall asleep, however. A position other than reclining is usually recommended.

There seem to be many similar elements in various cultures and
religions relating to these mental processes. It should be noted that
there may be several roads to the relaxation response; it is an individual response.

Benson also relates additional results of utilizing the relaxation response. Individuals with high blood pressure have found it has decreased, and there has also been a decrease in the use of drugs (i.e.,
marijuana, amphetamines, LSD, smoking).

Benson reports that this experience will vary in different people.
The consistent factor seems to be that subjects feel it is beneficial and
can be reclaimed. It can be utilized by setting time aside and consciously using the technique. It is also felt that a belief that the system
will work may be an important factor in eliciting relaxation.

This last statement is true for a great deal of success with patients.
Our encouragement and suggestion that a technique may help often
will give patients an extra boost which allows them to perform more
appropriately. Patient motivation is extremely important.

The therapist's attitude and manner can do much to facilitate relaxation. Therapists must strive to achieve a calm, relaxed atmosphere
and develop good rapport when dealing with a tense patient. The therapist should speak quietly and at a slow pace, almost monotonous and

reassuring. Care should be taken not to speak too softly so that the patient cannot hear well. This would become irritating and counter-productive.

EXERCISE

The last techniques to be discussed are rhythmic exercise and mobilization exercise. These general exercises are familiar to the physical therapist and are cited as a review with emphasis on the approach to the tense patient. The following exercises should be done slowly and rhythmically.

1. Arm swings.
   Bilaterally forward and backward.
   Out to the sides.
   Alternately forward and backward.
   Across the front and out to the sides.
2. Arm circles.
   The arms circumscribe small circles and then form progressively larger and larger circles.
3. Swimming movements.
   The patient pantomimes a swimmer doing the backstroke, alternately reaching and stretching each arm up, back and forward.
4. Arm swings in a forward bending position.
   The patient bends at the waist while standing and swings arms forward, backward, to the sides and crosswise.
5. Sitting on a table.
   The patient swings his legs slowly forward and backward (there should be a towel roll under each knee).
6. Sitting on a table.
   The patient circumscribes circles with his legs.
7. Standing.
   Holding onto a stationary object, the patient puts his weight on one leg and swings the other from the hips—forward, backward, sideways and across the front.
8. Standing.
   On one leg as above, the patient makes a circle with his free leg in both directions.
9. On hands and knees (all fours position).
   Hunch back up, hold, relax (don't allow back to relax to a lordotic position).

10. On hands and knees.
    Sway in a circular pattern in both directions.
11. Sitting.
    Rotate the head through the complete range—drop head forward, to the side, back, side and forward *slowly!* Change direction.
12. Head and neck.
    Inscribe *X's* with the head and neck. Look down at the right hip, turn and look up and over the left shoulder. Reverse. Then look at the left hip and turn and look over the right shoulder. Reverse. Do several times.
13. Eyes.
    Look at 12, 3, 6, and 9 o'clock. Hold at each point for a few seconds.
14. Shoulders.
    Shrug shoulders up, hold for a few seconds. Relax.
15. Shoulder rolls.
    Push shoulders forward, up, back, down and forward. Reverse directions *(slowly)*.
16. Shoulder blades.
    Pull shoulder blades together, relax, allow shoulders to drop.
    In these exercises, when the patient is asked to hold and then relax (or let go), a longer time should be spent in relaxing than in holding. For example, shrug shoulders (hold 3 seconds, relax 10 seconds). This allows time for and emphasis on relaxation rather than contraction. It follows the concept of Jacobsen's contract relax principles.
    A combination of several techniques may be used. Techniques may be modified. Patients need to try various methods and techniques and learn to adapt those that are most beneficial to themselves.

GUIDED IMAGERY OR VISUALIZATION

Guided imagery, also referred to as visualization, is a process that enables an individual to make contact with various aspects of his or her physical, mental, emotional, and spiritual self. Imagery is really a form of daydreaming with direction and purpose. It is a conscious experience in which an individual is able to maintain a focus on one object of concentration through involving perceptual and emotional participation.

Guided imagery and visualization have been successfully used to relieve intractable pain, to improve vision, and to restructure negative images surrounding childbirth. Authors have mentioned that the use of imagery can aid in diagnosis by allowing information about a person's internal world to surface. Individuals using imagery have reported feeling a sense of control over their lives establishing a more positive outlook on a variety of topics, being able to set goals, increasing the ability to establish positive expectations, and being able to practice new behaviors.

Imagery

Take a comfortable position, and close your eyes. Take three breaths as you let go of the day's tension. Relax your body from toe to head.

Imagine yourself in a green field on a warm, spring day. You begin to walk up a grassy hill. After a few steps, you pause, and leave your worries behind. You continue walking up the hill until you reach the top. You rest on the lush grass. You notice that the field is full of clover, with occasional dandelions. The leaves on the trees rustle in the gentle wind. The soft breeze blowing over your skin soothes and relaxes you. In the air are the pleasant scents of grass and flowers. Nearby are lilac trees—the breeze carries their fragrance to your nostrils. Billowy white clouds spot the bright blue, sunny sky. A few birds circle lazily in the sky, others are singing in the trees. You are peaceful and happy. All is right with the world.

Stay here for a few moments. This is your safe place and you can return here to rest each day if you wish. You can feel happy, relaxed, and confident when you leave here to continue your day's activities.

Mental Imagery

Take three deep diaphragmatic breaths, close your eyes, and relax. Imagine you are on a bank of a glorious flowing river—visualize as only you can—see blue ships reflected on shimmering currents—breathe in and really smell nature's beauty around you—all favorite trees and flowers are within your reach—hear only sounds you adore—be it birds, water rustling, or wind in the trees—hear it, really hear it—move gracefully to edge of water holding tight to a beautiful tree beside you—put your toes in river—the current suddenly tries to pull you to its flow—cling desperately to the tree, deeply fearing unknown waters—suddenly realize you want to let go, really want to give in to natural flow and you release fearful grip, trusting that life will carry you or right your course—flowing with river, behold splendor above and around you—you are completely relaxed and confident when river leads to fork. Know it will take you in the right direction, so free yourself of fear and anxiety.

The Blue Sky

Picture a beautiful blue sky without any clouds in it. As you picture the clear blue sky, feel that your body is growing lighter and lighter. Close your eyes and keep the image of the blue sky in your mind. There are no limits to the blue sky. It stretches endlessly in every direction, never beginning and never ending. As you visualize the blue sky, feel that your body has become so light that you have floated up into the clear blue sky. Feel that you are floating in the sky and that all tension, fatigue, worry, and problems have left you. Relax your mind and allow your breathing to seek its own level. Feel yourself floating gently in the clear blue sky that stretches endlessly in every direction, never beginning and never ending.

After several minutes have passed and you feel yourself relaxing, then picture that your entire body is merging with the blue sky. Your body is merging with the peace of the blue sky . . . Your mind is merging with the tranquility of the blue sky . . . Feel that you have actually become the blue sky. You have become the infinite blue sky that stretches endlessly in every direction, never beginning and never ending. Feel that you have become the perfect peace and tranquility of the blue sky. Completely let go and experience total relaxation.

When you feel that you have relaxed for as long as you like, then open your eyes. You will now have a new and deeper sense of peace, relaxation, and poise. This renewed energy, joy, and calm will stay with you as you resume your normal activities.

The Rain: Autogenic and Mental Imagery

It is early in the morning and you slowly wake to the sound of rain falling on the roof. You can imagine the cold and wet outside, but you are warm and snug in your bed. You pull the soft blue comforter up around your ears and sink deeper and deeper into the soft bed. Your body feels very warm and relaxed as you listen to the sound of the rain.

Your house is very quiet except for the steady pattering of rain. No one else has awakened and you feel very peaceful. What a wonderful morning to lie silently in bed listening to the rain's rhythmical sound.

You can feel the soft blue comforter pressing lightly over your legs. Allow your legs to feel heavier and heavier as a deep warmth and tingling sensation settles over your legs.

You can feel your hips sinking deeper and deeper into the soft bed. Allow your hips to give with the freedom of total relaxation.

As your breathing slows, watch the soft blue comforter rise and fall with each breath. Your abdominal and chest muscles sink deeper and deeper into your soft bed with each exhalation. Slow the exhalation phase of your breathing pattern and enjoy sinking deeper and deeper into your soft comfortable mattress.

Allow your arms to feel warmer and heavier and under the soft blue comforter. Even your fingers are feeling warm and very loose.

As your head sinks deeper into your pillow, you can still hear the sound of the rain. The rain is gradually slowing until there is only an occasional dripping sound from the roof. The sun begins to spread its warming rays through the clouds. Other people in the house are beginning to stir and you know it is time for you to arise and begin a new day. You feel grateful for the rain and solitude you enjoyed. Slowly and peacefully stretch your arms overhead as you greet the day with renewed optimism.

The Beach and a Friend

Picture yourself walking leisurely along a cool sandy beach. It is dawn. The beach is empty. An occasional seagull and tiny sandpiper play on the beach.

You notice the waves quietly and peacefully sweeping the beach. Each wave is different with a subtle shape and sound.

You can smell the cool sea air as it blows over the incoming waves. You feel content and at peace.

Gradually, the sun spreads its warming rays over the water and beach. You can feel its warmth spreading throughout your body. The sunlight glistens on each wave. Tiny fish leap from the sea to greet the rising sun. They also glisten in the sunlight.

In the distance you can see a human figure approaching. As you approach each other, you recognize your best friend. You warmly greet each other with surprise and continue together down the beach. You share important details of your lives and each person understands. Friends are important for caring, giving, and receiving. Someone close whom you can trust and with whom you share your deepest thoughts and desires. Take care of your friendship. Protect that trust.

Associative Relaxation

Lie down on your back. Take a deep breath and slowly exhale. Relax. Think of the color green for a moment. Imagine that your feet, ankles, legs, knees, and thighs are being bathed in a beautiful green light. Now relax these parts of your body. Continue relaxing them until all tension has left.

Think of the color purple. Imagine that your stomach, abdomen, lower back, and lower ribs are being filled with purple light. Now consciously relax these areas of your body until they are completely relaxed.

Visualize your chest, upper torso, back, and ribs. Feel that they are being bathed in a beautiful light-blue light. Now relax these parts of your body until all stress and tension has left them.

Feel the area of your shoulders, neck, face, and head. Imagine that they are surrounded with a beautiful golden light. Now consciously relax these parts of your body until they are completely relaxed.

After you have completed this process, then imagine that your whole body is being bathed in a glowing white light. Now relax your entire body until all signs of tension have left you.

After you have practiced this technique a number of times, you will be able to use it to relax specific sections of your body at any time. For example, if you find that your stomach is tense while you are driving or at a meeting, then imagine that it is being filled with purple light. Your muscles should relax quickly. If you develop a headache or a tight neck, imagine that this area of your body is being bathed in golden light. If you feel a tightness around your chest, then imagine that your chest is being bathed in a light-blue light, and so on. The more you practice, the better and more quickly the technique will work. Eventually you should be able to relax any part of your body within moments of visualizing the color you associated with it.

SUMMARY

There are various techniques for relaxation. Patients need to be exposed to several alternatives, so they may try them and choose techniques beneficial to them.

REFERENCES

Periodicals
Benson H, Beary JF, Carol MP: The relaxation response. *Psychiatry* 1974; 37:37.
Canter A, Kondo CY, Knott JR: A comparison of EMG feedback and progressive muscle relaxation training in anxiety neurosis. *Br J Psychiatry* 1975; 127:470.
Coursey RC: Electromyographic feedback as a relaxation technique. *J Consult Clin Psychol* 1975; 43:825.

Crampton M: Answers from the unconscious. *Synthesis* 1975; 1(2):140–149.

Goyeche JR, Abo Y, Ikemi Y: Asthma: The yoga perspective. Part II: Yoga therapy in the treatment of asthma. *J Asthma* 1982; 19(3):189–201.

Lefer L: The blossoming of the rose. *Synthesis* 1977; 3(4):124–128.

Nusser M: Biofeedback. *Calif Nurse* 1984; Dec 1985, Jan 1980; 7(10):7.

Sitzman J, Kamiya J, Johnston J: Biofeedback training for reduced respiratory rate in chronic obstructive pulmonary disease: A preliminary study. *Nurs Res* 1983; 32(4):218–223.

Books

Benson H: Your innate asset for combatting stress. *Nursing Digest* 1975; May-June, 38–41.

Blattner B: *Holistic Nursing.* Englewood Cliffs, New Jersey, Prentice Hall, 1981.

Bressler D: *Free Yourself From Pain.* New York, Simon and Shuster, 1979.

Bry A: *Visualization—Directing the Movies of Your Mind.* New York, Barnes and Noble, 1979.

Gawain S: Creative visualization. *The Holistic Health Handbook.* Berkeley, California, And/Or Press, 1978.

Gendlin E: *Focusing.* New York, Exerest House, 1981.

Flynn P: *Holistic Health.* Bowie, Maryland, Robert J. Brady Co, 1980.

Fuller G: *Biofeedback: Method and Procedures in Clinical Practice.* San Francisco, Biofeedback Press, 1977.

Mason LJ: *Guide to Stress Reduction.* San Francisco, Peace Press, 1980.

McKay S: *Holistic Health.* In press.

Samuals M, Bennet H: *The Well Body Book.* New York, Random House, 1973.

Samuals M: *Seeing With the Mind's Eye.* New York, Random House, 1975.

Tapes

Bressler Center, 12401 Wilshire, Los Angeles, CA 90024. "Meditation and Relaxation."

Source, Box W, Stanford, CA 94304 1-800-227-1617 Ext. 514. "Letting Go of Stress."

Whatever Publishing, 158 E. Blithedale, Suite 4, Mill Valley, CA 94941. "Creative Visualization."

Windham Hill Records, Box 9388, Stanford CA 94305. "Balancing—Music for Meditation."

9

Respiratory Muscle Fatigue

Maureen Shekleton, D.N.Sc., R.N.

Roussos and Macklem[1] support the notion of a two-part respiratory system made up of the lungs which are the gas exchanging organs and a pump which ventilates the lungs. The pump is composed of the chest wall, the respiratory muscles, and the nerves and centers in the nervous system that control the respiratory muscles. The respiratory muscles are expected to function continuously throughout life to provide the appropriate level of ventilation for meeting the body's metabolic needs.

Citing the analogy of the heart as the circulatory pump and the consequences of heart failure, Macklem[15] maintains that the respiratory pump can fail, leading to a condition characterized by hypoventilation and hypercapnia that may ultimately progress to ventilatory failure and death. Causes of respiratory pump failure can be grouped in two major categories: (1) those in which the respiratory drive is decreased or the sensitivity and function of the respiratory center is altered, i.e., those that affect the central nervous system control; and (2) those in which the ventilatory response is decreased through impairment of the mechanics of respiration, i.e., those that affect the chest wall or musculature.[2]

The focus of this chapter is on the latter category, and more specifically, on the role of weakness and fatigue of the respiratory muscles as a pathophysiologic mechanism seen in many clinical conditions. The view of respiratory muscle fatigue as a cause of ventilatory failure is an idea becoming more widely accepted among pulmonary clinicians.[3] Respiratory muscle fatigue is postulated to be the final common pathway to respiratory failure in all conditions in which the respiratory musculature is affected.[4-10]

While both the inspiratory and expiratory respiratory muscles are susceptible to fatigue, clinically, concern centers on the inspiratory muscles, particularly the diaphragm since under normal conditions expiration is a passive process and the inspiratory muscles are responsible for the work of breathing. Presented initially in this chapter is an analysis of the phenomenon of inspiratory muscle fatigue. This is followed by a discussion of the identification and management of inspiratory muscle fatigue and its possible prevention through training of the inspiratory muscles.

THE CONCEPT OF INSPIRATORY MUSCLE FATIGUE

It is important to differentiate between muscle weakness and muscle fatigue, although both may lead to hypoventilation.[11] Muscle weakness refers to failure to *generate* an expected force or a chronic reduction in contractile force. Muscle fatigue refers to failure to *maintain* an expected force with repeated or sustained contraction. Fatigue is an acute loss of contractile force wherein, despite constancy of stimulation, force declines from the initial value. If fatigue is the inability of a muscle to continue to generate a required force, then in the respiratory system, fatigue will be manifested by the inability of the inspiratory muscles to continue to generate the force required to maintain the necessary level of alveolar ventilation to meet the body's metabolic needs. Inspiratory muscle fatigue occurs when inspiratory effort exceeds the capacity of the inspiratory muscles to sustain that effort.[12]

Physiologically, fatigue can be classified as central or peripheral, depending on its site of origin. Central fatigue is due to the loss of or inadequate neural drive which decreases the number or firing frequency of motor units. The resulting force generated by voluntary effort is less than that which can be achieved by electrical stimulation of the motor nerves. If electrical stimulation can restore contractile force or if stimulation and force decline in parallel, central fatigue is present.

Peripheral fatigue is present if force is decreased, but electrical stimulation is constant. Peripheral fatigue can be further categorized according to the selective loss of contractile force that occurs at varying stimulation frequencies. High frequency fatigue is a selective loss of contractile force at high stimulation frequencies; low frequency fatigue is the selective loss of force at low stimulation frequencies. High frequency fatigue is thought to be the result of impaired neuromuscular transmission and/or propagation of the muscle action potential. This type of fatigue is seen in myasthenia gravis, during ischemic exercise, with muscle cooling, and with partial curarization. It is reversible in minutes. The mechanism underlying low frequency fatigue is thought to be impaired excitation-contraction coupling. Recovery from this type of fatigue may take hours to days and possibly longer. Intense dynamic and static muscular activity can lead to low frequency fatigue.[13, 14]

MECHANISMS AND ETIOLOGY OF FATIGUE

The major mechanisms thought to be responsible for inspiratory muscle fatigue include an imbalance between energy supply and demand and impaired excitation-activation. Edwards[14] has proposed a model that accounts for the interaction of both mechanisms in the development of muscle fatigue. He has also proposed the idea that fatigue serves a protective function in that serious irreparable damage may be prevented if the muscle is unable to continue performing beyond a critical point.

The energy demands of the inspiratory muscles are determined by the work of breathing, the strength and endurance of the respiratory muscles, and the efficiency of the muscles. The work of breathing is the total amount of effort required to expand and contract the lungs. It is determined by the degree of compliance of the lung tissue, the resistance of the airways, the presence of active expiration (normally a passive process), and use of the accessory muscles of respiration. The work of breathing is increased by decreased pulmonary compliance, increased airway resistance, active expiration, and use of the accessory muscles.

Strength and endurance are the fundamental properties of muscle. Strength is defined as the maximum force that a muscle can develop with maximal stimulation. Contractile force is governed by the force-length (length-tension), force-velocity, and force-frequency relationships. Contractile force will be diminished in conditions characterized by increased lung volume (hyperinflation) since the muscles are stretched beyond the optimal length to generate maximum force. Strength is also determined by the number and size of individual fibers in a muscle. Strength is adversely affected in conditions in which the size of the fibers is reduced (atrophy) or the number of fibers is reduced (such as in malnutrition).

Endurance is defined as the ability to maintain a contraction against a given load and is determined by muscle fiber type, blood supply, and the force and duration of the contraction. Normally, the inspiratory muscles are fatigue resistant. Approximately 75% of the muscle fibers in the adult diaphragm are of the high oxidative, fatigue resistant type. In contrast, the diaphragm of the neonate contains a relative paucity of Type I fibers which have the greatest endurance capacity, and this pattern of fiber distribution is most pronounced in the premature infant. This condition exists in infants for up to a year after birth.

The energy supply to the muscles depends on an intact oxygen transport system, adequate oxygen carrying capacity of the blood, blood flow, substrate stores and availability, and the efficiency of oxygen uptake and utilization by the muscles. The energy supply to the inspiratory muscles will be compromised when cardiac output is reduced, the hemoglobin content of the blood is low, blood flow to the muscles is decreased, or energy substrates are lacking.

Excitation-activation depends on intact, functioning, neuromuscular pathways. Impaired excitation-activation is probably the primary mechanism underlying respiratory muscle weakness and fatigue in the patient with a neuromuscular disorder. Disruption of excitation-activation can occur at any point along this pathway which Edwards[14] refers to as a "chain of command" for muscular contraction. Presented in Figure 9–1 is a list of the possible mechanisms that may lead to fatigue by disrupting the neuromuscular pathway. Impaired excitation of the muscle membrane is probably interrelated with energy metabolism. For example, if the ATP supply to the Na^+-K^+ pump is compromised, an alteration in the Na^+ and K^+ concentrations in the transverse tubular system may result in impaired excitation-contraction coupling.

In summary, those patients who are at risk for the development in inspiratory muscle fatigue are those in whom energy demands are increased, energy supplies are compromised, or whose neuromuscular chain of command has been disrupted at some point. Patients at highest risk for the development of inspiratory muscle fatigue are those in whom the work of breathing is increased, thus increasing the demands for energy, and those who are experiencing hypoxemia, acidosis, low cardiac output, or any other condition in which the blood supply to the muscle is diminished and therefore energy supply is reduced. Patients whose nutritional status is poor or who are experiencing a catabolic state such as stress or fever will have reduced energy stores and may experience muscle fatigue during times of high need.

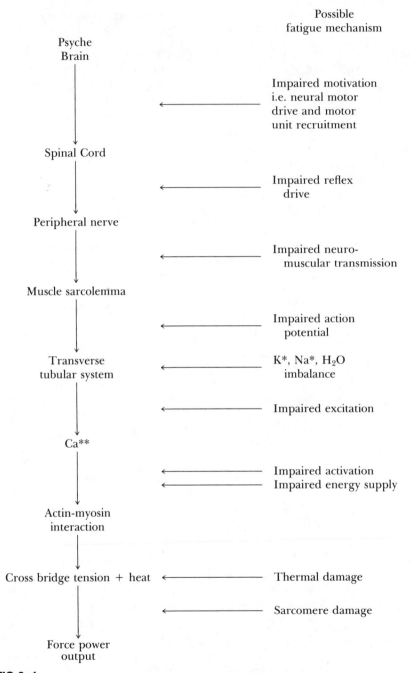

FIG 9–1.
Chain of command for muscular contraction and the possible mechanisms underlying fatigue. (From Edwards RAT: Biochemical basis of fatigue in exercise performance: Catastrophe theory of muscular fatigue, in Knuttgen H, Vogel J, Poortmans J (eds): *Biochemistry of Exercise*. Champaign, Ill, Human Kinetics Publishers, 1983, pp 3–28. Used by permission.)

ASSESSMENT OF FATIGUE

The clinician will most often have to rely on physical signs exhibited by the patient in order to recognize inspiratory muscle fatigue. Two other methods that would yield more objective evidence of inspiratory muscle fatigue include power spectral analysis of the electromyelogram (EMG) and identification of the force-frequency curve. The use of these two methods at the bedside, however, is not feasible at the present time.

The physical signs indicative of inspiratory muscle fatigue are listed below in their characteristic order of appearance:

1. Tachypnea.

2. Decreased tidal volume.

3. Development of a discoordinated respiratory pattern characterized by inward abdominal movement on inspiration (a sign referred to as abdominal paradox) and alternating abdominal and thoracic respiratory patterns (a sign referred to as respiratory alternans).

4. Increased P_{CO_2} (which is a late sign).

5. Bradypnea and decreased minute ventilation.

In animals in whom inspiratory muscle fatigue has been experimentally induced, the fall in respiratory rate and minute ventilation immediately precedes respiratory arrest and death.[1, 5]

This sequence of events has been observed following an initial change in the EMG power spectrum indicative of muscle fatigue in normal subjects exercised to fatigue, in patients experiencing difficulty being weaned from mechanical ventilation as well as in animals in whom fatigue was experimentally induced.[1, 15] When fatigue is present, the ratio of high to low frequency power, which can be detected by EMG, shifts as low frequency power increases and high frequency power decreases. The difficulty in obtaining an EMG at the bedside and in analyzing the results makes its use in most clinical situations unrealistic at this time.

Based on studies completed to date, it is believed that the physical signs described above are reliable and can be used in the clinical situation to determine whether the patient is experiencing inspiratory muscle fatigue. Macklem[15] states that abdominal paradox is pathognomonic of weak diaphragmatic contraction since it has only been observed in bilateral diaphragmatic paralysis and in diaphragmatic fatigue. The abdomen must be palpated in order to differentiate between abdominal contraction and true abdominal paradox. Detection of the signs, abdominal paradox and respiratory alternans, will most often depend on the techniques of observation and palpation until reliable respiratory monitors that can detect chest and abdominal muscle contraction become generally available for use in clinical practice.

TREATMENT OF FATIGUE

The goals of treating inspiratory fatigue are as follows: (1) restore the balance between energy supply and demand; (2) improve diaphragmatic contractility; and (3) increase the strength and endurance of the inspiratory muscles. The last goal is obviously a more long-term preventive approach while the first two goals apply in the more acute situation when inspiratory muscle fatigue is present.

Energy demands in the patient experiencing fatigue can be decreased by reducing the work of breathing through activities intended to promote compliance, decrease resistance in the lung and chest wall, and promote normal lung volumes and pressures. Energy supplies can be enhanced by ensuring maximal oxygen transport to the tissues and the availability of adequate amounts of oxygen and other energy substrates. Oxygen transport is enhanced by promoting adequate cardiac output, blood flow to the tissues, and oxygen carrying capacity of the blood. Various forms of respiratory therapy are available to supplement oxygen supplies. Losses of organic and inorganic energy in substrates must be replenished and adequate levels maintained. Nutritional supplementation and administration of electrolytes and inorganic phosphate may be necessary to augment energy supplies. Mechanical ventilation may be required to allow the fatigued muscle to rest and recover while energy supplies and demand are brought into balance.

Much current research is being done in the area of pharmacologic interventions to improve diaphragmatic contractility. Aminophylline has been shown to increase the contractile force of the diaphragm at any given level of activation, shorten the duration of fatigue when given before fatigue develops, and restore force within 20 minutes when given after fatigue develops.[12] In addition to the methyl xanthines, another class of drugs with inotropic properties are the beta agonists. Clinical investigation of the potential usefulness and application of these pharmacologic agents in inspiratory muscle fatigue is ongoing.

The last goal, that of increasing the strength and endurance of the inspiratory muscles, can be accomplished by training the inspiratory muscles in much the same way that athletes train and condition their muscles. Inspiratory muscle training may represent a useful clinical approach to prevent the development of inspiratory muscle fatigue in those patients who are at risk.

INSPIRATORY MUSCLE TRAINING

A promising direction for breathing exercises, which is more directly related to the phenomenon of inspiratory muscle fatigue, is conditioning and training of the inspiratory muscles for strength and endurance. General principles of skeletal muscle training that must be considered when designing and evaluating an inspiratory muscle training program for respiratory patients include overload, specificity, and reversibility. In order to train a muscle to improve its functional ability, the muscle must be subjected to a stress greater than its usual load (overload), the training must be directed at developing specific functional attributes (such as strength or endurance) of the muscle (specificity), and the training must be maintained or function will revert back to pretraining levels (reversibility).[16, 17] The effects of strength and endurance training generally include an increase in the size (hypertrophy) and number of the muscle fibers, an increase in the proportion of fatigue-resistant fibers in the diaphragm, an increase in the metabolic capability of the muscle, and a reduction in the susceptibility of muscle fibers to the deleterious effects of exercise. Strength training to increase the size and number of myofibrils requires a high load and a slow rate of repetition. Endurance training to increase the metabolic capability and circulation of the muscle requires exercise of a sufficient load, speed, and duration such that cellular concentrations of energy producing substrates drop to minimum levels.[16] Endurance training of skeletal muscle has been found to be most effective when brief periods of fatiguing exercise are alternated with periods of rest.[18]

Improvement in the strength and endurance of the inspiratory muscles through training has the twofold effect for patients of enhancing the resistance to inspiratory muscle fatigue and improving ventilatory function. The work of breathing is reduced and respiratory reserves are increased. As the clinical signs and symptoms are diminished, the ultimate outcome for the patient is an improved quality of life. Kim[16] has developed a model (Fig 9–2) that outlines the relationship between the effects of respiratory muscle training and potential patient outcomes.

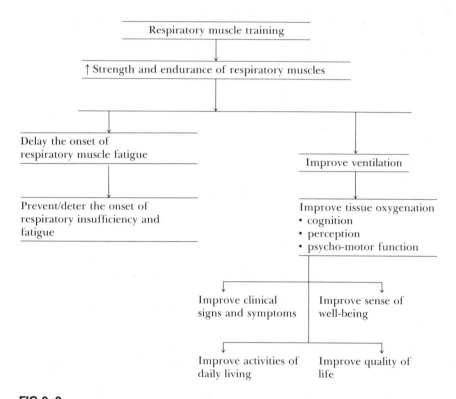

FIG 9–2.
Conceptual framework for respiratory muscle training. (From Kim M: Respiratory muscle training: Implications for patient care. *Heart Lung* 1984; 13(4):333–340. Used by permission.)

Respiratory muscle training has been used to successfully increase muscle strength and endurance in healthy volunteers[19, 20] and in patients with COPD,[21–25] with chronic air flow limitation,[26, 27] with cystic fibrosis,[19] and who are quadriplegic.[28] In patients experiencing acute respiratory failure, improved function of the muscles and fatigue resistance should facilitate the process of weaning these patients from mechanical ventilation. In conditions requiring full ventilatory support, the respiratory muscles may contract at minimum levels for a period of time possibly leading to the development of disuse atrophy. As their strength and endurance decrease, the inspiratory muscles will be more prone to fatigue due to the interaction of disuse, the underlying pathophysiologic state, and catabolic effects of stress. The ultimate effect of these interacting processes will be difficulty in weaning the patient from the ventilator.[29] An EMG pattern of fatigue has been documented in the ventilatory muscles of neonates who experienced difficulty in weaning.[9] Grassino et al.[7] found an EMG fatigue pattern in a patient being weaned from mechanical ventilation. Cohen et al.[5] found an EMG pattern of fatigue in 7 of 12 patients who experienced difficulty during discontinuation of mechanical ventilation. Resolution of the fatigue pattern was observed in those neonates who recovered[9] and in adult patients who were successfully weaned. Andersen et al.[4] studied the latter group of patients and found that thoracoabdominal discoordination was also resolved. Three recent reports indicate that respiratory muscle training may prove to be an important adjunct therapy to facilitate weaning in the patient who requires mechanical ventilation for acute respiratory failure.[30–32]

Two techniques have been used for inspiratory muscle training: isocapnic hyperventilation (also called isocapnic hyperpnea) and inspiratory resistive or resistance breathing. Isocapnic hyperventilation is dynamic and is used to increase the endurance of the inspiratory muscles. Expiratory muscles will benefit as well with this technique. Patients are asked to breathe at the highest rate they can manage for 15 to 30 minutes. A rebreathing circuit or the addition of CO_2 to the inspired air must be used with this technique in order to prevent hypocapnia. Because of this requirement, the usefulness of this technique with patients will be limited until portable, inexpensive, easy-to-use equipment for home use is developed.

Inspiratory resistive breathing allows both strength and endurance training since it incorporates both isometric and isotonic exercises. Patients inspire through a narrow tube that offers alinear airway resistance for one to three daily periods of 15 to 30 minutes. The size of the orifice through which the patient inspires is adjusted to provide a level of resistance that the patient can tolerate without becoming immediately exhausted. Currently, two inspiratory resistive breathing training devices are commercially available. Both provide six different levels of fixed inspiratory resistance, are hand held and portable, and are easily used and maintained by patients (Fig 9–3).

Potential outcomes of a training program geared toward increasing inspiratory muscle strength and endurance might include any of the following, depending on the individual patient's conditions and goals of treatment: (1) prevent acute deterioration of respiratory status and ventilatory failure; (2) improve ventilatory function and decrease the work of breathing which may lead to an increase in general exercise tolerance and an improved quality of life as tissue oxygenation improves and signs and symptoms are attenuated; and (3) facilitate the weaning process in acute respiratory failure patients who are being mechanically ventilated.

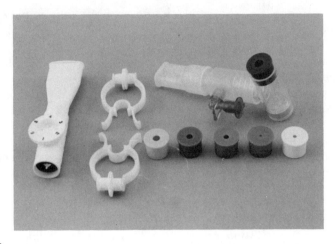

FIG 9–3.
Handheld resistive breathing training devices. **A,** P-Flex; resistance level is altered by changing settings on dial. **B,** DHD device; resistance level is altered by inserting stopper with different size orifice into inspiratory port.

SUMMARY

Inspiratory muscle training and conditioning is a new area of treatment for the respiratory patient. As such, further validation of its efficacy in treatment is needed if it is to become an accepted component of pulmonary rehabilitation programs. At this time, respiratory muscle training looks promising as a means of offering the respiratory patient one possible method of control over disease processes that are most often very debilitating and unrelenting in their course.

REFERENCES

1. Roussos C, Macklem P: The respiratory muscles. *N Engl J Med* 1982; 307:786–797.
2. Groer M, Shekleton M: *Basic Pathophysiology: A Conceptual Approach.* St Louis, CV Mosby Co, 1983.
3. Sharp J: Respiratory muscles, in Simmons D (ed): *Current Pulmonology,* vol 5. New York, John Wiley & Sons, 1984, pp 1–51.
4. Andersen J, Kann T, Rasmussen J, et al: Respiratory thoracoabdominal coordination and muscle fatigue in acute respiratory failure. *Am Rev Respir Dis* 1978; 117 (pt 2):89.
5. Cohen C, Zagelbaum G, Gross D, et al: Clinical manifestations of inspiratory muscle fatigue. *Am J Med* 1982; 73:308–316.

6. Derenne J, Macklem P, Roussos C: The respiratory muscles: Mechanics, control, and pathophysiology, Part III. *Am Rev Respir Dis* 1978; 118:581–601.

7. Grassino A, Gross D, Macklem P, et al: Inspiratory muscle fatigue as a factor limiting exercise. *Bull Eur Physiopathol Respir* 1979; 15:105–111.

8. Macklem P, Roussos C: Respiratory muscle fatigue: A cause of respiratory failure? *Clin Sci Mol Med* 1977; 53:419–422.

9. Muller N, Gulston G, Cade O, et al: Diaphragmatic muscle fatigue in the newborn. *J Appl Physiol* 1979; 46:688–695.

10. Roussos C, Fixley M, Gross D, et al: Fatigue of inspiratory muscles and their synergic behavior. *J Appl Physiol* 1979; 46:897–904.

11. Bryant S, Edwards R, Faulkner J, et al: Respiratory muscle failure: Fatigue or weakness. *Chest* 1986; 89(1):116–124.

12. Rochester D: Fatigue of the diaphragm, in Fishman A (ed): *Update: Pulmonary Diseases and Disorders.* New York, McGraw Hill Book Co, 1982, pp 87–100.

13. Edwards RHT: The diaphragm as a muscle: Mechanisms underlying fatigue. *Am Rev Respir Dis* 1979; 119(2 pt 2):81–84.

14. Edwards RHT: Biochemical bases of fatigue in exercise performance: Catastrophe theory of muscular fatigue, in Knuttgen H, Vogel J, Poortmans J (eds): *Biochemistry of Exercise.* Champaign, Illinois, Human Kinetics Publishers, 1983.

15. Macklem PT: The diaphragm in health and disease. *J Lab Clin Med* 1982; 99(5):601–610.

16. Kim MJ: Respiratory muscle training: Implications for patient care. *Heart Lung* 1984; 13(4):333–340.

17. Sharp J: Therapeutic considerations in respiratory muscle function. *Chest* 1985; 88(2) Suppl:118S–123S.

18. Aldrich T: The application of muscle endurance training techniques to the respiratory muscles in COPD. *Lung* 1985; 163:15–22.

19. Keens T, Krastens I, Wannamaker E, et al: Ventilatory muscle endurance training in normal subjects and patients with cystic fibrosis. *Am Rev Respir Dis* 1977; 116:853–860.

20. Leith D, Bradley M: Ventilatory muscle strength and endurance training. *J Appl Physiol* 1976; 41:508–516.

21. Belman M, Mittman C: Ventilatory muscle training improves exercise endurance in patients with chronic obstructive pulmonary disease. *Am Rev Respir Dis* 1980; 121:273–280.

22. Jardim J, Mayo S, Godoy I, et al: Inspiratory muscle conditioning training in chronic obstructive pulmonary disease (COPD) patients. *Am Rev Respir Dis* 1982; 125(pt 2 of 2):132.

23. Larson M, Kim MJ: Respiratory muscle training with the incentive spirometer resistive breathing device. *Heart Lung* 1984; 13(4):341–345.

24. Martin L: Respiratory muscle function: A clinical study. *Heart Lung* 1984; 13(4):346–348.

25. Sonne L, Davis J: Increased exercise performance in patients with severe COPD following inspiratory resistive training. *Chest* 1982; 81:436–439.
26. Williams M, Kim MJ, Larson J, et al: The effects of resistive breathing training on the strength and endurance of the respiratory muscles. *Am Rev Respir Dis* 1984; 129(4) pt 2 of 2:128.
27. Pardy R, Rivington R, Despas P, et al: The effects of inspiratory muscle training on exercise performance in chronic airflow limitation. *Am Rev Respir Dis* 1981; 123:426–433.
28. Pardy R, Rivington R, Despas P, et al: Inspiratory muscle training compared with physiotherapy in patients with chronic airflow limitation. *Am Rev Respir Dis* 1981; 123:421–425.
29. Gross D, Ladd H, Riley E, et al: The effect of training on strength and endurance of the diaphragm in quadriplegia. *Am J Med* 1980; 68:27–35.
30. Rochester D, Braun N: The respiratory muscles. *Basics RD* 1978; 6(4):20–25.
31. Aldrich T, Karpel J: Inspiratory muscle resistive training in respiratory failure. *Chest* 1984; 86(2):302.
32. Aldrich T, Karpel J: Inspiratory muscle resistive training in respiratory failure. *Am Rev Respir Dis* 1985; 131(3):461–462.
33. Belman M: Respiratory failure treated by ventilatory muscle training: A report of two cases. *Eur J Respir Dis* 1981; 62:391–395.

BIBLIOGRAPHY

Black L, Hyatt R: Maximal respiratory pressures: Normal values and relationship to age and sex. *Am Rev Respir Dis* 1969; 99:696–702.
Braun N: Respiratory muscle dysfunction. *Heart Lung* 1984; 13(4):327–332.
Braun N, Faulkner J, Hughes R, et al: When should respiratory muscles be exercised? *Chest* 1983; 84(1):76–84.
Derenne J, Macklem P, Roussos C: The respiratory muscles: Mechanics, control, and pathophysiology, Part I. *Am Rev Respir Dis* 1978; 118:119–133.
Nickerson B, Keens T: Measuring ventilatory muscle endurance in humans as sustainable inspiratory pressure. *J Appl Physiol* 1982; 52:768–772.
Roussos C: Function and fatigue of respiratory muscles. *Chest* 1985; 88(2):124S–132S.
Roussos C, Macklem P: Diaphragmatic fatigue in man. *J Appl Physiol* 1977; 43:189–197.
Sharp J: Respiratory muscles: A review of old and newer concepts. *Lung* 1980; 157:185–199.
Tenney S, Reese R: The ability to sustain great breathing efforts. *Respir Physiol* 1968; 5:187–201.
Wyndham C, Strydom N, van Graan C, et al: Walk or jog for health. *S Afr Med J* 1971; 45:53–57.

10

Breathing Exercise and Retraining, Chest Mobilization Exercises

Donna Frownfelter, P.T., R.R.T.

Breathing exercise is a controversial and ironic term. It is generally used, it seems, for lack of a better phrase. It is ironic because it denotes increased work to breathe on the part of a patient who already has increased exertion in breathing. Breathing control, breathing retraining or controlled breathing are probably more appropriate phrases, but due to the common use of "breathing exercise," we will be using it in this chapter.

It is appropriate to refer to the "work of breathing" concept in discussing methods of improving breathing patterns. Everyone must expend energy to perform adequate respiration. A healthy person uses approximately 5% of his total oxygen consumption for the work of breathing. Generally, 250 ml/min is the rate of oxygen consumption. Another "normal" measurement is the percentage of the vital capacity used for tidal volume (see Chapter 2). At rest, a person will use approximately 10% of his vital capacity for his tidal volume. Taking these figures as normal, we see an increased work (or energy) of breathing if the oxygen consumption is increased and the patient is using a larger percentage of his vital capacity for his tidal volume. One may test this experimentally by taking several breaths at normal tidal volume, and then increasing tidal volume to endeavor to breathe with 50% of one's vital capacity. It will quickly be realized that it is extremely fatiguing and much more energy is expended. One may then understand more fully the plight of a patient who has a low vital capacity, pain, copious secretions, bronchospasm and other symptoms, and his increased energy expenditure.

One may note several indications for controlled breathing or breathing exercise. Generally, any patient with an abnormal pattern of breathing or increased work of breathing should be treated. Breathing exercise should be emphasized in conjunction with postural drainage and respiratory therapy treatments such as ultrasonic nebulizers (USN). The results of USN will be determined by how well the patient breathes and whether they are able to cough up mucus after treatment. Proper breathing will allow the patient to increase his exercise tolerance and his state of relaxation. Relaxation is one of the most important aspects of proper breathing. We often find the patient needs to be instructed in relaxation techniques before breathing exercise can be performed. If a patient is extremely nervous and tense, it is impossible for him to breathe properly. The converse is also true. There are some patients who improve their breathing dramatically just by relaxation with very little breathing exercise. (Relaxation techniques are discussed in Chapter 8.)

There is a specific vocabulary to define specific abnormal breathing patterns. The most common are listed here.*

1. Eupnea: Normal breathing, repeated rhythmic inspiratory-expiratory cycles.

2. Hyperpnea: Increased breathing, usually refers to increased tidal volume with or without increased frequency.

3. Polypnea, tachypnea: Increased frequency of breathing.

4. Hyperventilation: Increased alveolar ventilation in relation to metabolic rate (an increase in alveolar ventilation seen is a decrease in arterial P_{CO_2}).

5. Apnea: Cessation of respiration in the resting expiratory position.

6. Apneusis: Cessation of respiration in the inspiratory position.

7. Apneustic breathing: Apneusis interrupted periodically by expiration.

*Adapted from Comroe JH, Jr: *Physiology of Respiration,* ed 2. Chicago, Year Book Medical Publishers, Inc, 1974, p 26.

8. Cheyne-Stokes respiration: Cycles of gradually increasing tidal volume followed by gradually decreasing tidal volume (usually followed by an apneic period).

9. Biot's respiration: Sequences of uniformly deep gasps, apnea and then deep gasps.

As one works in any specialized field, he becomes increasingly aware of the need to communicate effectively and learn the language of the specialty area. It is also of great importance to communicate why we are treating a patient and what we are trying to accomplish. Abnormal breathing patterns may be due to several factors. Thus, we need to discuss the specific indications and purposes for breathing exercise.

INDICATIONS FOR BREATHING EXERCISE

1. Pain: From surgery or trauma.

2. Nervousness, apprehension.

3. Surgical procedures such as thoracic surgery or abdominal surgery.

4. Bronchospasm.

5. Airway obstruction.

6. Atelectasis.

7. Restriction due to musculoskeletal abnormalities, obesity, pregnancy, increased gas in the stomach, pulmonary pathology such as fibrosis, or secondary pulmonary effects such as in scleroderma.

8. Central nervous system deficit.

9. Narcotic medications or drug overdose.

10. Pulmonary disease, either primary or secondary.

11. Neurologic patients with muscle weakness and/or uncoordination, such as myasthenia gravis, Guillain-Barré or spinal cord injuries.

12. Pulmonary emboli.

13. Pulmonary edema, congestive heart failure.

14. Ventilatory insufficiency or failure.

15. Metabolic disturbances (acidosis, alkalosis) with a compensatory respiratory response.

16. Patients on ventilators often will have uncoordinated diaphragmatic movement.

17. Pleural reactions: Pain, effusion.

18. Debilitated or bedridden patients that tend to hypoventilate and retain secretions.

This list is not inclusive but gives an overall idea of the subject. Whatever the reason for the abnormal breathing pattern, it becomes an indication for breathing exercises.

Before one discusses improvement of breathing patterns, one must note the normal patterns. As discussed in Chapter 1, the diaphragm and external intercostals are used in quiet breathing. As one increases his work and exercise, the accessory muscles tend to come into play. These are primarily the sternocleidomastoid, trapezius, scalenes, pectoralis major and serratus anterior. Normal expiration is passive, with the internal intercostals possibly playing a role. In forced expiration, the abdominal muscles are involved. These muscles are the rectus abdominus, transversus abdominus, and internal and external obliques.

There is also a normal sequence of inspiration which the therapist should observe:

1. The diaphragm contracts, therefore the upper abdomen rises.

2. Lateral costal expansion—also due to the diaphragm, the ribs move up and out to the side.

3. The upper chest rises.

In relaxed breathing, the diaphragm and external intercostals are used and a 1, 2, 3 sequence is observed. Generally, the upper chest moves little in quiet breathing. If it does rise, it should rise after the abdomen and ribs flare.

GOALS OF BREATHING EXERCISE

1. To improve ventilation.

2. To prevent atelectasis.

3. To decrease the work of breathing.

4. To increase cough efficiency.

5. To increase strength, coordination and efficiency of respiratory muscles.

6. To correct abnormal breathing patterns.

7. To teach the patient what to do in case of an "attack" of shortness of breath.

8. To reinforce the patient's determination to help himself and gain confidence in his ability to control his breathing.

9. To help the patient relax.

10. To mobilize and maintain mobility of the chest wall.

PROCEDURE FOR BREATHING EXERCISE

In order to determine the specific therapy indicated, one must properly assess the patient's breathing pattern. It is found that observation may be effectively done while the patient is either aware or unaware that he is being observed. When observing the patient unaware, the therapist obtains much significant information. Does he appear relaxed or tense? Is he short of breath? Is he using accessory muscles? What position does he favor? Is he smoking? Does he seem to have a chronic, ineffective cough? Does he appear to be uncomfortable? Does he talk in full sentences or need to take a breath in between? Is his coloring good—are his nail beds or lips cyanotic? Are his fingers clubbed? Does he need to sit up high in bed or lie flat? The list could go on and on. Patients often will try to seem either better or worse than usual if they know a therapist is evaluating them, and this can be avoided by observing with the patient unaware.

When the patient is aware he is being observed and evaluated, additional points, such as the following, may be noted. How well can he relax consciously? Can he cooperate with the exercise? On manual exam, are both sides moving symmetrically? Can he position himself and move about well? What is his level of motivation?

As we begin to discuss specific breathing exercises, it is important to make a few generalizations. Positioning of the patient is extremely important. One strives for a relaxed, comfortable symmetrical position that allows freedom of abdominal and thoracic movement. The position will be changed to gradually progress the patient to activities of daily living (ADL) as tolerated. If the patient is unable to relax, specific relaxation procedures such as Jacobsen's relaxation exercises may be encouraged prior to breathing exercises. The room atmosphere and rapport with the therapist and staff will also assist in relaxing the patient.

In general, the patient should breathe in through his nose and out through his mouth. However, this should not be made a prime point. Many patients are mouth breathers by habit or necessity (such as those with nasal polyps or obstruction). These patients may often concentrate so hard on breathing in through their noses that they are unable to concentrate on proper breathing patterns. Often the most helpful procedure is to give the patient audible clues and ask him to follow your breathing. The therapist then breathes aloud to guide the patient. This will usually have much more impact than explaining, "Breathe in through your nose," etc. The patient needs simple, short commands. It becomes confusing to a patient to be instructed to: "(1) relax; (2) push your abdomen into my hand, or swell up around your waist; (3) breathe in through your nose and out through your mouth; (4) relax; (5) slow down." A patient has difficulty performing and understanding such a variety of verbal inputs. *Example* is easier to follow than verbal commands. This is seen frequently in patients that do not speak the language of the therapist and a pantomime ensues. Generally, these patients do *quite well as they simply "follow the leader."*

Finally, patient tolerance must be emphasized. Many short periods are often more effective than long sessions.

With this background, we now discuss specific breathing exercises. Usually the patient will first be instructed in diaphragmatic breathing. Either unilateral or bilateral costal breathing will be initiated later. Segmental breathing to emphasize selected areas may be used, as well as a number of total patterns and diaphragm strengthening exercises.

DIAPHRAGMATIC BREATHING

Diaphragmatic breathing is the normal mode of respiration. The diaphragm and external intercostals are the normal muscles of inspiration. If, in evaluating a patient's breathing pattern, the therapist observes the use of accessory muscles, the patient needs to be instructed in relaxation of accessory muscles and proper use of the diaphragm. The exception to this would be a patient with neuromuscular weakness (i.e., spinal cord injury, postpolio) that would need to utilize accessory muscles (see Chapter 21).

The author generally utilizes a sequential approach to diaphragmatic breathing. Generally, the sequence is taught with the patient in different positions which increase the difficulty and coordination of the procedure. The position sequence is:

1. Supine and well supported at about 45 degrees with knees flexed and hips in external rotation (Figs 10–1 and 10–2).

2. Sitting in a chair or at bedside (Fig 10–3).

3. Standing (Fig 10–4).

4. Walking (Fig 10–5).

5. Stairs (Fig 10–6).

6. Other activities such as lifting heavy objects, making a bed, carrying groceries or playing golf. These are done when the patient and therapist discuss specific breathing problems and try to find solutions.

Procedure for Teaching Diaphragmatic Breathing

1. *Explain* the purpose and goals of a breathing exercise.

2. *Position* the patient supine at a 45-degree angle in a relaxed, well-supported position, usually at the start of the sequence.

3. *Demonstrate* the technique and continue explaining the reasoning.

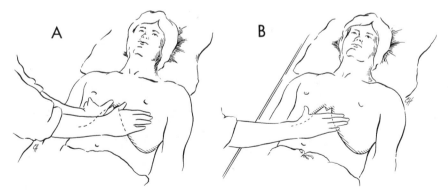

FIG 10–1.
A, placement of hands for diaphragmatic breathing (especially for a large patient where one hand is inadequate). **B,** therapist's hand placement for diaphragmatic breathing.

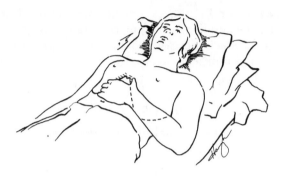

FIG 10–2.
The patient is encouraged to continue practicing diaphragmatic breathing to become aware of his breathing pattern. This is usually the first position of the diaphragmatic breathing teaching sequence.

4. *Place hand or hands* at the costophrenic angle as shown. Follow the patient's breathing: ask him to breathe as he usually does. Do not "invade" the patient's breathing pattern. Rather, gently squeeze down and inward during exhalation. Allow him to breathe in against your hand during inspiration.

5. After following several respiratory cycles, as exhalation proceeds, squeeze more firmly and say, "*Now! Push* into my hand." (The short command should be stated just at the end of exhalation. The verbal command prepares the patient for action. The stretch will facil-

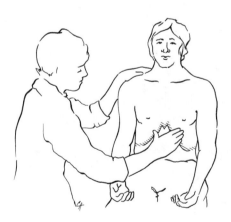

FIG 10–3.
The patient advances to the sitting position for breathing retraining. Note the relaxed position of the patient's shoulders and hands.

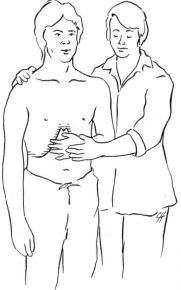

FIG 10–4.
The third position in the sequence is standing. Full-length mirrors are helpful at this point.

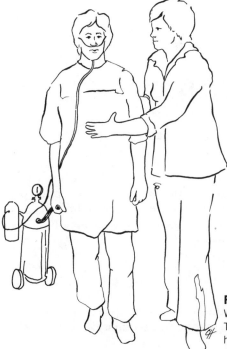

FIG 10–5.
Walking is the fourth stage of retraining. The patient is encouraged to relax, control his breathing, take long steps and *slow* down.

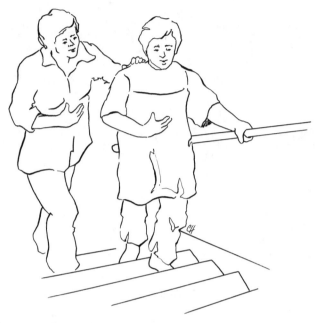

FIG 10–6.
Stairs are important, especially if the patient has them at home. He is instructed to pause slightly as he breathes in and to exhale as he climbs one to two stairs.

itate the muscular response.) Nothing was said to the patient regarding breathing in through his nose. Initially, the most important factor is understanding the diaphragmatic movement.

6. The therapist will follow several cycles of stretching the costo-phrenic angle and asking the patient to push into his hand.

7. The patient should then be asked if he feels the difference between the breathing he is doing now with the therapist as opposed to his previous pattern. If he feels no difference, the procedure needs to be repeated and reinforced. Perhaps an additional explanation of what he should be feeling needs to be included.

8. When the patient "feels" the proper breathing, he is asked to continue to try to perform the maneuver independently. His hands should be placed appropriately and time should be allowed to concentrate on the procedure. Initially, the therapist can place his hand atop the patient's to help him feel the rhythm and sequence.

Note: a few things to check and observe at this point are:

1. Forced expiration should be avoided as this will promote airway collapse. A slow, relaxed, pursed-lip breathing may be encouraged.

2. Greatly prolonged expiration should be discouraged. Often chronic lung patients try to "squeeze" every bit of air from their lungs. This makes them virtually gasp for their next breath and their pattern becomes irregular.

3. Observe the patient's trunk carefully to make sure he isn't hyperextending his back to give the appearance of "pushing" his abdomen out.

4. Also observe the abdomen so that the patient is not "bloating" his lower abdomen out.

5. Some patients will also tend to overuse their upper chest. The upper chest should be relatively relaxed.

6. The patient should be reminded to breathe at about the same volume that he usually does. Frequently, patients will try to breathe very deeply and may hyperventilate. The patient should concentrate on breathing for only short periods of time to avoid hyperventilation. Signs to observe are patients complaining of dizziness and tingling in their fingers.

When discussing the diaphragmatic breathing in sequence with patients, they say overwhelmingly that it is necessary to teach breathing in several positions and activities. If breathing is taught only with patients supine or sitting, when they get up and walk or use stairs they are unable to control their breathing. Thus, we are emphatic about working through various activities. Much of this seems to be common sense but it is observed over and over that in times of stress, it is difficult to think clearly and reason what to do. Breathing is generally automatic, yet patients with respiratory difficulty need to think ahead and plan to conserve energy.

When the patient seems to be understanding and performing diaphragmatic breathing well, he should be advanced to the sitting position. The increase in difficulty with sitting comes from the fact that in a supine, supported position, the patient has to concentrate only on breathing. When sitting, he must balance himself, relax his shoulders, and breathe.

In the standing position, the patient needs to relax, breathe and balance his stance. However, much more difficulty is involved in walking and climbing stairs because now the patient must learn not only to control his breathing but also to coordinate it with his activity.

In walking, breathing is "patterned" to be regular. Generally, our inspiratory:expiratory (I:E) ratio is 1:2. This ratio is utilized in walking by trying to count steps and breathe in coordination. For example, the patient may breathe in for two steps and blow out for four steps. He may breathe in for three and blow out for six steps. *There is no set pattern.* The only rule of thumb is that the I:E ratio should be one that can be continued for a long period. Sometimes patients try to take very long inspiration and prolong expiration unduly. For example, breathing in for four steps and blowing out for eight is common. Usually, this becomes too tiring and should be discouraged. The goal is for the patient to develop a pattern of breathing that will increase exercise tolerance. Actually, a patient should think of blowing out for longer than he breathes in, or at least equal to the inspiration. Generally, patients will tend to have irregular, almost gasping inspirations when they are walking or under stress. Patient education is necessary to help them understand what they usually do and what method is more efficient. Most patients find their walking tolerance greatly improved by controlling and patterning their breathing.

Stair climbing also presents great difficulty for many patients. Generally, patients will take a deep breath and hold it while they try to climb several stairs. They will then blow the air out in exhaustion (whew!) and become short of breath. Some simple principles help in this situation. First, gain breathing control at the base of the stairs, then breathe in while standing still and exhale while climbing one or two stairs. Patients should pause slightly during inspiration and continue to climb as they exhale. As the patient learns the patterning, the movement becomes smoother, but initially it does help to make a definite pause for inspiration (see Fig 10–6). The ascent of the stairs should be slow. The patient should make sure his entire foot is on the stair so he has firm support and balance. He should also hold the railing if one is available. If he does become quite short of breath, he can put his foot up a stair or two and lean forward on his knee or on the railing to relax and gain breath control.

Other special cases for consideration with the patient are instances when he becomes short of breath. A general statement may be made that when the normal breathing sequence is interrupted, the patient becomes short of breath. The situation should be analyzed and discussion centered on how to prevent the problem in the future. Several common instances are generally cited for triggering attacks of shortness of breath. Among these are lifting a heavy object, talking, eating, being nervous, having a bowel movement, mowing the lawn, carrying shopping bags and making a bed. Each patient needs to evaluate factors causing his own shortness of breath.

To demonstrate to a patient how he should do this, let us take two of these examples and follow them through. When a patient complains of shortness of breath while eating, usually it is because of habit or fear of shortness of breath (SOB) that he eats quickly and tries to "beat" it. He is obviously interrupting his breathing pattern because the epiglottis must close to prevent aspiration. If he eats quickly, he cannot have much time to breathe. By slowing his eating and pausing between every few bites, he will be less short of breath and enjoy his meal more.

In lifting a heavy object or having a bowel movement, the patient will perform the Valsalva maneuver due to the strain. Patients should be aware of this and be encouraged not to hold their breath or bear down unduly. If they must, they should relax and take several deep breaths in between the bearing down phases.

Patients learn quickly how to analyze their breathing problems and in many instances will surprise the therapist with ideas to suggest to other patients.

In this discussion, we have covered breathing retraining and instruction in proper use of the diaphragm. There are many instances when a more specialized technique may be necessary to emphasize specific problem areas in the lungs. Some examples of these could be atelectasis, pneumonia, muscle splinting from pain and thus hypoventilation, after cardiovascular or thoracic surgery, tight chest walls, and scoliosis or kyphoscoliosis, to name a few. The technique of choice in these instances is segmental or lateral-costal breathing, emphasizing the problem lung area. The therapist's hand placed over the surface area of the lung being emphasized delivers proprioceptive input for selected muscular movement. The therapist places her hands on the chest wall and follows several respiratory cycles, "squeezing" the chest during exhalation and allowing the patient's chest to move during inspiration. Then, at the end of an expiration, she squeezes the chest and asks the patient to push up against her hands. The therapist continues to assist in exhalation and also gives some resistance to inspiration to make the patient inhale more fully.

The selected areas for hand placement are: lateral costal either unilateral or bilateral, anteriorly at the lower ribs for the lower lobes, mid chest (midaxillary area) for right middle lobe or lingula, upper chest for upper lobes and posteriorly at the lower chest and mid chest (Figs 10–7 to 10–16).

Physical therapists familiar with proprioceptive neuromuscular facilitation (PNF) techniques can also apply them to segmental breathing. Repeated contractions are especially helpful. The patient is asked to take a deep breath and hold it. He is then asked to breath more, more, more, while repeated stretch is given. This is especially effective if administered over the sternum or in the lateral-costal area. The coordination of commands and stretch are very important. Most therapists find a slower stretch helpful with chronic lungers since a very rapid stretch may make the patient more tense and make relaxation difficult. The pressure given in stretch techniques needs to be evaluated as many patients have tight barrel chests that are inflexible. It would not be appropriate to try to give much pressure to a patient with a barrel chest.

For therapists and nurses, a modification of these techniques is also helpful. The patient is told to think of a sneeze in which he takes a breath, holds it, then ah-ah-ah-ah-choo! The patient usually can relate to the "stretching" of his lungs and chest in this maneuver to increase vital capacity. It is often helpful to do this exercise three or four times

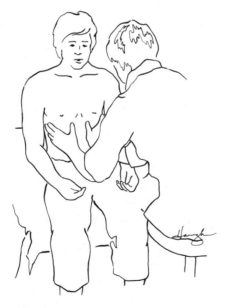

FIG 10–7.
Bilateral lower lobe expansion (this also facilitates diaphragmatic movement).

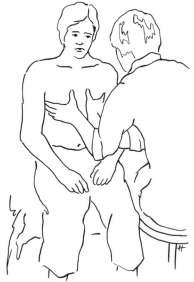

FIG 10–8.
Bilateral midchest expansion exercise.

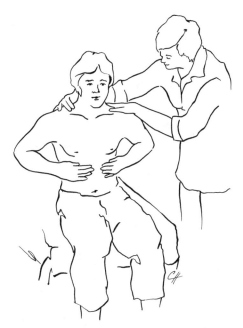

FIG 10–9.
Bilateral chest expansion exercise. Keep the patient's shoulders relaxed.

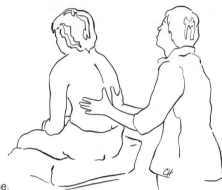

FIG 10–10.
Bilateral posterior chest expansion exercise.

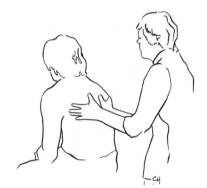

FIG 10–11.
Bilateral posterior chest expansion exercise.

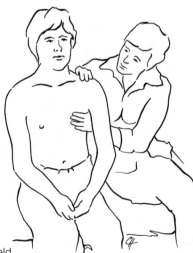

FIG 10–12.
Unilateral (segmental) breathing, left mid-lung field.

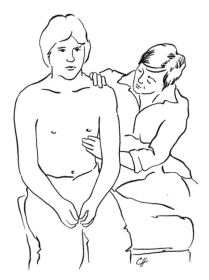

FIG 10–13.
Unilateral (segmental) breathing emphasizing the left lower lobe. Note that the patient's shoulder must remain down, with hands placed on ulnar border or palm up in his lap.

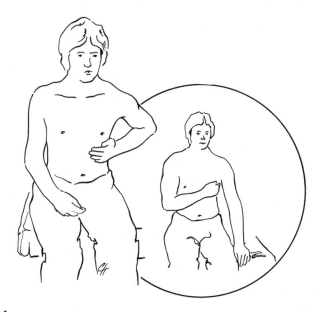

FIG 10–14.
The patient can perform unilateral (segmental) breathing by placing either hand on the side of the chest to be emphasized. The patient can also perform mid-chest expansion by moving his hand up.

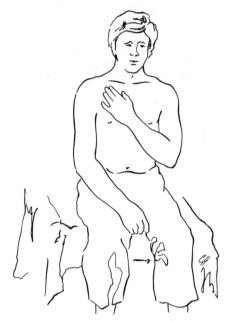

FIG 10–15.
Segmental right upper lobe expansion exercise.

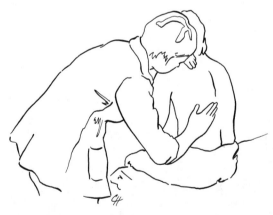

FIG 10–16.
Unilateral (segmental) posterior chest expansion (left lower lobe).

prior to coughing to increase distribution of ventilation and "loosen" mucus. The therapist can also give hand contact and direct the patient to push against her hand as he repeats the breathing to selectively aerate the emphasized area.

Total patterns, or the use of a movement of the entire body, may be used very effectively with breathing exercise. In this exercise, the patient reinforces one movement with another. For example, as a patient flexes his trunk, the abdominal viscera compress the diaphragm and will facilitate expiration. When a patient extends his trunk, inspiration is facilitated. A few examples will be discussed.

Patient Sitting. The patient is asked to exhale as he bends forward to touch the floor. His arms should come to the midline. As he extends, he inspires and lifts his arms up and out to a "V" above his head (Fig 10–17).

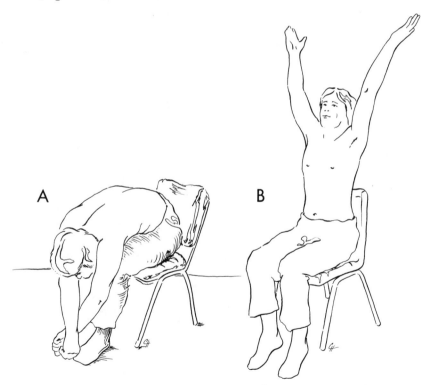

FIG 10–17.
A, chest mobilization. Total pattern exercise. Patient exhales during flexion. **B,** patient stretches and breathes in during the extension phase.

Patient Sitting. The patient again is instructed to exhale but rather than flex forward, he rotates to the right side to touch the floor at the lateral condyle of the right ankle. (This stretches the left lateral and posterior chest.) He then inspires as he extends and rotates to the opposite side as in the illustration. This procedure is then reversed to mobilize the right lateral and posterior chest (Fig 10–18).

Both of the above methods can be performed with a cane or wand and often this gives the patient better guidelines for movement. One should also give visual clues for a total pattern, such as looking down as you bend forward and looking up as you extend.

Patient Lying Supine. To strengthen abdominal muscles, the patient can do modified or conventional sit-ups. The patient flexes his

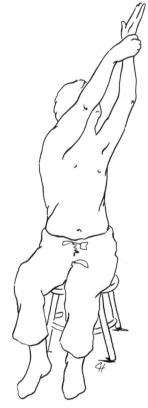

FIG 10–18.
Chest mobilization using trunk rotation and PNF (chopping and lifting) patterns.

knees, takes a breath, lifts his head and pulls his knees toward his chest during exhalation. He inspires while extending back to a supine position. A patient who is quite weak can try to lift only his head and shoulders and exhale, or even just lift his head. Minimum work for abdominal muscles is simply to practice "blowing out" while supine. The patient must be monitored to prevent hyperventilation. Often a few relaxed breaths will be needed between sit-ups or pulling in abdominal muscles. Many patients are unable to do sit-ups in one breath in and out. They may do the exercise in two breaths. Breathe in while supine, then exhale while flexing. Take a breath in and out while holding knees; then breathe in during extension. The patient should then rest and take several breaths while supine. As with any difficult exercise, patient tolerance needs to be considered, and repetitions and difficulty of exercise need to be graded carefully.

Patient on Hands and Knees.   The hands and knees position has been found particularly helpful for many patients with respiratory problems. The reasons for this may be that there is a reflex contraction of abdominal muscles in this position, the abdominal viscera fall away from the diaphragm (gravity eliminated position), and also because the shoulder girdle is stabilized. Thus, in a chronic lung patient who ordinarily has difficulty in exhalation and uses accessory muscles, there is automatic relief of symptoms.

Variations of Hands and Knees Position.   The patient can rock forward to extension as he inspires and rock back to heel-sitting with head and neck flexed during exhalation. This should be slow, relaxed and rhythmic, pausing in the flexed position for an additional one or two breaths. Then the patient rocks forward during inspiration and continues the cycle.

Modified Push-ups.   The patient is instructed to place his hands on a wall and exhale as he lets his arms bend and lowers himself to the wall. He inspires as he pushes away and extends his body. As general strength improves, he may choose to use a lower, stable object such as a heavy table or sink to lower himself. Few patients are able to do complete floor push-ups. The patient must be monitored closely in this instance so that he *does not* do the Valsalva maneuver due to the strain of the exercise.

General Exercise.   General conditioning exercise will be covered under pulmonary rehabilitation but at this point it will suffice to say the patient needs to get his musculature in tone. Usually exercise such as swimming, bicycling, walking, mowing the lawn, doing general housework and shopping will help keep the patient fit, if done regularly. We try not to give a calisthenics program to patients to remind them of their disability, but rather we try to increase their activities of daily living and concentrate on their abilities.

Other Chest Mobilization Exercises.   Any exercise that affects the upper extremities or trunk will help to mobilize the chest (Figs 10–17 to 10–22).

Incentive Spirometers.   Figures 10–23 and 10–24 illustrate the use of these devices.

INCENTIVE SPIROMETRY

When utilizing these devices, the patient is asked to breathe in and hold the balls (floats, bellows) up for three seconds (inspiratory hold). The

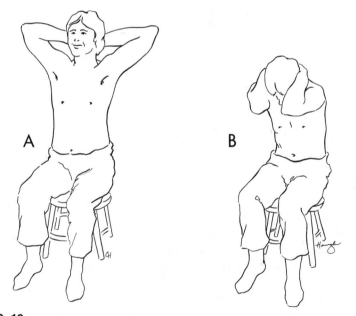

FIG 10–19.
A, chest mobilization exercise; breathe in during extension. **B,** chest mobilization; breathe out during flexion.

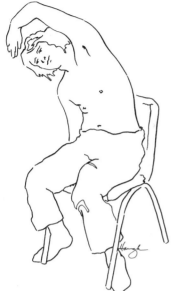

FIG 10–20.
Chest mobilization, lateral flexion; patient exhales during lateral bending.

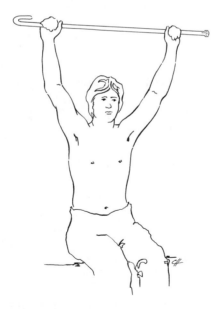

FIG 10–21.
Cane exercise. Patient may do flexion-extension or rotation exercise (all coordinated with proper breathing patterns).

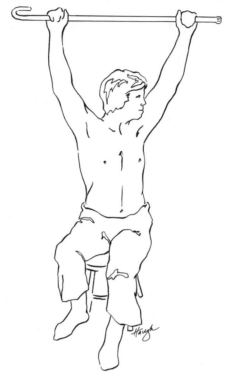

FIG 10–22.
Cane exercises for chest mobilization. Patient exhales as he rotates his trunk.

purpose of the inspiratory hold is to allow time for collateral ventilation to occur in the alveoli. When the patient takes a deep inspiration, air will follow the path of least resistance. If small airways leading to the alveoli are plugged with mucus, little ventilation goes to the alveoli. When the patient performs a slow inspiration (15–30 lpm) and an inspiratory hold, the well-ventilated alveoli will donate air to the underventilated alveoli through the pores of Kohn.

It is important to emphasize a slow, deep inspiration and inspiratory hold when instructing the patient to use the incentive spirometer. Patients often try to "blow" into the incentive spirometer. It is also important to emphasize breathing from the diaphragm. The patient should be instructed to breathe from the lower ribs and upper abdomen rather than the upper chest when using the incentive spirometer. The therapist can place his/her hands on the patient's ribs to facilitate the breathing pattern. A patient having difficulty utilizing the device

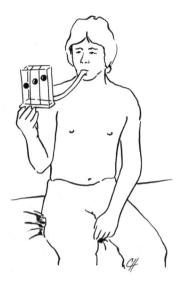

FIG 10–23.
Incentive spirometer is a simple device that will often greatly encourage the patient to take deep breaths (especially following surgery). He is encouraged to hold the spheres up for a few seconds to permit better distribution of ventilation.

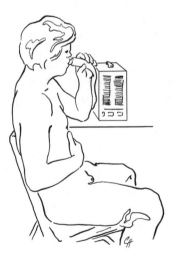

FIG 10–24.
The patient is encouraged to perform diaphragmatic breathing independently with an incentive spirometer.

may have success if he is reminded to exhale fully (blow out the air) before initiating the inspiration with the incentive spirometer. As a follow-up to the treatment session, the patient is asked to use the incentive spirometer hourly, 10–15 times per hour.

Hyperventilation is a potential side effect if patients overuse or try too hard with the device. They will usually complain of dizziness or having tingling in their fingers. If this happens, patients should be told to use fewer repetitions on the device or to rest in between breaths instead of doing 20 consecutive breaths.

INSPIRATORY RESISTANCE BREATHING EXERCISE

As noted in the previous chapter, inspiratory resistance exercise has been shown to be beneficial with patients with chronic obstructive lung disease, neurological dysfunction, and secondary respiratory problems.

The training starts at the largest orifice with the patient maintaining his mouth around the mouthpiece (preferably with a noseclip) for the total time of the exercise. The hardest thing for a patient to get used to is learning how to swallow saliva while keeping the mouthpiece in place. The goal is to work up to sessions breathing with the device for 15–30 minutes. When the patient is able to do the largest hole, the next smaller hold is utilized until the patient can accomplish 15–30 minutes at that setting. This method continues until the smallest pinhole orifice is reached. If difficulty is experienced when the patient goes to a smaller orifice, he should stay there and continue to work at that level rather than going back to a larger orifice. It is better to use the smaller orifice and go to a shorter time period and work up to 15–30. A negative inspiratory force manometer can be utilized to note progress in inspiratory muscle force. The training effect will only be maintained if the patient continues to utilize inspiratory resistance breathing or becomes more physically active so he ventilates to a higher level to accomplish the same level of use of the inspiratory muscles. It is the old adage of "use it or lose it." The patient can be encouraged to do inspiratory resistance breathing while watching TV, listening to the radio, or just giving their spouse a chance to talk for an uninterrupted 30 minutes!

This device may have real benefit preoperatively with patients that are high risk for surgery in order to help them improve their respiratory strength and endurance before surgery.

REFERENCES

Periodicals

Barach A: Breathing exercises in pulmonary emphysema and allied chronic pulmonary disease. *Arch Phys Med Rehabil* 1955; 36:379.

Barach A: Chronic obstructive lung disease: Postural relief of dyspnea. *Arch Phys Med Rehabil* 1974; 55:494.

Barach A: Effect of abdominal compression on minute ventilation of patients with chronic obstructive lung disease and bronchial asthma. *Ann Allergy* 1976; 36:231.

Barach A, Seamon A: Role of the diaphragm in chronic pulmonary emphysema. *NY State J Med* 1963; 63:415.

Bartlett R, Gazzaniga A, Geraghty T: Respiratory maneuvers to prevent postoperative pulmonary complications: A critical review. *JAMA* 1973; 224:1017.

Donaldson A, Gandevia B: The physiotherapy of emphysema. *Aust J Physiother* 1962; 8:55.

Egbert L, Battit G, Bartlett M: Reduction of postoperative pain by encouragement and instruction of patients. *N Engl J Med* 1964; 270:825.

Gaskell D: Physiotherapy in obstructive airways diseases. *Physiotherapy* 1976; 62:53.

Grimby G: Aspects of lung expansion in relation to pulmonary physiotherapy. *Am Rev Respir Dis* 1974; 110:145.

Harmony W: Segmental breathing. *Phys Ther* 1956; 36:106.

Innocenti D: Breathing exercises in the treatment of emphysema. *Physiotherapy* 1966; 52:437.

Innocenti D: Chest conditions. *Physiotherapy* 1969; 52:437.

Johnston R, Lee KH: Myofeedback, a new method of teaching breathing exercises in emphysematous patients. *Phys Ther* 1976; 56:826.

Jones J: Physical therapy—present state of the art. Part II. *Am Rev Respir Dis* 1974; 110:133.

Martin C, et al: Chest physiotherapy and the distribution of ventilation. *Chest* 1976; 69:2.

McNeil R, McKenzie J: An assessment of the value of breathing exercise in chronic bronchitis and asthma. *Thorax* 1955; 10:250.

Motley H: The effects of slow deep breathing on the blood gas exchange in emphysema. *Am Rev Respir Dis* 1963; 88:484.

Petty T, Guthrie A: The effects of augmented breathing maneuvers on ventilation in severe chronic airway obstruction. *Respir Care* 1971; 46:104.

Pfeiffer V, Wilson N, Wilson R: Breathing patterns and gas mixing in patients with pulmonary emphysema. *J Am Phys Ther Assoc* 1964; 44:331.

Quimby G: Aspects of lung expansion in pulmonary physiotherapy. *Am Rev Respir Dis* 1974; 110:145.

Roe B: Prevention and treatment of respiratory complications in surgery. *N Engl J Med* 1960; 263:547.

Rottenburg C, Holaday D: Lung physiotherapy as an adjunct to surgical care. *Surg Clin North Am* 1964; 44:219.

Sharp J, et al: Respiratory muscle function in patients with COPD: Its relationship to disability and respiratory therapy. *Am Rev Respir Dis* 1974; 110:154.

Shearer M, et al: Lung ventilation during diaphragmatic breathing. *Phys Ther* 1972; 52:139.

Stein M, Cassara E: Preoperative-pulmonary evaluation and therapy for surgical patients. *JAMA* 1970; 211:787–790.

Thoren L: Postoperative pulmonary complications: Observations on their prevention by means of physiotherapy. *Acta Chir Scand* 1954; 107:193.

Warren A: Mobilization of the chest wall. *Chest Disord Child* 1968; 48:582.

Watts N: Improvement in breathing patterns. *Chest Disord Child* 1968; 48:563.

Watts N: Improvement of breathing patterns. *Phys Ther* 1968; 48:563.

Webber B: Current trends in the treatment of asthma. *Physiotherapy* 1973; 59:388.

Williams T, Prater D: The physiotherapist and abdominal operations. *Physiotherapy* 1950; 36:248.

Books

Gaskell D, Welsher B: *The Brompton Hospital Guide to Chest Physiotherapy*, ed 2. Philadelphia, FA Davis, 1973.

Knott M, Voss E: *Proprioceptive Neuromuscular Facilitation*, ed 2. New York, Harper & Row, 1968.

Rusk H: *Rehabilitation Medicine*, ed 3. St Louis, CV Mosby Co, 1971.

Miscellaneous

Asthma Research Council: *Physical Exercises for Asthma*, ed 8. London, His Majesty's Stationery Office, 1949.

Breathing Exercises

Carrieri VK, Janson-Bjerklie S, Jacobs S: The sensation of dyspnea: A review. *Heart Lung* 1984; 13(4):436–447.

Casciari RJ, Fairsbter RD, Harrison A, et al: Effects of breathing retraining in patients with chronic obstructive pulmonary disease. *Chest* 1981; 79(4):393–398.

Craig DB: Postoperative recovery of pulmonary function. *Anesth Analg (Cleve)* 1981; 60(1):46–52.

Cserhati EF, Gegesi Kiss A, Poder G, et al: Thorax deformity and asthma bronchial. *Allergol Immunopathol (Madr)* 1984; 12(1):7–10.

Evans TW, Howard P: Whistle for your wind. *Br Med J (Clin Res)* 1984; 289(6443):449–450.

Grassinoa-Bellemare F, Laporta D: Diaphragm fatigue and the strategy of breathing in COPD. *Chest* 1984; 85(6 Suppl):515–545.

Greenwood BS: The before and after of good postop pulmonary care. *Nursing (Horsham)* 1982; (12):68–69.

Kulpati DD, Kamath RK, Chauhan MR: The influence of physical conditioning by yogasanas and breathing exercises in patients of chronic obstructive lung disease. *J Assoc Physicians India* 1982; 30(12):865–868.

Mahler DA, Weinberg DH, Wells CK, et al: The measurement of dyspnea. *Chest* 1984; 85(6):751–758.

Ratnam KV, Sim MK: Treatment of disease without the use of drugs. IV. Self-treatment of asthma by thought control and breathing exercises. *Singapore Med J* 1980; 21(3):604–608.

Risser NL: Preoperative and postoperative care to prevent pulmonary complications. *Heart Lung* 1980; 9(1):57–67.

Shaffer TH, Wolfson MR, Bhutani VK: Respiratory muscle function assessment, and training. *Phys Ther* 1981; 61(12):1711–1723.

Williams IP, Smith CM, McGavin CR: Diagraphmatic breathing training and walking performance in chronic airways obstruction. *Br J Dis Chest* 1982; 76(2):164–166.

Anderson JB, Falk P: Clinical experience with inspiratory resistance breathing training. *Int Rehabil Med* 1984; 6(4):183–185.

Asher MI, Pardy RL, Coates AL, et al: The effects of inspiratory muscle training in patients with cystic fibrosis. *Am Rev Respir Dis* 1982; 126(5):855–859.

Belman MS, Dendregan BA: Physical training fails to improve ventilatory muscle endurance in patients with chronic obstructive pulmonary disease. *Chest* 1982; 81(4):440–443.

Chen H, Dukes R, Martin BJ: Inspiratory muscle training in patients with chronic obstructive pulmonary disease. *Am Rev Respir Dis* 1985; 131(2):251–255.

Larson M, Kim MJ: Respiratory muscle training with the incentive spirometer resistance breathing device. *Heart Lung* 1984; 13(4):341–345.

Pardy RL, Leith DE: Ventilatory muscle training. *Respir Care* 1984; 29:278–284.

Pardy RL, Rivington RU, Despas JP, et al: Inspiratory muscle training compared with physiotherapy in patients with chronic airflow limitation. *Am Rev Respir Dis* 1981; 123 (4 pt 1):421–425.

Reid WD, Loveridge BM: Ventilatory muscle endurance training in patients with chronic obstructive airways disease. *Physiother Can* 1983; 35:197–205.

Sonne LJ, Davis JA: Increased exercise performance in patients with severe COPD following inspiratory resistive training. *Chest* 1982; 81(4):436–469.

11

Cough

Donna Frownfelter, P.T., R.R.T.

"Cough truly serves many purposes: a therapeutic technique, a diagnostic signpost, and a social necessity. If it didn't already exist, we would have to invent it."

Glen A. Lillington, M.D.

A cough may be thought of as a "housekeeping" device necessary for maintenance of bronchial hygiene during unusual conditions in the respiratory system. Generally, one coughs when there are either abnormal kinds or quantities of material in the airways. Under normal circumstances, one coughs very little because the mucociliary escalator is mainly responsible for mucus clearance.

The cough mechanism functions to promote airway clearance of excess mucus and foreign bodies in the tracheobronchial tree. The impairment of the cough mechanism will result in retained mucus secretions and bronchial obstruction.

A cough may be either a reflex or a voluntary action. The mechanism of a cough is described as: (1) a deep inspiration; (2) the closure of the glottis; (3) contraction of the muscles of the chest wall, abdomen and pelvic floor (in order to increase intrathoracic and intra-abdominal pressure); (4) opening of the glottis and (5) a rapid expulsive exhalation phase (Fig 11–1). During a cough, pressures (alveolar, pleural and subglottic) may rise as much as 200 cm/H_2O.

The cough is often taken for granted. Many people are unaware of their coughing. (Consider the number of people with a "smoker's" cough who are unaware that they cough.) It is important that patients be made aware of both their reflex and voluntary coughs.

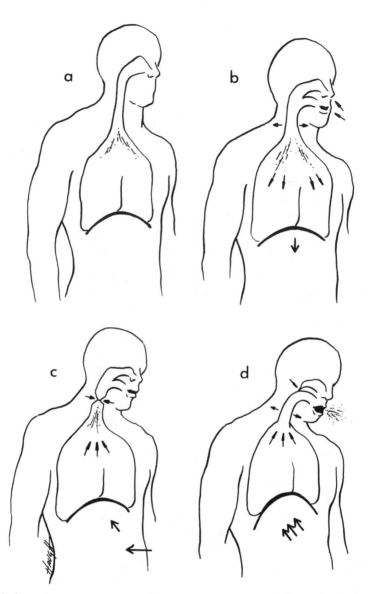

FIG 11–1.
Cough mechanics. **A,** deep inspiration. **B,** glottis closes, causing a buildup of intrathoracic and intra-abdominal pressure. **C,** glottis opens. **D,** rapid expulsion of air occurs as a result of forceful abdominal contraction.

Often patients deny coughing even though they may be coughing frequently during your evaluation. Frequent throat clearing is a form of coughing very typical in patients with asthma and/or postnasal drip. If the patient is chronically coughing, an evaluation of the precipitating factor is needed. Most patients with a chronic cough have chronic bronchitis. Other causes may be bronchogenic carcinoma, pneumonia, asthma, psychogenic origins, smoking, or postnasal drip. This list is not exhaustive. Any factor that causes irritation in the tracheobronchial tree could cause a cough. One thing to consider as well is dehydration of the mucociliary blanket. Basically the mucociliary escalator clears mucus from the airways. When it is not functioning properly, the cough mechanism will attempt to rid secretions from the airways.

The intricacy of the cough mechanism may be appreciated by looking at its pumplike effect. Mucus must literally be pumped up a series of branching tubes against gravity. It should be obvious that much energy is required to perform that function.

A few important points should be made regarding the cough mechanism which will have great clinical significance in teaching patients how to cough. First, the cough is most effective at high expiratory flow rates and at high volumes. Generally, high volumes are necessary to generate high expiratory flow rates. Second, the cough is of limited value beyond the sixth or seventh generation of branching. Therefore, if a patient has lower lobe pneumonia or atelectasis or bronchiectasis, coughing alone will be unable to clear the retained secretions. (Postural drainage must be performed first to move secretions upward and allow the mucociliary escalator to carry them to regions where the cough is effective.)

If a cough is associated with eating, swallowing disturbances should be evaluated. Simply observing the patient as you ask him to swallow will give you clues that there is a dysfunction present. The head and neck should be neutral or slightly flexed. The mouth should be closed. Then the larynx moves upward and backward, then downward. If there seems to be a dysfunction and coughing noted with eating or drinking, an x-ray fluoroscopic study should be done to document the dysfunction. A swallowing training program should be instituted to teach the patient the proper swallowing mechanisms and improve cognition of the process and retraining of the musculature. If the patient is not able to comprehend and cooperate, alternate means of nutrition should be utilized.

The very act of coughing can cause enough irritation to the airways to provoke more coughing spasms (feedback loop). If a patient's cough is unproductive and dry sounding, he should not be encouraged to continue to cough. If there is evidence of retained secretions (i.e., expiratory wheezing, rhonchi, chest x-ray atelectasis, etc.), it is more effective to do postural drainage, breathing exercises, and hydration (or aerosol) to mobilize secretions. Continued coughing will cause airway narrowing and can precipitate bronchospasm, especially in asthmatics.

Some questions to ask a patient about his cough are: How long have you been coughing like this? Did it come on with a cold or infection? What seems to increase your coughing? i.e., eating, drinking, cold weather, noxious inhalation, exercise? The last question is particularly helpful as many patients know what is causing them to cough.

FAILURE OF THE COUGH MECHANISM

A failure of the cough mechanism may be an impairment of any step in the previously listed cough sequence. For example, the patient may be: (1) unable to take a deep breath, (2) unable to close his glottis, (3) unable to build up intra-abdominal and intrathoracic pressure, and so on. It is important to seek the cause of the inappropriate cough. When the cause is known, appropriate therapy to improve the cough may be initiated. As an example, if the reason a patient coughs poorly is that he cannot take a deep breath, deep breathing instructions are initiated in conjunction with "cough" instruction. On the other hand, if a patient has weak abdominal muscles and cannot forcibly exhale, abdominal strengthening exercises will be included, or in the case of a quadriplegic, coughing is assisted by pushing upward and inward against the diaphragm (also compressing the lateral chest in a side-lying position) during the expulsive phase to act as abdominal muscles (Fig 11–2). Specific clinical suggestions for improving a patient's cough are listed later in this chapter and in Chapters 21 and 22.

Further assessment of failure of the cough mechanism may be divided into one of three areas. First, the energy source for coughing may be disturbed. Examples of this are neuromuscular diseases, skeletal deformities (kyphoscoliosis, trauma such as flail chest), anesthesia, drug overdose, cachexia, depression or lack of motivation. Second, the "feed" system may be disrupted; for example, ciliary action is paralyzed by smoking, secretions may be distal to the ciliated mucous blanket. Mucus may be too thick to be moved easily by the mucociliary escalator. Therefore, the cough is ineffective because mucus is below the sixth or seventh mucus generation. Third, there may be some structural abnormality in the airways or lung parenchyma. Examples of this are bron-

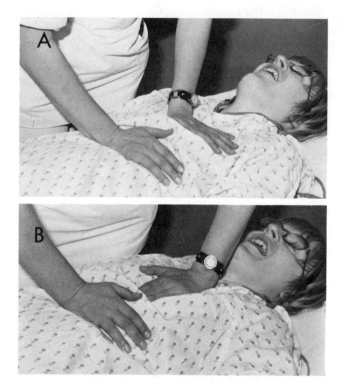

FIG 11–2.
Quadriplegic (or severe neuromuscular weakness) cough techniques. See chapters 21 and 22 for details.

chiectasis, tracheomalacia, partial obstruction by tumor, or artificial airways such as endotracheal or tracheostomy tubes.

SUGGESTIONS FOR TEACHING PATIENTS TO COUGH

In interviewing the patient initially, several questions may be asked: How do you feel you are coughing? Is your cough productive? If so, how much, what color and what consistency? If not, why do you think you are not coughing up any mucus? Several responses may be given and chest physical therapy treatment (and other treatment coordination) will depend on the patient's responses. For example: the patient relates he has a poor cough that is unproductive. He states he has a great deal of pain in his incision and the mucus is so thick it is great work to mobilize it. The therapist could suggest at least two specific treatment plans. First, an ultrasonic nebulizer or aerosol would help to thin the secretions. The patient would also be encouraged to drink more fluid (providing this is not contraindicated). Second, the therapist and nurse could coordinate the patient's treatment sessions with his pain medication.

If the patient with neurological deficit (i.e., spinal cord injury) said his cough was poor because he was weak, one may think of utilizing IPPB or glossopharyngeal breathing (see Chapter 22) to assist deep breathing and coughing. The patient may take a deep inspiration from the IPPB machine, hold it, take the mouthpiece out of his mouth and "cough" with the increased volume from the IPPB. The patient will also receive instructions in deep breathing and possibly abdominal exercise, if appropriate.

Another helpful technique with a weak patient (or a patient with a low vital capacity) is to have the patient draw several breaths in, holding each until a larger volume is attained. The instructions to the patient for this maneuver are: Take a deep breath, hold it (don't let it out) now! a little more, a little more, a little more, and *cough!* It may be likened to a sneeze—ah, ah, ah, ah-choo!

The therapist needs to learn to "hear" where a cough is coming from and whether it is effective. He also needs to know how to cough well *himself* if he expects to teach the patient a proper cough. The sound of a cough should be low pitched and deep. The patient's head and neck should be in a relatively neutral or flexed position (hyperextension of the neck makes coughing very difficult). Flexion of the head and neck will facilitate a cough. The patient can be asked to protrude his tongue while coughing to clear the airway and have less resistance to expulsion of air. He may be encouraged to make a K sound (especially if he has difficulty opposing his cords). The patient should also be aware that the abdominal muscles should "pull in" during the cough. This can be demonstrated easily by having the patient place his hands flat across his abdomen and blow out several times, feeling the abdominal muscles pull in. He is then instructed to blow out with more force, then to cough and feel the muscles tighten. If a patient is unable to oppose his cords or build up pressure for a cough, he may be encouraged to "huff" to try to mobilize secretions. This also works well for patients that try too hard to cough and show obvious signs of strain.

Clinically, therapists and nurses often find little tricks to help patients cough. A few of the author's favorite tricks will now be discussed.

Two general factors should be kept in mind for all patients treated for coughing problems. First, the patient's position is very important. Generally, patients cough best sitting up straight or leaning forward.

This pushes the diaphragm upward and puts the patient in a position that facilitates exhalation. Each patient should be considered individually, however, and the appropriate position for maximum efficiency and patient comfort should be utilized. Some other examples are: patients with median sternotomies may cough better in a high side-lying position that helps to stabilize the chest, and quadriplegics may cough better in a side-lying, head-down position (see Fig 11–2).

Second, any patient with an incision or pain should first be instructed on splinting the area prior to coughing. Splinting may be done with the hands supporting or a pillow or blanket held firmly over the area.

Series of Three Coughs. The patient is asked to start a small breath and small cough, then a bigger breath and harder cough, and finally a really deep breath and hard cough. This is especially good for postoperative patients who tend to splint from pain and are relieved not to always have to give a maximum effort. By this technique, they can *focus* on the final cough and not cause undue pain and tiring.

Cough Twice in One Breath. The patient is asked to take a deep breath and cough twice with the air from that breath. The second cough seems to be the more effective and powerful expulsive force.

Don't Cough—Say "Ha-Hahaha" or "Aha" in a Low Tone. Many patients, especially asthmatics, tend to prolong the expiratory phase of coughing almost into a wheeze. By having them interrupt with ha-ha-ha-ha, it prevents the wheeze, yet contraction of the abdominals and interruption of the expiratory air stream facilitate cough effectiveness.

Tracheal Tickle. The "tracheal tickle" is poorly named as it is an uncomfortable maneuver designed to elicit a reflex cough. The therapist places the index and middle finger flat in the sternal notch and gently massages inward in a circular fashion over the trachea. This may be used in obtunded patients or patients coming out of anesthesia. This is inappropriate with alert, cooperative patients or patients with artificial airways (Fig 11–3). It must be used judiciously or not at all with young children and the frail, elderly patient.

Emphysema Patients. With their tendency to trap air, these patients will generally cough more effectively with lower volumes and less stressful techniques. If they are asked to take a really deep breath and cough hard, they may tend to increase air trapping and unduly exhaust themselves.

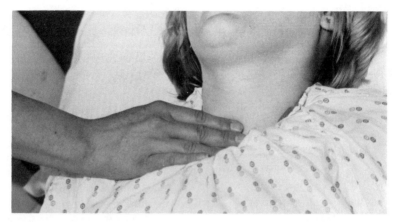

FIG 11–3.
Tracheal tickle (see text).

"Pump" Coughing. In patients with air trapping, i.e., emphysema or hypersensitive airways, i.e., asthma, trying to take a deep breath and give a maximum cough may cause more problems with air trapping or bronchospasm rather than facilitate removal of secretions.

A "pumping" technique has been found to be very beneficial clinically. The patient is asked to give three short easy coughs (kuh) (kuh) (kuh), then three "huffs" (huh) (huh) (huh) in a very breathy manner. In an alternating fashion, this is repeated 3–4 times. Often secretions will be mobilized effectively. If not, it is better not to stress hard coughing but encourage more deep breathing or postural drainage to get secretions to the segmental bronchi where they may be coughed out.

Coordination of Therapies. The patient will generally be able to cough more effectively following USN and IPPB treatments. Ideally, aggressive coughing should always follow these treatments. Many benefits are lost when a therapist or nurse turns off the machines and says "Don't forget to cough" while walking out of the room.

Cough Simulation. Patients with artificial airways cannot cough normally since the tube is either between the cords (endotracheal tubes) or below the cords (tracheostomy tubes). Adequate pressure cannot be built up without approximation of the cords. These patients may have a cough simulated by inflating the cuff on the tube, giving a large, rapid inspiration by manual resuscitation bag, holding the breath for 1–2 seconds and rapidly allowing the bag to release and exhalation to ensue. This is ideally performed with two persons and is made more effective by one therapist/nurse performing vibration and chest compression from the time of the inspiratory hold, all during exhalation (Figs 11–4 and 11–5).

The alternatives to coughing may need to be discussed briefly. Often patients will say they will cough the next day when they have less pain. But tomorrow will never come. Therapists and nurses should not threaten patients with pneumonia or atelectasis. Patients may be told they may develop pulmonary congestion or infection and retained secretions that will be *more* difficult to clear if they are deeper in the lungs. If they cough now, it will be much less traumatic than the alternative of more aggressive treatment when complications arise. Prophylactic treatment should be emphasized primarily rather than therapeutic regimes.

The other alternative to coughing is suctioning. This is indicated for all patients with artificial airways. It is also indicated (nasotracheal suction) for patients who are too weak or unable to cough effectively. It is a relatively simple procedure that will effectively remove secretions from the trachea and main-stem bronchi. Suctioning has limitations and should be done by trained, capable individuals. (Ideally, *all* therapists and nurses working with chest physical therapy *should* be capable

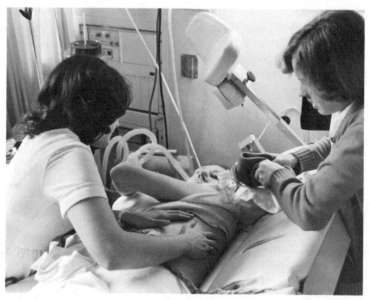

FIG 11–4.
Simulated cough using self-inflating bag and chest compression with vibration.

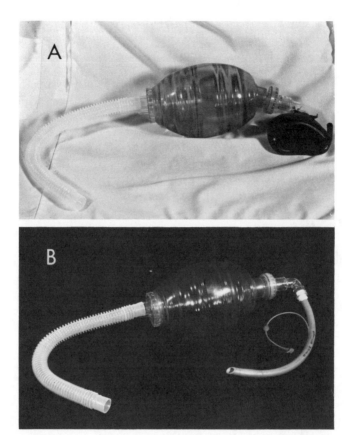

FIG 11–5.
The self-inflating bag may be used to simulate cough by attaching it to either a mask **(A)** or an artificial airway **(B)** (the mask results are less effective).

of suctioning effectively.) The dangers of suctioning are hypoxemia, cardiac arrhythmias (particularly bradycardia due to vagal stimulation) and lung collapse (see Chapter 30).

In conclusion, one may say that the cough is actually one of the most important aspects of any respiratory treatment. To perform postural drainage or give a USN treatment without aggressive coughing is ridiculous. Coughing is not without hazards, however, and several warnings need to be made. Patients with obstructive airway disease may find that intrathoracic pressure may become so high, for so long, that venous return to the heart is impeded. This makes the cardiac output fall and the patient may become dizzy to unconscious. This is referred to as *tussive syncope*. Patients should not be allowed to exert and put forth continued maximum effort. They must be monitored closely during coughing. Certain types of patients should not be encouraged to cough. These patients can be taught to "huff" to clear their upper airways; for example, preoperative patients with aneurysms. The high pressures of coughing may elicit severe problems. Patients with the possibility of cerebrovascular injury or CVA should also be carefully treated and monitored. Some patients may become cyanotic during periods of uncontrollable cough spasms. This should be avoided. Experienced therapists learn to guide their patients into effective coughing with control and decreased energy expenditure.

REFERENCES

Periodicals

Barach A, Beck J: Physical methods simulating cough mechanisms. *JAMA* 1952; 150:1380.

Irwin RS, Pratter MR: Postnasal drip and cough. *Clin Notes Respir Dis* 1980; 18(4):11–12.

Irwin RS, Rosen MJ, Braman SS: Cough: A comprehensive review. *Arch Intern Med* 1977; 137:1186–1191.

Lagerson J: The cough—its effectiveness depends on you. *Respir Care* 1971; 18:434.

Leith DE: Cough. *Phys Ther* 1968; 48:439.

Loudon G: Finding the cause of cough: Ask, listen, and look. *J Respir Dis* 1985; January, 97–107.

Loudon RG: Cough: A symptom and a sign. *Basics Respir Dis* 1981; 9(4):1–6.

Ross BB, Gramiak R, Rahn H: Physical dynamics of the cough mechanism. *J Appl Physiol* 1955; 8:264.

Books

Bendixen HH, et al: *Respiratory Care.* St Louis, CV Mosby Co, 1965.

Cherniak RM, et al: *Respiration in Health and Disease,* ed 2. Philadelphia, WB Saunders Co, 1972.

Leith DE: *Cough, Chest Disorders in Children.* Hislop HJ, Sanger JO (eds). New York, American Physical Therapy Association, 1968.

Shapiro B, Harrison R, Trout C: *Clinical Application of Respiratory Care.* Chicago, Year Book Medical Publishers, Inc, 1975.

12

Postural Drainage

Donna Frownfelter, P.T., R.R.T.

Postural drainage is classically defined as a method of removing secretions from the lungs by using gravity. It is essential that the therapist understand the anatomy of the tracheobronchial tree in order to effectively perform postural drainage. Emphasis, then, will be placed on learning the lung segments and thus determining the drainage position by placing the segmental bronchus in the most vertical position. In this manner, gravity will have its fullest effect.

The importance of the technique can be understood by remembering that as one goes down into the lungs, he discovers there are fewer cartilaginous rings and few to no mucus-producing glands and cilia (see Chapter 1). Therefore, with secretions in the depths of the lungs, it is difficult and sometimes impossible to raise secretions without moving them to a larger airway that has a good mucous blanket and cilia (mucociliary escalator).

Another consideration is that the cough mechanism will clear only the segmental bronchi. Therefore, in the distal parts of the lung, the two main clearing mechanisms (the mucociliary escalator and the cough mechanism) are ineffective in raising retained secretions. The purpose and need for postural drainage thus become obvious.

INDICATIONS FOR POSTURAL DRAINAGE

To Prevent the Accumulation of Secretions (Prophylaxis)

1. Any patient on a continuous ventilator (providing his condition is stable enough to tolerate treatment) as they are prone to atelectasis and pneumonia (see Chapter 26).

2. Any patient on prolonged bed rest, especially a high-risk patient such as a chronic lunger or postoperative patient who is immobilized or has an abdominal or thoracic incision.

3. Any patient who has an increased sputum production, such as a bronchiectatic or cystic fibrosis patient.

4. Any patient who tends to splint from pain and thus hypoventilate. Generally, patients in this category would also have an ineffective cough.

5. Any patient with greatly increased work of breathing. Usually they will fatigue and have difficulty maintaining bronchial hygiene.

To Mobilize Retained Secretions (Therapeutic)

1. Any patient with atelectasis caused by retained secretions occluding air entry causing the collapse.

2. Any patient with a draining lung abscess. (Care should be taken to also drain areas that could possibly be cross-contaminated by the purulent secretions.)

3. Any patient with pneumonia. Although antibiotics are the most important, drainage will help clear the consolidation more quickly and effectively.

4. Any patient needing pre- and postoperative secretion control. In particular, heavy smokers, patients with abnormal pulmonary functions, obese or aged patients and those with abdominal or thoracic incisions should be considered (see Chapter 18).

5. Any obtunded patient such as from a drug overdose, a brain stem tumor or coma.

6. Any neurologic patient with general weakness and/or uncoordinated swallowing or cough mechanisms.

7. Any patient with an artificial airway who is unable to maintain clear lungs.

Note: The following comment must be made prior to discussing the precautions and general contraindications for postural drainage. It is essential that the therapist and physician communicate and decide on treatment priorities. At times, there may be a decision to treat a patient although there seems to be a contraindication and/or a concern that the patient may not tolerate the procedure. For example, generally one does not "tip" a patient soon after neurosurgery head down until a specific order is written, as the tipping would increase intracranial pressure. However, if the patient develops atelectasis and/or pneumonia, the stress of respiratory embarrassment may also increase intracranial pressure. In this instance, the decision may be made to tip the patient to clear the atelectasis and then subsequently return to a modified conservative regime.

As rapport between therapist and physician develops, the therapist will be given more difficult and critical patients to treat as confidence is established in the therapist's skill. Clinical experience will dictate how aggressive one can be in individual circumstances. Patient tolerance is of the utmost importance. Ironically, most patients can tolerate more than one would assume!

GENERAL PRECAUTIONS AND CONTRAINDICATIONS FOR POSTURAL DRAINAGE

1. Untreated tension pneumothorax. This is an acute emergency and we offer no treatment. It is caused by positive pressure in the pleural space. When a chest tube has been inserted, treatment, if indicated, may proceed when the patient is stable.

2. Hemoptysis.

3. Unstable cardiovascular system, such as hypotension or hypertension, acute myocardial infarction and arrhythmias.

4. Postoperatively following:
    a. neurosurgery: positioning may cause increased intracranial pressure.
    b. esophageal anastomosis: gastric juices may affect the suture line.
    c. certain orthopedic patients who are limited in positioning.
    d. specific instances where there were surgical problems, such as a tear in the pericardial sac.

5. Aneurism or decrease in the circulation of main blood vessels.

6. Pulmonary edema, congestive heart failure.

7. Aged or nervous patients who become agitated or upset with therapy.

8. Pulmonary embolism. There is a question (which is *controversial*)

whether there may be a recurrence with aggressive movement to position for postural drainage versus allowing the patient to lie still and develop further venous stasis.

9. Recent laminectomy. The patient may be treated but should be log-rolled, and care must be taken to properly align the vertebrae during positioning.

10. Large pleural effusion. This is a compression of the lung from fluid in the pleural space. The lung will not be able to expand fully due to the fluid. Postural drainage will not be beneficial.

PREPARATION FOR POSTURAL DRAINAGE

Obtain All Pertinent Information

1. *Where* is the lung area to be emphasized? This information may be obtained from a thorough chest evaluation, the patient's chart, conferring with the physician, and looking at the patient's x-rays.

2. *What* is the patient's general medical condition? Vital signs, especially relatively stable pulse and blood pressure, arrhythmias, level of sensorium, ability to tolerate treatment, any acute or chronic medical condition that may pertain to treatment and positioning precautions should all be taken into account.

3. *When* is the best treatment time? Obviously, one cannot treat each patient at an ideal time when there is a busy schedule, but good timing will make a more efficient treatment session, particularly with *difficult* patients. One should consider meals or tube feedings: generally, a treatment should not be given immediately after a meal, rather 1½–2 hours after the ingestion. This is very important with tube feedings since if one followed the idea that the feedings are at 9 A.M., 1 P.M., 5 P.M., 9 P.M., etc., it may *start* then but won't be finished for another ½–1 hour. This may present specific problems especially since the nasogastric tube passes through the gastric sphincter and in positioning the patient will allow easy reflux of gastric contents. If, however, the patient has an artificial airway, the cuff can be inflated and head down positions used without problems. However, each patient must be evaluated individually. Another important consideration is pain. If pain is hampering treatment, coordinating therapy following pain medication (usually about 20 minutes later is maximal dose efficiency) will be beneficial. We are utilizing transcutaneous nerve stimulators (TNS) to decrease postoperative pain as well as in selected pa-

tients who seem to have extreme postoperative pain. This has been used quite extensively in chronic pain but seems to be adaptable to acute pain as well.

4. *How* can I best treat the patient? Which positions are indicated? What will the patient tolerate? Are position modifications necessary? What coordination with nursing and respiratory therapy is appropriate?

Prepare the Patient

1. Loosen any tight or binding clothing, especially around the neck or waist.

2. Explain the treatment to the patient, simply but completely.

3. Seek to develop a relaxed atmosphere and rapport with the patient.

4. Observe any tubes and connections attached to the patient (jokingly called the "tube index"), things such as IVs, ECG monitor, artificial airway, ventilator, Foley catheter, arterial lines, central venous pressure lines, aortic balloon, etc. Determine how each of the connections will move as the patient is positioned.

5. Adjust any tubes that would not move properly *before* positioning patient.

6. Make sure there are enough personnel to position patient with as little stress to both patient and staff as possible.

7. With a critically ill patient or one who is of questionable stability, check the pulse and blood pressure to establish baselines before treatment begins.

8. Have the patient either cough or be suctioned prior to positioning if he tends to have a large amount of secretions. This should be repeated before changing positions if more than one position is to be utilized.

TREATMENT

1. The therapist should be positioned in *front* of the patient during postural drainage in order to observe any changes quickly. Care should be taken not to have the patient cough directly at the therapist,

with proper covering of his mouth, utilizing tissue, and other precautions.

2. Position patient in proper postural drainage position or modify position as indicated (Figs 12–1 to 12–6). Modified positions are utilized if there is a precaution or relative contraindication to the ideal position. For example, if the bed should not be tipped due to the patient's unstable blood pressure, a flat bed may be utilized while maintaining proper body alignment.

3. Position should be maintained at least 5–10 minutes if tolerated, and may be maintained longer if a large amount of secretion is present or if secretions are thick. (*Note:* If secretions seem thick and difficult to mobilize, an ultrasonic nebulizer (USN) should be considered (see Chapter 29). The patient should also be encouraged to drink more fluids unless this is contraindicated.) If several positions are used, it is best to limit the total treatment time to 30–40 minutes as this may become extremely fatiguing to the patient. One may treat certain lung areas in the morning and others in the afternoon rather than doing everything in one treatment. If this is done, the most important areas should be treated in the morning.

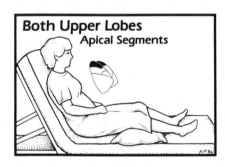

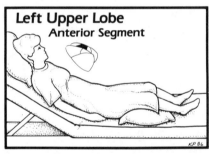

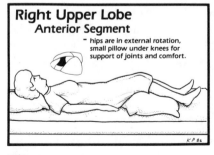

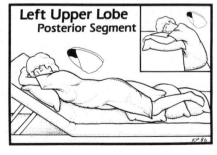

FIG 12–1.
Upper lobes.

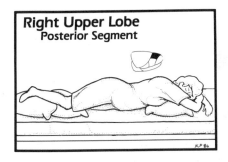
Right Upper Lobe
Posterior Segment

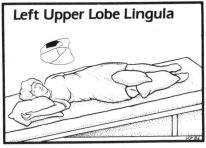
Left Upper Lobe Lingula

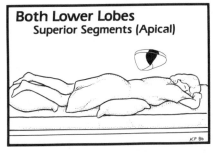
Both Lower Lobes
Superior Segments (Apical)

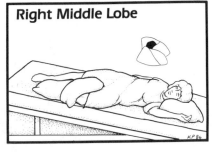
Right Middle Lobe

FIG 12–2.
Upper, middle, and lower lobes.

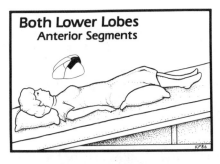
Both Lower Lobes
Anterior Segments

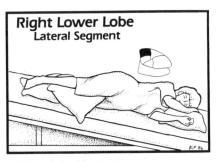
Right Lower Lobe
Lateral Segment

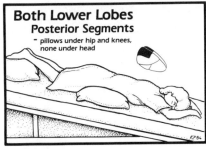
Both Lower Lobes
Posterior Segments
- pillows under hip and knees, none under head

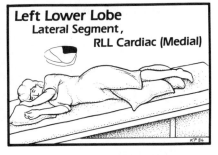
Left Lower Lobe
Lateral Segment,
RLL Cardiac (Medial)

FIG 12–3.
Lower lobes.

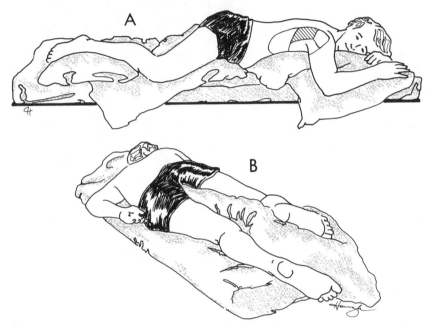

FIG 12–4.
A, right upper lobe—posterior segment (anterior view—patient positioned three-fourths prone). **B,** right upper lobe—posterior segment (posterior view). *Note:* Upper extremities toward prone, underneath arm pulled free from under patient's body. This position may also be a modified position for right lower lobe posterior segment.

4. Generally, percussion, vibration and breathing exercises will be included in the treatment if there are no specific contraindications (see Chapter 13 for such contraindications).

5. Intermittent positive pressure breathing (IPPB) may be included with patients who have a decreased vital capacity, muscle weakness, in-

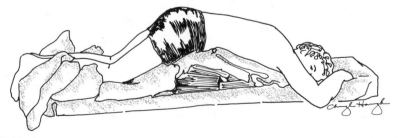

FIG 12–5.
Both lower lobes—posterior segments (shown using telephone books or pillows for home use). A beanbag chair is also helpful for home treatments.

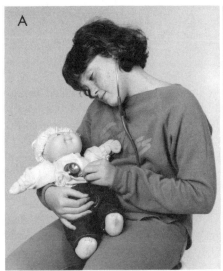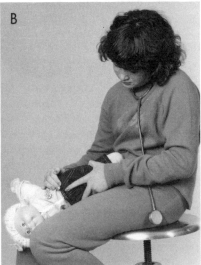

FIG 12–6.
A and **B,** if children are able to role play the treatment, they will better understand what is expected and be more cooperative with therapy.

creased airway resistance or increased work of breathing. The sequence for this procedure is to first position the patient comfortably, then begin IPPB. When the patient is stable and breathing well, percussion and vibration may be started. The patient may be asked to take a deep breath with the machine so that vibration will be more effective.

6. The patient should sit up slowly after the treatment to take some deep breaths and cough. Secretions mobilized may not be raised at the time of treatment but possibly ½–1 hour later. The patient should be thus informed and requested to clear secretions then. The nurse should be included in this aspect of treatment, especially with difficult patients who need such encouragement.

7. The therapist may determine to have the patient stay in the postural drainage position for a prolonged time. This may be accomplished by instructing a trustworthy patient in adjusting his bed back to normal, requesting the nurse to check the patient and return his bed to position at a given time; or if the therapist has other patients on the floor, he can return to the patient when finished on the floor. *Caution:* The decision to leave a patient in a head-down position should not be taken lightly. The patient should be alert and able to reposition himself quite well. A comatose patient, a stroke patient, an aged patient or one

with an unstable cardiovascular system, cervical spinal cord injury, severe arthritis or other special problem should not be left unattended for obvious reasons; he needs close monitoring. One may leave the patient in the same body alignment but return the bed to flat or slightly head up as necessary.

8. Notes regarding positioning and effectiveness of treatment should be recorded and communicated to physician, nurses and therapists. In this way, a positional rotation may be set up to accentuate and emphasize areas that are difficult and productive.

ASSESSMENT OF TREATMENT

1. On *auscultation,* are breath sounds increased and more equal bilaterally? (Sometimes it seems the lungs sound worse after a treatment. The reason is that there has been more air introduced and therefore there may be an increase in bronchi or expiratory wheezes!)

2. On *manual chest examination,* are both sides of the chest moving equally well? Is there a discrepancy, a lag, muscle splinting from increased pain, and so on?

3. Was the *cough productive?* How much mucus was raised? Are the secretions too thin or too thick? Is any respiratory therapy equipment indicated? Is the coordination between the therapies appropriate? Could it be improved? Does the patient need more instruction in coughing? Has the patient's nurse been involved in continuing the instruction?

4. How did the *patient feel* about the treatment? Was he exhausted, feeling better, work of breathing decreased, pain increased?

5. What effect was seen on the *patient's vital signs?* Was there an increase or decrease in the patient's temperature and pulse, in blood pressure or arrhythmias?

6. Has the *chest x-ray* improved?

7. At the next treatment, is the *patient happy* to see the therapist? Does he feel it is a waste of time, or groan at the aspect of increased pain?

8. *Compare findings* with physicians, other therapists and nurses working with the patient. They may realize improvements or problems of which the therapist may be unaware. For example, typically, little

mucus is initially raised following treatment. The nurse may report that 30 to 40 minutes after treatment the patient was productive and that the patient took two hours to recover from treatment.

DISCONTINUING POSTURAL DRAINAGE

As a general rule, the treatment should be discontinued when the reason for initiating it is reversed. For example, in a postoperative thoracic surgery patient, when he is deep breathing and coughing well, afebrile, ambulating and has good range of motion in the shoulder of the affected side, his treatment should be discontinued. On the other hand, a chronic lung patient with copious secretions would not have treatment discontinued but rather would be instructed in a home program. He would have his sessions with the therapist discontinued but would continue his sessions independently.

The following are general criteria for discontinuing treatment:

1. Patient is *afebrile* for 24–48 hours.

2. *Auscultation* of the lungs shows good breath sounds at least "relatively clear" or "normal" for the patient (a chronic lung patient will *never* have *good* breath sounds).

3. Relatively clear *chest x-ray.*

4. *Ambulation*—at least up in a chair regularly.

5. *Patient's ability* to deep breathe and cough independently or to position himself if indicated for home program.

Note: All these criteria may not be met and the patient's treatment may be discontinued at the discretion of the therapist and doctor. On the other hand, even though some patients may meet the criteria, they may be continued if there is a question of prognosis in order to prevent future problems or maintain respiratory status.

HOME PROGRAMS

Home programs are a means of teaching patients to care for themselves or become involved and responsible for their own care. In the past, chronic lung patients often were seen week after week for therapy. By teaching patients first of all to understand the concept of postural drainage and then the appropriate positions to use, we make them a part of the "team."

Candidates for home programs are any chronic patients with increased mucus secretions, patients with an acute respiratory exacerbation of a disease (either primary or secondary lung pathology), patients who are high-risk surgical candidates seen before surgery to insure optimal respiratory status, and others.

In general, *home postural drainage:*

1. Should not last longer than 30–45 minutes for the entire program sequence. If it is longer, the patient becomes fatigued and may lose interest.

2. Usually should be performed *in the morning before breakfast.* If it is required more often, it may be done *in the evening* also, but not too close to bedtime as secretions may loosen when the patient is trying to sleep. The exercise before bedtime may make the patient tense rather than relaxed. Ideally, the treatment may be scheduled 1–1½ hours before retiring for the night.

3. Positions for therapy should be chosen according to the patient's individual needs. Usually a chronic lunger is involved in the lower lobes. Therefore, a simple four-position rotation is helpful. Each position is held 5–10 minutes. The patient will be taught self-percussion and breathing exercises while draining. If the patient is bronchiectatic, the involved lobe and lobes that may be contaminated are drained. Only the patient with cystic fibrosis has all lobes drained at home.

4. The patient should be instructed in *aids* for positioning, such as using pillows, magazines or newspapers tied in a stack, a slant board, a foam wedge, a beanbag chair or a sofa cushion. These are a few helpful modalities. This should be discussed and the patient should give the therapist a return demonstration to show the positioning and understanding of the treatment.

5. A *family member or friend* should also be instructed in case the patient is ill or needs more aggressive care. This should also be a source of encouragement.

6. The patient should be checked at intervals (perhaps 1–2 weeks after discharge from the hospital and then monthly or when the patient visits his physician). This is important to evaluate the effectiveness of treatment and the need for upgrading the program and maintaining contact with the patient. Patients often have numerous questions when

they try the therapy at home rather than in a supervised hospital setting.

7. The physician should be informed of the patient's progress and/or problems at home.

8. Patients should be aware of the usual amount, color and consistency of mucus produced. If there is a change, he should note and report this to the therapist and physician.

SUGGESTIONS FOR COORDINATION OF RESPIRATORY TREATMENTS

Clinically, it becomes obvious with experience that the optimal coordination of therapies yields a superior treatment program. Nursing care, respiratory therapy and chest physical therapy need to be integrated in such a way as to have the least stress on the patient and also to achieve optimal goals. In order to accomplish this, all personnel need to understand each other's role and strive to cooperate to the fullest extent.

Some general principles pertaining to *postural drainage* will be discussed at this time. Priorities need to be set for when nursing care such as a bath or medications need to be done. When does the patient receive his ultrasonic nebulizer (USN; see Chapter 29) or intermittent positive pressure breathing (IPPB) treatment? When should chest physical therapy be done? This becomes more and more of a problem as the patient is more critical and more tests and procedures are indicated.

To simplify a complicated procedure, one may say that most nursing procedures such as a bath or linen change are quite flexible. Procedures such as medications, intravenous feedings and so on are important and need to be attended to promptly. The bath, or procedures that are tiring, ideally will not be done just prior to therapy as the patient will be too fatigued to obtain maximum benefits.

If the patient has *very* thick secretions, the USN prior to postural drainage may prove helpful. Often the patient may also receive a bronchodilator before postural drainage as this insures more open airways and maximum use of the patient's lungs. This helps the patient take deeper breaths and may help mobilize the secretions more quickly. It is particularly helpful in a weak patient with a poor vital capacity, such as a quadriplegic or neuromuscular weakness or a recent postoperative patient. Patient tolerance is obviously a prime concern. This procedure is not necessary in the majority of patients (in the author's opinion) but is helpful in difficult patients. In patients with an artificial airway, the patient may be "ambued" while receiving treatment.

Ideally, when chest physical therapy follows the respiratory therapy treatments, the patient may remain in position or repositioned more comfortably. The nurse then resumes responsibility for encouraging deep breathing, coughing and general bronchial activity for the majority of the day.

A positional rotation should be instituted which modifies the usual nursing positions. The positions generally utilized are side to side, on the back with head flat or sitting. If the nurse thinks in terms of lung segment drainage in these positions only, the lateral segments and the upper lobe anterior segments will be drained. A modified system of approximately eight positions may be used to completely drain all lung segments. They are as follows:

1. Supine, flat—drains anterior segments and upper lobes.

2. Supine, head elevated—drains anterior and apical segments and upper lobes.

3. Lying on right side—drains left lower lobe lateral segment and right lower lobe cardiac segment.

4. Lying on right side, three-fourths prone—drains left lower lobe posterior and apical segment.

5. Lying on right side, three-fourths supine—drains lingula and left lower lobe anterior segment.

6. Lying on left side—drains right lower lobe lateral segment.

7. Lying on left side, three-fourths prone—drains right upper lobe posterior segment and right lower lobe apical and posterior segments.

8. Lying on left side, three-fourths supine—drains right middle lobe and right lower lobe anterior segment.

Note: the positional rotation system is a modified set for postural drainage. Ideally, if the patient could be head down in positions 3–8, it would be more appropriate. The positions then require a physician's order. But using the modified flat bed positions, the nurse can initiate this as part of the routine nursing care. This can become the most important part of a good respiratory program as the patient will not have dependent lung areas for a long period of time. Usually, positions will be changed every 1–2 hours. In critical patients, this may be done 24 hours a day if necessary, or until the patient is settled for the night.

Coordination will be discussed later in more depth as it is extremely important and the hub of a good total respiratory care program.

REFERENCES

Periodicals

Barach A, Beck G: Ventilatory effects of head-down position in pulmonary emphysema. *Am J Med* 1954; 16:55.

Barach A, Dulfano M: Effect of chest vibration on pulmonary emphysema: A preliminary report. *Ann Allergy* 1968; 26:10.

Bateman JRM, Newman SP, Daunt D, et al: Is cough as effective as chest physiotherapy in the removal of excessive trachiobronchial secretion? *Thorax* 1981; 36:683.

Bateman JRM, Newman SP, Daunt KM, et al: Regional lung clearance of excessive bronchial secretions during chest physiotherapy in patients with stable chronic airway obstruction. *Lancet* 1979; 1:294–297.

DeCesare J, Babchyck BM, Colten HR, et al: Radionuclide assessment of the effects of chest physical therapy on ventilation in cystic fibrosis. *Phys Ther* 1982; 62(6):820–827.

Desmondk J, Schwenk WF, Thomas E, et al: Immediate and long-term effects of chest physiotherapy in patients with cystic fibrosis, *J Pediatr* 1983; 103(4):538–542.

Dreisin RB, Albert RK, Talley PA, et al: Flexible fiberoptic bronchoscopy in the teaching hospital, yield and complications. *Chest* 1978; 74:144.

Falk M, Delstrup M, Anderson JB, et al: Improving the ketchup bottle method with positive expiratory pressure, PEP in cystic fibrosis. *Eur J Respir Dis* 1984; 65(6):423–432.

Finer NN, Morairtey RR, Boyd J, et al: Postextubation atelectasis: A retrospective review and a prospective controlled study. *J Pediatr* 1979; 94(1):110–113.

Haas A, Cardon H: Rehabilitation in chronic obstructive pulmonary disease. *Med Clin North Am* 1969; 53:593.

Hallb"o"ok T, Lindblad B, Lindroth B: Prophylaxis against pulmonary complications in patients undergoing gall-bladder surgery: A comparison between early mobilization and physiotherapy with or without bronchodilation. *Ann Chir Gynaecol* 1984; 73(2):55–80.

Howell S, Hill J: Acute respiratory care in the open heart surgery patient. *Phys Ther* 1972; 52:3.

Innocenti D: Chest conditions. *Physiotherapy* 1969; 52:437.

Johnson MC, et al: Bronchopulmonary hygiene in cystic fibrosis. *Am J Nurs* 1969; 69:320.

Jones L: Physical therapy—present state of the art. *Am Rev Respir Dis* 1974; 110:133.

Kigin CM: Chest physical therapy for the postoperative or traumatic injury patient. *Phys Ther* 1981; 61(12):1724–1736.

Kimbel P: Physical therapy for COPD patients. *Clin Notes Respir Dis* 1970; 8:3.

Lorin M, Denning C: Evaluation of postural drainage by measurement of sputum volume and consistency. *Am J Phys Med* 1971; 50:215.

MacKenzie CF, Shin B, Hadi F, et al: Changes in total lung/thorax compliance following chest physiotherapy. *Anesth Analg* (Cleve) 1980; 59(3).

March H: Appraisal of postural drainage for chronic obstructive pulmonary disease. *Arch Phys Med Rehabil* 1971; 52:528.

Matthews LW, et al: A therapeutic regimen for patients with cystic fibrosis. *J Pediatr* 1964; 65:558.

Oldenberg FA, Dalovich MB, Montgomery JM, et al: Effects of postural drainage: Exercise and cough on mucus clearance in chronic bronchitis. *Am Rev Respir Dis* 1979; 120:739.

Plumstead A: Modified slant board and vibrator for independent bronchial drainage. *Chest Disorders Child* 1972; 52:178.

Pryor JA, Webber BA, Hodson ME, et al: Evaluation of the forced expiration technique as an adjunct to postural drainage in treatment of cystic fibrosis. *Br Med J* 1979; 2(6187):417–418.

Remolina C, Khan AV, Santiago TV, et al: Positional hypoxemia in unilateral lung disease. *N Engl J Med* 1981; 304:523–525.

Rochester DF, Goldberg SK: Techniques of respiratory physical therapy. *Am Rev Respir Dis* 1980; 122 (5 pt 2):133–146.

Rottenburg C, Holaday D: Lung physiotherapy as an adjunct to surgical care. *Surg Clin North Am* 1964; 44:219.

Shrader DL, Lakshminarayan S: The effect of fiberoptic bronchoscopy on cardiac rhythm. *Chest* 1978; 73:821.

Sutton PD, Parker RA, Webber BA, et al: Assessment of the forced expiration technique of postural drainage and directed coughing in chest physiotherapy. *Eur J Respir Dis* 1983; 64(1):62–68.

Sutton PP, Pavia D, Bateman JR, et al: Chest physiotherapy: A review. *Eur J Respir Dis* 1982; 63(3):188–201.

Tecklin JS: Physical therapy for children with chronic lung disease. *Phys Ther* 1981; 61(12):1774–1781.

Tecklin J, Holsclaw D: Evaluation of bronchial drainage in patients with cystic fibrosis. *Phys Ther* 1975; 55:1081.

White DJ, Mawdsley RH: Effects of selected bronchial drainage positions and percussion on blood pressure of healthy human subjects. *Phys Ther* 1983; 63(3):325–330.

Windsor HM, Harrison GA, Nicholson TJ: Bag squeezing: A physiotherapeutic technique. *Med J Aust* 1972; 2:829.

Zack MB, Pontoppidan H, Kazemi H: The effect of lateral position on gas exchange in pulmonary disease. *Am Rev Respir Dis* 1979; 110:49.

Zadai CC: Physical therapy for the acutely ill medical patient. *Phys Ther* 1981; 61(12):1746–1754.

Zausmer E: Bronchial drainage. *Phys Ther* 1968; 48:586.

Books

Bendixen HH, et al: *Respiratory Care.* St Louis, CV Mosby Co, 1965.

Cash J: *Chest, Heart and Vascular Disorders for Physiotherapists.* London, Faber and Faber, 1975.

Frownfelter D: Massage in chest physical therapy, in Wood E: *Beard's Massage Principles and Techniques,* ed 2. Philadelphia, WB Saunders Co, 1974.

Gaskell D, Welsher B: *The Brompton Hospital Guide to Chest Physiotherapy,* ed 2. Philadelphia, FA Davis Co, 1973.

Rie MW: Chest physiotherapy, in Young J, Crocker D (eds): *Principles and Practice of Respiratory Therapy,* ed 2. Chicago, Year Book Medical Publishers, 1976.

Shapiro B, Harrison R, Trout C: *Clinical Application of Respiratory Care.* Chicago, Year Book Medical Publishers, 1975, pp 199–209.

Storey G: *Thoracic Surgery for Physiotherapists.* Philadelphia, JB Lippincott Co, 1955.

Thacker WC: *Special Problems in Postural Drainage and Respiratory Control,* ed 3. Chicago: Year Book Medical Publishers, 1973.

13

Percussion and Vibration

Donna Frownfelter, P.T., R.R.T.

Chest physical therapy utilizes three techniques in conjunction with postural drainage—breathing exercise, percussion, and vibration. The patient is placed in the appropriate drainage position and the adjunctive techniques are performed to mechanically loosen secretions, attempt to improve the distribution of ventilation and assist in the movement of secretions cephalad to larger airways.

BREATHING EXERCISES

Breathing exercises are discussed in Chapter 10. Here it suffices to say that the goals are to have lung areas selectively emphasized (segmental breathing) and to have air delivered distal to retained secretions. Air will tend to follow the path of least resistance, and therefore in patients with excessive secretions, airways that are obstructed tend to be hypoventilated. Consequently, atelectasis may occur. The therapist attempts to correct this situation with local expansion breathing exercises in conjunction with postural drainage.

The combined techniques of postural drainage with percussion and vibration for mobilization of secretions have been likened to a person attempting to extract ketchup from a bottle. First, the bottle is turned upside down (postural drainage). Second, several blows are made to the bottom of the bottle (percussion). Third, the bottle is vigorously shaken (vibration). Generally, mobilization of ketchup occurs after the shaking. In working with patients, we virtually perform the same regime.

PERCUSSION

Percussion is applied to the chest wall over the surface landmark of the lung segment being drained. The purpose of the technique is to mechanically jar and dislodge retained secretions. Percussion initiates waves of mechanical energy which are applied to the chest wall and transmitted to the lungs. A picture in one's mind should liken this to a stone dropped in water, with circles spreading outward from where the stone falls.

Percussion is performed with cupped hands, fingers and thumbs adducted. The hand position is more easily and successfully achieved by first adducting the fingers and thumbs, then forming the cup. This will help to prevent air leaks between fingers and thumbs. Cupping the hands provides a cushion of air between the hands and the chest wall to eliminate irritation and discomfort. While performing percussion, the therapist's shoulders, elbows and wrists must be loose and flexible, but the hands must maintain a cupped position (Fig 13–1).

The hands rhythmically and alternately strike the chest wall, maintaining equal force. The relaxing effect on the patient is derived from the monotonous rhythm and rate of the procedure. The speed of the technique is also controversial. Some therapists feel that only a rapid technique is effective. The author's opinion tends to favor a slower, more relaxing technique. Patients seem to tolerate a slower rate better and results seem more beneficial. If a therapist has one hand performing well while the other nondominant hand seems uncoordinated, he

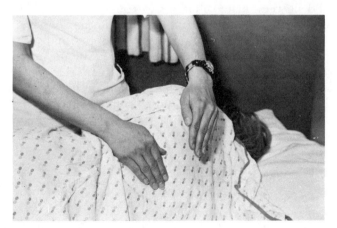

FIG 13–1.
Chest percussion.

should attempt to regulate both hands equally. For example, lightening the pressure on the dominant hand and trying to slow the rate to a speed the nondominant hand can tolerate are helpful. Another helpful technique is to *start* with the nondominant hand and let the dominant hand match the nondominant.

The technique need not be extremely forceful to be effective. There should be no pain or discomfort to the patient. It is not the force but the cupping that is effective. The force of the percussion must be determined for each individual patient. Factors to consider are the anatomical site, age of the patient, condition of the chest, pain, secretion density and amount, and tolerance of the patient.

The therapist will mold her hand to fit the contour of the bony thorax. The hand is made flatter over flatter surfaces such as the posterior chest. The hand is made more cupped to fit areas such as the lateral surfaces and the upper chest region.

The therapist should determine a pattern for percussion. One should not stay in one particular spot for an extended period. The hands may proceed back and forth or in a circular pattern, but not wander aimlessly around the patient's chest wall. This is not relaxing but irritating. Once the technique is begun, it should be continued for approximately 3–5 minutes rather than starting and stopping erratically. If the therapist loses rhythm or fatigues, or if the patient begins to cough, some vibration and chest compression can be done. Then the sequence can return to percussion.

There should not be an erythema following the treatment. If there is, and the patient complains of discomfort, the technique of the therapist should be reevaluated. Things to consider are that the patient may have extremely sensitive skin, the technique may have been improper, or if percussion was done on bare skin, perhaps a thin towel or hospital gown should have been used to cover the patient's skin. There are two views in regard to treatment on bare skin or over a sheet or gown. It seems there are times that patients prefer the technique be applied directly to the skin to prevent the shirring effect between fabric and skin. Some patients insist on a layer of cloth. Usually patients asking for covering are thin and relatively bony, whereas muscular, stocky patients may prefer direct treatment. It seems there is room for professional preference. However, nothing heavier than a sheet should be used (such as a terry towel or a blanket). If heavy material was used, the percussion would be absorbed by the material rather than transmitted through the chest wall.

Practically speaking, percussion is useless at times, as in the example of an extremely obese patient where, again, the fatty layer absorbs the mechanical action.

Surface areas over bony prominences, such as the clavicles, vertebrae and spine of the scapula, should be avoided. Percussion should not be done over the floating ribs and special care should be taken over the anterior and lower lateral chest wall areas. The ribs in those areas are more loosely attached or not attached bilaterally as in the case of the floating ribs.

Areas over breast tissue should also be treated carefully. The breasts should be avoided in young girls with developing breast tissue as this would be uncomfortable to the patient. Large breasts may be gently moved aside if areas such as the middle lobe or lingula need treatment. If necessary, the therapist may percuss with one hand, while retracting the breast that is causing obstruction of the surface area being emphasized. This should not be a cause for embarrassment to either the therapist or patient. The therapist's approach to the patient in a serious and sensitive manner will set the stage for the treatment. These women are well aware of the special problems associated with their anatomy. They are used to the chest examination procedures and will usually be cooperative and not present a problem. If there is discomfort or percussion is not tolerated, vibration alone will generally be satisfactory.

Indications for Percussion

Percussion is routinely done with patients receiving postural drainage. This is especially true if the patient has thick secretions that are difficult to mobilize. Therefore, any indication for postural drainage is also a general indication for percussion.

Precautions to Observe

1. Flail chest or fractured ribs.

2. Conditions prone to hemorrhage, i.e., platelet count below 30,000.

3. Conditions that lead to fragile ribs, such as metastatic bone cancer or brittle bones.

4. Nervous and aged people who do not tolerate the procedure.

5. Recent postoperative patients who have greatly increased pain and splinting following the treatment.

6. Subcutaneous emphysema of the neck and thorax.

7. Poor or unstable cardiovascular condition.

8. Recent spinal fusion.

9. Recent skin grafts or flaps.

10. Fresh burns, open wounds, skin infections in thoracic area.

11. Pulmonary emboli (one is worried about moving the patient and possible recurrent embolization).

12. Resectable tumors—usually percussion is not done over the tumor area.

13. Untreated tension pneumothorax.

In general, precautions may be put aside if there is a life-threatening situation that demands treatment. The therapist does not have to make this decision alone but needs proper medical direction in this matter.

VIBRATION

Vibration is generally administered following percussion. During postural drainage, therapists generally alternate between percussion and vibration techniques. The percussion technique, as discussed above, mechanically jars loose the mucous plugs. Vibration with chest compression moves mucus toward a larger airway.

Vibration is administered only during exhalation. The patient is asked to take in a deep breath, and chest compression and vibration are initiated at the peak of inspiration and continue throughout expiration. Patients unable to take a deep breath can be assisted with an IPPB treatment or with an ambu bag (if the patient has an artificial airway). The IPPB machine and ambu bag are excellent for use in conjunction with postural drainage and percussion and vibration. Clinically, we have seen more rapid clearing of atelectasis and retained secretion using the combined, coordinated techniques. When the ambu bag is used, an attempt is made to simulate a cough. The patient is given a deep inspiration. The breath is held for a few seconds, vibration begins at the breath hold and proceeds all during expiration. If this equipment is not available, the therapist can simply follow the patient's breathing pattern and vibrate during exhalation. If the pattern is extremely rapid, vibration can be done on every other breath. This will also help to slow the rate of breathing.

The technique of vibration is performed by tensing all muscles in

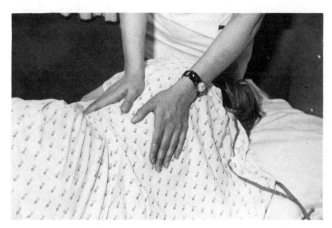

FIG 13–2.
Vibration—hands positioned on both sides of the chest.

a cocontraction from the shoulders to the hands. Chest compression is done simultaneously, being mindful of normal chest wall mechanics. Normally, during inspiration the lower ribs move up and out to the side. The sternum also moves upward to expand the anterior-posterior diameter of the chest. During expiration, the ribs move downward and inward. Vibration with compression should follow the normal chest movement. Care should be taken if a patient has a stiff, inelastic chest wall as pathologic fractures may occur.

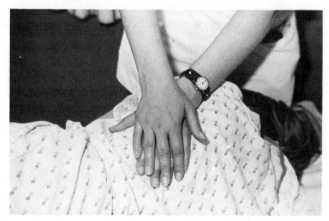

FIG 13–3.
Vibration—hand placement one on top of the other.

The hand position for vibration is variable. Some therapists position hands on either side of the chest, while others place one hand over the other for vibration (Figs 13–2 and 13–3). Generally, the author prefers the hands on either side of the chest as better compression is achieved.

RIB SPRINGING

There are clinical conditions that necessitate more aggressive treatment. If the patient has a mobile chest wall and is able to tolerate treatment, rib springing may be indicated.

Rib springing is done similarly to vibration, but more pressure is exerted on the chest wall. The ribs are "pumped" in a springing fashion three to four times during exhalation. The more forceful compression will result in more rapid and efficient mobilization of secretions.

Patients must be evaluated carefully before trying this technique. It should not be used for patients with tight chest walls, increased A-P diameters and pain. If there is a question in the therapist's mind whether to use the treatment or not, it probably should not be done!

REFERENCES

Rivington-Law BA, Epstein SW, Thompson GL, et al: Effect of chest wall vibrations on pulmonary function in chronic bronchitis. *Chest* 1984; 85(3):378–381.

Sutton P, Lopez-Vidriero MT, Pavia D, et al: Assessment of percussion, vibratory shaking and breathing exercises in chest physiotherapy. *Eur J Respir Dis* 1985; 66(2):147–152.

Torrington KG, Sorenson DE, Sherwood LM: Postoperative chest percussion with postural drainage in obese patients following gastric stapling. *Chest* 1984; 86(6):891–895.

14

Pulmonary Rehabilitation

Donna Frownfelter, P.T., R.R.T.

Rehabilitation was defined in 1942 by the Council of Rehabilitation as the restoration of the individual to the fullest physical, medical, mental, emotional, economic, social and vocational potential of which he is capable. One can sense the scope of rehabilitation as being all inclusive, touching every aspect in a patient's life.

Pulmonary rehabilitation is necessary for patients who are incapacitated due to their respiratory status. Any patient with symptomatic COPD should be considered. Patients with mild or severe COPD may not have as comprehensive a program as patients that have moderate to moderately severe COPD. The mildly involved patient may not be motivated to participate as he may not be very limited in his activities of daily living. Whereas the severely involved patient may not physically be able to participate in strenuous exercise, the moderately involved patient with COPD seems the ideal candidate.

A vicious cycle occurs in patients with chronic pulmonary disease. Shortness of breath from primary or secondary lung disease results in a decrease in activity tolerance. As the patient decreases his activity levels, muscular tone and efficiency decline, leading to more rapid fatigue and increased dyspnea. The patient strives to have as little activity as possible to avoid shortness of breath. The less he does, the less he is able to do. This downward spiral will continue unless intervention reverses the trend (Fig 14–1).

The goal of pulmonary rehabilitation and physical training is not to make athletes out of invalids but to prevent the problems of immobility. To stress this point, the goal is not just to increase muscle

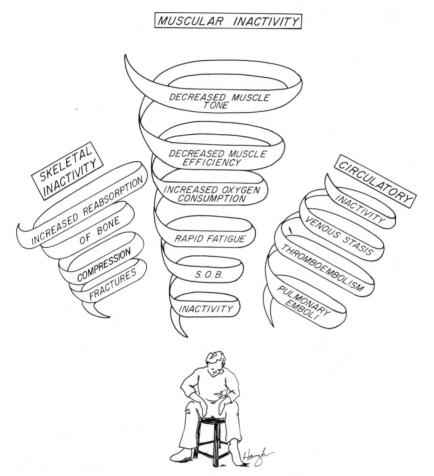

FIG 14–1.
The effects of inactivity. *S.O.B.* = shortness of breath.

strength but rather to allow patients to carry out their activities of daily living with less fatigue and more enjoyment; in short, to improve their quality of life.

The patient is encouraged to attain the maximum degree of physical fitness of which he is capable. Physical fitness may be described as physiologic and perceptual well-being. Physiologically, physical fitness is the ability to maintain cardiopulmonary functions as close as possible to those of a resting state while performing strenuous activities. It is also the ability to return promptly to the resting state following exercise if these functions are disturbed.

The exercise capacity of most healthy persons is determined by the muscles, not the heart and lungs. However, most patients with COPD find that the lungs (ventilatory mechanics) play the critical role in limiting their activity. Another way of stating this is that physical fitness is the ability to carry out daily tasks with vigor and alertness, without undue fatigue, and with ample energy to enjoy leisure time pursuits and meet unforeseen emergencies (Nancy Allard notes, NUPT class, May, 1986).

The patient's perception of how he feels and his state of well-being is also very important. He needs to feel capable of performing activities that are important and necessary. Physical fitness improves a patient's feeling about himself. It enhances self-worth, motivation, and ability to relate to others.

There has been much controversy regarding pulmonary rehabilitation. Perhaps some of it comes from a misunderstanding of what is actually involved. The American College of Chest Physicians adopted a definition of pulmonary rehabilitation in 1971. It reads:

> Pulmonary rehabilitation may be defined as an act of medical practice wherein an individually tailored, multidisciplinary program is formulated which through accurate diagnosis, therapy, emotional support, and education, stabilizes or reverses both the physio- and psychopathology of pulmonary diseases and attempts to return the patient to the highest possible functional capacity allowed by his pulmonary handicap and overall life situation.

When one relates to this definition, it is easy to understand why a program of pulmonary rehabilitation is difficult. The scope is from physical to emotional problems, from muscle weakness to motivation. Numerous allied health fields may need to be involved. Costs may be prohibitive, and third-party payers frequently will not recognize the program as valid. Equipment may be needed and vocational counseling and training may be indicated. These considerations only begin to scratch the surface of other areas and problems that arise. This is not meant to discourage those ready to embark on initiating a pulmonary rehabilitation service but rather to increase the therapists' awareness of the considerations.

The positive results of successful pulmonary rehabilitation should be understood. These are helpful in discussing the program with physicians and patients. Even the most skeptical physician may be willing to remain neutral (rather than negative) concerning rehabilitation after reading these studies, and he may allow the therapist to try to help his patients. When the patients know the results, they have hope and motivation. Some results of pulmonary rehabilitation are:

1. Decrease in frequency and duration of hospitalization.

2. Socioeconomic advantages.

3. Reduction in anxiety levels, depression and fewer complaints of a somatic nature.

4. Possible return to gainful employment and the ability to make a contribution to the work force.

5. Increase in self-esteem.

6. Slower rate of pulmonary function deterioration.

7. Improved exercise tolerance.

8. Increased survival.

Pulmonary rehabilitation is often criticized for being "psychological" in its effect. The author's opinion is that if it is indeed mainly psychological, it is still significant in that patients are able to perform their activities of daily living, enjoy life more and feel their quality of life improved. However, much research has been done in this field and many physiologic studies have been performed to designate the effects of the program. These will now be discussed.

It has been shown repeatedly that patients with chronic lung disease who continue to maintain physical fitness remain in better health than those who live a sedentary existence. The parameters that were measured and compared before and after training were heart rate (HR), respiratory rate (RR), minute volume (MV), oxygen consumption and CO_2 production as well as level of exercise. Heart rate was found to decrease an average of 24%, and respiratory rate and minute volume had an average decrease of 40%. Oxygen consumption and CO_2 production decreased 23%. The level of exercise increased along with the comfort in exercising. All functions returned more rapidly to baseline levels following exercise after training. These programs mainly involved the use of a treadmill so there was no new skill involved (Fig 14–2). The patients had been accustomed to the use of the treadmill for several days *before* baselines were established. Motivation and anxi-

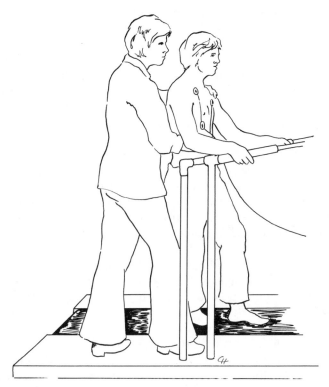

FIG 14–2.
The treadmill provides an objective, reproducible level of exercise. The patient should be monitored and well guarded. A mirror in front of the treadmill helps to keep the patient aware of his breathing as well as prevents the patient from watching his feet!

ety were not felt to be extreme as this was a conditioned exercise *before* data were recorded.

Even in normal subjects, the exact mechanisms for benefits received from physical training are unknown. Things to consider are better coordination, improved cardiopulmonary function, increased efficiency of muscles and improved motivation. Therapists should note, however, that often a patient's maximum exercise tolerance may be seen immediately following the training program.

If the patient continues to exercise at the same level, he should maintain his gains. If, however, he does not continue to exercise, his exercise tolerance will go back down to what it was before the program. Although the patient with pulmonary dysfunction may not continue to greatly increase his exercise tolerance following a rehab program, just maintaining the higher level of exercise is progress as COPD is a progressively deteriorating disease. This actually is still a good sign as the pulmonary disease is progressively deteriorating, and without the rehabilitation program the patient would be functioning at a lower level.

Decrease in activity may also be due to other conditions. This should be evaluated before sending patients as candidates for a pulmonary rehabilitation program. Physical deformities, peripheral vascular disease, obesity, cardiovascular disturbances and neuromuscular weakness may all lead to inactivity and shortness of breath with exercise. These patients need to have their primary disease dealt with rather than undergoing aggressive pulmonary rehabilitation. For example, if a patient has a tendency toward heart failure, ankle edema and shortness of breath, his symptoms should be dealt with by proper medication, *not* by exercise, which would aggravate the condition. The patients must be medically stable prior to entering a pulmonary rehabilitation program.

Patients needing pulmonary rehabilitation usually fall into two categories—those with restrictive lung disease, in which inadequate lung volumes inhibit ventilation during activity, and those with obstructive disease who cannot exhale sufficiently to meet exercise demands. Both types of patients also have ventilation-perfusion mismatching or diffusion-perfusion impairment. In the early stages of disease, there may be an inability of the lungs to deliver sufficient oxygen to the blood during exercise. These patients will be seen to desaturate with exercise. (Oxygen is carried on the Hb molecule. It is saturated with 97.5 % + when the Hb molecule is "saturated" with oxygen). During heavy exercise or when oxygen demand is great, oxygen is released in greater quantities to meet the demand. Normally, individuals do not desaturate with exercise. These patients will benefit from supplemental O_2 during exercise. An exercise test (functional) with titrated O_2 can determine the proper level of O_2 to be administered during exercise.

Toward the end stages of the disease, there may be an inability to provide enough oxygen even at rest and also an inability to remove CO_2. Most patients we treat will be found somewhere between these extremes but caught in a downward incapacitating spiral unless an intervention is made.

PATIENT ASSESSMENT

A thorough assessment should be made prior to admitting a patient into a pulmonary rehabilitation program. This should include evaluation of the patient's personal medical history both past and present, his familial medical history, and his level of motivation.

PERSONAL MEDICAL HISTORY

The patient's present state of health is extremely important as it designates the baseline level of activity. Other factors do enter the picture, however, such as the patient's general health history (i.e., chronically ill or just ill for a few months but previously well). Often a patient will relate, "I was fine until I had a bad cold six months ago and I haven't been able to do much since," or he may state that "slowly over the last two years," he has done less and less.

Considerations in the medical history are generally concerned with the cardiovascular, respiratory, gastrointestinal, genitourinary and nervous systems. The present state of the patient's exercise tolerance should be tested. Each system will be evaluated and no grave deficiency should be noted in any system if a patient is to be a *good* rehabilitation candidate.

Cardiovascular System

Dyspnea may be caused by cardiovascular (CV) disturbances. If a patient complains of orthopnea, it may be an indication of left-sided ventricular failure. Ankle edema and jugular vein distention are signs of right ventricular failure—a disorder secondary to lung disease.

Pleurisy-like chest pain may indicate a pulmonary embolism or pneumonia and should be pursued. Any patients with cardiac arrhythmias before exercise should be considered high-risk patients for exercise training. Blood pressure and pulse should be observed at rest and in response to exercise. Most patients with COPD that have mild arrhythmias at rest do not tend to have increased arrhythmias during exercise. At times the arrhythmias may disappear with exercise and increased perfusion.

Respiratory System

A thorough chest exam should be performed to evaluate the patient's lungs. A recent chest x-ray should be read, and chest mobility and breathing pattern should be observed. If an improper breathing pattern is noted, i.e., breathing with accessory muscles, it is appropriate to initiate relaxation and breathing retraining before continuing with the rehab program.

The patient should be asked about his cough and sputum production in amount, color and consistency. His symptoms, such as shortness of breath and fatigue, should be evaluated in terms of their frequency and duration. The effects of changes in position should be noted. For example, if the patient reports a production of sputum while lying on his left side, there are secretions mainly in the right lung field. Methods that allow the patient to get relief, i.e., catch his breath, relax or mobilize sputum, should also be analyzed.

Gastrointestinal System

Anorexia is one notable symptom seen commonly in respiratory patients. Weight loss is found in many patients due to shortness of breath and anxiety, which prevent good nutrition. This is also common in patients with tuberculosis or bronchogenic cancer.

Diarrhea and bowel upsets are also common due to suppurative pulmonary disease and medications. Nausea is seen in patients taking several medications, especially frequent or prophylactic antibiotics. Frequently, patients do not drink enough water (or have cardiac conditions that prevent them from increasing fluids). These patients are poorly hydrated and this can adversely affect lung clearing mechanisms (decrease mucociliary escalator function).

Nutritional Consult

A dietary consult is also an important part of a rehab program. COPD may alter a client's eating habits (i.e., SOB prevents eating full meals). A good nutritional state will provide for maintenance of muscle metabolism for daily activities. An improved nutritional state may also provide for increased resistance to infections. The dietician will take a nutrition survey of eating habits, calories consumed, fluid intake, protein fats and carbohydrate intake, and identify any special dietary needs. Nutritional problems will be documented as well as an ideal client weight. A diet can be designed for weight gain, loss, or stabilization. Behavior modification techniques can be introduced to alter eating habits. It is often helpful to work with the client's spouse and discuss nutritional problems and needs.

Genitourinary System

Tuberculosis may cause dysuria and hematuria, or amenorrhea in women.

Nervous System

Physicians will assess hypoventilation as being from the disease process versus neurogenic in origin.

Hypoxemia and CO_2 retention may be associated with any of the following symptoms: headaches, dizziness, double vision, fainting, confusion, restlessness, insomnia, depression, or personality changes.

Musculoskeletal System

Muscle tone should be evaluated as well as general chest mobility (see Chapter 1) and activity tolerance.

Clubbing of the fingers may be noted due to chronic lung disease and decreased oxygen level in the arterial blood. A sudden change may be seen with malignancies. Early changes are first seen at the base of the nail (nailbed). A quick test for early clubbing is to ask the patient to put his index fingers crooked (bent forward), then place the index fingernails together. Normally a diamond shaped air space will be noted. Even in early clubbing, this air space will disappear as the fingernail of a patient with clubbing is 180 degrees.

Personal Habits

The patient's personal living habits, migration, occupational history, hobbies, smoking, drinking, allergies, childhood diseases, recurrent diseases (i.e., recurring right middle lobe pneumonia), and socioeconomic history should all be evaluated. Familial tendencies toward respiratory disease should be noted.

Preprogram Evaluation

Prior to entrance in a pulmonary rehabilitation program, the patient should have the following workup: (1) diagnostic tests, which include pulmonary function tests, chest x-ray, ECG, arterial blood gases, sputum analysis, and blood theophylline levels; and (2) behavioral motivational/psychological assessment, which includes motivation, present mental status, i.e., depressed, angry, ability to learn, concentrate, and cooperate, motivational level. If the behavioral state seems to be inappropriate, i.e., extreme depression or anger, the patient will probably need further professional evaluation and counseling prior to entrance into a rehab program. The clinical psychologist may also be very helpful in helping the therapist know how to deal more effectively with the patient based on his personality and how he may learn best.

Setting Goals

The rehab team and the patient need to discuss and jointly set up realistic goals for rehabilitation. It is extremely important to include the patient at this level because if a patient sets his own goal he will be more motivated to achieve it. Often a physician-oriented or therapist-oriented goal is not necessarily important to the patient. It is then difficult to motivate patients. *Motivation* of the patient is the most important beginning of a successful program. Goals are generally both short and long term. The patient should determine what can be completed in 1–2 months and what may be accomplished in six or more months. The key is to be *realistic*. If patients ask for something unrealistic, they should not be negatively handled but should not be encouraged to reach that goal in a short time. It may be thought of as a long-term goal. Generally the patient himself will realize the goal is inappropriate during the course of therapy. It is important that the patient can see some immediate short-term goals met in order to be motivated to work for long-term goals. Examples of short-term goals such as these are being able to catch his breath, walking up a few stairs without getting exhausted, coughing effectively to mobilize mucus, getting to the bathroom and so on.

Goals must be determined individually according to the patient's baseline activity levels. If a patient has led a very active life, playing 18 holes of golf, working full time and maintaining a house, he will feel greatly incapacitated if he can play only nine holes of golf and work part time. However, a patient who has a desk job and minimal exercise—perhaps only watching sports on television—may not feel incapacitated until he is almost bedridden. This patient would not have been able to attain the first patient's activity in his prime, and it would be grossly unrealistic to set the same goals for both patients. Therefore, goal setting is one of the keys to patient motivation and program success. Goals must be reasonable and compatible with the patient's personality, ability, situation and life style, both medical and socioeconomic.

Guidelines for general goals may be:

1. Improve the patient's ability to achieve symptomatic control both in acute episodes and on a chronic long-term basis.

2. Teach the patient means of achieving optimal physical capacity to perform activities of daily living (ADL).

3. Teach the patient trouble-shooting techniques (i.e., what to do if there is a change in sputum color or if he has increased shortness of breath).

4. Teach the patient to analyze episodes of shortness of breath, increased dyspnea, and other symptoms, and evaluate ways of coping to prevent them in the future.

These are all general goals; they become more specific as patient input is added. For example, a housewife wants to be able to go back to shopping and carrying grocery bags, to make beds and do general housework. A working woman or man needs to walk a block to the train and climb several stairs at work, or even have enough "breath" to talk in long sentences and communicate effectively as well as having endurance to make it through the workday.

In physical activity, patients need to control and coordinate activity with breathing.

COMPONENTS OF PULMONARY REHABILITATION

A systematic program flow seems to be beneficial, beginning with proper testing and assessment, and ending with a thoroughly educated, trained patient who maintains himself at home with occasional calls and follow-up with the rehab team.

A sequence is suggested to prevent putting the cart before the horse; patients will often want to exercise first, but if proper bronchial hygiene, breathing retraining and relaxation have not preceded exercise, the patient will not have the capacity to perform. The usual order of flow is as follows:

1. Patient testing: ECG, x-ray, PFTs, arterial blood gases, medical checkup and medical history.

2. Therapist assessment: breathing patterns, cough, sputum, relaxation state, activity level, chest mobility and motivation.

3. Patient and family education.

4. Bronchial hygiene.

5. Breathing and relaxation training, chest mobilization.

6. Physical conditioning.

7. Home program.

8. Reevaluation and follow-up.

Each component of this flow builds on the former component in this manner. When the airways are clear of mucus, the patient then breathes more effectively in order to increase his exercises and begin a conditioning program. Patient education permeates all therapeutic techniques. As the therapist performs a treatment, teaching should be incorporated with the idea the patient is learning self-care. Patient testing and therapist assessment have already been discussed; emphasis will not be directed toward the actual treatment.

Patient and Family Education

Education is begun initially to help the patient understand his disease, why he is short of breath, why he is raising sputum and why he is generally unable to do what he wishes. It also should explain the rehabilitation process, the role of the therapist and especially the responsibility of the patient. It should be informative, but also encouraging that something can be done if the patient is willing to work and accomplish his goals (see Chapter 15). We will now deal with education specific to pulmonary rehabilitation. Specific areas to cover are:

Respiratory Anatomy and Physiology.   There should be a general discussion of the ciliary clearance mechanism and the cough. The patient should see the tracheobronchial lung segments and the different angles they take off from the mainstem bronchus. This will help in explaining postural drainage. Methods of oxygen transport as well as the interdependency of the heart and lungs should also be covered.

The mechanics of diaphragmatic breathing should also be discussed and demonstrated. In addition to the general overview, the patient should have an explanation of his particular respiratory problem (disease, dysfunction). In personalizing his situation and relating it to the therapy being taught, the patient is able to see the "total picture."

Environmental Factors.   This may be personal or external. Subjects such as smoking, air pollution, paint fumes, cold or hot weather extremes, altitudes, air travel and humidifiers should be discussed.

Avoid Infection.   Patients should take preventive injections (flu shots) at their physician's discretion. They should realize they should avoid friends with colds or viruses and not allow themselves to get overly tired or run down.

Fluid Intake.   Most respiratory patients do not drink enough water. The relationship between good hydration and proper mucociliary transport should be stressed. Patients who are limited in fluid intake should be encouraged to drink whatever they are able to consume. The patient may not always count the number of glasses of water he drinks, but should be taught to check the color of his urine as well as its consistency. Urine should be only light yellow (lemon colored) and very clear. When urine has a deep gold or yellow color and seems cloudy, the patient should have more fluid to be better hydrated.

They should be encouraged to increase their fluid intake to 10–12 glasses per day (2⅓–3 quarts) *unless* there are cardiac problems where their fluid intake should be limited. (*Note:* This will also increase their exercise to the bathroom!) Generally, fluids should not be extremely hot or cold as this can cause irritation in the airways. They should observe any ankle edema or sudden weight gains and report this immediately to their physician.

Nutrition.   A dietitian is helpful to the patient to assist in planning meals that are high in protein and avoiding fatty foods and gas-producing foods that cause discomfort. When gassy foods (i.e., raw apples, beans, onions) are eaten, gas expands and fills the stomach. The stomach "bubble" can elevate the left diaphragm and limit its effectiveness. This can cause a great deal of discomfort to a compromised patient's breathing. It is helpful to teach patients to eat small meals several times a day rather than large meals three times a day. If they are to be very active, patients would be better to have easily digested foods rather than heavy proteins, fats, and gassy foods.

Many respiratory patients lose their appetite and weight; anorexia is a common complaint. Often patients that are dyspneic swallow air. This combined with irritating medications can lead to nausea. Being short of breath at meals makes patients less motivated to eat as it is too much work. Often several small meals and snacks will provide better nutrition than the usual "three square meals" a day. Supplemental vitamins should also be encouraged.

Review of Patient Medications

Often patients come in with a plastic bag filled with many medications that several different physicians have given them. There are many sympathomimetic drugs that additively cause many side effects. It is important to write down every drug a patient is taking and, with the physician working with the pulmonary rehab unit, determine what the drug regimen should be. The relationship in the rehab unit is usually one of a consulting role, so the pulmonary rehab physician will usually call the patient's attending physician to clear changes in the drug regimen.

Patients need to know what they are taking and the potential synergistic effects and side effects. Symptoms to watch for are particularly related to *bronchodilators*. These include heart palpitations, insomnia, tremor, nausea, vomiting, urinary retention, anorexia, irritability and personality changes. The most bizarre symptoms may be related to a toxic level of medication. General respiratory pharmacology is covered in Chapter 31.

Bronchodilators

Pharmaceutical agents are employed in the treatment of obstructive airways disease. They exert a direct effect on smooth muscle tone of the airways. They are particularly beneficial in asthma, but are frequently used with other obstructive lung diseases.

The bronchial tree can be altered by other factors as well as smooth muscle contraction. Therefore, if there is mucosal edema (i.e., swelling secondary to inflammation or edema) or excessive secretions from the goblet cells and mucus gland, the lumen of the bronchial tree will be affected. Corticosteroids may be used with patients exhibiting these characteristics.

Common oral bronchodilators include ephedrine, theophylline, and aminophylline (may be given IV). Metered dose inhalation bronchodilators include Bronkosol, Alupent, Isuprel, and Tornalate (newer and longer acting).

Inhaled Powder or Aerosol

Cromolyn-sodium can be inhaled on a regular basis to prevent bronchospasm (it coats the receptor sites in the bronchial tree to prevent a reaction to an allergen by blocking the site of action).

Corticosteroids

Oral, inhaled, or IV; prednisone, beclomethasone. Inhaled steroids may have less systemic affect and a more local effect. Digitalis strengthens contraction of heart muscle.

Corticosteroids may be beneficial to patients with intermittent attacks of bronchial obstruction or blood or sputum eosinophilia. They are sometimes administered in short courses, other times as long-term, low-dose steroids. The difference is the objective—whether to get the patient over an acute episode or to provide a long-term, relatively symptom-free patient.

Side effects may be cushingoid features, osteoporosis, bruising, glucose intolerance, peptic ulcers and electrolyte imbalance related to potassium loss.

Expectorants

Specific *expectorants* are generally not indicated. Some can produce gastric irritation, skin rashes or swelling of the salivary glands (and may precipitate hypothyroidism). Water is the best expectorant.

Antibiotics

Antibiotics are generally given to treat respiratory tract infections. They should be started 24 hours after an increase in sputum, corresponding with a sputum color change to yellow or green, and they are continued for 7–10 days. They may cause much gastrointestinal distress, mainly nausea and vomiting. This can be counteracted by suggesting that patients eat yogurt or drink buttermilk while taking antibiotics if it is not contraindicated. Patients taking antacids or milk may have interference with the absorption of tetracycline from the intestinal tract.

If a patient remains febrile and demonstrates symtoms not responding well to the given antibiotic, a sputum culture should be done to ascertain a more appropriate antibiotic.

Ionotropic Cardiotonic Agent (Digitalis)

Digitalis strengthens contraction of heart muscle.

Beta Blockers

Beta blockers such as Inderal slow conduction through the AV node, which can slow pulse rate and decrease the work load of the heart. Beta blockers will not allow the patient to have the normal cardiac response to exercise. Consequently, exercise needs to be monitored more carefully and the patient's response evaluated carefully.

Diuretics

Diuretics are usually given for left- or right-sided heart failure. Patients must remember to take bananas, orange juice or other potassium supplements to avoid hypokalemia.

A family member or friend who is to be involved in the patient's care should also receive basic education in these areas. In addition, they need to know how to recognize and assist the patient if a crisis occurs.

The chapter on cardiopulmonary pharmacology will have an in-depth discussion of the medications utilized by patients with cardiopulmonary dysfunction. It is important that the patient's condition be stabilized prior to starting the pulmonary rehabilitation. If the patient is jittery and nervous normally due to his condition and also overloaded on sympathetic nervous system stimulants given to him by three different physicians, he will not be able to comply with the therapy. During the rehab program, education regarding his medication and a schedule for how to take it and possible side effects are essential.

Bronchial Hygiene

Bronchial hygiene is the first therapy technique utilized. It is necessary to mobilize retained secretions to allow the lungs to function optimally. Generally, all patients should try postural drainage for at least 2–3 days even if they claim they produce no sputum regularly. Often patients who do not feel they are productive will raise mucus with this technique. Most patients who are sputum producers will have an increase in the amount of sputum raised. Many times it will be noted that there is an initial increase in the amount of sputum raised with postural drainage, then it levels off to a set amount per day. The patient should be aware of the amount as well as the color and consistency of sputum normally raised.

Areas emphasized for postural drainage in patients with chronic lung disease are mainly the lower lobes, although some patients may also need the right middle lobe, lingula, or apical segments of the lower lobes drained. The areas should be emphasized according to results of postural drainage, x-ray and auscultation. The patient should be made aware of the most important areas. In this way if he has to rush and can only concentrate on one or two drainage positions, he knows which ones to do.

In general, the patient is taught drainage positions lying head down, prone and on the sides (see the discussions on home program and postural drainage in Chapter 12).

The patient can be instructed in self-percussion and can usually reach all chest surfaces easily except the posterior lower lobes. He can perform the technique with one hand rather than coordinating both hands.

Vibration is somewhat difficult to do independently but the patient can do chest compression in a modified manner.

Bronchial hygiene should be stressed as a regular routine, *not* just for when the patient feels poorly. It is a prophylactic measure to prevent retained secretions leading to pneumonia and respiratory failure.

Relaxation and Breathing Training

Relaxation and proper breathing go hand in hand. Even in normal people, breathing is inhibited if one is nervous and tense or rushed in a stressful situation. The specific techniques are discussed in Chapter 8. The relaxation exercise precedes breathing retraining. Generally, breathing exercise is done in sequence from supine progressing to stairs as noted in Chapter 8. Finally, coordination of breathing with various activities is taught. Chest mobilization is routinely done from the start of treatment for the duration of the program by the physical therapist and taught to the patient. The goal is to obtain and maintain proper function of the therapy.

The depressed flat diaphragm is a poorly functioning muscle. It is not the "cause" of bad breathing, but rather a consequence of pulmonary disease. The therapist strives to develop a breathing pattern as close to the "normal" pattern as possible. The inspiratory muscles can be trained to improve strength and endurance (see Chapter 9).

Cough

The sequence and purpose of a normal cough should be discussed. Patients should be instructed not to waste energy by constant ineffective coughing. If the cough is nonproductive, it is better to work on deep breathing exercises. Continued coughing can narrow the airways and cause bronchospasm. The cough should not be forced, but controlled. A rapid expiratory airflow (tussive blast) is most important. If the patient's FEV_1 is less than 700 cc, the tussive blast is ineffective. A "tussive squeeze" may be used by gently pushing on the lower chest while coughing. Other manual techniques are discussed in Chapter 21. If the patient is receiving oxygen, he should be encouraged to keep on it during coughing. The oxygen should be removed only to expectorate sputum if necessary.

Physical Conditioning and Training

Conditioning should be started as early as possible in the course of a patient's disease. The later in the disease progression rehabilitation is started, the less can usually be done. At times all a therapist can offer is to teach the patient how to live with limited resources and how to utilize energy conservation methods. A thorough assessment should be made of a patient that has not exercised in years prior to an aggressive

exercise program. The therapist needs to be aware of potential orthopedic injuries that could occur in these patients during start-up of
exercise and as the exercise program is advanced. Proper footware
should be used, and the importance of stretching and warm-up before
getting into aerobic exercise should be emphasized.

Any physical activity greater than resting level results in an increase
in oxygen consumption and CO_2 production by the exercising tissue.
These increased demands will cause secondary increases in ventilation
and cardiac output. The increased ventilation and work load may
cause dyspnea in chronic lung patients. In addition, depending on
the ventilation-perfusion relationships, the arterial oxygen saturation
and PO_2 may fall. In patients with severe obstructive airway disease,
the pulmonary artery pressure may rise during exercise and markedly increase the work of the right ventricle. Even so, patients need
to perform a certain amount of activity in order not to become bedridden.

Two types of training are noted—horizontal and vertical. *Horizontal
training* occurs when exercise training increases muscle efficiency as
noted by a decrease in physiologic stress and oxygen consumption at
the same workload. *Vertical training* also includes an increase in the efficiency of muscles and involves an increase in work capacity. Our goal
optimally is to strive first for horizontal training, then to progress further to vertical training. (When a patient has become conditioned to a
level of exercise and is performing well, the level is then increased
gradually. This is an example of horizontal training progressing to vertical training.)

Exercise begins at the baselines of the patient. A totally dependent
patient on a ventilator receives exercise in an attempt to maintain muscle tone and joint range of motion. Following weaning from the ventilator, progressive exercise will be initiated to increase exercise tolerance. The conditioning programs ideally will continue on an outpatient
basis followed by a comprehensive home care program.

Patient A: Severely Debilitated.   Two general exercise programs
will be discussed using fictitious patient cases. Patient A is a severely
involved, debilitated patient. Patient B demonstrates the progression of
a less advanced, more active patient capable of more aggressive exercise.

Patient A, with chronic obstructive lung disease, is generally first
seen for evaluation in the hospital with pneumonia and impending or
actual ventilatory failure. Following the acute episode, he has minimal
exercise tolerance. He relates that he has been able to do less and less

over the last 5 years and was virtually housebound prior to this hospital admission. He is on oxygen at 2 L/min via a nasal cannula. He can barely walk to the door of his room (approximately 10 ft) without severe dyspnea. He uses accessory muscles and has an abnormal pattern of breathing. He is anxious and depressed. He feels weak (states his knees are buckling) and has no appetite to encourage better nutrition. His pulse rate at rest is 96 beats per minute, his respiratory rate is 20 per min, BP 130/86.

Patient assessment, education, relaxation, breathing training and bronchial hygiene are all dealt with in depth in other chapters. In this chapter, we will consider these evaluations and treatments to have been initiated (in the order listed above) previously and now the exercise testing and physical conditioning are beginning.

The therapist should explain to the patient that he will take portable oxygen and try to take a short walk. During this time, the therapist will be monitoring his pulse and BP, trying to estimate a comfortable work load. The patient should try to do as much as he feels capable of, but should not try to be a "hero." Walking should stop when the patient feels it is necessary and chairs should be available for him to sit on and rest. (The therapist makes *sure* these are available *before* starting the walk or another person may pull a chair.)

A maximal HR for the individual should be calculated. The following simple equation is utilized.

$$220 - \text{patient age} = \text{maximal predicted HR}$$

Generally, with COPD patients, we try to get their HR to 75%–85% maximum predicted HR. Example: patient 60 years old, MP HR = 220–60 = 160 × 75% = 120 × 85% = 136. Therefore, we will aim to exercise the patient at a HR between 120–136/min.

The resting heart rate will determine how much more reserve the patient has available. For example, if the patient's resting heart rate is 96, it will not take much activity to increase that to 120–136 in that same patient given above. Drs. Hughes and Davidson in their article went so far as to say that resting heart rate should be no higher than 110 beats/min if the patient is to be exercised.

The therapist will have the patient sit on the side of the bed or on a chair and establish resting baselines. The BP, pulse, and respiratory rates should be measured. General guidelines for increase after exercise are:

1. BP and pulse increase 20%–30%.

2. BP and pulse return to the baseline level within 5–10 minutes after cessation of exercise.

3. Patient feels tired, possibly short of breath, but definitely exercised.

Before starting exercise, the oxygen (FI_{02}) should be increased (a written physician order is needed to increase the O_2). If the patient was receiving 2 L/min, this should be increased to approximately 3–5 L/min for the exercise period. (The oxygen should be returned to the baseline 2 L/min very shortly after exercise when the pulse returns to baseline, generally within 5 min after exercise.) The increase in oxygen during exercise is not harmful and should not diminish the *hypoxic drive* to breathe as there is increased oxygen consumption during exercise and the increased FI_{02} is simply providing for this. An order for increased FI_{02}, with exercise needs to be written by the physician prior to increasing the O_2.

Hypoxic drive refers to a phenomenon that generally occurs when the PO_2, at rest is less than 55–60 mm Hg and the PCO_2 is elevated. The patient's major drive to breathe changes from a CO_2 stimulus to hypoxemia. If a patient receiving oxygen has a PO_2 of more than 60 mm Hg, it may remove the hypoxic drive to breathe. This leads to increased hypoventilation and respiratory failure (acidosis) or respiratory decompensation.

Given during exercise, oxygen will decrease the cardiovascular work by minimizing the cardiac output necessary for the work load. Oxygen may decrease ventilation, respiratory rate and heart rate in patients with severe ventilatory insufficiency. Patients who are chronically hypoxemic may have multiple PVCs during exercise if supplemental O_2 is not given. The oxygen will decrease the work of breathing and help the patient meet the additional exercise stress. The PVCs with exercise in these patients usually result from increased pulmonary artery pressure caused by an increased workload and a hypoxic myocardium. By administering O_2 the arterial oxygen saturation becomes more normal, and there is a decrease in cardiac output for a given PO_2 as well as a decrease in pulmonary hypertension.

Oxygen supplementation during exercise should be thought of as a *tool* rather than a crutch. Patients should be informed that we are not trying to give them continuous oxygen that they need for the rest of their lives but rather a means to an end, the end being a faster, more intense exercise program. Usually oxygen will allow 3–5 times more exercise then breathing room air. It is also interesting to note that in studies done by Pierce, Paez and Miller, after exercise with oxygen, patients performed better on room air.

Some patients may need home oxygen. This should be given in specific instances and *not* as a routine for chronic lung patients. Miller lists criteria for oxygen administration as a maximum voluntary ventilation (MVV) less than 20 L/min and an FEV_1 less than 500 cc. These patients generally need O_2 continuously just to walk from room to room. Other criteria are hypoxemia and pulmonary hypertension. Some physicians authorize the use of supplemental oxygen during the night, especially for patients complaining of sleeplessness, restlessness and irritability, and those that exhibit pulmonary hypertension. Additional indications are a PO_2 of less than 55 mm Hg, extreme shortness of breath while eating or during airplane flights, and arrhythmias which result from exercise. The therapist may suggest the use of oxygen for increased activity but it is used only under the physician's orders. Oxygen must be respected and utilized as a drug.

To summarize the procedure for patient A:

1. Baseline BP and pulse and respiratory rates are measured.

2. The patient may be started on oxygen (or O_2 is increased if the patient is on resting O_2).

3. The patient is asked to walk slowly with long strides until he feels he needs to rest. (A chair should be readily available.)

4. The BP and pulse are measured immediately as the patient stops (to get the peak pulse rate). The therapist will note the time (or use a stopwatch, as it is ideal for measuring elapsed time) and continue to take the patient's pulse each minute until it returns to baseline. The time interval from peak pulse to the *recovery pulse* (former baseline pulse) is the *recovery pulse time.* This should be 5–10 minutes. Generally, the pulse will return to approximately 10% of the baseline pulse within 5–7 minutes.

5. An estimate of the distance traveled should be made or a floor route can be marked out in feet to measure more exactly.

Charting should include the above parameters. A flowchart is helpful to see patient progression. The following may be charted: "Patient ambulated in hall, approximately 100 feet with O_2 by cannula at 5 L/min. Pulse at rest 92/min to 116/min following exercise. Pulse recovered in 8 min. No abnormal beats felt. Patient moderately short of breath but recovered quickly. Patient well motivated and cooperative. Will continue exercise b.i.d. Patient's objective: to increase distance and exercise tolerance."

If the therapist uses a flowchart, the objective data are available as well as a section for the patient's subjective feeling and goals. The week's therapy may be seen at a glance, and data are more concise and readily available.

General Considerations

1. The initial thrust of the exercise is to increase the work load (i.e., distance walked) to a "goal" load (based on pulse and BP increase to 20%–30%, recovery pulse time 5–10 minutes and patient feeling exercised).

2. When the optimal work load is obtained, it is held *constant.*

3. If the patient is on oxygen, the oxygen is the variable. The goal is to get the patient exercising *without* O_2.

4. The oxygen is decreased by 1 L/min when the pulse recovery interval is less than five minutes. Generally, this proceeds easily downward until the decrease from 1 L to room air. Many patients seem to do very well with exercise at 1–2 L/min oxygen but do poorly when exercised on room air. If the therapist has misgivings about taking the patient off oxygen to exercise, a physician or his designate should be present and an oximetry test done with exercise to test for desaturation.

5. At *no time* should a patient be exercised with less oxygen than he is receiving at rest. (For example, if the patient is on O_2 at 2 L/min, the O_2 would be *no* less than that during exercise.) If this instance ever arises, the therapist should refer to the patient's physician for direction. Generally, repeat arterial blood gases will be measured to reassess the patient's need for oxygen at rest and during exercise.

6. The patient should be asked *why* he needed to stop exercising. Often it is not shortness of breath but cramps in the lower extremities (caused by lactic acidosis or anaerobic metabolism).

7. The therapist should be optimistic and encouraging in regard to the patient's performance. This is not to be unrealistic and "sugar sweet." If the patient has a bad day and does poorly that should be acknowledged; a comment such as: "Well, *everyone* has a bad day once in a while, tomorrow should be better" is easier to live with than a comment such as, "Yes, you really did poorly; is that the best you can do?"

8. Patient motivation should be checked during therapy. There are times patients may not give maximum effort for personal reasons (diarrhea, a fight with spouse, a late lunch) or patients may be looking for

attention (negative reinforcement, i.e., I do poorly and you talk to me and feel sorry for me). *The therapist should not dwell on the patient's disability but rather on his present and potential ability.*

If a patient does well in floor ambulation in the hospital or if an outpatient with fair exercise tolerance is referred for rehabilitation, treadmill (or bicycle) exercise will generally be used. In presenting patient B, the more active patient, we will again consider that the patient has been evaluated and educated and is now receiving aggressive bronchial hygiene, breathing and relaxation training, including total patterns and chest wall mobilization.

Patient B: Generally Active With Decreased Tolerance to Exercise. Patient B gives a history of decrease in physical activity over the last few years. He may relate this decrease to a particular situation (i.e., "I was fine until two years ago when I had a bad cold and I haven't been the same since"). The patient states he can walk 3–4 blocks on a good day and can climb one or two flights of stairs. He used to play 18 holes of golf and now can play only nine holes and must use a cart. He gets short of breath if he tries to talk while walking or carries a suitcase or any load. This patient would be given an exercise stress test by the physician or therapist and started on treadmill exercise as well as a graded strengthening and endurance program of exercise. Treadmill exercise is ideal as it is much more objective than the more subjective walking in the hall. The parameters that can be measured during treadmill exercise are patient's BP, pulse, respiratory rate, ECG rhythm, speed of treadmill, incline of treadmill and time walked. Again, the flowchart is used.

There are a variety of ways to perform a stress test and a variety of data that can be collected, such as O_2 consumption, CO_2 production, at rest and exercise blood gases, ECG strips and so on. The author wishes to deal here with a clinical exercise test to set up an exercise program to increase patient tolerance and endurance.

We had utilized a metabolic cart for a few years but with our population of patients (more severely involved COPD), we found data collection inconclusive and frustrating as we rarely reached an anaerobic threshhold. Patients found it difficult to have a noseclip in place and try to breathe through the mouthpiece. We began to utilize a more functional clinical test which we will describe. The test is not a stress test as is done for cardiac patients with a strict protocol. Rather, there are regular procedures and guidelines, yet it is meant to assess the patient's ability and evaluate whether or not the patient desaturates with functional exercise. Based on the functional testing, an exercise pre-scription will be given. If the patient desaturates with exercise, the test will be repeated with O_2 being titrated to the appropriate level to pre-vent desaturation with exercise.

It is important for the therapist to know prior to exercising a pa-tient what medications are being taken. For example, if the patient takes a beta blocker such as Inderal, it will limit the CV response to exercise. If the patient takes bronchodilators orally or by metered dose inhaler (MDI), it is important to know how he takes them and when the last dose was taken. It is important to gauge increased exercise with good bronchodilator coverage. If the blood level is low, a broncho-spasm could occur with exercise, especially in patients with exercise in-duced asthma. In these patients, it is helpful to take their bronchodi-lators by MDI 20–30 minutes prior to exercise and then perform some mild stretching and warm-up exercise prior to more high work load exercise. In this manner, they may avoid bronchospasm with exercise.

Procedure for Functional Exercise Testing

Prior to the exercise test, an ECG should be performed and an arterial blood gas drawn for baselines. The oximeter is put in place (either ear or fingertip). The patient will have ECG and BP monitoring as well as oximetry during the exercise test. All emergency equipment should be checked for readiness. There should be a well-understood emergency procedure that will be immediately instituted if necessary.

Set Up Client

The client should have proper skin preparation with electrodes put in place. Baseline ECG strips are run. Baseline BP sitting and standing are also taken as well as an oximetry reading.

The client is then shown the proper use of a treadmill or bicycle. If an aerobic measurement system is demonstrated and a three-minute baseline used, breathing is done initially.

The client should be instructed how to give a sign if the test should be stopped and why he should stop. He is instructed not to be a "hero," but only to do as well as possible. He can terminate the test at any time, but the usual endpoints patients reach are: (1) intolerable dyspnea, (2) extreme fatigue, (3) leg cramps, (4) feeling faint or dizzy, and (5) chest pain.

Test Protocol

This is one modified test protocol that we have used for our pul-monary rehab clients. There will be many other types, and the important aspect is that it works for us and is a consistent method with which we are comfortable.

1. Start treadmill at 0 degree elevation 1 mph.

2. Allow patient to begin to ambulate and slowly increase speed to a comfortable stride length (usually 1.5–2 mph).

3. Levels will be changed at three-minute increments.

The heart rate and BP are recorded at the first and third minute. Any change in the ECG should also be noted.

4. If the client tolerated the first level well at three minutes, inform the client and increase the elevation by 2.5 degrees. (This will continue for each level; speed remains constant and incline increases 2.5 degrees with each three-minute interval.)

5. The elevation increase continues until an end point is reached.

The test endpoint is symptom limited. The symptoms may be subjective or objective.

Subjective Endpoints

1. Severe intolerable dyspnea.

2. Chest pain.

3. Extreme fatigue.

4. Leg cramps.

5. Fainting or dizziness.

Objective Endpoints

1. More than 6 PVCs per minute.

2. Paired PVCs.

3. Bigeminy.

4. PVC falling on T wave.

5. ST-segment depression of 1 mm or more.

6. Bradycardia.

7. More than 85% maximal heart rate.

8. Systolic BP in excess of 210 mm Hg.

9. Systolic BP decrease of 25 mm Hg.

10. Mental confusion, nervousness, severe apprehension.

11. Sudden onset of pallor, diaphoresis.

12. Failure of ECG monitoring system.

When the endpoint is reached, the client is "wound down" to 0 degree elevation and 1 mph. They may walk or ride for a few minutes as they wind down. The treadmill or bicycle is stopped. BP and HR are recorded. The vitals are followed every two minutes until baselines are again reached.

The client should remain in the department at least 20–30 minutes to be observed and relax following the test. The client should be informed of how well he performed the test and what the implications are for therapy and follow-up.

The treadmill or bicycle test is used to determine an exercise load for general exercise conditioning during therapy. For example, if a client walked up to a 7.5% incline for 10 minutes at 2 mph at 75% maximal heart rate, this could be his conditioning work load. The patient would then exercise 10 minutes at 7.5%, 2 mph at 75% maximal heart rate. As the patient becomes more conditioned and exercises at a lower heart rate, he can have his work load increased either by an increased incline (usually) or increased time.

An exercise prescription for independent exercise is made for each client based on his treadmill or bicycle exercise. This level is progressively increased according to patient tolerance. The length of time is usually 20 minutes. The patient is instructed to walk a certain distance in 20 minutes. He is taught to take his pulse and to shoot for a target heart rate. When he is comfortably performing the exercise at a lower heart rate, he can increase his speed or distance to maintain conditioning effects.

During subsequent visits, he should be questioned specifically about his exercise. A diary may be helpful to document specific exercise and heart rates. Clients are often more compliant if they feel they have to account to a therapist for their program follow-up.

Patient education at this point should involve the importance of maintaining physical fitness, exercising at least 4–5 times per week, alternatives to use if it is raining and they can't walk outside, etc. Many clients are given an exercise prescription for both a walking schedule and comparable stationary bicycle exercise. They can exchange modes of exercise as they feel or as the weather permits.

An excellent adjunct to graded exercise is inspiratory resistance exercise, which is helpful for patients with severe COPD. Exercise is usually limited in these patients by their ventilatory capability. Respiratory muscle endurance has been found to be increased in patients with COPD by inspiratory muscle training. These devices are now readily available and are an excellent home therapeutic modality (see Chapter 9 for more information).

If the client desaturates with exercise, an appropriate oxygen prescription should be given. Proper maintenance and use of oxygen should be taught along with the hazards of increasing oxygen above the prescribed dosage. The client should give a return demonstration of all oxygen appliances to be used at home to determine his competency.

Home Programs

An individually tailored home program should be implemented with the patient. Generally, this may consist of bronchial hygiene daily in the morning with a few breathing exercises, including stretching and pacing techniques. An exercise prescription has been given, and exercise should become a daily routine (at least 4–5 times a week). Diet and fluid intake should be considered and goals set for the return visits. The patient should understand his medications and take them appropriately.

Goals should be jointly set and things to accomplish before the next follow-up session discussed. Generally, a client comes to the rehab program 2–3 times a week for 2–3 weeks. Then a follow-up is set for a week later, then two weeks, then a month. Depending on a client's condition and needs, a two- to three-month follow-up, for a checkup is all that is necessary. A client that has been well-educated will know the signs and symptoms of impending problems and will call earlier if he is having trouble. The client should always feel free to call when he has a question or need. A rehab program is complete when the client is caring for himself, making his own decisions, and assuming responsibility for his situation. We need to work ourselves out of a "job" to be successful in rehabilitation.

The literature documents the need for proper assessment and treatment of the COPD patient. It is difficult to pinpoint the reason for the successful rehabilitation of a client. There are few objective parameters that can be measured to show improvement. For example, chest x-rays, pulmonary functions, and arterial blood gases usually do not change significantly. However, patients often increase their exercise tolerance and endurance dramatically. This is sometimes referred to as a psychological improvement. The client is said to be more motivated and not as afraid of being short of breath. There have been some changes seen clinically in increased ability for oxygen consumption. This may lead to a better understanding of efficiency of muscles in a trained COPD client.

There is, however, a dearth of specific articles explaining the reason for successful COPD rehabilitation. Most articles note how the rehabilitation program is designed, the role of the physical therapist, and the necessity for early intervention, rather than end-stage disease involvement. (A comprehensive pulmonary rehabilitation bibliography is included.)

WHAT DO WE NEED TO KNOW?

Future investigation of pulmonary rehabilitation could delve into the role of motivation, finding specific tests that note objective improvement, following rehab and designing programs that are cost effective and yet meet client's needs. Often programs have several members on a "team." This can become very expensive in that rehabilitation is time consuming and scheduling is always a problem. A means of designing a "team" that can be as simple as possible with overlapping roles so that one or two people can meet most of the patient's needs, rather than 10 individuals seeing each client, seems desirable. The care team could make referrals to other specialists if there is a need, but for the most part could handle most of the client's rehab program.

The failure of a rehabilitation effort may be due to any number of factors. Among them are:

1. Patient lack of motivation.

2. Personality conflict between patient and therapist.

3. Poor understanding of what is expected of the patient.

4. Lack of proper goals—an overly enthusiastic patient and/or therapist, unrealistic goals (when goals are not accomplished patients get discouraged).

5. Poor motor coordination of patient.

6. Patient very nervous, unable to relax.

7. Skepticism of family, friends or hospital staff.

8. *Skepticism of attending physician.*

The last point cannot be overemphasized. If the patient senses his physician does not think rehabilitation will work, he picks this up quickly. It is almost to prove that his doctor was right. Patients feel physicians have all the answers and will not listen and cooperate well with the therapist and program under these circumstances.

The reason the failures are pointed up is to try to gear our programs to meet the patient's needs. If we are aware of potential problems, we can strive to correct them and achieve success. Success may be measured in many ways: to a patient unable to walk across the room without dyspnea, a one-block walk is a miracle; others are happy just being able to get through a meal with their families. *We need to plan for patient success, not therapist success.* A program is complete when the patient is his own therapist and nurse, caring for himself, making decisions and assuming responsibility for himself. Therapists are consultants, listeners, go-betweens and, it seems, anything else under miscellaneous in our job descriptions!

Clinical practice has demonstrated that the increase in the maximum exercise tolerance is greater than should be accounted for by just increased muscle efficiency. This may be accounted for by an increase in motivation or increased cardiopulmonary function. Generally, a decrease in heart rate and respiratory rate is seen with exercise training. Patients also feel more worth, have an increase in self-esteem and are motivated to do more. A successful rehabilitation "graduate" is generally self-motivated and feels a definite improvement in his quality of life.

REFERENCES

Periodicals

Agle D, et al: Multidiscipline treatment of chronic pulmonary insufficiency: Psychologic aspects of rehabilitation. *Psychosom Med* 1973; 35:41.

Bass H, Whitcomb J, Forman R: Exercise training: Therapy for patients with chronic obstructive pulmonary disease. *Chest* 1970; 57:116.

Bergofsky E: Rehabilitation medicine and prospects for the prevention of disability from COLD. *Prev Med* 1973; 2:43.

Blessey R, et al: Metabolic energy cost of unrestrained walking. *Phys Ther* 1976; 56:109.

Bobbert AC: Energy expenditure in level and grade walking. *J Appl Physiol* 1961; 15:1015.

Brundin A: Physical training in severe chronic obstructive lung diseases, I. Clinical course. *Scand J Respir Dis* 1974; 55:25.

Brundin A: Physical training in severe chronic obstructive lung disease, II. Observations on gas exchange. *Scand J Respir Dis* 1974; 55:37.

Cherniack R, Handford R, Svanhill E: Home care of chronic respiratory disease. *JAMA* 1969; 208:821.

Christie D: Physical training in obstructive lung disease. *Br Med J* 1968; 2:150.

Degre S, et al: Hemodynamic responses to physical training in patients with chronic lung disease. *Am Rev Respir Dis* 1974; 110:395.

Emmanuel GE, Moreno F: Distribution of ventilation and blood flow during exercise in emphysema. *J Appl Physiol* 1966; 21:1532.

Fishman D, Petty T: Physical, symptomatic and psychological improvement in patients receiving comprehensive care for chronic airway obstruction. *J Chronic Dis* 1971; 24:775.

Fuhs M, Stein A: Better ways to cope with COPD. *Nursing* 1976; 6:28.

Gilbert R, Auchincloss JH: Arterial blood gases and the acid-base balance at the exercise breaking point. *Arch Intern Med* 1970; 125:820.

Guthrie A, Petty T: Improved exercise tolerance in patients with chronic airway obstruction. *Phys Ther* 1970; 50:1333.

Haas A, Cardon H: Rehabilitation in chronic obstructive pulmonary disease. *Med Clin North Am* 1969; 53:593.

Haas A, Rusk H: Rehabilitation of patients with obstructive pulmonary diseases. The role of enriched oxygen. *Postgrad Med* 1966; 39:612.

Hodgkin J, et al: Chronic obstructive airway diseases. Current concepts in diagnosis and comprehensive care. *JAMA* 1975; 232:1243.

Hudson L, Tyler M, Petty T: Hospitalization needs during an outpatient rehabilitation program for severe chronic obstructive lung disease. *Chest* 1976; 70:606.

Keighley J, Mithoefer J: The management of arterial hypoxia in chronic obstructive pulmonary disease. *Chest* 1972; 62(suppl):45.

Kimbel P, et al: An in-hospital program for rehabilitation of patients with chronic obstructive pulmonary disease. *Chest* 1971; 60(suppl):65.

Lefcoe N, Paterson N: Adjunct therapy in chronic obstructive pulmonary disease. *Am J Med* 1973; 54:343.

Lertzman M, Cherniak R: Rehabilitation of patients with chronic obstructive pulmonary disease. *Am Rev Respir Dis* 1976; 114:1145.

Levine E, et al: The effect of long-term oxygen administration on pulmonary hypertension, polycythemia, and exercise tolerance in chronic airway obstruction with hypoxia. *Am Rev Respir Dis* 1966; 94:487.

Lorber B: Bad breath: Presenting manifestation of anaerobic pulmonary infection. *Am Rev Respir Dis* 1975; 112:875.

Lustig F, Haas A, Castillo R: Clinical and rehabilitation regimen in patients with chronic obstructive pulmonary disease. *Arch Phys Med Rehabil* 1972; 53:315.

Marcus H, et al: Exercise performance in relation to the pathophysiological type of chronic obstructive pulmonary disease. *Am J Med* 1970; 49:14.

McIlroy M: Respiratory response to exercise in sick and healthy people. *Chest Disorders Child* 1968; 48:749.

Miller W: Rehabilitation of patients with chronic obstructive lung disease. *Med Clin North Am* 1967; 51:349.

Miller W, Taylor H: Exercise training in the rehabilitation of patients with severe respiratory insufficiency due to pulmonary emphysema: The role of oxygen breathing. *South Med J* 1962; 55:1216.

Nicholas J, et al: Evaluation of an exercise therapy program for patients with chronic obstructive pulmonary disease. *Am Rev Respir Dis* 1970; 102:1.

Paez PN, et al: The physiologic basis of training patients with emphysema. *Am Rev Respir Dis* 1967; 95:944.

Pande JN, Gupta SP, Guleria JS: Effect of exercise on ventilation and gas exchange in normal subjects and in patients with chronic obstructive lung disease. *Ind J Med Res* 1974; 62:3.

Petty T: Ambulatory care for emphysema and chronic bronchitis. *Chest* 1970; 58(suppl 2):441.

Petty T: Does treatment for severe emphysema and chronic bronchitis really help? (A response). *Chest* 1974; 65:124.

Petty T: Pulmonary rehabilitation. *Basics Respir Dis* 1975; 4:10.

Petty T: Pulmonary rehabilitation. *Respir Care* 1977; 22:199.

Petty T, Nett L: Patient education and emphysema care. *Med Times* 1969; 97:117.

Petty T, et al: A comprehensive care program for chronic airways obstruction. *Ann Intern Med* 1969; 70:1109.

Petty T, et al: Objective functional improvement in chronic airway obstruction. *Chest* 1970; 57:216.

Pierce A, et al: Responses to exercise training in patients with emphysema. *Arch Intern Med* 1964; 113:28.

Pierce A, Pedro N, Miller W: Exercise training with the aid of a portable oxygen supply in patients with emphysema. *Am Rev Respir Dis* 1965; 91:653.

Saltin B, et al: Response to exercise after bed rest and after training. *Circulation* 1968; 38(suppl 7):78.

Suero T, Woolf CR: Decrease in pulmonary diffusing capacity during exercise in chronic obstructive lung disease. *Am Rev Respir Dis* 1970; 101:608.

Vyas MN, et al: Response to exercise in patients with chronic airway obstruction. Effects of exercise training. *Am Rev Respir Dis* 1971; 103:390.

Wasserman K, Whipp B: Exercise physiology in health and disease. *Am Rev Respir Dis* 1975; 112:219.

Woolf C: A rehabilitation program for improving exercise tolerance of patients with chronic obstructive lung disease. *Can Med Assoc J* 1972; 106:1289.

Woolf CR, Svero JT: Alterations in lung mechanics and gas exchange following training in chronic obstructive lung disease. *Dis Chest* 1969; 55:37.

Books

Berland T, Snider G: *Living with Your Bronchitis and Emphysema.* New York, St Martin's Press, Inc, 1972.

Dudley D: *The Psychophysiology of Respiration in Health and Disease.* New York, Appleton-Century-Crofts, 1969.

Petty T: *Intense and Rehabilitative Respiratory Care.* Philadelphia, Lea & Febiger, 1972.

Petty T, Nett L: *For Those Who Live and Breathe. A Manual for Patients with Emphysema and Chronic Bronchitis,* ed 2. Springfield, Illinois, Charles C Thomas, Publisher, 1972.

Miscellaneous

Shapiro B, et al: A Special Report from the Josephine Rubloff Pulmonary Rehabilitation Clinic of the Rehabilitation Institute of Chicago: A Two-Year Prospective Study.

The Nebraska COPD Rehabilitation Project—A Program to Identify the Factors Involved in the Rehabilitation of Patients With Chronic Obstructive Pulmonary Diseases—A Multidisciplinary Study of 140 Cases. Regional Chest Center, University of Nebraska Medical Center. In press.

Pulmonary Rehabilitation Bibliography

Alison JA, Anderson SD: Comparison of two methods of assessing physical performance in patients with chronic airway obstruction. *Phys Ther* 1981; 61(9):1278–1280.

Alison JA, Samios R, Anderson SD: Evaluation of exercise training in patients with chronic airway obstruction. *Phys Ther* 1981; 61(9):1273–1277.

Ambrosino N, Pagglaro PL, Macchi M, et al: A study of short-term effect of rehabilitation therapy in chronic obstructive pulmonary disease. *Respiration* 1981; 41(1):40–44.

Bagg LR: The 12-minute walking distance; its use in the preoperative assessment of patients with bronchial carcinoma before lung resection. *Respiration* 1984; 46(4):342–345.

Braun SR, Fregosi R, Reddan WG: Exercise training in patients with COPD. *Postgrad Med* 1982; 71(4):163–173.

Bundgaard A, Ingemann-Hansen T, Schmidt A, et al: Effect of physical training on peak oxygen consumption rate and exercise—induced asthma in adult asthmatics. *Scand J Clin Lab Invest* 1982; 42(1):9–13.

Bundgaard A, Ingemann-Hansen T, Schmidt A, et al: Exercise-induced asthma after walking, running, and cycling. *Scand J Clin Lab Invest* 1982; 42(1):15–18.

Burdon JG, Killian KJ, Jones NL: Pattern of breathing during exercise in patients with interstitial lung disease. *Thorax* 1983; 38(10):778–784.

Butland RJ, Pang J, Gross ER, et al: Two, six, and 12 minute walking tests in respiratory disease. *Br Med J (Clin Res)* 1982; 284(6329):1607–1608.

Bye PT, Anderson SD, Wollcock AJ, et al: Bicycle endurance performance of patients with Interstitial lung disease breathing air and oxygen. *Am Rev Respir Dis* 1982; 126(6):1005–1012.

Bye PT, Farkas G, Roussos C: Respiratory factors limiting exercise. *Ann Rev Physiol* 1983; 45:439–451.

Calverly PM, Leggett RJ, Flenley DC: Carbon monoxide and exercise tolerance in chronic bronchitis and emphysema. *Br Med J (Clin Res)* 1981; 283(6296):878–880.

Cerny FJ, Pullano TP, Cropp GJ: Cardiorespiratory adaptation to exercise in cystic fibrosis. *Am Rev Respir Dis* 1982; 126(2):217–220.

Cerny FJ, Cropp GJ, Bye M: Hospital therapy improves exercise tolerance and lung function in cystic fibrosis. *Am J Dis Child* 1984; 138(3):261–265.

Chetty KG, Brown SE, Light RW: Improved exercise tolerance of the polycythemic lung patient following phlebotomy. *Am J Med* 1983; 74(3):415–420.

Coates AL, Boyce P, Shaw DG, et al: Relationship between the chest radiograph and clinical condition in cystic fibrosis. *Arch Dis Child* 1981; 56(2):106–111.

Cockcroft A, Beaumont, A, Adams, L: Arterial oxygen desaturation during treadmill and bicycle exercise in patients with chronic obstructive airway disease. *Clin Sci* 1985; 68(3):327–332.

Cockcroft AE, Saunders MJ, Berry G: Randomized controlled trial of rehabilitation in chronic respiratory disability. *Thorax* 1981; 36(3):200–203.

Connelan SJ, Gough SE: The effects of nebulized salbutamol on lung function and exercise tolerance in patients with severe airflow obstruction. *Br J Dis Chest* 1982; 76(2):135–142.

Dantzker DR, Patten GA, Bower JS: Gas exchange at rest and during exercise in adults with cystic fibrosis. *Am Rev Respir Dis* 1982; 125(4):400–405.

Davido J: Pulmonary rehabilitation. *Nurs Clin North Am* 1981; 16(2):275–283.

Delgado HR, Braun SR, Skatrud B, et al: Chest wall and abdominal motion during exercise in patients with chronic obstructive pulmonary disease. *Am Rev Respir Dis* 1982; 126(2):200–205.

Dempsey J, Hanson P, Pegelow D, et al: Limitations to exercise capacity and endurance: Pulmonary system. *Can J Appl Sports Sci* 1982; 7:4–13.

Elliott CG, Morris AH, Cengiz M: Pulmonary function and exercise gas exchange in survivors of adult respiratory distress syndrome. *Am Rev Respir Dis* 1981; 123(5):492–495.

Grassino A, Gross D, Macklem PT, et al: Inspiratory muscle fatigue as a factor limiting exercise. *Bull Eur Physiopathol Respir* 1979; 15:105–111.

Green JM, Coggings D: A movement and exercise group for asthmatics. *Practitioner* 1982; 222(1367):961–964.

Guyatt GH, Pugsley SO, Sullivan MJ, et al: Effect of encouragement on walking test performance. *Thorax* 1984; 39(11):818–822.

Henricksen JM, Nielsen TT: Effect of physical training on exercise-induced bronchoconstriction. *Acta Paediatr Scand* 1983; 72(1):31–36.

Horvath SM: Exercise in a cold environment. *Exerc Sport Sci Rev* 1981; 9:221–63.

Horvath SM: Impact of air quality in exercise performance. *Exerc Sport Sci Rev* 1981; 9:265–296.

Hughes RL, Davison R: Limitations of exercise reconditioning in COLD. *Chest* 1983; 83(2):241–249.

Kanarek DJ, Hand RW: The response of cardiac and pulmonary disease to exercise testing. *Clin Chest Med* 1984; 5(1):181–187.

Jawad I, Kinhal V, Boudoula H: Respiratory arrest after treadmill exercise stress testing. *Postgrad Med* 1984; 75(5):241–242, 248.

Keogh BA, Lakatos E, Price D, et al: Importance of the lower respiratory tract in oxygen transfer. Exercise testing in patients with interstitial and destructive lung disease. *Am Rev Respir Dis* 1984; 129(2 Pt 2):S76–80.

Killian KJ, Jones NL: The use of exercise testing and other methods in the investigation of dyspnea. *Clin Chest Med* 1984; 5(1):99–108.

King JT, Bye MR, Demopoulas JR: Exercise programs for asthmatic children. *Compr Ther* 1984; 10(11):67–71.

Loke J, Mahler DA, Man SF, et al: Exercise impairment in chronic obstructive pulmonary disease. *Clin Chest Med* 1984; 5(1):121–143.

Mallinson BM, Cockroft C, Burgess DA: Exercise training for children with asthma. Outpatient program and a residential experiment. *Physiotherapy* 1981; 67(4):106–108.

Mathews JI, Hooper RG: Exercise testing in pulmonary sarcoidosis. *Chest* 1983; 83(1):75–81.

McFadden ER, Jr: Exercise performance in the asthmatic. *Am Rev Respir Dis* 1984; 129(2 Pt 2):584–587.

Mohsenifar Z, Horak D, Brown HV, et al: Sensitive indices of improvement in a pulmonary rehabilitation program. *Chest* 1983; 83(2):189–192.

Moser KM, Bokinsky GE, Savage RT, et al: Results of a comprehensive rehabilitation program. Physiologic and functional effects on patients with chronic obstructive pulmonary disease. *Arch Intern Med* 1980; 140(2):1596–1601.

Morgan AD, Peck DF, Buchanan DR, et al: Effects of attitudes and beliefs on exercise tolerance in chronic bronchitis. *Br Med J (Clin Res)* 1983; 15:286(6360):171–173.

Nery LE, Wasserman K, Andrews JD, et al: Ventilatory and gas exchange kinetics during exercise in chronic airways obstruction. *J Appl Physiol* 1982; 53(6):1594–1602.

O'Reilly JF, Shaylor JM, Fromings KM, et al: The use of the 12-minute walk test in assessing the effect of oral steroid therapy in patients with chronic airways obstruction. *Br J Dis Chest* 1982; 76(4):374–382.

Orenstein DM, Franklin BA, Doershuk CF, et al: Exercise conditioning and cardiopulmonary fitness in cystic fibrosis. The effects of a supervised three-month running program on exercise tolerance, pulmonary function, cardiorespiratory fitness (peak oxygen consumption), and respiratory muscle endurance in CF patients. *Chest* 1981; 80(4):392–398.

Pardy RL, Hussains NA, Macklem PJ: The ventilatory pump in exercise. *Clin Chest Med* 1984; (5):35–49.

Pardy RL, Rivington RN, Despas PJ, et al: The effects of inspiratory muscle training on exercise performance in chronic airflow limitation. *Am Rev Respir Dis* 1981; 123:426–433.

Pineda H, Haas F, Axen K, et al: Accuracy of pulmonary function tests in predicting exercise tolerance in chronic obstructive pulmonary disease. *Chest* 1984; 86(4):564–567.

Reid WD, Loveridge BM: Physiotherapy management of patients with chronic obstructive airways disease. *Physiother Can* 1983; 35:183–195.

Ries AL, Fedullo PF, Clausen JL: Rapid changes in arterial blood gas levels after exercise in pulmonary patients. *Chest* 1983; 83(3):454–456.

Scano G, Van Meerhaeghe A, Willeput R, et al: Effects of oxygen on breathing during exercise in patients with chronic obstructive lung disease. *Eur J Respir Dis* 1982; 63(1):23–30.

Shepherd RJ: On the design and effectiveness of training regimes in chronic obstructive lung disease. *Bull Eur Physiopathy Respir* 1977; 13:457–469.

Shepherd RJ: Training and the respiratory system therapy for asthma and other obstructive lung disease. *Ann Clin Res* 1982; 14 (Suppl 34):84–96.

Singh BS, Lewin T: Predictors of initial and final work capacity in a chronic obstructive airways disease rehabilitation program. *Aust NZ J Psychiatry* 1983; 17(4):321–327.

Smidt U, Worth H, Busch A: Limitation of ergometric work and respiratory muscle fatigue. *Bull Eur Physiopathol Respir* 1980; 16; 211–212.

Sue DY, Van Meter LR, Hansen JE, et al: Exercise gas exchange in asthmatics after beta-adrenergic blockade. *J Appl Physiol* 1983; 55(2):529–533.

Svenonius E, Kautto R, Arborelius M, Jr: Improvement after training of children with exercise-induced asthma. *Acta Paediatr Scand* 1983; 72(1):23–30.

Tydeman DE, Chandler AR, Graveling BM, et al: An investigation into the effects of exercise tolerance training on patients with chronic airflow limitation. *Physiotherapy* 1984; 70(7):261–264.

Unger KM, Moser KM, Hansen P: Selection of an exercise program for patients with chronic obstructive pulmonary disease. *Heart Lung* 1980; 9(1):68–76.

Wasserman K: The anaerobic threshold measurement to evaluate exercise performance. *Am Rev Respir Dis* 1984; 129(2 pt 2):S35–40.

Webber BA: Living to the limit: exercise for the chronic breathless patient. *Physiotherapy* 1981; 67(5):128–130.

Young A: Rehabilitation of patients with pulmonary disease. *Ann Acad Med Singapore* 1983; 12(3):410–416.

Zach M, Oberwaldner B, Hausler F: Cystic fibrosis: Physical exercise versus chest physiotherapy. *Arch Dis Child* 1982; 57(8):587–589.

APPENDIX

Response Letter to Answer Patient Inquiry Re: Pulmonary Rehabilitation

Dear M_____:

Thank you for inquiring about our pulmonary rehabilitation services.

Our program consists of a team of health specialists assisting private physicians in the management of respiratory difficulties.

A description of the goals and techniques used by our pulmonary rehabilitation team is to be found in the attached brochure.

Please note that the techniques as well as the amount of time spent in the various activities are individualized according to the patient's needs. On the average, a patient is expected to spend in our department, three to four hours at a time, two to three times weekly for two to four weeks.

Should you be interested in our program, please contact your family physician. It is only at his request by phone or mail that we will be able to send the information as to how you may be accepted.

Sincerely yours,

Donna Frownfelter, P.T., R.R.T.
Patricia Adney, P.T., R.R.T.

mb

attachment

Welcome to our Pulmonary Rehabilitation Program!

This program has been especially designed for you, a person with chronic obstructive pulmonary disease, that is, emphysema, bronchitis, or chronic asthma.

Our goal is to help you feel better and to live your life more fully.

Prior to admission to the program, you will have an evaluation to determine if you would be able to benefit from the program. This will consist of a medical evaluation, including history, electrocardiogram, chest x-ray, pulmonary function tests, complete blood count, arterial blood gas analysis, and physical assessment. (If some of these tests have been done in the last three months, they won't need to be repeated.) You will also be evaluated by a physical therapist and a nurse from our program prior to admission.

These evaluations will help us to outline a plan most likely to fit in with and help you with your daily activities. The program as such will have four parts:

1. Education—to help you and your family learn more about lung disease.
2. Bronchial hygiene—to help clear your lungs of mucus (if you cough and produce mucus daily.
3. Breathing exercises and relaxation—to help you cope better with tension and stress and to decrease episodes of shortness of breath, this will include individual and group discussions about living with COPD as well as training in relaxation techniques to help reduce tension.
4. Exercise—simple arm and leg exercises, plus walking and/or bicycling to improve muscle tone and stamina.

You will spend 2–3 hours a day in our clinic, usually three days a week. In addition, we will ask that you spend 45 minutes to an hour on nonclinic days at home working on the various exercises. If you have any questions, give us a call at 942–6690.

Patient Questionnaire

In order to help us plan your program, we would like to know what your interests and concerns are.

Circle one number under each statement to indicate your interest.

After hearing about pulmonary rehabilitation, I would like to learn more about:

1. How to keep my lungs free of extra phlegm or mucus.
   least interested 1–2–3–4 most interested
2. How to control my breathing when I feel short of breath.
   least interested 1–2–3–4 most interested
3. How to cope with stress or tension in my life.
   least interested 1–2–3–4 most interested
4. How my medications help my lungs.
   least interested 1–2–3–4 most interested
5. How to exercise properly.
   least interested 1–2–3–4 most interested
6. How to make everyday tasks or jobs easier.
   least interested 1–2–3–4 most interested
7. How to eat properly.
   least interested 1–2–3–4 most interested
8. How my lungs work.
   least interested 1–2–3–4 most interested

9. What is wrong with my lungs.
   least interested 1–2–3–4 most interested
10. Knowing when I'm sick and when I'm not.
    least interested 1–2–3–4 most interested

After each of the following statements, please circle yes or no.

After finishing this program I would like to . . .

1. Be able to go out more.	Yes	No
2. Cough less.	Yes	No
3. Sleep better.	Yes	No
4. Stop smoking.	Yes	No
5. Lose weight or gain weight.	Yes	No
6. Return to work.	Yes	No
7. Improve my sexual activity.	Yes	No
8. Feel better about myself.	Yes	No
9. Take care of myself without help.	Yes	No
10. Join a support group.	Yes	No

If there is anything else you would like to learn or do, please indicate by finishing the following statement.

I would like to _____
_____
_____
_____

Pulmonary Rehabilitation Unit Exercise Report

Name: _____
Age: _____
Height: _____

Date	Heart rate	MPH	% Grade	BP	% Saturation
Rest	_____			_____	_____
Warm-up					
_____min	_____	_____	_____	_____	_____
Exercise					
_____min	_____	_____	_____	_____	_____
_____	_____	_____	_____	_____	_____
_____	_____	_____	_____	_____	_____
_____	_____	_____	_____	_____	_____

___	___	___	___	___
___	___	___	___	___
___	___	___	___	___
___	___	___	___	___
___	___	___	___	___
	___	___	___	___

Slow down
_____min_____   _____   _____   _____

Rest after exercise

Min	Heart rate	Resp rate	BP	% Saturation
___	___	___	___	___
___	___	___	___	___
___	___	___	___	___
___	___	___	___	___
___	___	___	___	___

Summary: Max. HR _____ After _____ minutes exercise
Max. BP _____ After _____ minutes exercise
Degree of fatigue:
Degree of dyspnea:
Other symptoms:
Comments:

Pulmonary Rehabilitation Discharge Summary

Name _____ Date _____

Subjective _____
_____
_____

Objective
Bronchial hygiene _____
_____

Relaxation _____
_____

Breathing exercises _____
_____

Physical conditioning _____
_____

Diet _____
_____

Medications _____
_____

Assessment _____

_____

_____

_____

Plan
Home program _____

_____

Follow-up _____

_____

Pulmonary Rehabilitation Worksheet

Name

Date					
Aerosol Duration Type of BD used					
PD					
Cough and secretions					
Breathing exercises Type Performance					
Lower extremity trunk exercises Number of rep. Pounds used					
Treadmill or bicycle exer. Duration Tolerance Oxygen used					
Patient education Areas covered					
ABGs					

Spirometry					
Oximetry					
Weight					
Relaxation					

Pulmonary Rehabilitation Patient Questionnaire

Please indicate how helpful the Pulmonary Rehabilitation Program was to you by circling a number for each item. Number *one* means *least helpful*, and number *four, most helpful*.

Overall, do you feel this program has been a help to you?

What parts have been most helpful?

1. Teaching about your disease 1–2–3–4
2. Bronchial hygiene (postural drainage, percussion and vibration) 1–2–3–4
3. Relaxation exercises 1–2–3–4
4. Breathing exercises 1–2–3–4
5. Medication instruction 1–2–3–4
6. Nutrition instruction 1–2–3–4
7. Exercise—walking and bicycling 1–2–3–4

What else would you like to see included?

What was least helpful to you?

Other comments:

15

Patient Teaching

Kim Litwack, N.D., Ph.D., R.N.

The goal of the health care team is to assist clients to achieve optimal levels of functioning. Optimal functioning is a state of being a client strives to attain, regain, or maintain. It may not involve the absence of disease. One mechanism available to health care providers in assisting clients to move toward optimal functioning is patient teaching.

PLACE OF PATIENT TEACHING

Throughout this book, information has been presented to assist you, the health care professional, in providing patient care. Much of the information, however, must be shared with the clients with whom you are working to be effective. It is the goal of this chapter to briefly present an introduction to teaching-learning theory, with major emphasis placed on assisting you, the health care provider, to develop, implement, and evaluate a teaching plan.

The teaching-learning process is an interpersonal and collaborative process designed to bring about knowledge, comfort, control, or other change in the learner. It requires knowledge and skill on the part of the teacher, who communicates this knowledge and skill to the learner. Thus, we have identified some elements essential to the teaching-learning process: a learner, a teacher, communication, and a goal. These four elements shall be presented in greater detail with emphasis placed on the importance of each to the process of patient teaching.

Learning Theory

No discussion of patient teaching would be complete without reference to learning theories as they have contributed to the teaching-learning process. The mention of learning theory is by no means a complete presentation of the subject. The reader interested in the subject would do well to consult works by the learning theory authors.

Primarily, learning theories can be divided into two theoretical frameworks: behavioral and cognitive. Behavioral theories of learning have been developed by Skinner, Hull, and Thorndike. Behavioral learning theories developed the concepts of classical and instrumental conditioning. In its simplest form, behavioral learning theory involves an individual in need performing a behavior to satisfy this need. Satisfaction of this need may be reinforced from external or internal sources.

Application of behavioral theory into the clinical setting involves a client, motivated by a need to know or fear from not knowing, seeking information about his disease, in an effort to reduce the anxiety felt by not knowing. By obtaining requisite knowledge, the client reduces the anxiety, thereby reinforcing the information-seeking behavior. Cognitive learning theories have been developed by Piaget, Bandura, and Gestalt psychology. Contributions from cognitive theories of learning include assessment of learner understanding, development of a learning environment, and cognitive ability, skill development, and mastery.

Learning can be defined as a relatively permanent change in behavior that occurs as a result of experience. Teaching acts to guide or facilitate the experience. Effective teaching is a planned process with identified goals. The teaching-learning process can be broken down into four steps, each of which shall be detailed: *assessment, plan, implementation,* and *evaluation.*

The steps of the teaching-learning process are not unlike those employed in the formulation of nursing care plans or physical therapy treatment plans.

Assessment

Assessment is an active gathering of facts and information from the client, his family, his health care team, and his chart, with the goal being the identification of learning needs. It is essential for the health care provider to identify what it is a client (or family) *wants* to learn or *needs* to learn to reach the goal of optimal functioning. The assessment establishes a point of reference for learning. It is an opportunity for the health care provider to identify knowledge deficits and incorrect knowledge. It is an opportunity for the development of trust and rapport, essential as the teaching-learning process is an interpersonal one developed through communication.

Learning needs may be defined by the client or family, by the situation, and/or by the health care provider. The client or family may identify wanting to know how to take care of a ventilator-dependent person at home. A mother may state she wants to learn how to do chest physical therapy for her child with cystic fibrosis. A patient with a tracheostomy may want to know how to manage his tracheostomy, so as to return home and ultimately to work. Clients can be helped to diagnose their own needs for learning. They need to be encouraged to feel some responsibility for their own learning. The teaching-learning process is an active one, by both the health care provider and the patient.

The situation may dictate learning needs as well. A patient who is acutely ill and physiologically unstable will be incapable of learning skills for self-management. Teaching at this time may involve little more than the providing of basic information, i.e., "I am going to suction out your breathing tube to make it easier for you to breathe." A patient preparing for discharge to home or long-term care setting will have different needs and is likely to have a greater capacity and ability to learn.

Finally, learning needs are identified from the expertise and skills of the health care provider, given an understanding of the nature and limitations of the existing physical condition of the client. For the client with COPD, the need to provide information about developing effective breathing patterns, postural drainage, and energy conservation would be identified. A patient who is about to undergo thoracic or cardiac surgery needs to learn how to cough while protecting the chest wall. A child with asthma must learn breathing retraining and relaxation techniques to help effectively manage the onset of acute episodes.

Once the need for learning has been identified, a detailed assessment of the learner's abilities must be made. This includes consideration of the client's age and educational/developmental level, physical status, and emotional readiness. Situational variables unique to the client must also be identified to include assessment of support systems, financial resources, home and work environments, and other intervening variables. Only after a thorough *assessment* has been made can the health care provider begin to formulate a plan.

Plan

The purpose of developing a plan is to clarify what it is to be taught, what it is to be learned, and how it is to be evaluated. Objectives for the teaching-learning plan represent the goals of the teaching-learning process. Objectives are behavioral goals that serve as a standard from which to plan activities and evaluation.

An objective is made up of two parts. The first part is an action word, or verb. For example, demonstrate, perform, state, or set-up. This action word joins with the second part of the objective—the identification of content, i.e., demonstrate postural drainage, perform coughing/deep breathing exercises, state three ways to conserve energy, set up an IPPB machine to provide treatment.

Objectives must be realistic in consideration of client and family needs and abilities. By stating them in behavioral terms, the objective lends itself to evaluation, for the outcomes of learning will be objective, countable, testable, and/or measurable.

INTERVENING VARIABLES—DEVELOPMENTAL NEEDS

While it is possible to identify detailed objectives to guide the teaching-learning process, part of developing a plan includes the identification of how information will be taught. The teaching methods will be selected as to their appropriateness to the audience and type of material to be taught.

Age Factor

The development of a teaching plan must consider the age and developmental level of the person to be taught. While this will in no way represent a complete discussion of learning principles as they relate to various age groups, unique factors will be introduced. A health care practitioner who is expecting to work with pediatric patients would do well to review the developmental levels and age-appropriate behaviors for children. Likewise, a practitioner with a geriatric case load should review and become familiar with developmental tasks of the elderly.

The Pediatric Patient

Obviously, very little direct teaching can be done to the infant or toddler. The main target of teaching will be directed toward the parents or care provider. A sick child is a crisis in any parenting experience. It is important to assist the parent in crisis to reach a manageable level of anxiety and relative comfort *before* any teaching can be attempted. *Mild anxiety is a stimulator for action. Panic is a barrier.*

Prior to beginning patient teaching to parents, it is important to make assessments in three areas:

1. *Can* the parent learn the required information?

2. Is the parent *physically able* to perform care?

3. Is the parent a *responsible and accountable* adult?

The answer to all three questions must be yes if the parent is to become the primary care giver for the child. Additionally, it would behoove the practitioner to evaluate or seek assistance from someone skilled in evaluating the nature of family relationships and the degree of parental involvement with the child.

Preschoolers are taught with one main objective: to decrease the anxiety experienced in the frightening world of the hospital. Explanations should be simple and direct. Any questions asked by the preschooler should be answered. Parents can assist in providing information as well as comfort. The pediatric patient, particularly the preschooler, will regress developmentally upon admission to the hospital. The regression is a normal, valuable coping mechanism for the child and should be permitted and expected.

School-agers are able to learn about and participate in their own care. Erikson identified the developmental task of the school-aged child as the development of a sense of industry versus inferiority. The major theme for this period of psychosocial development is the child's determination to master what he is doing. Skill mastery should be encouraged in preparing to meet the child's learning needs.

The adolescent patient is capable of being an active participant in his own care. The need to know and to maintain control is vital. Identity issues for the adolescent patient are paramount. Teaching strategies designed to give the adolescent patient control, as appropriate, will hasten trust and help the adolescent to develop effective coping mechanisms, problem-solving skills, and mastery.

Teaching the adult patient also requires assessment of individual learning capabilities. Adult learners vary in their intellectual skills and their coping mechanisms, and situational variables may impact upon the individual learners. Many of the patient teaching guidelines presented thus far are applicable to the adult learner. Adults, in general, are growth-oriented, personal, and professional. Learning must facilitate and maintain this growth. Interfering variables must be kept at a minimum.

The Older Adult

Perhaps no greater variation in intellectual and physical abilities in an age group can be identified than in the 65 and older age group. As a result, this age group is frequently subdivided into three groups: the young-old, aged 65–75, the old, age 75–85, and the old-old, aged 85 and above. Due to the great variation across these three groups, individual assessments are crucial.

Contrary to popular belief, the intellectual ability of the older adult does *not* decline or deteriorate. It does, however, *change*. Skills based on past experience and knowledge are rapidly assimilated. Decreased short-term memory and increased processing time may be present, requiring the need for repetition in teaching. Test anxiety or a fear of failure may be present. Therefore, it is important to provide an environment that is supportive and conducive to learning.

Methodology

Choosing appropriate teaching methods comes as a result of an assessment of the patient and the material to be presented. The content to be taught will frequently suggest the method. Teaching methods vary according to the degree of involvement required by both the teacher and the learner. A general rule of thumb is, the less active the learner participation, the less sensory involvement, the less effective the learning.

Teaching methods requiring little involvement from the learner include lecturing, use of written instructions, and use of pictures or other visual aids. Methods that require increased involvement and participation from the learner include use of exhibits, demonstrations and return demonstrations, and repeated planned experiences.

In patient teaching, the most frequently utilized method is the demonstration-return demonstration. The method allows for active learner participation. The health care provider can easily recognize mastery and deficiency. In planning for the demonstration-return demonstration, it is important to outline performance expectations clearly. Each step in the process should be clearly identified. It is important for patients to use the same equipment in the demonstration that they will use at home. It is necessary to provide sufficient time for patients to practice and to ask questions. Written information to support what has been demonstrated may be helpful.

The methodology must be selected as to its appropriateness in meeting identified objectives. If the objective calls for the patient to correctly set-up an IPPB machine, the demonstration method with hands-on experience is an obvious choice. If a patient is to be able to state three means of conserving energy, it may be possible to share the information through lecture or discussion.

Implementation

Implementation, simply stated, is the actual process of putting a teaching plan into action. A need for teaching has been established, learner objectives have been identified, and the content to be taught has been organized, all as a result of a careful assessment of learner needs, abilities, and limitations. It is possible to identify factors likely to foster the teaching-learning process as well as barriers that may interfere with the process.

SUPPORTIVE MEASURES FOR PATIENT TEACHING

Commitment/Coordination. During the course of patients' hospitalizations, they come in contact with a number of health care team members, each providing unique contributions to their care. Often there exists little coordination of effort between disciplines, particularly as it relates to discharge planning and patient teaching. It is essential that *one* person assume responsibility for coordination of any discharge planning and patient teaching that needs to be done. Many may contribute to the process, but *one* person must assume the ultimate responsibility.

Optimal Environment. Too often left to chance, the environment in which patient teaching is to be done should be attended to by the health care provider. Privacy, ample space, and freedom from noise and other distractors are essential.

Use of Materials. If the patient teaching experience is to involve the use of equipment, it is important to gather the necessary items prior to beginning any session. Equipment should be readily usable and in good working order.

Individual Versus Group Teaching. Frequently, situations may arise where several patients require the teaching of the same information at the same time. For example, three or four patients scheduled for cardiac bypass surgery may all need to be taught how to cough and deep breathe. Group teaching may be an option, provided that the learning needs of each patient can be attended to by the instructor. Given the kinds of patients that have been presented throughout the text, it is more likely that patient teaching will focus on one individual, with the "group" being the individual's support person or family.

BARRIERS TO PATIENT TEACHING

It is possible to identify barriers to teaching that may affect you, the health care professional, and barriers to learning that may affect your patient or client.

Barriers to Teaching

Time. There never seems to be enough, so patient teaching does not get done.

Communication. There is little communication between members of the health care team. As a result, no one is able to assist the patient to pull it all together. A patient may be medically cleared for discharge after his tracheostomy, but no one has taught him how to suction or clean his tracheostomy.

Language Barrier. If a careful assessment has been made of a client and/or family's learning needs, language and other communication problems should be identified and planned for accordingly.

Attitudes and Values. As individuals, we bring to our practice attitudes and values about people and health. These may act to facilitate our interactions or may act as barriers. For example, if I believe that smoking is unhealthy and that individuals who smoke deserve any lung problems that may develop, I am not likely to be effective in teaching a COPD patient how to best live with his limitations. These biases may exist, however, and be placed aside by the health care provider in order to provide objective patient care.

Documentation. Documentation prevents duplication of effort and omission of information. Unless teaching and a patient's response to it have been documented, it cannot be assumed to have been done. There is no better mechanism for the coordination of patient care and patient teaching than thorough documentation.

Barriers to Learning

Psychosocial. Before patients are able to accept teaching, they must first acknowledge the need. This necessitates the development of an awareness of their disease and its limitations. A patient who refuses to acknowledge the fact that he is to undergo lung surgery is unlikely to acknowledge a need to learn how to cough and deep breathe. Only after a patient has accepted his diagnosis and/or prognosis can teaching be implemented.

Physical Status. For effective learning to take place, a patient must be physiologically stable and in no acute distress. A patient in status asthmaticus needs immediate treatment, not teaching. A patient in pain cannot be expected to generate effective coughs. Basic physical needs must be attended to *before* higher level learning needs can be addressed.

Trust and Rapport. For patients to place their trust in the health care professional, patients must feel as though the health care professional is acting in consideration of their interests. Patients must feel a part of a relationship with the professional, a relationship built upon trust, openness, and caring. If trust cannot be established, efforts at patient teaching are likely to fail.

Motivation. Motivation relates back to the importance of establishing a need to know in patients. Not only must a patient feel a need to learn about his disease and treatment intervention, he must be capable of learning. His ability to learn must be reinforced.

EVALUATION

While the evaluation is the final step in the patient teaching process, evaluation has been an ongoing and integral part of the entire process. Based on your assessment of a patient situation, you concluded that there existed a need for teaching. Your conclusion was based on the evaluation of data collected during your assessment.

In formulating a plan, there was a need to establish objectives. Objectives were created to guide learning and to provide for measurable or observable changes in behavior. A patient's learning, and ultimately, your teaching will be evaluated according to the objectives.

While you were doing the teaching, you were constantly evaluating the teaching-learning process. Are you being understood? Did the patient understand what you said or was it necessary to change your vocabulary or method of presentation? By watching your patient, you were able to recognize fatigue and draw the teaching session to a close.

Finally, it is important to evaluate the entire process, with your patient and independently. Were the objectives met? Were there any problems or suggestions for the future identified by the patient? Did you feel successful? Were there ways you could improve? Essentially, you are evaluating two components: patient learning and the patient teaching process itself.

FOLLOW-UP

An important part of concluding any patient teaching situation includes making formal arrangements for follow-up. A patient should not feel abandoned by the health care system simply because he has mastered the skills of tracheostomy care. Follow-up phone calls, clinic or home visits, and/or return demonstrations may be appropriate. Providing the patient with a phone number of an appropriate resource person will help to maintain the trust relationship felt between the patient and the health care system.

SUMMARY

The four step process of patient teaching: *assessment, plan, implementation,* and *evaluation,* has been presented in this chapter. The patient teaching process is a method available to the health care provider to assist patients and their families to regain, attain, and maintain optimal functioning.

REFERENCES

Periodicals

Acee S: Helping patients breathe more easily. *Geriatric Nurse* 1984; 5:6:230–233.

Kopacz, MA, Moriarty-Wright R: A multidisciplinary approach for the patient on a home ventilator. *Heart Lung* 1984; 13:3:255–262.

Marion RJ, Creer TL, Burns K: Training asthmatic children to use the nebulizer correctly. *J Asthma* 1983; 20:3:183–188.

Rachelefsky GS: The wheezing child. *Pediatrics* 1984; 47:941–947.

Walson PD: Coughs and colds. *Pediatrics* 1984; 74(5):937–940.

Books

Bandura A: *Social Learning Theory.* Englewood Cliffs, New Jersey, Prentice-Hall, 1977.

Belle D (ed): *Practical Approaches to Patient Teaching.* Boston, Little, Brown & Co, 1981.

Frownfelter D: *Chest Physical Therapy and Pulmonary Rehabilitation,* ed 2. Chicago, Year Book Medical Publishers, 1987.

Hergenhahn B: *An Introduction to Theories of Learning,* ed 2. Englewood Cliffs, New Jersey, Prentice-Hall, 1982.

Maslow A: *Motivation and Personality.* New York, Harper & Row, 1970.

Redman B: *The Process of Patient Teaching in Nursing,* ed 3. St Louis, CV Mosby Co, 1976.

Patient Education

Passero MA, Remor B, Salomon J: Patient-reported compliance with cystic fibrosis therapy. *Clin Pediatr (Phila)* 1981; 20(4):264–268.

Perry JA: Effectiveness of teaching in the rehabilitation of patients with chronic bronchitis and emphysema. *Nurs Res* 1981; 30(4):219–222.

Rifas EM: Teaching patients to manage acute asthma: The future is now. *Nursing (Horsham)* 1983; 13(4):77–80, 82.

Vaughan P: A teaching guide for patients with chronic lung disease. *Crit Care Nurse* 1981; 1(6):64–68.

PART THREE

Guidelines for the Delivery of Chest Physical Therapy

16

The Intensive Care Unit: Monitoring Systems

Elizabeth Dean, Ph.D., M.C.P.A.

The primary goal of the intensive care unit (ICU) team is the achievement of stable cardiopulmonary function. This chapter presents an introduction to monitoring systems used in the evaluation of cardiopulmonary status and describes some related elements of cardiopulmonary regulation that are relevant to assessment and treatment in physical therapy.

Intensive care units are becoming more specialized. In larger hospital centers, units are often exclusively designed and staffed for the management of specific types of conditions, e.g., medical, surgical, trauma, burns, and coronary and neonatal care. Although monitoring priorities may differ among intensive care units, the principles are similar and relate either directly or indirectly to the foremost goal of optimizing cardiopulmonary function.

Cardiopulmonary status is often jeopardized in the ICU patient by fluid and electrolyte disturbances and acid-base imbalance. Regulation of these systems and the clinical implications of imbalance are described first with special reference to the ICU patient. The principles of monitoring systems used in assessing cardiopulmonary sufficiency are presented including the ECG monitor, monitors related to left- and right-sided heart function utilizing arterial and venous lines, and the intracranial pressure (ICP) monitor. The intra-aortic counter pulsation technique used to augment myocardial efficiency is also described.

349

Familiarity with the extensive monitoring facilities in the ICU helps to allay some of the apprehensions the therapist may have working in a critical care area. On introduction to the unit, the physical therapist is immediately struck by the high technology atmosphere and may initially feel insecure. These feelings can be replaced with professional competence and self-assurance. Quality performance in this setting is achieved once the therapist harnesses the potential of the monitoring equipment in optimizing assessment, treatment selection and effectiveness, as well as reducing untoward risk for the patient.

Figure 16–1 illustrates a general view of a typical ICU. A closer view of the patient at bedside indicates to the therapist the parameters that are being monitored, and the types of lines, catheters, and leads in place (Fig 16–2). A closer view with the patient's gown removed demonstrates precisely where the various lines, leads, and catheters are positioned, and identifies where caution must be observed. Treatments are modified according to the types and positions of the lines and leads for each individual patient (Fig 16–3).

FLUID AND ELECTROLYTE BALANCE

When the normal regulation of fluid intake, utilization, and excretion are disrupted, fluid, electrolyte, and acid-base imbalances result. Essentially all medical and surgical conditions threaten these life-dependent

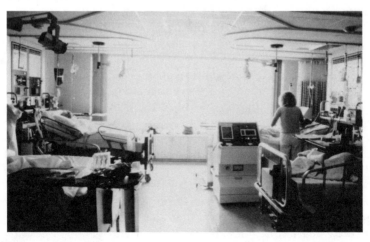

FIG 16–1.
General view of a typical ICU.

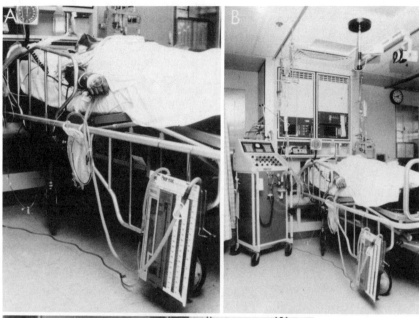

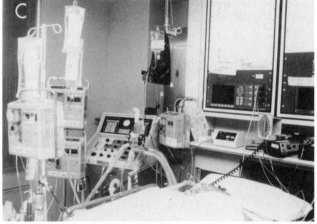

FIG 16–2.
A and **B,** closer bedside views of patients in an ICU. Note that with all the equipment, the patient is almost lost. **C,** note two IV lines with flow monitors. Blood infusion is also being received. *(Continued.)*

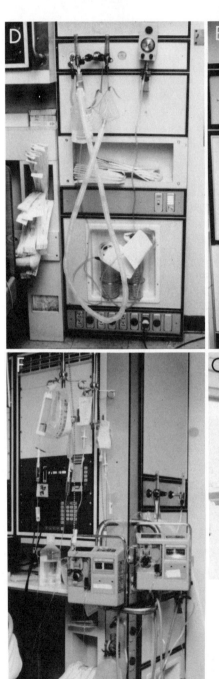

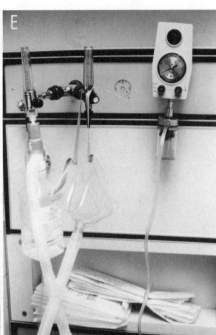

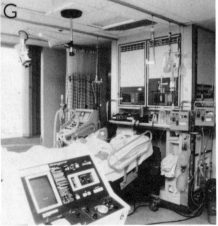

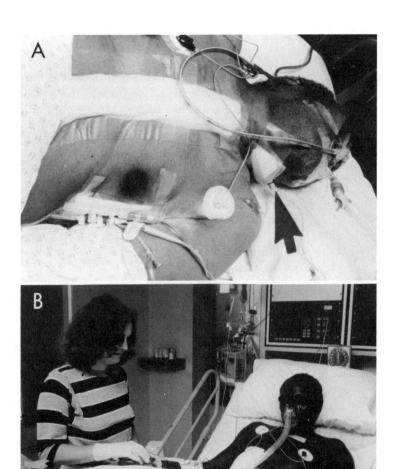

FIG 16–3.
A, patient after open heart surgery. Note insert of Swan Ganz, CV tubing connection taped to left chest. On ventilator with oral endotracheal tube, oral airway is in place. Note the nasogastric tube, EKG leads, and dressing covers sternal split incision site. **B,** patient after open heart surgery. Note EKG leads. Patient is now weaned from ventilator and endotracheal tube; pacemaker wires are held intact at upper abdomen in syringe area. Patient has arterial line in right forearm; Swan Ganz, CVP also removed. Patient is almost ready to leave ICU; he is receiving an aerosol treatment.

← FIG 16–2 (cont.).
D, bedside oxygen and suction set-up. **E,** close-up piped in O_2 and suction units. **F,** close-up IVs and drip monitoring flow devices (IMED). **G,** note IABP, ventilator, IVs, organization of unit at the head of the bed, EKG unit overhead, suctioning and airway care equipment at the right of the patient, and "Ambu" bag at bedside.

mechanisms to some degree. Minor imbalances may be corrected by modification of the patient's nutrition and fluid intake. More major imbalances can be life threatening and necessitate prompt medical attention.

Imbalances are reflected as excesses, deficits, or as an abnormal distribution of fluids within the body. Excesses result from increased intake and decreased loss of fluid and electrolytes. Deficits result from abnormal shifts of fluid and electrolytes among the intravascular and extravascular fluid compartments of the body. Excesses occur with kidney dysfunction promoting fluid retention and with respiratory dysfunction promoting carbon dioxide retention. Deficits are commonly associated with reduced intake of fluids and nutrition. Diaphoresis and wounds can also contribute to significant fluid loss. Diarrhea and vomiting drain the gastrointestinal tract of fluid stores. Hemorrhage is always responsible for fluid and electrolyte loss. Deficits may be secondary to fluid entrapment and localized edema within the body, making this source of fluid unavailable for regulation of homeostasis.

Moderate to severe fluid imbalance can be reflected in the systemic blood pressure and jugular venous pressure (CVP). Elevated blood pressure can be indicative of fluid overload, but an intravascular fluid deficit of 15% to 25% must develop before blood pressure drops. The jugular vein becomes distended with fluid overload. Normally the jugular pulse is not visible 2 cm above the sternal angle when the individual sits at a 45-degree angle. If the jugular pulse is noted, this can be a sign of fluid overload.

Fluid replacement is based on a detailed assessment of the patient's needs. Whole blood is preferred to replace blood loss. Plasma, albumin, and plasma volume expanders such as dextran can be used to substitute for blood loss and to help reestablish blood volume. Albumin and substances such as dextran increase plasma volume by increasing the osmotic pressure of the blood, hence the reabsorption of fluid from the interstitial space. Low molecular weight dextran has the added advantage of augmenting capillary blood flow by decreasing blood viscosity, and therefore is particularly useful in treating shock.

Clinical Picture

Excesses and deficits of fluids and electrolytes can be determined on the basis of laboratory determinations of serum levels of the specific electrolytes. Electrolyte levels and hematocrit are decreased with fluid excess (hemodilution) and increased with fluid loss (hemoconcentration).

Excess fluid can be managed by controlled fluid intake, normal diuresis, and diuretic medications. Replacement of fluid and electrolyte losses can be achieved by oral intake, tube feeding, intravenous infusion, and parenteral hyperalimentation.

Assessment of fluid and electrolyte balance is based on both subjective and objective findings (Table 16–1). At the bedside, the therapist must be alert to complaints of headache, thirst, nausea; and changes in dyspnea, skin turgor, and muscle strength. More objective assessment is based on fluid intake, output, and body weight. Fluid balance is so critical to physical well-being and cardiopulmonary sufficiency that fluid input and output records are frequently maintained at bedside. These records also include fluid volume lost in wound drainage, gastrointestinal output, and fluids aspirated from any body cavity, e.g., abdomen and pleural space.

A patient's weight may increase by several pounds before edema is apparent. The dependent areas manifest the first signs of fluid excess. Patients on bed rest show sacral swelling; patients who can sit over the bed or in a chair for prolonged periods will tend to show swelling of the feet and hands.

Decreased skin turgor can indicate fluid deficit. Tenting of the skin over the arterior chest in response to pinching may suggest fluid depletion. Wrinkled, toneless skin is more common in younger patients.

Weight loss may be deceptive in the patient on intravenous fluids

TABLE 16–1.

Assessment of Fluid and Electrolyte Imbalance*

AREA	FLUID EXCESS/ELECTROLYTE IMBALANCE	FLUID LOSS/ELECTROLYTE IMBALANCE
Head and neck	Distended neck veins, facial edema	Thirst, dry mucous membranes
Extremities	Dependent edema "pitting," discomfort from weight of bed covers	Muscle weakness, tingling, tetany
Skin	Warm, moist, taut, cool feeling when edematous	Dry, decreased turgor
Respiration	Dyspnea, orthopnea, productive cough, moist breath sounds	Changes in rate and depth of breathing
Circulation	Hypertension, jugular pulse visible at 45-degree sitting angle, atrial arrhythmias	Pulse rate irregularities, arrhythmia, postural hypotension, sinus tachycardia
Abdomen	Increased girth, fluid wave	Abdominal cramps

*Adapted from Phipps WJ, et al: *Medical Surgical Nursing: Concepts and Clinical Practice.* St Louis, CV Mosby Co, 1983.

who can be expected to lose a pound a day. This sign should therefore not necessarily be interpreted as underhydration.

The cardiopulmonary assessment can reveal changes in fluid balance. Lung sounds are valuable in identifying fluid overload. Vesicular sounds may become more bronchovesicular in quality. Rales may increase in coarseness. In the presence of fluid retention involving the pleurae, breath sounds diminish to the bases. Dyspnea and orthopnea may also be symptomatic of fluid excess.

An early sign of congestive heart failure with underlying fluid overload is an S_3 gallop (Ken-tuck-ee) caused by rapid ventricular filling.

CHEST TUBE DRAINAGE AND FLUID COLLECTION SYSTEMS

Chest tubes are large catheters placed in the pleural cavity to evacuate fluid and air. A typical chest tube drainage and collection system is shown in Figure 16–4. The removal of thick fluids such as blood and organized exudates with chest tubes is often indicated to prevent entrapment and loculation. Chest tubes are commonly inserted in the sixth intercostal space in the mid or posterior axillary line. Chest tubes inserted into the pleural space are used to evacuate air or exudate. Chest tubes can also be inserted into the mediastinum after open heart surgery, for example, to evacuate blood. Conventionally a one-, two-, or three-bottle system has been used. Bottles are being replaced in many centers with more compact plastic units partitioned into separate reservoirs. The complete unit attaches to the side of the bed or stands on the floor.

Any collection system is designed to seal the drainage site from the atmosphere and offer minimal resistance to the drainage of fluid and gas. This is accomplished by immersing the end of the collection tube under water (see Fig 16–4). This is referred to as an underwater seal system. Additional reservoirs are included to decrease the resistance to fluid leaving the chest. This resistance is greater in a single reservoir system in which the reservoir serves both as the collection receptacle and underwater seal. A third reservoir can be added to the system that is attached to the suction and serves as a pressure regulator. The more elaborate drainage systems are used for open heart surgery, i.e., for precise measuring of fluid loss.

The amount of exudate collected in the reservoir is estimated every several hours or more frequently if the patient is losing considerable

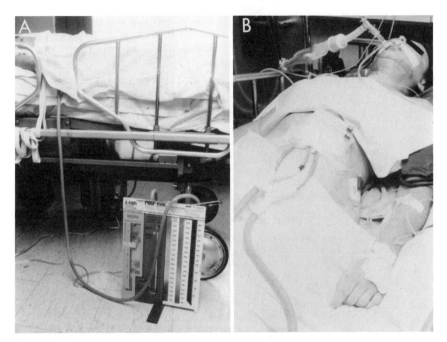

FIG 16–4.
A. chest tube drainage. **B,** anterior view, mediastinal drains.

amounts of fluid or less than the amount predicted. This information is incorporated into the overall fluid balance assessment. In addition, changes in the quantity and quality of exudate should be noted by the physical therapist before, during, and after changes in position and therapeutic interventions.

ACID BASE BALANCE

Control of acid base balance in the body is achieved by regulation of hydrogen ion concentration in the body fluids. The pH of the body is normally maintained within a range of 7.35 to 7.45, or slightly alkaline. When pH of the blood drops below 7.35, a state of acidosis exists; above 7.45, a state of alkalosis exists. Regulation of pH is vital because even slight deviations from the normal range will cause marked changes in the rate of cellular chemical reactions. A pH below 6.8 and above 8 are incompatible with life.

Acid base balance is controlled by several regulatory buffer systems; primarily carbonic acid-bicarbonate, phosphate, and protein buffer systems. These systems act very quickly to prevent minute-to-minute changes in pH. In compensation, pH is returned to normal primarily by altering the component not primarily affected. If the primary cause is respiratory, the compensating mechanism is metabolic. If the primary cause is metabolic, the compensating mechanism is respiratory. The lungs compensate for metabolic problems over hours whereas the kidneys compensate for respiratory problems over days.

Normal pH is a function of carbon dioxide and bicarbonate. The role of carbon dioxide in acid base balance is illustrated in the following equation:

$$H_2O + CO_2 \rightleftharpoons H_2CO_3 \rightleftharpoons H^+ + HCO_3^-$$

Hydrogen and carbon dioxide combine to form a weak acid, carbonic acid. Carbonic acid then dissociates into hydrogen ions and bicarbonate ions. The pH is derived from the Henderson-Hasselbalch equation as follows:

$$pH = pK + \log \frac{[HCO_3^-]}{[CO_2]}$$

where pK is a constant equal to 6.10. The term $[HCO_3^-]$ refers to the concentration of bicarbonate and the term $[P_{CO_2}]$ refers to the concentration of carbon dioxide. The body attempts to maintain the ratio of HCO_3^- to CO_2 at 20:1. Normal HCO_3^- concentration equals 24 mEq/liter; P_{CO_2} equals 40 mm Hg or 1.2 mEq/liter which equals a ratio of 24:1.2 or 20:1. Therefore, substituting normal values of carbon dioxide and bicarbonate into the equation gives a pH of 7.4:

$$pH = 6.10 + \log \frac{[24 \text{ mEq/liter}]}{[1.2 \text{ mEq/liter}]}$$
$$pH = 6.10 + \log 20$$
$$pH = 6.10 + 1.3$$
$$pH = 7.4$$

The four principal mechanisms by which acid base imbalance occurs include increased P_{CO_2}, decreased P_{CO_2}, increased bicarbonate and decreased bicarbonate.

Respiratory acidosis results from increased P_{CO_2} and decreased pH. This in turn reduces the $HCO_3 : P_{CO_2}$ ratio. Respiratory alkalosis results from decreased P_{CO_2}, and increased pH. The $HCO_3 : P_{CO_2}$ ratio is increased. This condition is commonly caused by hyperventilation secondary to lesions of the respiratory center, obstruction of the airways, loss of lung surface for ventilation, weakness of the respiratory muscles, increased metabolism, overventilation, and anxiety.

Metabolic acidosis results from a reduction in HCO_3 which in turn reduces the HCO_3:PCO_2 ratio and pH. Metabolic acidosis is associated with acid accumulation in the blood as a result of uncontrolled diabetes mellitus, starvation, following prolonged strenuous physical exercise, and as a result of hypoxia secondary to shock or heart failure. Bicarbonate deficits may also result from the loss of alkaline secretions in the gastrointestinal tract, e.g., diarrhea or a fistula, and from renal failure.

Metabolic alkalosis results from an excess of HCO_3 which increases the HCO_3:PCO_2 ratio and pH. Principal causes of this condition are loss of hydrochloric acid from the stomach, loss of potassium, excessive ingestion or infusion of alkaline substances, and diuretic therapy.

Base excess is often reported along with acid base balance. Base excess mainly reflects the concentration of bicarbonate and is affected only by metabolic processes. Positive values, therefore, reflect metabolic alkalosis, and negative values reflect metabolic acidosis. The normal range of base excess is $+2$ to -2.

Respiratory and metabolic acid base imbalances often coexist. Therefore, a careful analysis of the acid-base status for each patient must be performed to insure optimal treatment response.

Clinical Picture

A guide to the clinical presentation of acid base imbalances is shown in Table 16–2. Besides the major distinguishing characteristics of acid base imbalance described in this chapter and elsewhere in this volume, potassium excess (hyperkalemia) is associated with both respiratory and metabolic acidosis, and neuromuscular hyperexcitability is associated with both respiratory and metabolic alkalosis.

BLOOD GASES

Analysis of the composition of arterial and mixed venous blood provides vital information about respiratory, cardiac, and metabolic function. For this reason, blood gases are usually analyzed daily in the ICU. In cases where the patient's condition is changing for better or worse over a short period of time or a specific treatment response is of interest, blood gases may be analyzed several times daily. With an arterial

TABLE 16–2.

Signs and Symptoms of Common Acid Base
Disturbances

Respiratory Acidosis	*Metabolic Acidosis*
Hypercapnia	Bicarbonate deficit
Hypoventilation	Hyperventilation
Headache	Headache
Visual disturbances	Mental dullness
Confusion	Deep respirations
Drowsiness	Stupor
Coma	Coma
Depressed tendon reflexes	Hyperkalemia
Hyperkalemia	Cardiac arrhythmias
Ventricular fibrillation	(secondary to
(secondary to	hyperkalemia)
hyperkalemia)	
Respiratory Alkalosis	*Metabolic Alkalosis*
Hypocapnia	Bicarbonate excess
Lightheadedness	Depressed respirations
Numbness/tingling of digits	Mental confusion
Tetany	Dizziness
Convulsions	Numbness/tingling of digits
Hypokalemia	Muscle twitching
Cardiac arrhythmias	Tetany
(secondary to	Convulsions
hypokalemia)	Hypokalemia
	Cardiac arrhythmias
	(secondary to
	hypokalemia)

line in place, frequent blood gas analysis is feasible and not traumatic for the patient.

Arterial saturation (SaO_2) can be readily monitored noninvasively with an ear oximeter. The ear lobe is initially warmed by rubbing prior to attachment of the oximeter. Within a couple of minutes, the SaO_2 can be directly read from the monitor. Ear oximetry is a useful adjunct for routine evaluation of the effectiveness of artificial ventilation, the effect of anesthesia and treatment response. Continuous estimation of SaO_2 is particularly useful during exercise, before and after position change, and following therapeutic interventions. The SaO_2 may appear to be reduced in patients who are anemic, jaundiced, have heavily pigmented skin, or have reduced cardiac output.

HYPOXEMIA

Hypoxemia refers to reduced oxygen tension in the blood. Some common signs and symptoms of various degrees of hypoxemia in adults appear in Table 16–3. Older adults tend normally to have slightly lower arterial oxygen levels. Although the brain is protected by autoregulatory mechanisms, an arterial oxygen tension of 60 mm Hg produces signs of marked depression of the central nervous system reflecting the extreme sensitivity of cerebral tissue to hypoxia.

Hypoxemia is compensated primarily by increased cardiac output, improved perfusion of vital organs, and polycythemia. Secondary mechanisms of compensation include improved unloading of oxygen as a result of tissue acidosis and anerobic metabolism.

The progressive physiologic deterioration observed at decreasing arterial oxygen levels will occur at higher oxygen levels if any of the

TABLE 16–3.

Signs and Symptoms of Hypoxemia

PaO$_2$	SIGNS AND SYMPTOMS
80–100 mm Hg	Normal
60–80 mm Hg	Moderate tachycardia, possible onset of respiratory distress
50–60 mm Hg	Malaise
	Lightheadedness
	Nausea
	Vertigo
	Impaired judgment
	Incoordination
	Restless
	Increased minute ventilation
35–50 mm Hg	Marked confusion
	Cardiac dysrhythmias
	Labored respiration
25–35 mm Hg	Cardiac arrest
	Decreased renal blood flow
	Decreased urine output
	Lactic acidosis
	Poor oxygenation
	Lethargy
	Maximal minute ventilation
	Loss of consciousness
<25 mm Hg	Decreased minute ventilation (secondary to depression of respiratory center)

major compensating mechanisms for hypoxemia is defective. Even a mild drop in PaO_2, for example, is poorly tolerated by the patient with reduced hemoglobin and impaired cardiac output. Alternatively, the signs and symptoms of hypoxemia may appear at lower arterial oxygen levels, e.g., in patients with chronic obstructive lung disease who have adapted to reduced PaO_2 levels.

HYPEROXIA

Mean tissue oxygen tensions rise less than 10 mm Hg when pure oxygen is administered to a healthy subject under normal conditions. Therefore, the function of nonpulmonary tissues is little altered. In the lung, high concentrations of oxygen replace nitrogen in poorly ventilated regions. This results in collapse of areas with reduced ventilation perfusion matching. Lung compliance is diminished.

High concentrations of oxygen (inspired oxygen fractions greater than 50%) directly injure bronchial and parenchymal lung tissue. The toxic effect of oxygen is both time and concentration dependent. Very high concentrations of oxygen can be tolerated for up to 48 hours. High concentrations of oxygen in combination with positive pressure breathing can predispose the patient to oxygen toxicity. At concentrations of inspired oxygen less than 50%, clinically detectable oxygen toxicity is unusual, however, long-term oxygen therapy is indicated.

HYPOCAPNIA

Acute reductions in arterial carbon dioxide levels (hypocapnia) result in alkalosis and diminished cerebral blood flow. The major consequences of abrupt lowering of $PaCO_2$ are altered peripheral and central nerve function. Mechanical ventilation may initially cause an abrupt decrease in arterial PCO_2 and lead to a life-threatening situation.

HYPERCAPNIA

Carbon dioxide, the principal end product of metabolism, is a relative benign gas. Carbon dioxide has a key role in ventilation and in regulating changes in cerebral blood flow, pH, and sympathetic tone. Acute increases in CO_2 (hypercapnia) depress level of consciousness secondary to the effect of acidosis on the nervous system. Similar but slowly developing increases in CO_2, however, are relatively well tolerated. A high $PaCO_2$ is suggestive of alveolar hypoventilation which causes a reduction in alveolar and arterial PO_2. Some patients with severe chronic airflow obstruction have been reported to be able to lead relatively normal lives with $PaCO_2$ in excess of 90 mm Hg if hypoxemia is countered with supplemental oxygen. Acute administration of oxygen to patients with chronic lung disease, however, may be hazardous because it interferes with the hypoxic drive to breathe observed in these patients.

Acute hypercapnia enhances sympathetic stimulation, causing an increase in cardiac output and in peripheral vascular resistance. These effects may help to offset the effect of excess hydrogen ion on the cardiovascular system, allowing better tolerance of low pH than with metabolic acidosis of a similar degree. At extreme levels of hypercapnia, muscle twitching and seizures may be observed.

ECG MONITOR

A single channel ECG monitor with an oscilloscope, strip recorder, and digital heart rate display is typically located above the patient at bedside in the ICU (Fig 16–5). The ECG can often be observed both at bedside as well as at a central monitoring console where the ECGs of all patients being monitored can be observed simultaneously.

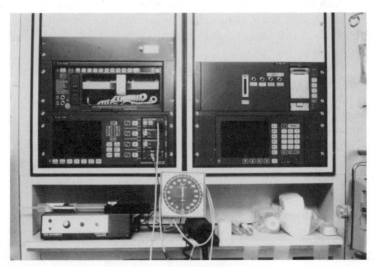

FIG 16–5.
ECG oscilloscope, printout for ECG. Note defibrillator paddles and BP cuff on shelf.

The ECG monitor allows for continuous surveillance of the patient regardless of activity. Low and high heart rates are determined below and above which the alarm will be triggered. For routine monitoring in the coronary care unit, a modified chest lead is often used. Three electrodes are positioned on the chest to provide optimal information regarding changes in rhythm and heart rate, and thereby ensure close patient monitoring. The positive electrode is positioned at the fourth intercostal space at the right sternal border. The negative electrode is positioned at the first intercostal space in the left midclavicular line. The ground electrode used to dissipate electrical interference is often positioned at the first intercostal space in the right midclavicular line, although the ground electrode may be positioned wherever convenient. Other electrode placements may be required, e.g., in patients with pacemakers or in patients with chest burns. The electrode wires are usually secured to the patient's gown.

Problems with the monitor usually result from faulty technique, electrical interference, and movement artifact. A thickened baseline can be caused by 60-cycle electrical interference. An erratic signal frequently results from coughing and movement. The cause of any irregularity must be explained and untoward changes in electrical activity of the myocardium ruled out. It is a dangerous practice for the therapist to turn off the ECG alarm system during treatment.

Cardiac arrhythmias can be broadly categorized into tachyarrhythmias and bradyarrhythmias. Tachyarrhythmias are subdivided into supraventricular and subjunctional tachycardias. Bradyarrhythmias are subdivided into sinus bradycardia, and those related to heart block and conduction abnormalities.

The characteristic features of arrhythmic ECG tracings are illustrated in Chapter 3. Therapists specializing in ICU management should be thoroughly familiar with ECG interpretation and the implications of the various arrhythmias for patient management.

The subjunctional tachycardias or ventricular arrhythmias are potentially life threatening. Ventricular tachycardia and ventricular fibrillation are medical emergencies requiring immediate recognition and treatment.

Clinical Picture of Common Arrhythmias

The clinical picture associated with arrhythmic activity of the heart depends on the nature of the arrhythmia, the age and condition of the patient, and specifically the absence or presence of underlying heart disease. Distinguishing clinical features of common atrial and ventricular arrhythmias are outlined in Table 16–4.

TABLE 16–4.

Clinical Picture of Common Arrhythmias

ARRHYTHMIA	IN HEALTHY INDIVIDUALS WITH NO UNDERLYING CARDIOVASCULAR DISEASE	IN INDIVIDUALS WITH UNDERLYING CARDIOVASCULAR DISEASE
I. Tachycardias		
A. Supraventricular tachycardia	No symptoms Abrupt onset palpitations, light-headedness, nausea, fatigue	May precipitate congestive heart failure, acute coronary insufficiency, myocardial infarction, pulmonary edema
1. Sinus tachycardia	Awareness of the heart on exertion or with anxiety	Secondary to some precipitating factor, e.g., fever, electrolyte imbalance, anemia, blood and fluid loss, infection, persistent hypoxemia in COPD, acute MI, congestive heart failure, thyrotoxicosis
2. Paroxysmal atrial tachycardia (PAT)	Prevalent, sudden onset, precipitated by coffee, smoking, and exhaustion	Common supraventricular tachycardia Spontaneous onset of regular palpitations that can last for several hours May be obscured by myocardial insufficiency and CHF in older patients Increased anxiety and report of fatigue
3. Atrial flutter	Rare May be difficult to distinguish from PAT May be precipitated by alcohol, smoking, physical and emotional strain	Rapid regular-irregular rate Suggests block at AV node Atrial flutter waves in jugular venous pulse
4. Atrial fibrillation	Rare, occasionally with alcohol excess in the young	Usually secondary to a variety of cardiac disorders
5. Paroxysmal atrial tachycardia with block	Rare	Common arrhythmia seen with digitalis toxicity
B. Subjunctional	Rare	Usually related to MI, pulmonary embolus, severe CHF Often unconscious, cyanotic, ineffective pulse, blood pressure and respiration
1. Ventricular tachycardia	Rare	Predisposed to ventricular fibrillation

(Continued)

TABLE 16–4. *(continued)*

Clinical Picture of Common Arrhythmias

ARRHYTHMIA	IN HEALTHY INDIVIDUALS WITH NO UNDERLYING CARDIOVASCULAR DISEASE	IN INDIVIDUALS WITH UNDERLYING CARDIOVASCULAR DISEASE
2. Ventricular fibrillation	Rare	Ineffective cardiac output, unconscious, dusky, cardiac arrest threatens
II. Bradycardias		
A. Sinus bradycardia	Physiologic in very fit young adults	In older patients may suggest sinus node and conduction system pathology; can produce syncope or congestive heart failure
B. Heart block	Rare	Hypotension, dizziness, light-headedness, syncope
		In chronic block with sustained bradycardia, congestive heart failure may be more frequent
		Most common arrhythmia iatrogenically produced with digitalis excess
		Associated with numerous cardiac conditions; commonly in age-related degenerative disease in conducting system, inferior and occasionally anterior MIs

The subjunctional or ventricular arrhythmias are typically associated with an extremely ill individual. Cyanosis and duskiness of the mucosal linings and periphery may be apparent. The patient is unresponsive, the pulse is ineffective, and spontaneous respirations are likely to be absent. Defibrillation is initiated to restore an effective more normal rhythm. The high incidence of myocardial conduction irregularities warrants a defibrillator being present at all times in the ICU for rapid implementation of this common cardioversion procedure by the medical personnel. Ventricular arrhythmias may be tolerated better if ventricular rate is low, thereby improving cardiac output. Even in this circumstance, however, these arrhythmias still present an emergency.

The ECG of a patient with a pacemaker will reflect either an imposed fixed or intermittent rhythm and rate depending on whether a fixed rate or demand pacemaker has been inserted.

Intra-Arterial Lines

An arterial line is established by direct arterial puncture, usually of the radial artery. Blood pressure can be measured directly from this line. A digital monitor displays systolic and diastolic blood pressures above the patient at bedside. High and low blood pressure levels are set, above and below which the alarm will sound. Blood gas analysis can be performed routinely with an intra-arterial line in place without repeated puncturing of a blood vessel (Fig 16–6).

Swan Ganz Catheter

The Swan Ganz catheter is designed to provide an accurate and convenient means of hemodynamic assessment in the ICU. The catheter is usually inserted into the internal jugular vein, the subclavian vein, or a large peripheral arm vein and directed by the flow of blood into the

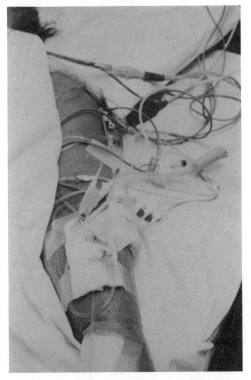

FIG 16–6.
Intra-arterial blood gas line.

right ventricle and pulmonary artery (see Fig 16–3, arrow). The catheter is securely taped to the patient's arm which is splinted with an armboard to prevent dislodging. The procedure is generally associated with little risk and discomfort. Some of the complications that have been associated with Swan Ganz catheterization, however, include infection, venous thrombosis, myocardial irritation, air embolism, and pulmonary ischemia or infarct to segmental lung tissue.

Complex catheters are available for monitoring a variety of parameters. In a two-lumen catheter, the first lumen is used to measure pulmonary artery pressure (PAP) and obtain mixed venous blood samples. The second lumen terminates in a balloon with a volume of less than 1 cc, which is inflated and deflated to obtain pulmonary artery wedge pressure (PAWP). The average range of the PAP is 15 to 30 mm Hg, and normally reflects right ventricular pressure (RVP). The average range of PAWP is 5 to 10 or 15 mm Hg and gives an estimation of mean left atrial pressure (LAP) and the pressure in the left ventricle (LVP). More elaborate catheters have pacing wires, thermistors for cardiac output determination, and sensors for arterial saturation. Figure 16–7 shows the normal cardiac pressures in each heart chamber. Abnormal pulmonary function may vary these readings.

The PAP increases as a result of elevated pulmonary blood flow,

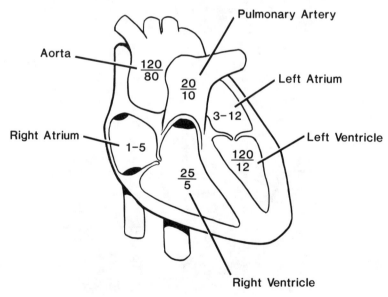

FIG 16–7.
Normal cardiac pressures in each heart chamber.

increased pulmonary arteriolar resistance secondary to primary pulmonary hypertension or mitral stenosis, and left ventricular failure. Measurement of PAP and PAWP in particular allows for more prudent management of heart failure and cardiogenic shock.

The PAP, PAWP, and end diastolic LVP are directly related. Impaired left ventricular contractility that compromises normal emptying, e.g., left ventricular failure, mitral stenosis, or mitral insufficiency, result in an elevated end diastolic LVP, which in turn elevates PAWP and PAP. An end diastolic PAP or PAWP greater than 12 mm Hg is considered abnormal.

The PAP and PAWP are low during hypotension secondary to hypovolemia. Infusion of normal saline, whole blood, or low molecular weight dextran elevates the blood volume and blood pressure. Restoration of blood volume returns end diastolic PAP and PAWP to normal.

Elevation of the end diastolic PAP secondary to heart failure with pulmonary edema can typically be reduced with appropriate medication. The effectiveness of a drug and its prescription parameters can be assessed by the observed changes in the end diastolic PAP.

Deterioration of cardiovascular status and worsening of the clinical signs and symptoms of heart failure elevate end diastolic PAP and PAWP, decrease cardiac output, decrease arterial and right atrial oxygen tension, and increase the oxygen difference between arterial and venous blood.

As the heart pump continues to fail, arterial oxygen tension decreases suggesting abnormal lung function and probably elevated LAP. Pulmonary dysfunction at this stage includes diffusion abnormalities, redistribution of pulmonary blood flow into the less well ventilated upper lobes, and right to left shunting. All patients with acute infarction or shock have reduced arterial oxygen tension. Pulmonary congestion must be cleared before the patient responds to oxygen administration.

INTRAVENOUS LINES

Intravenous (IV) lines are routinely established in the superficial veins of patients, e.g., in the hand, usually prior to admission to the ICU. These lines provide an immediate route for fluids, electrolytes, nutrition, and medications. The specific lines used depend on the patient's individual needs determined by the history, laboratory tests, and physical examination.

MEASUREMENT OF CENTRAL VENOUS PRESSURE

Central venous pressure (CVP) is monitored by means of a venous line or catheter inserted into the subclavian, basilic, jugular or femoral vein (see Fig 16–3,A). The catheter is advanced to the right atrium by way of the inferior or superior vena cava depending on the site of insertion. Minimal risk of phlebitis or infection is associated with this procedure.

Central venous pressure is the blood pressure measured in the vena cavae or right atrium. Normal CVP is approximately 0 to 5 cm H_2O and 5 to 10 cm H_2O if measured at the sternal notch and midaxillary line, respectively. Essentially the CVP provides information about the adequacy of right-sided heart function, including effective circulating blood volume, effectiveness of the heart as a pump, vascular tone, and venous return. Measurement of CVP is particularly useful in assessing fluid volume and fluid replacement. If the patient has chronic obstructive lung disease, ventricular ischemia, or infarction, the CVP will reflect changes in pathology rather than fluid volume.

Specifically, CVP provides an index of RAP. The relationship between RAP and end diastolic LVP is unreliable; therefore, end diastolic PAP and PAWP are used as the principal indicators of cardiopulmonary sufficiency in patients in failure and shock.

INTRA-AORTIC BALLOON COUNTER PULSATION (IABP)

Intra-aortic balloon counter pulsation (Fig 16–8) provides mechanical circulatory assistance with the use of an intra-aortic balloon. The balloon is inserted into the femoral artery. To maintain proper placement and good circulation, the leg must be kept straight. The presence of an intra-aortic balloon must be taken into consideration whenever the patient is being treated and positioned. Inflation and deflation of the balloon with helium is correlated with the ECG. The intra-aortic balloon is deflated during ventricular systole and assists the emptying of the aorta. Stroke volume is potentiated, afterload is reduced (hence, ventricular pressure), and myocardium oxygen consumption enhanced. The balloon is inflated during diastole, thereby restoring arterial pressure and coronary perfusion. Counterpulsation improves cardic output, reduces evidence of myocardial ischemia, and reduces ST-segment elevation. Intra-aortic balloon counterpulsation is commonly used after open heart surgery, for congestive heart failure, medically refractive myocardial ischemia, ventricular septal defects, and left main coronary

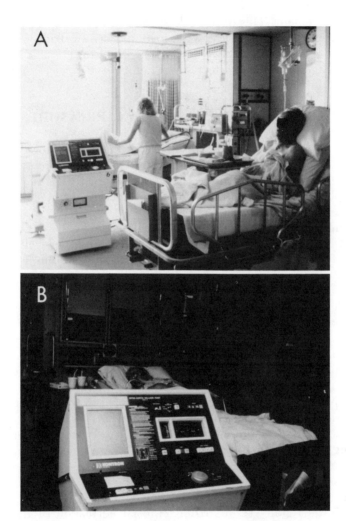

FIG 16–8.
A, patient near the window is receiving intra-aortic balloon pump (IABP) support. **B,** close-up of an IABP unit.

stenosis in patients who have shock. The intra-aortic balloon pump provides protection for the myocardium in many instances until surgery can be performed. Limb ischemia, the most frequent complication, occurs in 10% to 15% of patients.

A left ventricular assist device is being developed experimentally for use postoperatively in patients following open heart surgery who have developed cardiogenic shock and are unresponsive to conventional management. This device takes over the pumping action of the left ventricle and decreases the work load and myocardial oxygen consumption. This type of assistive device may have considerable potential in the management of refractory heart failure.

MEASUREMENT OF INTRACRANIAL PRESSURE

Increased intracranial pressure results from many neurological conditions including head injury, hypoxic brain damage, or cerebral tumor, and may require surgery. In the adult, the cranial vault is rigid and noncompliant. Increases in the volume of the cranial contents result in an elevated intracranial pressure.

Changes in consciousness are the earliest and most sensitive indicators of increased cranial pressure. Altered consciousness reflects herniation of the brainstem and compression of the midbrain. Compression of the oculomotor nerve and the pupillo-constrictor fibers results in abnormal pupillary reactions associated with brain damage.

The effect of cranial pressure on blood pressure and pulse is variable. Blood pressure may be elevated secondary to elevated cranial pressure and hypoxia of the vasomotor center. A reflex decrease in pulse occurs as blood pressure rises.

Herniation can produce incoordinate respirations that are correlated with the level of brainstem compression.

Compression of upper motor neuron pathways interrupts the transmission of impulses to lower motor neurons; progressive muscle weakness results. A contralateral weakened hand grasp, for example, may progress to hemiparesis or hemiplegia. The Babinski sign, hyperreflexia, and rigidity are additional motor signs that provide evidence of decreasing motor function as a result of upper motor neuron involvement.

Cerebrate rigidity results from tentorial herniation of the upper brainstem. This results in blocking of the motor inhibitory fibers and the familiar extended body posture. Seizures may be present. These neuromuscular changes may further compound existing cardiopulmonary complications in the ICU patient.

Clinically, increased intracranial pressure is best detected by altered consciousness, blood pressure, pulse, pupillary responses, movement, temperature, and respiration. The intracranial pressure monitor provides direct measurement of ICP. A hollow screw is positioned through the skull into the subarachnoid space. The screw is attached to a Luer-Lok, which is connected to a transducer and oscilloscope for continuous monitoring.

The prevention of further increase in ICP, hence increased brain damage, is a treatment priority. Measures to reduce venous volume are maintained until ICP has stabilized within normal range. Prudent body positioning is used to enhance venous drainage by elevating the bed 15 to 30 degrees and maintaining the head above heart level. Neck flexure is avoided. Fluid intake and output are carefully monitored; the patient may need to be fluid restricted. The Valsalva maneuver is avoided since intrathoracic pressure and ICP may increase correspondingly.

Normal range of ICP is 0 to 10 mm Hg for adults, and 0 to 5 mm Hg for patients under 6 years. The ICP may reach 50 mm Hg in the normal brain; typically, however, this pressure returns to baseline levels instantaneously. In patients with high levels of ICP and low cerebral compliance, extra care must be exercised during routine management and therapy. An ICP elicited by turning or suctioning up to 30 mm Hg may be acceptable provided the pressure drops immediately following removal of the pressure-potentiating stimulus. Patients may be mechanically hyperventilated to keep arterial PCO_2 at low levels since hypercapnia dilates cerebral vessels and hypocapnia constricts them.

EEG MONITOR

An electroencephalogram or EEG provides useful information about gross cerebral functioning and changes in level of consciousness. A single-channel EEG monitor can be readily used in the ICU to reveal evidence of posttraumatic epilepsy when the clinical signs may be inhibited by muscle relaxants. An EEG assessment may also be of some benefit to the therapist in assessing the role of passive movement and sensorimotor stimuli in altering EEG activity.

SUMMARY

Monitoring cardiopulmonary function is an essential component of the management of the patient in the ICU. Regulation of homeostasis is disrupted in disease or following medical and surgical interventions. Therapists working in the unit require a thorough understanding of homeostatic regulation and monitoring of fluid and electrolyte balance, acid base balance, and blood gases. Physical therapy has an essential role in restoring homeostasis in patients requiring intensive care, using conservative, noninvasive approaches, in addition to averting the musculoskeletal complications associated with immobility. The selection of treatment and the assessment of treatment response must be based upon quantitative evaluation of the parameters affecting cardiopulmonary functioning. Meticulous monitoring will contribute substantially to more rational management of the ICU patient; specifically, the optimization and efficacy of physical therapy, in addition to minimizing deleterious treatment outcomes.

REFERENCES

Periodicals
Barrell SE, Abbas HM: Monitoring during physiotherapy after open heart surgery. *Physiotherapy* 1978; 64:272.
Buchrinder N, Ganz W: Hemodynamic monitoring: Invasive techniques. *Anesthesiology* 1967; 45:146.
Burki NK, Albert RK: Noninvasive monitoring of arterial blood gases. *Chest* 1983; 4:666.
Davis FM, Stewart JM: Radial artery cannulation. *Br J Anaesthesiol* 1980; 52:41.
Fisher RD: Role of electrophysiologic testing in the diagnosis and treatment of patients with known suspected bradycardias and tachycardias. *Prog Cardiovasc Dis* 1981; 24:25.
Folk-Lighty M: Solving the puzzles of patients' fluid imbalances. *Nursing* 1984; 14:34.
Forrester JS, et al: Filling pressures in the right-left sides of the heart in acute myocardial infarction: A reappraisal of central venous pressure monitoring. *N Engl J Med* 1970; 285:190.
Hinterbuchner LP: Evaluation of the unconscious patient. *Med Clin North Am* 1973; 57:1363.
Puri VK, et al: Complications of vascular catheterization in the critically ill: A prospective study. *Crit Care Med* 1980; 8:495.
Snider GL: Interpretation of the arterial oxygen and carbon dioxide partial pressures. *Chest* 1973; 63:801.
Swan HJC: The role of hemodynamic monitoring in the management of the critically ill. *Crit Care Med* 1975; 3:83.
Thomas HM, et al: The oxyhemoglobin dissociation curve in health and disease. *Am J Med* 1974; 57:331.
Wiedemann HP, Matthay MA, Matthay RA: Cardiovascular-pulmonary monitoring in the intensive care unit. *Chest* 1984; 85:537.

Books
Andreoli KG, Fowkes VK, Zipes DP, et al: *Comprehensive Cardiac Care,* ed 5. St Louis, CV Mosby Co, 1983.
Cromwell L, Weibell FJ, Pfeiffer EA: *Biomedical Instrumentation and Measurements,* ed 2. Englewood Cliffs, Prentice-Hall, 1980.
DeGowin El, DeGowin RL: *Bedside Diagnostic Examination,* ed 4. New York, Macmillan Publishing Co, 1981.

Downie PA: *Cash's Textbook of Chest, Heart and Vascular Disorders for Physiotherapists,* ed 3. Philadelphia, JB Lippincott Co, 1983.

Dubin D: *Rapid Interpretation of EKGs,* ed 3. Tampa, Florida, Cover Publishing Co, 1974.

Guyton AC: *Textbook of Medical Physiology,* ed 6. Philadelphia, WB Saunders Co, 1981.

Marini JJ: *Respiratory Medicine and Intensive Care for the House Officer.* Baltimore, Williams & Wilkins Co, 1981.

Phipps WJ, Long BC, Woods NF: *Medical-Surgical Nursing: Concepts and Clinical Practice,* ed 2. St Louis, CV Mosby Co, 1983.

Shapiro BA, Harrison RA, Walton JR: *Clinical Application of Blood Gases,* ed 2. Year Book Medical Publishers, 1977.

Thorn GW, et al: *Harrison's Principles of Internal Medicine,* ed 8. New York, McGraw-Hill Book Co, 1977.

West JB: *Respiratory Physiology—The Essentials,* ed 2. Baltimore, Williams & Wilkins Co, 1979.

17

The Intensive Care Unit: Principles and Practice of Physical Therapy

Elizabeth Dean, Ph.D., M.C.P.A.

This chapter provides a general overview of the principles and practice of physical therapy in the intensive care unit (ICU). Profiles of some common categories of conditions are described. The categories of conditions included are obstructive and restrictive lung disease, adult respiratory distress syndrome, coronary artery disease, shock, postoperative intensive care, musculoskeletal trauma, central nervous system trauma, and burns. Special attention is given to the dying patient. Each category of condition is presented in two parts. First, related pathophysiology and aspects of the medical management of the condition are presented. This is followed by a description of the physical therapy management. Guidelines to management are not mutually exclusive for each category. Rather, considerable overlap may exist when conditions coexist.

Guidelines to patient management are provided in the following sections to sensitize physical therapists to their role in the ICU, and to alert them to what might be expected. The reader, however, is cautioned against applying general guidelines to patient management. No two patients are identical. Therapists are responsible for applying these guidelines prudently, taking each individual's condition, needs, and prognosis into consideration. Therapists are also responsible for monitoring treatment responses and bringing to the attention of the ICU team any possible contraindications to treatment or sudden changes in patients' conditions. Problem solving and rational management of patients are based upon a tripod approach: a knowledge of the underlying pathophysiology and basis for general care, the research evidence for treatment interventions, and clinical experience (Fig 17–1). Quality care is a function of these three areas of expertise and knowledge.

SPECIALIZED SKILLS OF THE ICU PHYSICAL THERAPIST

This chapter presents a problem-solving approach to the physical therapy management of the patient in the ICU. Effective problem-solving and practice in this specialized setting depend upon the following skills and expertise. The ICU physical therapist needs:

1. A thorough knowledge of cardiopulmonary physiology and pathophysiology, and familiarity with the related pharmacology of the cardiopulmonary system.

2. A working knowledge of the monitoring systems routinely used in the ICU with respect to treatment planning and modification.

3. Particular skill in assessment and optimal treatment selection in cardiopulmonary physical therapy, preferably a minimum of two to three years experience in general medicine and surgery.

4. An ability to practice effectively under pressure and in often apparently congested, suboptimal working conditions.

Knowledge of underlying pathophysiology
and basis for general care

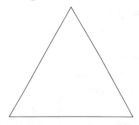

Clinical experience   Research evidence for
treatment interventions

FIG 17–1.
Tripod approach to patient management.

5. An ability to communicate effectively and work cooperatively with other members of the ICU team (Fig 17–2).

6. Familiarity with all emergency procedures including those for respiratory and cardiac arrest, equipment, or power failure.

7. Familiarity with the paging system used in the unit for contacting the physical therapist when she or he is out of the unit and out of the hospital. On-call service, 24 hours a day, seven days a week is a common practice, and should be considered in units without this service.

PRINCIPLES OF MANAGEMENT

Physical therapy management in the ICU is based on a treatment plan comprised of general and specific goals formulated from the findings of the assessment. The general goals relate to function optimization and prophylaxis. The specific goals relate first to the attainment of optimal cardiopulmonary function, and second to the attainment of optimal musculoskeletal and neurological function. In the ICU, the physical therapist must recognize the implications of cardiopulmonary insufficiency on neuromuscular status, and that apparent impairment of neuromuscular status is not necessarily indicative of primary neurological disease. Rather, reduced cardiac output and blood pressure, hypoxemia, hypercapnia, increased intracranial pressure (ICP) may be indirectly responsible for these changes.

Another important consideration in the ICU is the effect of position on cardiopulmonary function. Changing the position of the body from the erect to the supine position results in:

1. Reduced total lung capacity.

2. Reduced vital capacity.

3. Reduced functional residual capacity.

4. Reduced residual volume.

5. Decreased forced expiratory volume.

6. Altered regional ventilation and perfusion of the lung.

7. Increased closing volumes of small airways.

8. Restriction of chest wall and diaphragmatic excursions.

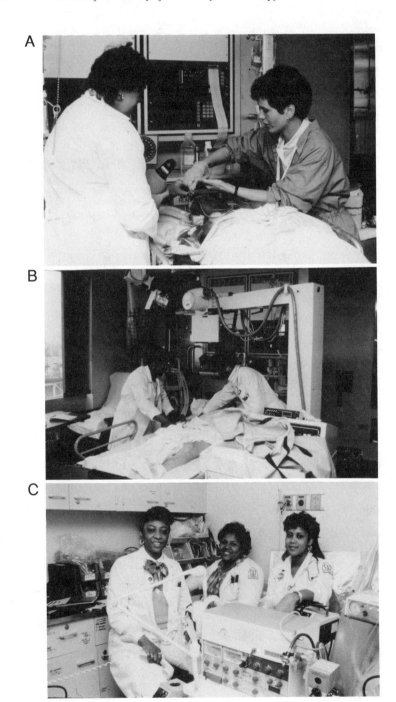

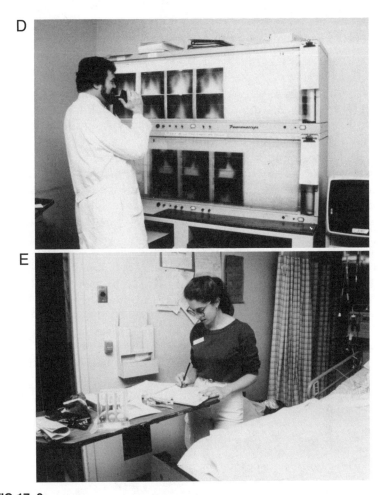

FIG 17–2.
Team work in the intensive care unit is essential to facilitate communication and patient treatment. **A,** physical therapist and nurse "bagging" and suctioning the patient. **B,** two persons positioning for dependent, heavy patients prior to portable chest x-ray. **C,** respiratory care practitioners. **D,** radiologist. **E,** nursing staff.

9. Reduced arterial oxygen levels.

10. Increased cardiac output.

11. Increased myocardial work load.

These physiological effects compound the superimposed factors of immobility, prolonged lying without the normal stimulation or will to turn the body, and underlying pathophysiology or trauma that may contribute to impaired lung function.

Physical therapy interventions must be specifically geared toward the management of each organ system taking into consideration the pathophysiologic basic for the signs and symptoms and rationale for each intervention, the scientific evidence supporting the usefulness of the technique, as well as the clinical experience of the therapist.

Physical therapy provides both therapeutic and prophylactic interventions for the ICU patient. The use of more conservative, noninvasive measures is the initial treatment of choice to avert the need for additional invasion monitoring and treatment, and the need for intubation and mechanical ventilation. The physical therapist can do a great deal to postpone for as long as possible or avert mechanical ventilatory assistance and its sequelae. In addition, the physical therapist helps to prevent the multitude of side effects of immobility and prolonged confinement to bed.

In general principles of physical therapy management in the ICU are based upon:

1. The patient's existing or potential medical instability.

2. Indications or necessity for intubation and mechanical ventilation.

3. The existence of or potential for complications and multisystem breakdown.

4. The presence of coma.

5. Elevated intracranial pressure (ICP) and the need for ICP monitoring.

6. The patient's vulnerability to infection and the presence of infection.

7. The availability of patient monitoring for assessment and ongoing evaluation.

8. The patient's past medical and surgical histories.

9. The patient's age.

10. The premorbid status of the patient.

11. Nutritional status of the patient; obesity or asthenia.

12. The recency of onset of the patient's present condition.

13. The patient's general intelligence, attitude, and emotional status.

Function Optimization

Function optimization refers to promoting optimal physiologic functioning at an organ system level as well as promoting optimal functioning of the patient as a whole. In critical care, primary goals related to function optimization are initially focused on cardiorespiratory function. With improvement in the patient's condition, increased attention is given to optimal functioning of the patient with respect to self-care, self-positioning, sitting up, and walking. Specific physical therapy goals related to function optimization include:

1. To assist in the maintenance and restoration of adequate ventilation in nonaffected and affected lung fields.

2. To prolong spontaneous breathing and thereby avoid or postpone mechanical ventilation.

3. To promote ventilation and perfusion matching.

4. To maintain or restore mobility, strength, endurance, and co-ordination, within the limitations of the patient's condition and consistent with the patient's anticipated rehabilitation prognosis.

5. To design a positioning schedule to maintain comfort and postural alignment, and optimize heart and lung function.

6. To strive for optimal involvement of the patient in a daily routine including self-care, changing body position, standing, transferring, sitting in a chair, and ambulating in patients for whom these activities are indicated.

7. To optimize treatment outcome by interfacing physical therapy with the goals of other team members, coordinating treatments with medication schedules where appropriate, and treating the patient specifically, based on results of objective monitoring available in the ICU.

Prophylaxis

General aspects of patient care related to physical therapy practice include the role of prophylaxis or prevention. The complications of immobility are described in Chapter 14, and relate primarily to the status of the cardiopulmonary and musculoskeletal systems. In the ICU, the negative physiologic effects of immobility are amplified in severely ill patients. A primary objective of the physical therapist is to avoid or reduce these untoward effects on the patient's recovery and length of stay in the ICU. Specifically these goals include reducing the deleterious effects of immobility and pathology on cardiopulmonary and neuromuscular function, and reducing the risk of deformity and decubiti.

Preparation for Treating the ICU Patient

Patients in the ICU are generally characterized by some degree of potentially life-threatening medical instability. In conjunction with treating a specific patient, the physical therapist must:

1. Be thoroughly familiar with the patient's history, including the differential diagnosis on admission to the ICU, and relevant past medical, surgical, and social histories.

2. Be knowledgeable about the medications administered to the patient, their indications, and side effects, especially those affecting response to physical therapy.

3. Be knowledgeable about the stability of vital signs since admission, including heart rate and rhythm, respiration rate and rhythm, blood pressure, skin color, core temperature.

4. Be familiar with the relevant findings of laboratory tests, procedures, and biopsies including arterial blood gases, blood analysis, fluid and electrolyte balance, ECG, x-ray, thoracentesis, central venous pressure (CVP), left atrial pressure (LAP), pulmonary artery wedge pressure (PAWP), microbiology and biochemistry reports, and urinalysis.

5. If the patient is ventilated, have an understanding of the rationale for the ventilatory parameters used.

6. (a) Conduct a thorough, detailed clinical assessment specific to the patient's condition(s) including inspection, palpation, percussion, and auscultation of the chest; as well as a neuromusculoskeletal assessment to rule out any secondary effects of cardiopulmonary dysfunc-

tion, and to establish rehabilitation prognosis. (b) Establish a physical diagnosis, problem list, and prioritize the treatment goals and overall treatment plan.

7. As treatment progresses report objective and relevant subjective changes in the patient on the chart and revise treatment goals as indicated by the patient's progress.

GENERAL CLINICAL ASPECTS OF THE MANAGEMENT OF THE ICU PATIENT

Assessment

The fundamental assessment procedures for the cardiorespiratory system are described in detail in Chapter 17. Laboratory reports, procedures, sputum culture, and x-rays supplement the findings of inspection, palpation, percussion, and auscultation of the chest. Of particular importance are the blood work, arterial blood gases, fluid and electrolyte balance, and ECG findings. These are the most commonly monitored parameters in the ICU in addition to vital signs; respiration rate, heart rate, temperature, and blood pressure.

The monitoring systems described in Chapter 17 provide invaluable information with respect to the management of the ICU patient. Information regarding acid/base and fluid and electrolyte balance helps to establish specific treatment goals. The Swan-Ganz catheter in situ gives the pressures for pulmonary artery pressure and wedge pressure which provide an index of myocardial sufficiency and specifically left heart function. Central venous pressure gives an indication of fluid loading and the ability of the right side of the heart to cope with changes in circulating body fluids. Pressures related to heart function give the therapist an indication of pulmonary status and help to determine whether heart dysfunction is affecting lung function, lung dysfunction is affecting heart function, or both. Existing cardiopulmonary stress alerts the therapist to appropriately modify work loads or the physical demands of treatment to keep the patient medically stable, avoid undue fatigue, and deterioration.

Changes in ECG may reflect heart disease, lung disease, altered acid/base, and electrolyte and fluid balance. The therapist is responsible for identifying the patient's heart rhythm and ECG changes that might be expected with improvement or deterioration, and secondary to drug intervention, to change in course of the disease and to treatment generally.

The physical therapist needs a thorough knowledge of the common pharmaceutical agents used in intensive care. With this knowledge, the physical therapist can work with these agents to optimize their effects, and to optimize physical therapy treatment response when treatments are coordinated with medication schedules. Most medications have optimal dosages for any given patient, optimal sensitivity, and peak response time. Most medications have side effects. Side effects may cause deterioration of some sort in the patient's condition, or create apparent signs and symptoms suggestive of other disorders. The physical therapist therefore needs to identify the medications each patient is taking and their side effects.

Certain medications such as bronchodilators, sedatives, mucolytic agents, antianginal medications, and analgesics help the patient to be able to cooperate during treatments. Special consideration must always be given to the different peak-response times of medications used in the ICU. The patient can and is willing to cooperate more actively in the treatment if pain is reduced; mucus is easier to clear, etc. A better treatment effect is therefore more likely. These advantages result in more effective use of the therapist's time, and often a shorter, more efficacious treatment.

Certain other medications may prevent close monitoring of patients during exercise and activity. Patients on beta-blocking agents, for example, will not show the normal changes in heart rate and blood pressure in response to exercise. Caution must therefore be observed when prescribing exercise for these patients. Another classification of drugs called vasopressor agents help regulate blood pressure and heart rate. Patients on these agents may also exhibit abnormal exercise responses. Hence, monitoring vital signs to assess treatment response may be of limited value for patients on drugs acting on the cardiovascular system.

Physical therapy treatments in the ICU must be prudently selected in a goal-oriented manner. Unlike other patient care areas, the frequency of treatments may range from one to several treatments daily. The frequency depends on the patient's specific treatment goals, the aggressiveness of treatment indicated, interfering related problems and their management, patient cooperation, and tolerance for the physical therapy treatments prescribed. Exercise tolerance is also important to the physical therapist in the ICU. Although dynamic exercise over prolonged periods of time is not an immediate priority in the ICU, the physical therapist needs to assess the patient's tolerance with respect to duration, intensity, and frequency of treatments as well as prescribed exercise. Objective and subjective measures of the patient's tolerance to the initial assessment and the observations of other members of the team help to establish this baseline. Even in the ICU, whenever possible, general body exercise is integrated into the treatment program to maintain optimal cardiopulmonary function in conjunction with traditional pulmonary physical therapy techniques.

Conventional treatment goals and techniques of chest physical therapy and pulmonary rehabilitation are described in Chapter 15. In brief, techniques frequently used in the ICU include those related to bronchial hygiene and adequate pulmonary ventilation such as deep breathing and coughing exercises, chest wall mobilization, postural drainage, percussion, vibration, shaking, rib springing, relaxation, body positioning, body alignment, and general body strengthening and mobilization exercises and ambulation. These techniques are the mainstay of cardiopulmonary physical therapy. Intensive care physical therapy demands particular skill in *selecting, priorizing and applying* the particular techniques that can effect the *optimal treatment outcome* in the shortest time in a given critically ill patient. For example, a common scenario in the ICU is the therapist's attempting to reduce or reverse the adverse changes observed in blood gases; that is, falling PaO_2 levels and increasing $PaCO_2$ levels, in the patient for whom intubation is being seriously considered if improvement is not observed soon. The focus of treatment for such a patient is delineated into two parts. The therapist first focuses on optimizing the pulmonary function of the involved lung fields, and second on maintaining optimal pulmonary function of the uninvolved lung fields.

Specific Treatment Goals

The specific goals of intensive care physical therapy that need to be implemented as soon as possible include:

1. To improve alveolar ventilation, and ventilation and perfusion matching; and thereby optimize arterial blood gases.

2. To improve breathing mechanics by body position and alignment at rest and during treatment, maintain or improve rib cage mobility.

3. To prevent joint, and muscle deformity by positioning, bed rolls, splints, turning schedule, turning technique.

4. To prevent the sequelae of immobility, e.g., decubiti, lesions, contracture, joint laxity, thromboemboli, deep vein thrombosis, pul-

monary embolism, orthostatic pneumonia, spinal deformity, stones in
urinary tract.

5. To encourage relaxation, reduce the work of breathing, increase
resistive breathing capacity, and optimize patient's effective functioning.

6. To reduce unnecessary myocardial oxygen consumption and
stress.

7. To maintain muscle strength and endurance and cardiovascular
endurance, as much as possible with respect to anticipated future reconditioning needs in rehabilitation.

8. To promote self-care as much as possible, e.g., grooming, washing, feeding, dressing, bed arrangement; access to tissue paper, water,
ice chips, access to call button.

Contraindications and the awareness of potential adverse effects of
chest physical therapy are particular concerns in the ICU. The physical
therapist needs to be well-versed about these and how treatments need
to be modified to achieve an optimal treatment effect without posing a
hazard to the patient. Herein lies one of the many challenges of intensive care physical therapy.

NONCLINICAL ASPECTS OF THE MANAGEMENT OF THE ICU PATIENT

Comprehensive patient care in the ICU includes some nonclinical activities. Team work is the essence of optimal patient care, particularly in
the ICU. The physical therapist interacts frequently with other team
members regarding observations and changes in the patient's condition, treatment goals, and treatment response (Fig 17–2). In addition
to providing therapy for patients, the physical therapist is often consulted regarding patient positioning, lifting, transferring, and self-care.

Personal hygiene and good hygienic practice on the part of the
physical therapist cannot be overemphasized. Patients in the ICU are
usually prone to infection. Meticulous hand washing with an antiseptic
detergent between patients is essential. Following contact with infected
wounds, saliva, wounds, pus, vomitus, urine, or stool, the therapist
must be particularly conscientious about washing immediately. Gown-
ing, gloving, capping, and masking may be indicated in situations
where a certain isolation technique has been implemented.

Pressure sores are largely preventable. Therapists and nurses need to examine routinely for sites of redness, pressure, and potential skin lesions in every patient regardless of expected length of stay in the ICU. The texture of bed coverings, their smoothness, bunching of the bed gown, or irritation from lines and catheters to the patient need to be routinely monitored.

Although constraints do exist in the high technology atmosphere of the ICU, the patient's dignity is observed as much as possible regardless of the reason for admission, the level of consciousness, or belligerent and objectionable behavior directed toward the ICU staff. Gestures such as using the patient's preferred name, explaining aspects of the patient's care, and continually orienting the patient to person, place, time, and day are widely practiced. A supportive caring atmosphere is created in which the patient is free to make choices and ask questions as much as possible.

Recent research suggests that the ICU environment can have a profound effect on the patient's recovery independent of the level of care received. Windows with pleasant views, for example, help to orient the patient, provide a sense of day and night and the passage of time (Fig 17–3). Other benefits observed included a reduction in the number and types of complications and reduced length of stay in the ICU and in hospital overall. Therapists who are involved in the designing

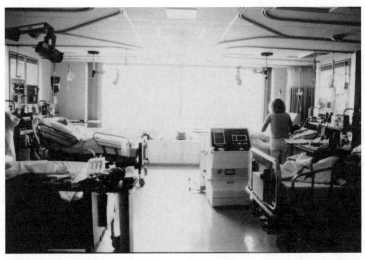

FIG 17–3.
An overview of an ICU room. Note large window area and openness of room. Windows help patients orient to day and night.

of ICUs are therefore advised to consider psychoenvironmental as well as technological and clinical factors.

THE PATIENT WITH OBSTRUCTIVE LUNG DISEASE

Obstructive lung disease can result in respiratory failure and admission of the patient to the ICU, or may complicate management if the patient was admitted for other reasons. If conservative management fails or is unlikely to improve or prevent further deterioration of alveolar ventilation, of gas exchange, and to adequately remove copious and tenacious secretions, intubation and mechanical ventilation may have to be implemented (see Chapter 26).

The goal of mechanical ventilation is to provide adequate alveolar ventilation which is usually assessed by arterial blood gas analysis. A tidal volume and respiration rate that provide satisfactory blood gas and pH values are established and maintained unless the clinical condition changes. The precise regulation of mechanical ventilation helps to restore more normal respiratory function, reduce the work of breathing, rest fatigued ventilatory muscles, and provide an optimal fraction of inspired oxygen (FIO_2) and humidification (Fig 17–4).

The physical therapist needs to be familiar with backup systems in the event of electrical failure, ventilator malfunction, tube disconnections, and leaks. A self-inflating breathing bag should be placed over each patient's bed. The alarm system should be constantly functioning to signal in the event of malfunction or disconnection. The alarm system should not be turned off during treatment.

Minute volume can be seriously impaired with a leak in the system. The tube connecting sites are often the sites of air leakage. Complete disconnection at the endotracheal or tracheostomy connection may occur in those patients with high pulmonary resistance. Close monitoring of the exhaled tidal volume will help ensure the patient is receiving sufficient ventilation.

Positive end-expiratory pressure (PEEP) is useful in promoting greater opportunity for gas exchange at end-expiration in ventilated patients. However, venous return and myocardial perfusion may be impaired during PEEP administration. Excessive stimulation to cough in these ventilated patients should be avoided as this amplifies the cardiovascular side effects of PEEP. Continuous positive airway pressure (CPAP) also helps to maintain airway patency during spontaneous ventilation. This mode of ventilation, however, seems to be preferred in children, whereas PEEP is used more commonly in adults.

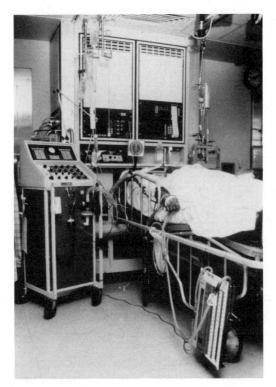

FIG 17–4.
Patient receiving mechanical ventilation.

Interference with the gag reflex in the patient with an endotracheal tube increases the risk of aspiration of the oropharyngeal and gastric contents and can result in pneumonia and pneumonitis. Risk of aspiration from the oropharyngeal cavity can be reduced by suctioning through the airway with the cuff of the airway inflated, in addition to suctioning the oropharynx following suctioning via the airway.

Repeated suctioning is more easily performed routinely in a patient with an artificial airway, and is less traumatic for the patient. Suctioning can produce significant desaturation (up to 60%), particularly in the ventilated patient. Administration of 100% oxygen for three minutes before and after suctioning can help reduce this desaturation effect. This is usually accomplished with a self-inflating bag prior to treatment. Risk of aspiration of gastric contents is reduced by the use of a nasogastric tube.

A common cause of acute respiratory failure is advanced chronic obstructive pulmonary disease (COPD) as a result of ventilation and perfusion mismatching, ventilatory muscle fatigue, reactive pulmonary hypertension, right ventricular failure, and impaired oxygen transport. Correcting the complications of respiratory failure, however, is often more problematic than treating the specific cause. Hypoxemia and hypercapnia are often present. Hypoxemia is usually improved with supplemental oxygen.

Cardiovascular complications are among the most prevalent observed with respiratory failure. Marked hypercapnia (increased arterial Pco_2) with acidemia (reduced pH) can produce extreme vasodilatation and hypotension due to the local action on blood vessels.

Mild hypercapnia can produce reflex vasoconstriction and hypertension. Occasionally systemic hypertension is observed during weaning from the ventilator with the presence of a moderate degree of hypercapnia.

Cor pulmonale is a well-known complication of chronic lung disease and occurrence of repeated episodes of congestive heart failure. Both hypoxia and reduced pH cause pulmonary vasoconstriction and an increase in pulmonary artery pressure. Consequently, reversing bronchospasm, hypoxemia, hypercapnia, and acidemia can often reduce pulmonary vasoconstriction, lower pulmonary artery pressure, and thereby improve hemodynamics.

The end stage of respiratory failure results in progressive increase in airway resistance, work of breathing, oxygen consumption, and carbon dioxide production. In areas of bronchial obstruction, marked alveolar hypoventilation results and ventilation and perfusion are severely mismatched. Hypoxemia and respiratory acidosis produce reactive pulmonary hypertension and further ventilatory failure. Profound carbon dioxide retention, refractory hypoxemia, and respiratory acidemia may terminate in a fatal arrhythmia.

Nutrition

Mechanically ventilated patients have specific nutritional needs. Without adequate nutrition, the patient will incur the effects of deconditioning faster, will be less capable of responding optimally to therapy, and will be more susceptible to bacterial invasion. Intravenous hyperalimentation or external hyperalimentation may be considered if ventilation is prolonged. In some centers, however, hyperalimentation is being initiated immediately in certain patients to maintain optimal nutritional status and to avoid excessive physical wasting and deterioration. If tracheostomy has been performed, the patient is able to eat normally.

Management

The principles of management of acute respiratory failure, regardless of etiology, involve maintenance of the airways, support of ventilation, provision of adequate oxygen transport, control of pH, provision of adequate carbon dioxide elimination, and maintenance of the circulation. The primary goals of physical therapy management are:

1. To prevent further decrease, maintain or improve arterial oxygen levels (PaO_2).

2. To prevent further decrease, maintain or improve arterial oxygen saturation (SaO_2).

3. To reduce or prevent further increase in arterial carbon dioxide levels ($PaCO_2$).

The means by which these goals are fulfilled depends on each patient's clinical presentation. If secretions are retained promoting airway closure and atelectasis, the patient is placed in specific postural drainage positions indicated by the pathology, x-ray, and clinical examination. The recommended positions related to involvement of specific bronchopulmonary segments should be approximated as closely as possible. Frequently, specific positioning in the ICU is compromised as a result of the patient's status, intolerance to lying flat or being tipped, or limitations imposed by monitoring apparatus or ventilator. Wherever possible, a schedule of four-point turning (supine, left side, prone, right side) is ideal and should be attempted if not contraindicated even in the ventilated patient.

A sequence including percussion, shaking, vibrating, and perhaps rib springing may be indicated in conjunction with postural drainage. The precise sequence, the duration, intensity, and frequency of treatment is based upon treatment outcome. Postural drainage may be contraindicated in patients with unstable vital signs, and usually contraindicated immediately after feedings and meals. In some institutions, however, patients on continuous 24-hour tube feedings are tipped after feeding has been discontinued for 15 minutes. The cuff in the artificial airway is inflated to avoid aspiration. Trendelenburg positioning and chest physical therapy have been associated with cardiac dysrhythmia and arrest; therefore, these techniques must be applied rationally and with attention to all monitoring systems and changes in signs and symptoms. If the patient is nonventilated or recently extubated, body positioning and breathing exercises are emphasized to promote bronchial hygiene, as well as decrease minute ventilation and respiratory rate, increase tidal volume, and improve arterial blood gases. Breathing exercises are most effective if pursed-lips breathing is performed in conjunction with mechanical pressure applied over the abdomen. Such breathing retraining has also been shown to improve exercise tolerance.

Positioning can be used to advantage to promote pulmonary function and gas exchange. Ventilation and perfusion are enhanced in the inferior lung fields. Thus, in postural drainage positions, the superior lung being treated is neither preferentially ventilated nor perfused. The less affected lung fields therefore may be contributing more substantially to improving arterial gases. Hence, the therapist must consider the goals of treatment with respect to pulmonary function in both the involved and less involved lung fields. During postural drainage, the length of time in a given position needs to be monitored to avoid drainage of secretions into the less involved, functional, inferior lung fields; and to avoid the possibility of physical restriction to expansion of lung fields on the underside.

Although positions can be predicted that will optimize ventilation-perfusion matching, each patient will respond differently depending on such factors as pathology, age, and specific disorders. Therefore, the patient's response to specific positioning must be observed and documented.

Positioning patients with obstructive lung disease in the head down position may have specific beneficial effects. The abdominal viscera are displaced upward and thereby elevate the typically flattened diaphragm. This effect may be mimicked in other body positions by manual abdominal compression, abdominal binders, or weights over the abdomen ranging from 15 to occasionally 40 to 50 pounds. Using weights in this range causes a marked decrease in FRC, which helps to reduce physiologic dead space and improve effective ventilation and ventilation/perfusion matching. Caution must be observed when applying weights to the abdomens of these patients.

Certain positions present a particular problem when a pressure-cycled ventilator is being used. The efficiency of the ventilator is greatly reduced when the patient's head is positioned below the hips because of an increase in total pulmonary resistance caused by the pressure of the abdominal contents.

The use of a self-inflating breathing bag may therefore be required to maintain pressure when changing from one position to another. Adequate tidal volume can be maintained by an assistant while the therapist aids the patient with bronchial drainage. With the use of the self-inflating bag, the therapist needs to ensure the patient is adequately ventilated and takes a larger than tidal breath every minute or so. As soon as possible, spontaneous breathing is encouraged in conjunction with postural drainage. The small airways dilate slightly on inspiration and cause mucus to peel away from the walls; thus, during expiration, mucus plugs are moved toward the trachea. Chest wall percussion, shaking, and vibration facilitate this movement. For the unconscious or paralyzed patient, the ventilator or self-inflating bag can be used to increase inflation volumes.

Supplemental oxygen is usually administered continuously whether the patient is ventilated or not, to maintain PaO_2 level within an optimal range. Oxygen concentrations can be increased prior to postural drainage and treatment to help compensate for any physical stress imposed by treatment. Oxygen, however, should always be increased to 100% and inspired for at least three minutes prior to and following suctioning. Should arterial desaturation be apparent with positioning and percussion, oxygen may need to be increased during treatment. If the patient is spontaneously breathing without oxygen, supplemental oxygen may also be indicated during treatment to avoid desaturation in some patients. Oxygen administration must be knowledgeably regulated by the ICU team based on arterial blood gas results. Severe hypoxemia is well-known to result in irreversible tissue damage within minutes, but hyperoxia can also produce harmful effects within hours. By maximizing alveolar ventilation, gas exchange as well as ventilation and perfusion matching, supplemental oxygen can be optimally utilized and the effects of acidemia minimized.

A common practice in some ICUs is "bagging." A self-inflating breathing bag is temporarily connected to the airway. The lungs are manually inflated for a few breaths. The purpose of bagging the patient is to provide some extra large breaths during treatment, to maintain some degree of positive end-expiratory pressure, to assess lung compliance, and to facilitate the effect of instillation of a small volume of saline solution into the tracheobronchial tree to loosen secretions. Bagging must be performed cautiously. Too aggressive bagging can produce bronchospasm. The use of bagging in conjunction with suctioning is controversial. Some clinicians prefer to bag the patient after suctioning to avoid the possibility of the positive pressure pushing the mucus distally. Others maintain that because of the adherent quality of the mucus to the walls of the airways and the dilatation of the airways in response to positive pressure, bagging does not propel the mucus distally. Rather, it is believed that bagging prior to suctioning promotes air entry distal to the mucus plugs, and promotes movement of plugs centrally on expiration. Research is needed to examine the role of bagging and the effect of this technique on mucus removal.

Instillation is another procedure that should be used selectively in certain patients. A mucolytic effect of saline has not been well established, although beneficial effects may be more apparent in neonates.

Treatment for respiratory acidosis is aimed at increasing alveolar ventilation rate in order to improve the exchange of carbon dioxide and oxygen. Because the respiratory center is depressed by increased amounts of carbon dioxide (carbon dioxide narcosis), the lowered oxygen tension of the blood becomes the stimulus for respiration. If the patient inhales high concentrations of oxygen, the stimulation for respiration may be removed. For this reason, oxygen is never given to patients with carbon dioxide narcosis.

Low flow oxygen (1 to 3 L/min) is given to a patient with chronic pulmonary disease who maintains a chronically elevated arterial P_{CO_2} in the presence of arterial hypoxemia. If intermittent positive pressure breathing is indicated, compressed or room air is used instead of oxygen in this situation.

Severe hypoxemia usually suppresses cardiac output to some degree. Cardiac output may be further compromised immediately after a patient is placed on a mechanical ventilator due to impaired venous return by the elevated transpulmonary pressure. An attempt is made to carefully balance ventilation with an optimal or adequate cardiac output by shortening inspiration time and by minimizing transpulmonary pressures by employing lower tidal volumes.

The patient in respiratory failure needs special attention to fluid balance in order to carefully regulate hydration. Inhaled humidified air is a significant additional source of body fluid. Normally the alveolar gas is saturated with water vapor. The lining of the tracheobronchial tree is therefore protected from erosion and potential infection. This is particularly important in the patient requiring frequent suctioning. The effect of humidification can be assessed by the consistency of the patient's secretions. Thick secretions suggest humidification may be inadequate and the patient may be systemically dehydrated.

General body activity and ambulation are requisite for normal physiologic functioning of the human body. Over recent years, this fact has been more appreciated in critical care settings. Patients in the ICU are encouraged more than ever before to move, exercise, sit up, stand, sit in chairs, take a few steps, and in some circumstances, ambulate across the unit even if they are ventilated. The upright position promotes improved cardiopulmonary function and gas exchange. Some have argued that reclining chairs should be available at the side of every ICU bed to provide greater opportunity to the patient to be upright. If not contraindicated, tremendous benefit can be gained from standing the ventilated patient in terms of both improving neuromuscular status and optimizing cardiopulmonary function. Standing and walking even a few steps can be extremely strenuous for the ICU patient, and this effort should in no way be minimized by the physical therapist. Standing and walking should be coordinated with other aspects of the patient's care. Monitoring of the patient's ECG is essential throughout any activity. Monitoring of the ECG or arterial saturation of the critically-ill patient performing activities such as standing or walking cannot be overemphasized. The therapist is working blindly and potentially dangerously by disconnecting these monitors because the leads do not reach or because of movement artifact. In anticipation of an increased work load, ventilatory parameters for the ventilated patients are likely to require adjusting. A greater concentration of oxygen should be delivered for at least three to five minutes prior to the activity and continued afterwards for ten minutes or so until the patient has recovered from the increased exertion and the heart rate and blood pressure have returned to within 5% to 10% of baseline values.

Exercising and in particular ambulating the ventilated patient can be extremely beneficial to the patient, both physiologically and psychologically. The potential risks, however, must be recognized. Thus, the physical therapist must include ambulation into the patient's regimen, intelligently, and responsibly.

Status Asthmaticus

Status asthmaticus is a potentially life-threatening situation. The pathophysiologic features include marked airway resistance secondary to bronchospasm and mucous secretion and retention. The work of breathing is increased resulting in marked respiratory distress. A cycle results in which the patient becomes more hypoxemic and hypercapnic secondary to alveolar hypoventilation, bronchospasm increases and reactive pulmonary hypertension may ensue.

The classical signs and symptoms of a severe asthmatic attack that may progress to status asthmaticus include tachypnea, dyspnea, labored breathing, audible wheezing, tachycardia, cyanosis, anxiety, and panic. If the patient is able to cooperate with spirometric testing, degree of reduced vital capacity, peak flow, and FEV_1 can provide an index of the severity of airway obstruction.

The prime objective of physical therapy is to help prevent the need for mechanical ventilation. If ventilation becomes necessary, prognosis for recovery is poorer. Medical management is aimed at administering drugs and fluids to reduce hypoxemia with oxygen, decrease airway inflammation and resistance, and hence reduce work of breathing and anxiety. Intravenous sodium bicarbonate helps to reverse respiratory acidosis and possibly metabolic acidosis.

Physical therapy can augment the medical management of the patient with status asthmaticus. In coordination with the patient's medications, the therapist helps to remove secretions, promotes relaxed, more efficient breathing, enhances ventilation-perfusion matching, reduces hypoxemia, and teaches the patient to coordinate relaxed breathing with general body movement. Caution needs to be observed to avoid stimuli that potentiate bronchospasm, and deterioration of the patient's condition, e.g., aggressive percussion, forced expiration maneuvers, aggressive "bagging," and possibly instillation. Certain body positions may have to be avoided, for example, because of the patient's intolerance and exacerbation of symptoms in those positions. Because of the relationship of altered lung function in different positions, positioning (especially in patients in respiratory distress) must be applied cautiously within the patient's tolerance.

A major problem in status asthmaticus is an ineffective cough. The therapist attempts to work in conjunction with the patient's medications to facilitate clearance of secretions with modified chest percussion and huffing or gentle coughing. Obtaining a productive cough without augmenting bronchospasm is a challenge. Deep breathing with pursed-lips expiration helps to prolong expiration and to maintain the patency of the small airways. Deep, slow, and relaxed breathing is emphasized along with periodic effective, controlled huffing as needed.

Weaning From the Ventilator

The physical therapist plays an important role in facilitating the weaning process of ventilated patients. Blood gas analysis and pulmonary function provide the baseline before weaning is attempted. Ideally, the patient's spontaneous tidal volume should approximate that of the ventilator. Forced vital capacity should be about two to three times the patient's required tidal volume (Fig 17–5). Weaning is not usually indicated if the patient requires PEEP or greater than 0.40 inspired oxygen on the ventilator. Minute ventilation and maximum voluntary ventilation can also be measured at bedside and contribute to the decision whether to wean.

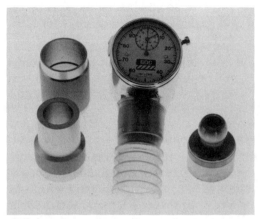

FIG 17–5.
Spirometer for bedside
measurement of TV, VC, and
minute volume.

General Steps in Weaning From the Ventilator

1. An individualized weaning schedule is designed for each patient in which periods of time are spent off the ventilator and on a T tube that delivers appropriate oxygen and humidity.

2. The initial time period off the ventilator is carefully selected; mornings are often good times.

3. (a) Physical activity should be at a minimum during this period, e.g., not during or following physical therapy, not after meals or following tests or procedures, not during family visits. (b) Supplemental oxygen and humidity are given.

4. The physical therapist offers support and reassurance.

5. Vital signs, and signs and symptoms of respiratory distress are monitored continuously during weaning.

6. The patient is not left unattended in the initial weaning sessions until periods off the ventilator are reliably tolerated well for several successive minutes.

7. (a) Deterioration of vital signs, blood gases and evidence of distress indicate that the patient will have to return to ventilatory assistance imminently. (b) Rest periods of at least an hour are strategically interspersed in the weaning schedule.

8. Blood gases are performed at regular intervals, e.g., 15, 30, 60, 90, 120 minutes, or more or less frequently as indicated.

9. If blood gases stabilize within acceptable limits during the weaning period and the patient is generally tolerating the procedure well, the time off the ventilator is increased.

10. Patients with underlying pulmonary disease and who are older can be expected to take longer to be completely weaned from the ventilator.

11. Weaning is generally faster in patients who have required a shorter period of mechanical ventilation.

12. To hasten the weaning process intermittent mandatory ventilation (IMV) has been reported to be useful in some patients. Others, however, have observed that the use of IMV tends to fatigue the patient and delay the patient's progress in weaning. Thus, IMV must be used cautiously, and individual variability must be considered in terms of its effectiveness.

Discharge From the ICU

To be recommended for discharge from the ICU, the patient should not require chest physical therapy more than every four to six hours. The patient should be breathing spontaneously and independently and elicit a cough with or without assistance, preferably one that is effective in clearing secretions. If alert, the patient should be moving purposefully in bed prior to transfer.

The physical therapist is responsible for documenting the physical therapy treatment priorities and frequent progress notes during the ICU stay in order that the team responsible for the patient following discharge is able to continue management with reduced risk of disruption of care or regression of the patient's condition. The patient should be consulted if possible, and informed at all times of his or her progress and plans made by the team and family. The patient should be given as many choices as possible about his or her care, and in long term planning.

THE PATIENT WITH RESTRICTIVE LUNG DISEASE

Acute respiratory failure can be associated with restrictive lung disease. Restrictive lung dysfunction may complicate the management of patients admitted to the ICU for reasons other than their pulmonary disease. The lung parenchyma, the chest wall, or both may be involved.

The underlying cause of respiratory failure may therefore reflect both impaired ventilation and impaired capacity for gas exchange. The specific restrictions to pulmonary function need to be identified and treated individually to optimize treatment.

Guillain-Barré syndrome, myasthenia gravis, and neuromuscular poisonings are common neuromuscular disorders that can be complicated by respiratory failure in the absence of underlying primary lung disease. If paralyzed, the patient will likely be dependent on ventilatory assistance.

Typically, in restrictive lung disease, all lung volumes and capacities may be reduced to some degree, but a relatively normal tidal volume may be present. In the presence of neuromuscular disease, forced expiratory capacities and forced expiratory volumes are reduced. Acidemia from respiratory causes with a pH of less than 7.25 is often harmful with respect to arrhythmia production. Conversely, hypoventilation is equally harmful, and pH elevations greater than 7.5 may cause neurologic cardiovascular complications.

In acute respiratory failure with profound acidemia, intravenous use of bicarbonate will be effective in buffering the hydrogen ion concentration until the underlying disorder is corrected. Bicarbonate infusion is guided by frequent pH measurements.

Transport of oxygen and carbon dioxide to and from the tissues is dependent on adequate circulation. Frequently, blood volume has to be restored by fluids or blood replacement or both. Inotropic agents are used in maintaining adequate circulation by augmenting myocardial contractility.

The techniques of bronchial hygiene that are so important in chronic airway obstruction are applicable to all situations in which secretions, mucosal edema, bronchospasm, or a combination of these factors occur.

Management

Restrictive ventilatory dysfunction is commonly associated with both medical and surgical conditions, but the principles of management of acute respiratory failure associated with these are similar. Regardless of whether mechanical ventilation is indicated, tissue oxygenation, carbon dioxide removal, regulation of blood pH, and an effective cardiac output are priorities. Supplemental oxygen is often effective in improving tissue oxygenation in conditions associated with restrictive lung disease.

A primary problem for patients with restrictive lung disease secondary to generalized weakness and neuromuscular disease is an ineffective cough. Cough facilitating techniques such as tracheal tickle can be effectively used in conjunction with manual abdominal support to increase intra-abdominal and intrathoracic pressures. A natural cough, although perhaps facilitated, is preferable and more effective in dislodging mucus from the sixth or seventh generation of bronchi than repeated suctioning is likely to be. Even a weak, facilitated cough may be effective in dislodging secretions to the central airways for removal by suctioning. Huffing, a modified cough performed with the glottis open and with abdominal support, may help to expectorate secretions in patients with generalized weakness or in pain. In some cases, suctioning may be the only means of eliciting a cough and clearing secretions simultaneously. Coughing attempts are usually exhausting for these patients. Thus, ample rest periods must be interspersed during treatment, particularly for the ventilated patient.

A patient with restrictive lung disease will be more adversely affected by the restriction placed on lung function in the lying position. The patient's body position and length of time in any one position therefore must be carefully monitored and records maintained regarding these two points. This is particularly important in the patient who is incapable of positioning him or herself, who is incapable of communicating a need to turn, and in whom body wasting, bony prominences, and thinning of the skin may predispose the patient to skin breakdown.

A judicious turning regime can also be designed to optimize cardiopulmonary function, even if the patient is artificially ventilated, reduce risks of cardiopulmonary complications, reduce musculoskeletal deformities, and promote comfort. Careful consideration should be given to the liberal use of sheepskins, soft bed covers, foam rubber, pillows, bed rolls, mattresses, and circoelectric and water beds. The risk of decubiti is a major concern in every bed-confined, immobile patient; thus, their prevention is always a primary treatment goal. Once decubiti have developed, healing is often slow because of the relatively poor condition of the patient, a portal of infection exists for the already vulnerable individual, and further constraints may have to be imposed on patient positioning and movement which increase the risk of cardiopulmonary complications.

As with routine positioning of any patient, the patient is not confined unnecessarily. Although lines, leads, and catheters may be used, these are anchored as securely as possible with sufficient length to allow the patient to move spontaneously, as well as to facilitate routine patient care.

General body movement is always a priority in the ICU, as much and as often as possible, *given* the patient's condition and safety considerations. Movements may be totally assisted, but more often are likely to be active-assisted and active. No matter how weak the patient may be, active-assisted and active movements are the mainstay of the movement interventions performed by the therapist particularly if these can be performed in near-upright positions. This point cannot be overemphasized. Therapists must guard against performing assisted or passive movements when these are not indicated. Even modest attempts at active-assisted movements with perhaps only a minimal number of repetitions benefit the patient considerably more both in terms of treatment goals related to musculoskeletal and cardiopulmonary function than assisted movements that in no way contribute to improve muscle strength, endurance, and coordination. Injudicious application of totally assisted movements will contribute to the patient's deconditioning and perhaps physical deterioration. Regardless of the type of movement being carried out, the patient is observed closely for discomfort, respiratory distress, cyanosis, fatigue, and extent of cooperation if assisted-active and active movements are being performed.

Assisted movements are indicated in cases of coma and extensive and local paralysis. The primary objective is the maintenance of joint range of motion and prevention of adaptive shortening of periarticular soft tissue in particular. In addition, the potential role of these movements in facilitating and increasing regional ventilation is an important therapeutic consideration that should not go unrecognized. Care must therefore be taken to perform these movements through the complete range of movement for each joint with special attention to rotatory components of joint movement. Lax joints can maintain range with one complete range of motion daily. Lax joints are unprotected and vulnerable to excessive strain. Protection may best be effected in these joints by moving the joint more slowly through the extremes of joint range, and perhaps just short of complete range. In the presence of spasticity or limb splinting due to discomfort, the involved joints will benefit from two or more excursions through full range daily.

Restriction of lung function secondary to morbid obesity is called the Pickwickian syndrome. In this syndrome, the weight of excess adipose tissue over the thoracic cage and over the abdominal cavity restricts chest wall movement and movement of the diaphragm and abdominal contents, respectively, during respiration. In very heavy individuals, lung function can be impaired considerably. In moderately heavy patients whose lung function normally is not apparently compromised, the condition of this patient with cardiopulmonary dysfunction may be worsened because of this additional load. Every effort needs to be made to work cooperatively with the patient during each treatment if the patient is able to do so. Treatments need to be intense, to the limits of the patient's tolerance provided this is not contraindicated. This approach is necessitated because the obese patient has a greater risk of deteriorating between treatments than other patients if all other variables are constant.

One approach that may be particularly beneficial is promotion of greater air entry through general body exercise and range of motion exercise particularly of the upper limbs. If the patient is able to assist, however, greater cardiopulmonary stress occurs with upper limb exercise; thus, blood pressure and heart rate need monitoring. Lower extremity movements such as hip and knee flexion may help to position the diaphragm for improved excursion. Lower extremity movements will also increase venous return which may or may not be desirable depending on the patient. The goals of upper or lower extremity work must therefore be clearly defined. Possible benefits and untoward effects must be identified to ensure the patient optimally benefits from the prescribed exercise (Fig 17–6).

THE PATIENT WITH ADULT RESPIRATORY DISTRESS SYNDROME

Adult respiratory distress syndrome (ARDS) results from major insult to the lung and injury to the alveolar-capillary membrane. Some of the causes of ARDS include shock, severe trauma or infection, overwhelming pneumonia, and inhaled toxins. Increased vascular permeability resembling that of the inflammatory response is a common feature. Fluid seeps into the interstitial spaces, overwhelms the alveoli, and potentiates pulmonary edema. Gas exchange is severely compromised; thus, the patient presents with severe dyspnea and hypoxemia. Pulmonary infiltrates appear on x-ray.

Fibrinogen in the fluids leaking into the alveoli contributes to fibrosis and reduction of lung compliance observed in ARDS. Lung surface tension and alveolar collapse tend to result from an inactivation of surfactant with the accumulation of fluid in the alveolar spaces. Thus, reduced lung compliance produces a reduced functional residual capacity (FRC) in the patient with ARDS.

The signs and symptoms of ARDS may take up to 48 hours to be fully manifested. The prognosis for survival of patients is 40% to 60%. Hypoxemia is a principal feature of the syndrome, and results from a right to left shunt whereby fluid-filled alveoli are ineffectively perfused. Hyperventilation and labored respiration can be expected in conjunc-

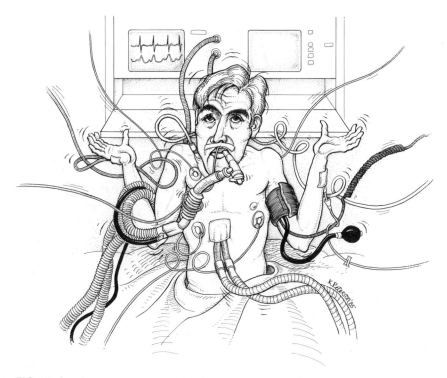

FIG 17–6.
When the patient is positioned and mobilized in the intensive care unit, all tubes and invasive lines must be carefully monitored to prevent untoward results.

tion with hypoxemia. Oxygen therapy has little effect in the presence of shunting. Hypercapnia is not usually a major problem in the ARDS patient.

Management

Intubation and ventilatory support are implemented if arterial blood gases are severely affected and respiratory distress worsened. An endotracheal tube can be placed through the nose, mouth, or tracheostomy. The tidal volume is set at about 10 ml per kg of the patient's body weight. The patient usually establishes the respiratory rate although it may be rapid. A positive end-expiratory pressure (PEEP) of around 12 cm H_2O helps to maintain the alveoli open and thereby helps to optimize gas transfer at end-expiration. Arterial oxygenation is usually improved with PEEP because the effect of shunting is reduced and a given FIO_2 tends to be more effective. As a result, the FIO_2 may be reduced which may help to reduce the possibility of oxygen toxicity.

Guidlines for weaning the patient with restrictive lung disease from mechanical ventilation are comparable to those described for the patient with obstructive lung disease.

Further monitoring of respiratory status in conjunction with arterial blood gases is essential for following the progress of the syndrome. The principal parameters monitored in ARDS are reduced lung compliance, tachypnea, and the concentration of inspired oxygen needed to maintain acceptable levels of the arterial blood gases.

The adult respiratory distress syndrome is characterized by a major pathophysiological restrictive component. Hence, the principles of management of restrictive lung disease can be effectively applied. Changes in lung compliance and FIO_2 requirements provide guidelines to treatment required, treatment response, and course of the syndrome. Patients with ARDS require close monitoring and often frequent treatments aimed at promoting optimal gas exchange because of the severity of the syndrome and high incidence of mortality associated with it. Special attention is given to positioning for postural drainage, to promote ventilation and perfusion matching, and to prevent mechanical restriction of diaphragmatic and chest wall excursion. Some patients, for example, benefit from sidelying in which excursion of the inferior hemidiaphragm is favored (Chapter 1). Other patients, however, seem to deteriorate from apparent restriction of the inferior lung in sidelying. Each patient's condition and specific areas of lung involvement must be taken into consideration when prescribing a turning regime. The effect of the patient's body position on blood gases helps to establish a suitable regime on a rational basis.

The sitting position optimizes lung capacity. The use of a reclining chair at bedside perhaps should be considered more often in the management of patients with ARDS. Theoretically, the potential function of all lung fields will be benefited with the lungs in a more upright position.

THE PATIENT WITH CORONARY ARTERY DISEASE

The initial priority of management in the acute phase of myocardial infarction (MI) is the correction of the immediate problems including arrhythmias and myocardial insufficiency, followed by implementation of a progressive rehabilitation program. Prior to admission to the unit, continuous monitoring of the heart rate and rhythm is established. An intravenous line is routinely started for the administration of medications and fluids. Pain medications are frequently used to minimize the patient's discomfort, at least initially. Drugs such as morphine serve to depress the respiratory drive; thus, the physical therapist must be aware of corresponding changes in vital signs. Less potent sedatives and tranquilizers are more routinely prescribed. Increased pain and anxiety potentially worsen the patient's cardiac status by increasing myocardial oxygen demand.

The primary purpose of oxygen in the cardiac patient is to help reduce myocardial work. Dyspnea, however, is commonly observed in the initial phases of myocardial infarction and can be effectively controlled by administration of supplemental oxygen administered by nasal cannulae or mask. Oxygen may also correct potential ventilation-perfusion mismatching and hypoxemia. Oxygen is always administered with humidity to avoid drying the airways.

Blood gas analysis is performed within an hour of initiating oxygen therapy to establish a baseline of arterial saturation. In this way, oxygen dose can be altered to regulate blood gases and acid base balance.

Management

A primary principle of the management of the patient following myocardial infarction is to reduce myocardial oxygen demand and work load. The myocardium needs rest to promote optimal healing.

Decreasing myocardial work load can be effected in the following ways:

1. A quiet environment without excessive noise and stimulation.

2. Bed rest until medical stability has been maintained and patient shows signs of physical improvement.

3. Progressive mobilization only begun in conjunction with patient's medical status, ECG stability, unchanging or resolving enzyme levels.

4. Reduce patient's anxiety about his or her condition, self-care activities, as well as family and work responsibilities.

5. Gentle mobilization exercises and deep breathing and coughing are usually begun immediately as a prophylactic measure although crepitations are frequently audible in the bases of the lungs of coronary patients; pulmonary congestion and cardiac stress are avoided.

6. Therapeutic exercise helps prevent cardiopulmonary complications, venous stasis, joint stiffness, and muscle weakness. Relaxation is often promoted with low-intensity activity. All levels of activity, including breathing exercises, are performed in a coordinated, rhythmic manner. Breath holding, Valsalva maneuvers, and isometric exercises are absolutely contraindicated during all activities in patients with coronary artery disease, and should not be performed in any stage of their rehabilitation program.

The physical therapist should be watchful at all times for signs of impending infarction including generalized or localized pain anywhere over the thorax, upper limbs, and neck, palpitations, dyspnea, light-headedness, syncope and sensation of indigestion, hiccups and nausea.

Depending on the degree of myocardial infarction and damage, varying lengths of bedrest with or without bathroom privileges may be recommended. During the bedrest period, the physical therapist concentrates on rhythmic breathing exercises, gentle coughing exercises or huffing, modified positioning with the bedhead elevated at least 15 degrees to facilitate the gravity-dependent mechanical action of the heart, and thereby reduce myocardial oxygen demand. The patient is encouraged to do the deep breathing and coughing routine every hour during the day. Bed exercises including rhythmic, unresisted, hip and knee, and foot and ankle exercises are usually performed every four hours or so, or when the patient turns in bed. The patient is cautioned to exercise one leg at a time in the supine position by sliding one heel up and down the bed, guarding against lifting the leg off the bed. These exercises performed correctly and coordinated with inspiration and expiration require relatively little effort or additional physical stress to the MI patient. Comparable to the management of the postoperative patient, these exercises are performed prophylactically to reduce the risk of venous stasis and formation of thromboemboli. In addition, they may help to regulate more coordinated breathing, encourage deep breaths, and reduce atelectasis.

Electrocardiographic monitoring of the cardiac patient is the responsibility of all members of the health care team involved in the patient's care. The physical therapist has a special responsibility to be proficient in ECG interpretation in the coronary care unit with respect to placing physical demands on patients. The physical therapist often has the responsibility of initiating new activities with the cardiac patient which might include sitting over the edge of the bed, engaging in self-care, particularly involving the arms being maintained in a raised position, getting in and out of bed, sitting in a chair, going to the bathroom, or walking around the room. Changes in the ECG must be watched for, particularly when introducing new activities and increasing the intensity of work load of activities. Careful attention to ECG changes and serum enzyme levels will contribute to enhanced physical therapy care of the acute MI patient by optimizing the treatments prescribed and the margin of safety with which activities are performed.

All cardiac patients are prone to anxiety about their conditions and prognosis. The patient is given realistic guidelines at each stage of recovery with respect to level of activity that can be safely performed that can potentially avert deterioration and promote recovery. Involving the patient in rehabilitation planning from the outset facilitates the patient's planning realistically for the future, and may help to reduce the depression often experienced by the acute MI patient. The initial rehabilitation program is planned with the long range rehabilitation goals in mind. The program designed for the cardiac patient is progressive in terms of types of activities, usually beginning with activities of daily living and with respect to the intensity, duration, and frequency of these activities. The patient's tolerance and changes in ECG and vital signs are used as indicators for establishing and modifying the treatment program. These physiological parameters must be observed carefully as the patient progresses to optimize the potential benefits of the therapeutic regimens as early as possible without endangering the patient.

Congestive heart failure may be unavoidable in cases of severe infarction or even milder infarction coupled with lung disease. Fluid intake and output measurements and daily weight help to prevent or to detect congestive heart failure as soon as possible. Routine fluid intake by an intravenous line should not exceed 20 to 30 ml per hour. Signs of imminent congestive heart failure include:

1. Development of tachyarrhythmias.

2. Development of a ventricular gallop.

3. Pulmonary rales and other persistent adventitiae.

4. Development of dyspnea.

5. Development of increased jugular venous pressure and jugular venous distention.

Patient education and prevention of infarction are particularly important for the cardiac patient. As soon as the patient is alert and able to cooperate, information about his or her condition with guidelines about activity and diet is given. The more involved and informed the patient is in self-management, the greater the likelihood of receptivity and adherence to a rehabilitation regimen following discharge.

THE PATIENT IN SHOCK

Shock is a potentially grave situation associated with a variety of precipitating conditions. Common causes of shock include hypovolemia, septicemia, heart failure, and direct insult to the central nervous system. Some of the classical features of shock are hypotension, reduced cardiac output, tachycardia, hyperventilation, diaphoresis, pallor, confusion, nausea, and incontinence. Inadequate tissue perfusion results in extracellular acidemia and loss of potassium ions from the cells. The pulmonary blood vessels constrict in response to hypoxemia tending to increase pulmonary artery wedge pressure (PAWP) and central venous pressure (CVP).

The pathology of shock and the effect on the respiratory membrane follow a similar course regardless of etiology. Swelling of the interstitial tissue disrupts the perfusion of the pulmonary capillaries. Congestive atelectasis and pulmonary edema ensue. In the advanced stages, hyaline membrane changes and pneumonitis may occur.

Management

Foremost, the physical therapist must become aware of the signs and symptoms associated with impending and frank shock. By recognizing and understanding the components of the different types of shock and the effect on the cardiopulmonary system, the physical therapist is in a better position to prescribe a rational treatment plan for the short- and long-term management of the patient.

Although physical therapy may be limited in reversing the signs and symptoms of shock, physical therapy can help to restore and maintain optimal pulmonary function, reduce the risk of complications associated with immobility, and maintain physical status at an optimal level as possible during the episode and in anticipation of the patient's recovery. Physical therapy judiciously applied is not likely to exacerbate the patient's condition.

Patients in shock are usually critically ill and not too responsive. The course of the shock episode is often complicated with the sequelae of immobility. The specific goals related to optimization of cardiopulmonary and musculoskeletal function and prevention of further complications associated with pulmonary function in particular are priorities. The details of physical therapy interventions related to these goals are presented in previous sections of this chapter.

Specific concerns for the patient in shock include the need for short, efficacious treatments and avoidance of unnecessary fatiguing of the patient. Treatment goals are therefore critically appraised and prioritized throughout each day in order to target physical therapy treatment only to the very immediate and essential needs of the patients. Prudent patient positioning is also a priority because of the relative immobility and reduced spontaneous movement observed in these patients.

Late stages of refractory shock leading to renal failure may necessitate peritoneal dialysis. A liter of fluid with a high osmotic fluid content is injected into the patient's abdomen to draw fluid out. The fluid is drained after about 30 minutes. Chest physical therapy is most effective if performed after the fluid has been completely drained from the peritoneum. Following drainage of the fluid the diaphragm is at a more optimal functional length for respiration which potentially can improve treatment response.

THE PATIENT WITH POSTOPERATIVE COMPLICATIONS

Respiratory failure in the postoperative patient is usually associated with a low PaO_2 and a high $PaCO_2$. This situation is likely to be more common than generally appreciated. If the patient is in good general health and is free from underlying lung disease, recovery is usually rapid. Otherwise, more severe complications and respiratory failure may result and progress to a life-threatening situation.

Anesthesia contributes to hypoventilation and atelectasis with physiologic shunting. The patient is difficult to arouse, respirations are slow and shallow, and the pulse is slow. Blood pressure may be elevated, initially reflecting hypercapnia. The administration of narcotics immediately postoperatively tends to further depress respiration. A common postoperative complication is hypoxemia secondary to hypoventilation. Adequate oxygenation, however, can be present despite hypoventilation when oxygen is being administered. The presence or absence of cyanosis may be an unreliable sign because peripheral cyanosis can occur despite adequate arterial PO_2.

Pain, in addition to the effects of anesthesia, is frequently responsible for reduced ventilation and atelectasis following abdominal or thoracic surgery. Rapid shallow breathing may be spontaneously adopted by the patient. Although minute ventilation is favored, alveolar ventilation is compromised by the increased ratio of dead space to tidal volume. Furthermore, in the absence of deep breaths, coughs, and sighs, atelectasis may develop in the underventilated portions of the lungs. The ventilation-perfusion ratio is disturbed because blood flow to underventilated lung segments is ineffective, physiologic shunting occurs, and arterial PO_2 tends to drop although PCO_2 may be unchanged.

Pulmonary Embolism

Pulmonary embolism is a potentially life-threatening complication. Pulmonary embolism usually results from a thrombus forming in the veins of the lower limbs, pelvis, in the right atrium, or in the right ventricle. Patients may be at risk if they have varicose veins, chronic heart failure, if they are obese, pregnant, or taking oral contraceptives.

The patient with a pulmonary thromboembolism usually has a sudden onset of tachypnea, radiating chest pain, and apparent anxiety. Occasionally, right heart failure follows. Enzymes are often elevated. Right heart strain may be evidenced on ECG. Right bundle branch block, peaked P waves, and inverted T waves may be seen. No abnormality may be noted on chest x-ray.

Treatment consists of primary ventilatory and circulatory support, with adequate oxygenation of peripheral tissues. Anticoagulants such as heparin are infused intravenously to help minimize further formation of thromboembolic substrates.

Management

Major changes in lung volume, mechanics, and gas exchange uniformly occur after anesthesia and tissue dissection. The extent and duration of these changes increase with the magnitude of the operative procedure and degree of anesthesia required. These abnormalities observed in the postoperative period are characterized by gradual and progressive alveolar collapse. Total lung capacity, FRC, and residual volume are significantly decreased. Because of the decrease in FRC, compliance is decreased, and therefore the work of breathing is increased. Hypoxemia secondary to transpulmonary shunting usually becomes maximal within 72 hours after surgery, and often is completely resolved with conservative management within seven days. The FI_{O_2} will depend on the mode of 100% oxygen administration. Low oxygen flows and low FI_{O_2}s tend to be delivered via nasal cannulae. Higher flows can deliver higher FI_{O_2}s via oxygen masks and masks with reservoir bags. The FI_{O_2} must always be taken into account when interpreting arterial blood gases. The FI_{O_2} is selected to provide adequate oxygenation with the lowest oxygen concentration possible.

Following surgery, the normal pattern of breathing is disrupted. Shallow, monotonous tidal ventilations without normal occasional, spontaneous deep breaths cause alveolar collapse to be potentiated within one hour. Within a few hours postsurgery, atelectasis becomes increasingly resistant to reinflation. This complication is exacerbated in patients receiving narcotics.

Tachypnea, tachycardia, and moderate fever are commonly observed with gross atelectasis secondary to hypoventilation. Breath sounds are decreased at the bases, and the coarse rhonchi associated with mucus obstructing air flow are heard on auscultation. Large areas of atelectasis are present. Left lower lobe atelectasis is common following cardiac surgery. Alveoli are likely to remain patent for one hour after reinflation. Hence, to sustain alveolar inflation and normal FRC, maximal inspiratory maneuvers should be performed minimally every hour, and preferably more frequently. Appropriate rest periods are interspersed within each session according to the patient's needs to avoid hyperventilation. Maximal expirations are avoided to prevent airway closure and potential increase of atelectasis. Huffing or forced expiration technique, however, beginning from mid-lung volume to low-lung volume can be especially effective in combination with postural drainage. There is less risk of bronchospasm than with coughing in which the glottis is closed, transpulmonary pressure is increased, and a compressive phase is involved. Forced expiration maneuvers are likely to be most effective in the sitting or slightly lean-forward position. Airway closure is position dependent; therefore, the degree of expiration encouraged by the therapist should be based upon the patient's position. Airway closure is potentiated in patients who are older and who are in horizontal as opposed to vertical body positions.

Mobilization and breathing exercises offer the greatest benefit to cardiopulmonary status and mucociliary clearance with the least risk to the patient compared with other more passive, invasive interventions. Each deep breath is performed to maximal inspiration to total lung capacity with a brief breath hold. This relatively simple maneuver has been consistently effective in reducing pulmonary complications by promoting alveolar inflation and gas exchange. If well taught and a comprehensible rationale is provided, the patient is capable of conducting deep breathing sessions independently every hour. This independence frees the therapist from having to be in attendance each session. In addition, the patient is able to assume some responsibility for his or her postoperative recovery.

If the patient is unable to cooperate due to pain, vigorous chest physical therapy and coughing exercises can often be well-tolerated and can be very effective after narcotic administration. If narcotics impair the patient's ability to participate in treatment, less potent sedatives or tranquilizers may be preferable. Intravenous administration prolongs the peak-effect time of analgesics, and therefore helps the patient tolerate a longer treatment. Oversedation is avoided. Transcutaneous electrical nerve stimulation (TENS) has been reported to be a useful adjunct in the management of postoperative pain. Pain control with TENS may enable the patient to participate more fully in deep breathing, coughing, and bed exercises. Research is needed, however, to evaluate this technique in the management of acute pain. A nonpharmacologic, noninvasive means of managing acute pain would be of tremendous benefit to patients, and would potentially enable them to participate more fully in physical therapy treatments in the absence of untoward side effects often associated with drug administration.

Incentive spirometry has been favored in some ICUs (Fig 17–7) (see Chapter 10). Postoperative hypoxemia has been shown to be reversed using this technique which employs the principle of sustained inspiration to achieve maximal inflating pressure in the alveoli and maximal inhaled volume. The use of the incentive spirometer can also be used independently by the patient. This technique helps to insure that each inspiration is physiologically optimal for the patient and is reproduced precisely from one inspiration to the next. For best results, patients who may be potential surgical risks are taught the use of the incentive spirometer during the preoperative teaching by the physical therapist.

The application of intermittent positive pressure breathing (IPPB) appears to be less effective for the postoperative patient than previously believed. The details of this modality are described in Chapter 29.

Restoration of alveolar ventilation is the foremost treatment objective in the postoperative patient threatened with respiratory failure. Nasal oxygen at low flow rate can help correct hypoxemia in the absence of hypercapnia and marked transpulmonary shunting.

Endotracheal intubation and mechanical ventilation may be indicated if blood gases fail to improve with conservative management. The treatment priorities for the ventilated patient before and during weaning are discussed in a previous section. Special attention in the postoperative patient is given to the pulmonary complications associated with

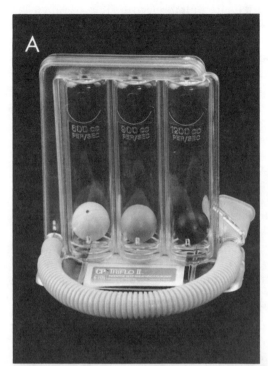

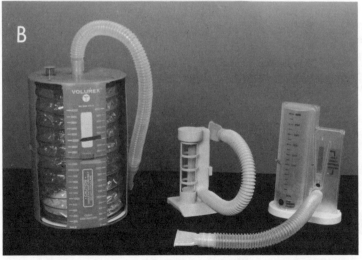

FIG 17–7.
Incentive spirometers.

surgical pain, restrictions to adequate pulmonary function secondary to dressings, binders, and diminished ability to cooperate, to move spontaneously, and to occasionally hyperventilate the lungs.

The importance of a thorough preoperative assessment and teaching by the physical therapist cannot be overstated. In cases of elective surgery, preoperative teaching includes a general description of the surgery to be performed, of the effect of anesthesia and surgery on lung function, and the effects of immobility and temporary confinement to bed. The lines, leads, and catheters usually associated with routine surgery are explained. The patient is instructed in lateral costal and diaphragmatic breathing exercises, in supported coughing, in mobility exercises for the limbs, in foot and ankle exercises, and in lying, sitting, and turning in bed as comfortably as possible postoperatively. The course of recovery postoperatively is described in general terms so the patient can anticipate this period knowledgeably. If the patient is well informed preoperatively, he or she will be able to cooperate more completely when waking up from the anesthetic as well as when more fully alert and oriented. The importance of frequent postural changes in the initial postoperative period and early ambulation are stressed. The patient is taught preoperatively how to move comfortably with a surgical incision.

Following surgery, all patients are detained in the recovery room until vital signs have stabilized, there is no apparent internal or external bleeding, and the patient is responding to his or her name. Patients recovering from minor surgery are usually transferred to the ward once discharged from the recovery room. Patients are transferred to the ICU postoperatively if complications arise during surgery, if the patient cannot be readily stabilized and requires close monitoring, or if the patient has had more serious surgery such as cranial, cardiovascular thoracic surgery, or emergency surgery such as that resulting from multiple trauma.

All patients considered for elective surgery are screened regarding their risk for potential postoperative complications. The physical therapist is often consulted by the surgeon to help make a poor-risk patient into a relatively better-risk patient. Patients with upper respiratory tract infections prior to surgery may have their surgery postponed depending on the type and extent of surgery to be performed, level of anesthesia indicated, other medical conditions including cardiopulmonary disease, age, and smoking history. Patients with lower respiratory tract infections preoperatively constitute a greater operative risk, hence these patients would be likely to have their surgery postponed until the infection had cleared up. Patients with chronic lung diseases require a prolonged period of preoperative physical therapy in preparation for surgery. Patients should also be as healthy and well as possible. Elective surgery is never considered during an exacerbation of the disease. Even minor surgery may be potentially hazardous for the patient with previous lung disease. The adverse effects of total anesthesia on these patients is magnified because of their reduced pulmonary reserve capacity. Smoking should be discontinued for as long as possible prior to surgery. The patient is placed on an exercise conditioning program, a regimen of bronchial hygiene, oxygen if necessary, and prophylactic antibiotics. This preoperative preparation may take one to several weeks depending on the patient and the indications for surgery.

Open Heart Surgery

Patients scheduled for open heart surgery are always treated as potentially high risk surgical candidates because of the nature and extent of the surgery required (Fig 17–8), regardless of their general level of

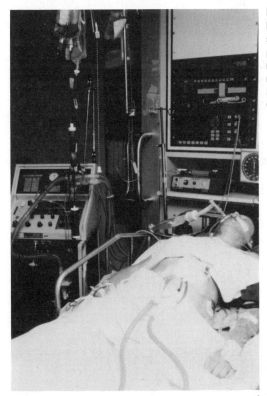

FIG 17–8.
Patient following open heart surgery (four hours postoperative). Note patient on mechanical ventilator, mediastinal drains, receiving blood, IVs, on EKG, CVP, Swan Ganz, Arterial Blood Gas lines.

health prior to surgery. Whenever possible, however, patients prepare for surgery in advance by decreasing or stopping smoking, by avoiding exposure to respiratory tract infections, by avoiding stress, by eating a balanced diet and sleeping adequately.

In the preoperative period, the physical therapist may spend additional time with patients scheduled for open heart surgery to provide good teaching in the basic anatomy and physiology of surgery to be performed, the effect of anesthesia, the role of intubation and mechanical ventilation, the incision lines to be expected over the chest and the legs if veins are to be removed for bypass surgery, the lines, leads, chest tubes, and catheters that will be in place after surgery, and the course of recovery the patient might expect barring complications. The emphasis on patient education in most open heart surgery units may contribute to the generally low incidence of complications and mortality.

The following guidelines to physical therapy management of the open heart surgical patient are to be used *cautiously* with regard to each specific patient's condition and observed recovery. These guidelines suggest the *upper limit* of intensity of physical therapy if all is progressing well initially, and should be reduced if warranted by the patient's condition. Therapists should remember that different institutions may advocate different practices depending on the adequacy of their facilities, experience of the surgical and ICU team, and the incidence of postoperative complications and survival for that institution.

Day 1.   Patient may be seen in the postanesthesia and recovery room for chest assessment; the patient is usually extubated within 36 hours after surgery. The patient must be permitted to rest as much as possible in the initial 24- to 36-hour period. Usually once extubated, the patient is positioned side to side for deep breathing and coughing at least four times in the first 24 hours. Medications are administered prior to treatment to assure optimal effect during treatment. Depending on the findings of x-ray, physical examination, and arterial blood gases, the patient may require vibrations and possibly percussion. Postural drainage positions are modified to avoid tipping the patient head-down and causing increased myocardial strain. A sputum sample for culture and sensitivity testing may be taken at this time. The patient can usually tolerate being dangled over the edge of the bed for a few minutes. Special care is taken for all heart patients to avoid the Valsalva maneuver, forced coughing and huffing, and to maintain a semirecumbent position for treatment. Blood pressure is checked before, during, and after treatment. Gentle mobilization is begun, including foot and ankle movements.

Day 2.   Two to three treatments of deep breathing and coughing with exercise are continued. Postural drainage, percussion, and vibration can be implemented if these procedures are indicated from the assessment. Upper limb and neck exercises are introduced. Neck exercises are withheld if central venous pressure lines are still in place in the neck veins. The patient can sit in a chair at bedside for a short period of time. The patient is encouraged to stand erect for a minute or so on transferring back and forth to the chair.

Day 3.   The patient can take two short walks. Mobilization is not begun until arterial lines and Swan-Ganz catheter have been capped or removed. Vital signs are monitored before and after standing and walking. Chest physical therapy continues twice daily unless more intense treatment is indicated. Deep breathing and coughing exercises are *not* discontinued even if the chest is clear, until the patient is up and about within reasonable limits as tolerated. The patient is encouraged in grooming and self-care.

Day 4.   Deep breathing and coughing should be done by the patient without supervision. The presence of atelectasis on x-ray or from assessment findings, however, would indicate the need for continuation of mobilization with breathing exercises. Ambulation is increased as tolerated.

Days 5 and 6.   Patient can participate in individual or class activities concentrating on trunk mobility, coordinated breathing activities, posture, biomechanics, and increasing the patient's endurance gradually.

Days 7 and 8.   The patient can attempt six to eight stairs if progress has been satisfactory. Aortic repairs in the first week or so are prone to rupture. Elevation of the blood pressure is therefore avoided to reduce the risk of breakdown of the aortic suture line.

Days 9 and 10.   The patient depends primarily on ambulation for maintaining a clear chest rather than breathing and coughing exercises. The patient is cautioned to balance a period of exertion with a period of rest. The patient may be discharged. The physical therapist insures the patient fully understands the specific details of the home exercise program. The emphasis of exercise for cardiac patients continues to be on rhythmic, coordinated dynamic movements on discharge, with the avoidance of isometric, static exercise. If possible, the patient is invited to participate in a reconditioning and health promotion program as an outpatient in a physical therapy department. Follow-up medical and physical therapy visits are arranged prior to discharge around four to six weeks postsurgery.

Note: The physical therapist must guard against excessively intense treatment of open heart surgical patients or other patients for whom prolonged periods of immobility (four to five days) are anticipated. These patients may be susceptible to soft tissue bruising from being on a prophylactic course of anticoagulants.

THE PATIENT WITH MUSCULOSKELETAL TRAUMA

Crush injuries involving the chest are commonly seen in the ICU. Damage to the chest wall and lung parenchyma contribute to the possibility of respiratory failure. Associated injuries of the head and abdomen may also contribute to respiratory failure.

Paradoxical motion of the chest wall associated with flail chest and rib fractures results from instability of portions of the rib cage following trauma to the chest. If severe, patients may require surgical stabilization of the ribs or stabilization by continuous ventilatory management.

The presence of blood or air in the chest cavity impairs ventilation, promotes retention of secretions, and interferes with effective clearance. Small effusions may completely resolve with chest physical therapy and reexpansion of any underlying atelectasis. The presence of a pneumothorax or hemothorax can severely compromise lung expansion. These disorders tend to be resistant to resolution with chest physical therapy alone. A tension pneumothorax results when air collects under tension in the pleural cavity. The tension pneumothorax promotes lung collapse on both the ipsilateral and contralateral sides which further threatens respiratory failure. Diaphragmatic injuries directly affect ventilation in two ways. First, the bellows action of the lungs is compromised. Second, the lung is displaced by herniation of the abdominal contents into the thoracic cavity.

Analysis of blood gases in the patient with posttraumatic injuries of the chest often shows severe hypoxemia and moderate elevations of arterial PCO_2. The presence of acidemia is common which may have both respiratory and metabolic components.

Management

Severe restlessness and dyspnea in a patient with chest injury are classic indications of respiratory failure. Auscultation and percussion can usually reveal an underlying pneumothorax or hemothorax. Tension pneumothorax is confirmed by chest x-ray or aspiration of the chest with a needle and syringe.

Flail chest refers to fractures involving the chest cage where there are two or more fractured ribs at two or more sites. This results in instability of the chest wall. The so-called flail segment is usually apparent on physical examination. Paradoxical movement of the flail segment can often be observed. The chest is depressed rather than elevated over the site during inspiration. Rib fractures are indicated by tenderness and crepitations on physical examination and from x-ray findings.

Nonventilatory management of chest injuries in the absence of severe hypoxemia is preferred in these patients.

Rib Fractures

Simple uncomplicated rib fractures may receive no specific treatment. More complicated fractures may be treated with intercostal nerve block and physical therapy to maintain good bronchial hygiene and avoid pulmonary complications. Strapping the chest is usually avoided, particularly in the patient with limited respiratory reserve.

The current method of therapy for flail chest is internal stabilization of the chest and use of a mechanical ventilator. Slight hyperventilation will usually reduce the respiratory drive of most patients to allow the ventilator to take over the full work of breathing. The flail segment is then stabilized by internal expansion of the lungs. The treatment assures adequate ventilation with the least pain possible. After two weeks, the flail segment is usually stable.

If the patient can maintain a reasonable tidal volume and normal blood gases, weaning is begun. As soon as tidal volume and forced vital capacity are within acceptable limits, oxygen can be administered through an endotracheal tube with a T tube assembly. Arterial blood gases are monitored closely after the ventilator has been discontinued. Once the blood gases are in acceptable ranges over a reasonable period of time, i.e., 12 to 24 hours, the endotracheal tube is removed.

Pneumothorax and Hemothorax

Air or blood in the pleural cavity following chest trauma must be removed through a chest tube. For a pneumothorax, the chest tube is positioned in the second or third intercostal space in the midclavicular line. For a hemothorax, the chest tube is positioned in the sixth intercostal space in the posterior axillary line. This tube is regularly milked or "stripped" free of blood clots so that it remains patent. Chest physical therapy has a significant role in facilitating chest tube drainage. Chest tubes should be "stripped" prior to treatment in order for drainage to be facilitated during the treatment. Care is taken to avoid kinking chest tubes during patient positioning and treatment. Usually the chest tubes are sutured and taped into position and therefore are not easily dislodged. If the tubes are pulled out, subcutaneous emphysema or a pneumothorax results. A pneumothorax will also result if the tube is disconnected from the underwater seal. This is the reason for securing the bottles of a chest tube drainage system with tape to the floor, or keeping the drainage containers in molded stands on the floor.

A bronchopulmonary fistula can be responsible for a major loss of the tidal volume delivered by the ventilator. Small leaks can be tolerated and are usually compensated for by an increase in tidal or minute ventilation.

Multiple Trauma

The management of multiple trauma is a major challenge for the ICU team. Multisystem involvement and complications often present a precarious situation in which priorities have to be defined for each individual situation. Problems associated with multiple trauma include head injury, chest wall injuries, fractures, lung contusions, diaphragm injury, pleural space disorders, internal injuries, thromboemboli, fat emboli, and so forth. Shock and adult respiratory distress syndrome may ensue. Positive end-expiratory pressure is frequently used to help reduce the effects of lung congestion secondary to shock or ARDS. Arterial blood gases are assessed to evaluate the effectiveness of PEEP in effecting improved oxygen transfer.

Multiple Fractures

Fixation, traction, and casting of fractures and dislocations of the limbs complicate the management of the trauma patient. Restrictions to body positioning are a primary concern of the therapist in the ICU. A strict routine of body positioning is maintained although severe limitations often exist with respect to degree of turning permitted. Lower limb traction can be maintained when the patient is positioned in a modified sidelying position. Percussion can often be performed relatively vigorously and longer in multiple trauma patients, particularly those who are young and who were previously healthy. Coordinating treatments with analgesic schedules helps to reduce the patient's fatigue and prolong the treatment. These patients usually tolerate tipping well, provided head injury does not complicate the clinical picture.

Frequent deep breathing and coughing exercises, positioning within the limits of the patient's traction and casts, and prescribing an exercise program that involves as many large muscle groups as possible constitute the most commonly used interventions in multiple trauma.

Relaxation techniques can be integrated into the treatment regime for the trauma patient. Every effort needs to be made to maintain the patient's spirits, reduce stress, and encourage a positive attitude toward active participation early in the rehabilitation program.

Care must be taken to avoid undertreating trauma patients. A clear chest can rapidly regress due to general immobility and limitations to body movement imposed by traction and pain. Treatments should *always* be coordinated with the patient's analgesics in order to optimize treatment response and for the patient's comfort. Whenever possible, the patient should be equipped with slings and pulleys and weights at bedside. Proprioceptive neuromuscular facilitation (PNF) patterns are often useful in preparation for slings and pulleys. The use of PNF techniques for trauma and postoperative patients has been reported to be well tolerated and associated with relatively little pain in these patients compared with nonresisted movements. All activities are taught in conjunction with breathing exercises and coordination with the respiratory cycle.

THE PATIENT WITH CENTRAL NERVOUS SYSTEM TRAUMA

Hypoxemia is observed in many patients with injury to the central nervous system. Arterial blood gases are therefore closely monitored in these patients.

Acute cerebral edema with sudden increase in intracranial pressure rapidly affects central control of respiration. Advancing cerebral edema is evidenced by deterioration in level of consciousness, pupillary reflexes, ocular reflexes, pattern of respiration, and exaggerated muscle tone and posture. The sequence of these clinical signs corresponds to intracranial pressure (ICP) progressively increasing from the cortex toward the medullopontine region. With involvement of the brainstem, respiration becomes variable and incoordinate. With loss of central control and imminent cessation of breathing, respiration is shallow and ataxic. The appearance of the jaw and laryngeal jerk with each inspiratory effort suggests a poor prognosis.

Spinal cord injuries above C_3 result in loss of phrenic nerve innervation, necessitating a tracheostomy and mechanical ventilation. All patients are at risk for developing atelectasis, pneumonia, and pulmonary emboli. Prophylactic low-dose heparin is used routinely unless the presence of pulmonary emboli is suspected and higher dosages are indicated.

Daily physical therapy and the patient's normal routine may have a dramatic effect on the ICP. Indirectly ICP can be elevated by an increase in intrathoracic pressure as a result of physical therapy or suctioning. Turning and positioning may produce obstruction to cerebral venous outflow. Noxious stimuli such as arterial and venous punctures or cleansing wounds can elevate ICP as well as relatively innocuous stimuli such as noise or pupil checks. Whether these factors elevate ICP depend on the patient's intracranial compliance and cerebral blood volume. On stimulation, a chain reaction is initiated. Cerebral activity is increased, which in turn elevates metabolic rate, blood flow; hence, volume and ICP.

The head of the bed is usually maintained at about 20 degrees to help reduce ICP. The patient's head and neck may be held in a fixed position by halo traction or sand bags positioned on either side (Fig 17–9). Hyperventilation is indicated if P_{CO_2} is above 20 mm Hg. Arterial blood gases are checked during or immediately following hyperventilation. Prolonged hyperventilation is to be avoided.

Management

Specific attention to cardiopulmonary function is an essential component of the assessment of *all* patients in the ICU, including the neurological patient. Physical therapy priorities include:

1. Prevention of cerebral hypoxia by maintaining a patent airway and reduced cerebral pressure.

2. Avoidance of activities and stimuli that increase ICP.

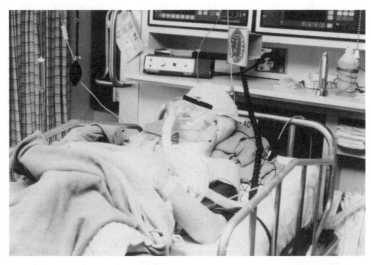

FIG 17–9.
Patient following neurosurgical procedure; head of bed elevated 20 degrees to help reduce ICP.

3. Reduced atelectasis, pooling of secretions, and possible risk of chest infection.

4. Reduce the work of breathing and improve the efficiency of the muscles of respiration, particularly if long-term disability is a risk.

5. Position the patient within the limits of fracture stabilization and elevated intracranial pressure to promote ventilation perfusion matching, to reduce pathological patterns of muscle synergy and thereby promote ventilation, and to reduce myocardial stress.

6. Perform assisted, active-assisted, and active movements as soon as possible to enhance cardiopulmonary function, reduce risk of thromboemboli, and optimally preserve musculoskeletal status.

In cases of abnormally elevated ICP, forced hyperventilation and maintenance of PCO_2 around 25 mm Hg are effective in reducing cerebral edema by reducing blood flow. Intracranial pressure may increase with treatment, and in particular with turning or suctioning. An ICP of up to 30 mm Hg may be acceptable provided the pressure returns to normal immediately after the removal of the pressure-potentiating stimulus. Prolonged elevation of ICP suggests low cerebral compliance and the possibility of potential brain damage unless pressure is reduced. Thus, all interventions must be performed guardedly with due consideration being given to corresponding changes in ICP. Typically, management of patients with central nervous system trauma includes judicious tracheal suctioning, a stringent turning regime, lung hyperinflation with the manual breathing bag in the nonventilated patient, or deep breathing with occasionally increased tidal volumes or "sighs" in the ventilated patients.

If the ICP is unstable and a risk of brain damage exists, physical therapy should follow sedation. Ideally, treatments should be performed when the ICP is low and intracranial compliance is satisfactory. The head is not tilted down for chest physical therapy. Noise should be kept to a minimum.

If the ICP is elevated, all noxious stimuli should be removed. In severe conditions, a decision may have to be made by the team to limit or withdraw chest physical therapy, suctioning, neurologic assessment, or turning.

Movement of the limbs is performed gently and in a relaxed manner. Patients in a comatose state may experience passive limb movement noxiously. Intracranial pressure may be elevated as a result. Passive movements, however, may have the added benefit of promoting improved tidal ventilation in the nonventilated patient by providing afferent stimulation to the respiratory center via peripheral muscle and joint receptors.

Neurophysiological facilitation of respiration has been suggested as a potentially beneficial means of improving ventilation, coughing, and breathing pattern in unconscious and conscious patients. Physiologically, these techniques have been based upon stimulation of reflexive involuntary respiratory movements. Neurophysiological facilitation techniques include cocontraction of the abdominal muscles, vertebral pressure, intercostal stretch, lifting the posterior basal areas of the lungs, and perioral stimulation. The rationale for and the role of these techniques in cardiopulmonary physical therapy, however, is unclear. Research is needed to objectively clarify these questions.

Patients with suspected spinal cord injuries usually undergo immediate spinal fixation on admission. Depending on the level of injury determined by clinical signs and x-rays, traction and fixation may be localized to the head and neck, or spinal support and casting may be required in the thoracic or lumbar regions. Although modified positioning can be achieved with these patients, the provision of optimal care under these restricted conditions is a singularly important challenge to the physical therapist, particularly with respect to the management of adequate pulmonary function while the patient is in the ICU.

Percussion and vibration techniques are applied cautiously depending on the severity of any complicating fracture-dislocation(s), the stability of fixation, the condition of the lungs, and the presence of chest wall injuries. Positioning, if done well despite the need in some cases for extensive modification, may help reduce the need for percussion and vibration by effecting good regional ventilation and perfusion to all lung fields over a given period of time.

The high frequency oscillating ventilator that has been gaining popularity in experimental trials may contribute to improved management of multiple trauma patients with spinal injuries who require ventilation. The advantages of the high-frequency oscillating ventilator include improved spontaneous mucociliary clearance and reduced incidence of atelectasis.

Weaning of quadriplegic patients off the ventilator requires special skill because of the lost function of the respiratory muscles. For these patients, weaning can be particularly fatiguing, frightening, and frustrating. Patients are weaned lying supine when they are alert and apparently willing to cooperate. Short periods off the ventilator on the T piece are used initially. Use of the accessory muscles of respiration and any other muscular reserves are encouraged to compensate for the loss of function of the respiratory muscles. In some centers, patients are started in the weaning period on respiratory muscle training. The physical therapist must be well versed and practiced in this procedure, however, prior to using it in conjunction with weaning the quadriplegic patient off the ventilator. Because of the potential risk of inappropriate application and of danger to the patient, respiratory muscle training must be effected knowledgeably to optimize its benefits for each individual patient.

Respiratory Muscle Training

Respiratory muscle fatigue is probably much more common in the ICU than appreciated. The combination of immobilization and respiratory involvement secondary to extensive injury may result in similar disuse atrophy of the diaphragm as observed in other skeletal muscles. Respiratory muscle fatigue has been identified as a component of both obstructive and restrictive lung diseases. Patients with neuromuscular weakness and paralysis do not have the advantage of performing coordinated general body activity and relaxation maneuvers to help reduce the work of breathing. There is a marked decrease of respiratory muscle strength and endurance resulting in decreased vital capacity, rib cage mobility, and the ability to cough. For these reasons, patients with neuromuscular paralysis are particularly well suited for respiratory muscle training. The quadriplegic patient has lost the function of the intercostal muscles that are important muscles of inspiration and are responsible for thoracic cage expansion. In addition, the absence of the abdominal muscles, which are the primary expiratory muscles, drastically reduces the ability to cough effectively and to perform a forced expiration. The diaphragm and the accessory muscles of inspiration, namely the scaleni and sternocleidomastoid muscles, then become the quadriplegic patient's respiratory muscles.

These factors as well as the effects of heat, humidity, and the vertical position all predispose the quadriplegic individual to the development of respiratory muscle fatigue. Respiratory muscle fatigue in turn may predispose the patient to acute respiratory failure. The physical therapist can help avert the effects of respiratory muscle fatigue with respiratory muscle training.

Respiratory muscle training with a regimen of progressive resistive breathing has been demonstrated to improve the strength and endurance of respiratory muscles and hence improve functional capacity in some patients. Resistive breathing is aimed at the prevention of respiratory failure by increasing the strength and particularly endurance of the key muscle of inspiration, the diaphragm. Because the diaphragm is skeletal muscle, it can be reconditioned using a series of inspiratory resistance maneuvers. A stronger, endurance-trained diaphragm will not fatigue nearly as quickly as an untrained diaphragm when exposed to such potentially fatiguing factors as eating a meal, talking, exposure to heat and humidity, sitting upright, overcoming a respiratory tract infection, and so on.

A candidate for respiratory muscle training is equipped with an individual resistive breathing package containing the valve, mouthpiece, noseclip, and a series of resistors that attach to the inspiratory side of the valve (see Fig 9–3).

An initial pretraining assessment is performed to determine the appropriate resistor with which to commence training. The progression to the next level of resistance is based on specific criteria of endurance on the current resistor.

Once the resistor has been chosen, a typical training session includes the following steps:

1. The patient is usually in the sitting or upright position for training initially unless sitting is not yet indicated.

2. The noseclip is attached snugly.

3. The mouthpiece is placed securely in the individual's mouth and allows him or her to select an individual rate and pattern of breathing.

4. Breathing is performed comfortably without force.

5. The patient is instructed to stop the exercise by letting go of the valve if the resistance becomes too difficult or if lightheadedness or dizziness occur.

6. When the individual has adjusted to the resistance in the initial training position, an attempt can then be made to train at the same load in other positions.

Measurements of maximum inspiratory mouth pressure and vital capacity can be easily done routinely with special apparatus to monitor change and evaluate strength of the diaphragm.

Evaluation of the patient's progress must be ongoing. The level of inspiratory resistance and the duration for which the patient can use each resistor are indications of the endurance of the inspiratory muscles. Measurement of vital capacity, maximum inspiratory and expiratory mouth pressures provide an index of the strength of the inspiratory muscles.

Certain precautions must be observed with respiratory muscle training. Each time a new resistance is tried, the therapist should be with the patient. The patient selects his or her own rate and pattern of breathing. Too shallow breathing is inefficient, and too slow, deep breathing may result in accumulation of CO_2. The patient is cautioned about avoiding hyperventilation. The physical therapist or the patient, when he or she is capable, should check the valving system on the respiratory muscle trainer prior to each training session to ensure it is functioning properly.

THE PATIENT WITH BURNS

Pulmonary complications are common in patients with moderately severe and severe burns; and are a major cause of death. Smoke and chemical inhalation produce bronchospasm, cough, and profuse secretions. Irritation of the alveoli and acute pulmonary edema can result in a condition resembling ARDS.

Medical stabilization of the patient is an initial priority. Depending on the severity and extent of the burns, treatment ranges from conservative medical interventions to multiple surgeries related to progressive debridement and skin grafting.

Both second- and third-degree burns have the potential to result in severe disfigurement and disability. Body positioning and limb splinting are therefore critical priorities for both optimal cardiopulmonary function and restoration of neuromuscular status. Positioning priorities in the burned patients therefore must consider both these aspects of management.

Treatment is directed at improving arterial saturation, maintaining fluid balance, and preventing infection. Hypoxemia is effectively treated with the administration of oxygen. If the patient is breathing spontaneously, oxygen is given via nasal cannulae or mask at flows of 1 to 5 L/min depending on the arterial oxygen saturation. Moisture can be administered through a face tent with a heated nebulizer.

Ventilatory assistance may be indicated in severe respiratory failure secondary to smoke inhalation. A nasotracheal tube is preferred to a tracheostomy tube because complications with a tracheostomy tube are greater in burned patients. Postburn pulmonary complications are generally related to fluid overload in the initial stage, or sepsis. Acute pulmonary edema and congestion are largely preventable with careful fluid therapy. Central venous pressure can be misleading in the burned patient because of severe fluid loss, and may remain at low values despite pulmonary edema. Pulmonary artery pressure more accurately reflects the status of the pulmonary circulation in these patients. Treatment of pulmonary edema consists typically of digitalis, diuretics, and assisted ventilation. Positive end expiratory pressure is usually indicated in the ventilated burned patient. Mist or aerosol inhalation is also used to help to reduce the thickness of lung secretions.

Management

On admission of the burned patient to hospital, the patency of the airway is assessed immediately. Inhalation injuries are common in burned patients and result from smoke inhalation, heat trauma, and chemical and gas inhalation. Oxygen and humidification are usually administered immediately. Heat may cause laryngeal and bronchial edema. If airway occlusion from impending edema threatens, intubation is performed. If indicated early, intubation may help to avoid respiratory distress within the critical 24-hour period after admission. Particular care is given to children and older adults with inhalation injury because these patients have a higher risk of developing secondary pulmonary complications. Chest physical therapy is often required immediately for the patient with inhalation damage, to maintain the patency of the airways, prevent atelectasis and retention of secretions, and improve or maintain gas exchange. Pulmonary function may be severely impaired as the net result of inhalation damage, burns to the chest wall, and generalized pain.

Chest physical therapy may have to be modified in the burned patient. Positioning may be achieved with care. Patients who have skin grafts will require particular care when moving or positioning. Sterile procedures must be observed at all times. The therapist is usually required to cap, gown, and glove prior to treating the patient, and to cover the chest with a sterile drape. Manual percussion of the chest wall may not be comfortably tolerated in the presence of first and second degree burns. Manual or mechanical vibration may have to substitute for more rigorous procedures.

Risk of aspiration is increased if tube feedings are not discontinued for at least one hour prior to treatment. A nasogastric tube is often used and should be correctly positioned particularly during treatment.

General mobilization is always preferable to manual chest physical therapy wherever possible in the maintenance of pulmonary function. Increased activity may initially consist of selected limb movements and dangling over the edge of the bed for a few minutes if this can be tolerated. As soon as the patient's tolerance increases, free unsupported sitting can progress to standing and walking. Ambulation during ventilator-assisted breathing should always be considered for any patient for whom this activity is not contraindicated. The upright position and physical activity in the upright position are likely to enhance markedly the patient's cardiopulmonary and neuromuscular function, and improve the patient's strength and endurance in preparation for more active rehabilitation. If sitting up and ambulation are not imminent, appropriate limb movements will help prepare the patient for these activities later on as well as enhance lung function to some degree in the meantime.

Certain precautions have to be observed in the management of the burned patient. First, large areas of skin loss increase the risk of infection; therefore, the therapist must be familiar with sterile technique. Second, skin loss can contribute to substantial fluid loss, often resulting in labile fluid and electrolyte imbalance. This situation may enhance myocardial irritability and the risk of arrhythmia. Whenever possible, ECG monitoring is done routinely during physical therapy treatment.

COMPLICATIONS OF RESPIRATORY FAILURE

Pulmonary Dysfunction

Complications of the pulmonary system during hospitalization may aggravate respiratory failure. Some of these relate to being mechanically ventilated. Certain technical problems related to the cuffs used in conjunction with artificial airways may occur, e.g., overinflation, distortion and herniation of the orifice of the tube. Mucous plugs can also occlude the tracheostomy or endotracheal tube and prevent ventilation. Physical therapists must be aware of these potential pulmonary complications. The common complications can be reduced if the tube is changed frequently and if minimal amounts of air are used for cuff inflation.

Prolonged endotracheal intubation can result in laryngeal edema, ulceration, and fibrosis. Mechanical ventilation may also rupture a bleb on the surface of the lung and produce a pneumothorax with rapid tension development. Chest tubes are inserted immediately to relieve the tension. Blebs occur when alveoli rupture, causing air to track to subpleural sites.

Mechanical ventilators can be a source of infection. The physical therapist can help minimize this risk by not directly handling the ventilator attachments that communicate with the air flow channels. Condensation from the hose should not be drained toward the ventilator or toward the patient. The therapist should be masked and gloved when connecting and disconnecting the patient to and from the ventilator.

Physical therapists are often responsible for collecting samples of secretions for culture and sensitivity tests. The lower respiratory tract is first suctioned according to sterile procedure. A sterilized sputum trap is interposed between the collection jar and the suction catheter. After the sample has been collected, the trap is removed and carefully labeled with the patient's name, bed number, date, and time the sample was collected.

Oxygen toxicity is a significant clinical complication of mechanical ventilation. Most contemporary ventilators have precise oxygen controls to deliver the lowest possible inspired oxygen concentration that will maintain arterial oxygen tensions between 65 and 75 torr. Excess oxygen above the patient's needs is never indicated.

Flow-directed pulmonary artery catheters commonly used in the ICU are also associated with some complications. Infection may lead to bacteremia and septicemia. Judicious selection and application of any invasive procedure is warranted to minimize undue hazard.

Electrolyte and Fluid Abnormalities

Any combination of acid-base imbalance may occur either acutely or chronically during respiratory failure. Severe alkalemia associated with potassium and chloride losses may occur after assisted ventilation and can precipitate serious cardiovascular and neurological complications.

Fluid retention can occur with prolonged mechanical ventilation in a patient with no evidence of cardiac failure. Pulmonary edema, weight gain, decreased pulmonary compliance, and reduced oxygen transport are common signs. Fluid overload is a common cause of this fluid retention. Mechanically ventilated patients are therefore usually maintained underhydrated. Because of a tendency for sodium retention (hence, fluid retention during mechanical ventilation), administration of intravenous saline solution is kept to a minimum. Humidifiers attached to mechanical ventilators are responsible for adding a considerable amount of water by absorption through the lungs.

Cardiac Arrhythmias

Cardiac arrhythmias are a common complication of respiratory failure. In addition, patients in respiratory failure tend to be older adults who as a group have a greater incidence of arrhythmias secondary to cardiac disease. Electrocardiographic monitoring is therefore essential for all patients requiring ventilatory assistance in addition to patients with overt or suspected heart disease. Both atrial and ventricular tachyarrhythmias are seen in acute respiratory failure. Sinus tachycardia and premature ventricular contractions, however, are particularly common types of arrhythmias associated with respiratory failure. With rapid lowering of arterial PCO_2, ventricular fibrillation or even death may occur.

In the presence of respiratory failure and in the absence of cardiac disease, the management of cardiac arrhythmias lies predominantly in the correction of blood gas abnormalities. Effective supportive management can usually be achieved with pharmaceutical agents. Intravenous injection of lidocaine followed by continuous infusion is useful in managing premature ventricular contractions which may be the precursor of potentially fatal tachyarrhythmias and cardiac arrest. Electrolyte replacement may also be required.

A thorough understanding of the clinical presentation, electrocardiographic diagnosis, and correct management of cardiac arrhythmias is fundamental to the optimization of physical therapy treatments in the ICU. Cardiac arrhythmias resulting from any cause necessarily require ongoing evaluation and therapy.

The physical therapist must be able to treat the patient optimally and safely within the restrictions of any arrhythmia in addition to other medical or surgical conditions. The implications of the arrhythmia on the patient's clinical presentation and on treatment selection and response must be recognized by the therapist and considered in designing the treatment plan.

Thromboembolism

A high incidence of pulmonary thrombosis or embolism exists in patients in acute respiratory failure. Diagnosis and management of pulmonary thromboembolism are difficult problems. Angiography has become the gold standard of diagnosis. Physical therapy has a key role in preventing the development of thromboemboli by promoting frequent changes in position and specific bed exercises, particularly of the lower limbs.

Myocardial Dysfunction

Acute myocardial infarction during the management of acute respiratory failure can occur as in any clinical situation. The probability of heart failure and associated arrhythmias is increased and significantly compounds the problems of the patient in respiratory failure.

Gastrointestinal Dysfunction

Peptic ulcer is commonly associated with chronic airway obstruction. The stress of respiratory failure predisposes the patient to peptic ulceration. Profound hemorrhage may occur and blood replacement is necessitated.

Gastric dilation may occur in patients who are receiving mechanical ventilation. Gastric dilation is best managed by means of a nasogastric tube and intermittent suction. Care must be exercised to avoid hypokalemia and hypochloremia caused by excessive gastric suctioning. Special care must also be taken to avoid fecal impaction, particularly in the paralyzed patient. This risk can be reduced with suitable fluid balance and possibly a frequent turning schedule in conjunction with appropriate trunk and lower limb assisted movements.

Neurological Dysfunction

A close correlation exists between the state of consciousness and the arterial PO_2 and PCO_2. In addition, changes occur in alertness, personality, memory, and orientation with altered blood gases. Motor changes also occur, including generalized or localized weakness, tremors, twitching, myoclonic jerks, gross clonic movements, convulsions, and flaccidity. Neurological complications of respiratory failure must be differentiated from those of nonpulmonary origin. The physical therapist must be aware of the spectrum of neurological complications that can result from respiratory failure and recognize that apparent improvement of neurological signs may reflect improved pulmonary status.

Renal Dysfunction

The development of renal failure greatly compromises the chances of the patient's survival. Renal failure can result from gastrointestinal bleeding, sepsis associated with shock, drug-induced nephrotoxicity, and hypotension. Urinary outputs are maintained with adequate fluid and diuretics, with care not to induce pulmonary edema. Dialysis may need to be instituted if more conservative management fails. If dialysis is anticipated, the physical therapist should review existing treatment goals to establish whether modification is appropriate.

THE DYING PATIENT

Dying and death are traumatic for the patient, family and friends, and health care team. There are phases of dying (Warner, 1978) that can be anticipated when caring for the dying patient:

1. Loss of strength, motion, and reflexes in the legs and then in the arms.

2. Failure of the peripheral circulation and profuse sweating causing body cooling.

3. The dying patient tends to turn toward the light.

4. Decreased sensitivity to touch, deep pressure, and pain tend to remain.

5. Often conscious until expires.

6. May experience pain, acute loneliness, and fear.

7. May increase spiritual needs, particularly at night.

8. An interval of quiescence just prior to death.

Management

The dying patient and his or her family and friends have special needs that must be included in and in fact constitute an integral part of the patient's overall care. In general, the physical comfort and personal hygiene of the patient as well as the quality of the immediate psychosocial environment are paramount concerns. Compassion, understanding, and respect for the patient and the family must be forthcoming from the ICU team. The ability to be attentive and comforting is an invaluable personal quality that needs to be developed to a high degree in the critical care area. The team needs to attend to how the patient, if sufficiently alert, is dealing with the possibility of dying, and take their cues from the patient with respect to the role they need to play. If requested by the patient or family, pastoral care services are summoned, preferably before death is imminent.

If life support systems are being continued, the physical therapist may provide treatment to keep the patient as comfortable as possible. Conservative prophylactic chest care may be provided to reduce the work of breathing. Treatments in general are kept to a minimum in terms of number and duration if death is inevitable. Range of motion exercises help to reduce the discomfort of immobility and facilitate nursing management and the basic care of the patient. Analgesics may be continued. If so, these are prudently timed with treatments if appropriate. In the presence of life supports, the patient's needs may have to be anticipated somewhat more than without life supports as these severely limit communication. The dignity and modesty of the patient continue to be observed even after death has occurred.

The patient who has had life supports removed receives the same level of palliative care as the patient with supports. Weakness and wasting may contribute to the fatigue induced by treatment and by coughing. Facilitated and supported coughing may help reduce the effort required to cough productively.

The use of human touch may be the single most important means of communicating with and providing support to the dying patient who may be unable or disinterested in communicating. Supportive touching and hand holding may be even more important to the patient on life support systems where these may be experienced as a physical barrier between the patient and those around him or her.

SUMMARY

This chapter described the principles and practice of physical therapy for several common categories of conditions seen in the intensive care unit. Categories included are obstructive and restrictive lung diseases, adult respiratory distress syndrome, shock, coronary artery disease, postoperative complications, trauma to the musculoskeletal system, trauma to the central nervous system, and burns. Common complications of respiratory failure and the special needs of the dying patient are also described.

The general goals of critical care are function optimization and prophylaxis. Specific primary goals are defined by the underlying cardiopulmonary pathophysiology. Specific secondary goals are defined by the presence of or the potential for neuromuscular dysfunction.

Physical therapy treatments in critical care areas are typically short, frequent, and should always be efficacious. That is, each treatment should produce some demonstrable positive treatment outcome either immediately or in the longer term, although long-term benefits may be more difficult to evaluate in the short term. The physical therapist also needs to prioritize treatment goals in order that cardiopulmonary function is optimally maintained, perhaps postponing or avoiding acute respiratory failure and mechanical ventilation.

Physical therapy treatments can be optimized by utilization of the monitoring systems available in the intensive care unit. Monitoring systems can be effectively used to:

1. Determine the necessity for, suitability of, and response to a specific intervention.

2. Assess the need for supplemental oxygen before, during, and after treatment if indicated and prescribed.

3. Determine appropriate patient positioning between, during, and after treatments.

4. Help define treatment intensity, duration, and frequency for optimal treatment outcome.

5. Help decide to avoid or discontinue a treatment if a negative objective response is observed.

A thorough knowledge and routine use of monitoring systems for each patient in the intensive care unit cannot be overemphasized in terms of contributing to improved quality of care with less potential risk to the patient.

REFERENCES

Periodicals

Alvarez SE, Peterson M, Lunsford BR: Respiratory treatment of the adult patient with spinal cord injury. *Phys Ther* 1981; 61:1737.

Bake B: Effects of shape changes of the chest wall on distribution of inspired gas. *Am Rev Resp Dis* 1976; 114:1113.

Barach AL: Chronic obstructive lung disease: Postural relief of dyspnea. *Arch Phys Med Rehabil* 1974; 55:494.

Barach AL, Chusid EL, Wood L: Ventilatory effect of decreasing functional residual capacity in pulmonary emphysema. *Ann Allergy* 1967; 25:211.

Bartlett RH, et al: Respiratory maneuvers to prevent postoperative pulmonary complication: A critical review. *JAMA* 1973; 224:1017.

Bateman JR, Newman SP, Daunt KM, et al: Regional lung clearance of excessive bronchial secretions during chest physiotherapy in patients with stable chronic airway obstruction. *Lancet* 1979; 1:294.

Bethune D: Neurophysiological facilitation of respiration in the unconscious adult patient. *Physiother Can* 1975; 27:241.

Bindslev L, Hedenstierna G, Santesson J: Ventilation-perfusion distribution during inhalation anaesthesia: Effects of spontaneous breathing, mechanical ventilation and positive end-expiratory pressure, *Acta Anaesthesiol Scand* 1981; 25:360.

Bjore D: Postmyocardial infarction: A program of graduated exercises. *J Can Physiother Assoc* 1972; 24:22.

Boyd JM: A new program for thoracotomy patients. *Physiother Can* 1976; 28:274.

Byrd RB, Bruns JR: Cough dynamics in the postthoracotomy state. *Chest* 1975; 67:654.

Casciari RJ, Fairshter RD, Morrison JT, et al: Effects of breathing retraining in patients with chronic obstructive pulmonary disease. *Chest* 1981; 79:393.

Cherniack RM, Hakimpour K: The rational use of oxygen in respiratory insufficiency. *JAMA* 1967; 199:178.

Cheshire DJE: Respiratory management in acute traumatic tetraplegia. *Paraplegia* 1964; 1:252.

Clauss RH, Scalabrini BY, Ray JF, et al: Effects of changing body position upon improved ventilation-perfusion relationships. *Circulation* 1968; 37(*Suppl* 2):214.

Connors AF, Hammon WE, Martin RJ, et al: Chest physical therapy: The immediate effect on oxygenation in acutely ill patients. *Chest* 1980; 78:559.

Craven JL, Evans GA, Davenport PJ, et al: The evaluation of the incentive spirometer in the management of postoperative pulmonary complications. *Br J Surg* 1974; 61:793.

Dalrymple D: Setting up for thoracic drainage. *Nursing* 1984; 84:12.

Didier EP: Some effects of anesthetics and the anesthetized state on the respiratory system. *Respiratory Care* 1984; 29:463.

Douglas WW, et al: Improved oxygenation in patients with acute respiratory failure: The prone position. *Am Rev Resp Dis* 1977; 115:559.

Etsen B, Proger S: Operative risk in patients with coronary heart disease. *JAMA* 1955; 159:845.

Fell T, Cheney FW: Prevention of hypoxia during endotracheal suction. *Ann Surg* 1971; 174:24.

Froeb HF: On relief of bronchospasm and the induction of alveolar ventilation. A comparative study of nebulized bronchodilators by deep breathing and intermittent positive pressure. *Dis Chest* 1960; 38:483.

Gallagher TJ, Civetta JM: Goal directed therapy of acute respiratory failure. *Anesth Analg* 1980; 59:831.

Gayrard R, Becker M, Bergofsky EH: The effects of abdominal weights on diaphragmatic position and excursion in man. *Clin Sci* 1968; 35:589.

Gibson GJ, et al: Pulmonary mechanics in patients with respiratory muscle weakness. *Am Rev Resp Dis* 1977; 115:389.

Grabenkort WR: A cardiopulmonary physiologic profile for use with the Swan-Ganz catheter. *Resident and Staff Physician* 1983; 29:80.

Graham WGB, Bradley DA: Efficacy of chest physiotherapy and intermittent positive-pressure breathing in the resolution of pneumonia. *N Engl J Med* 1978; 299:624.

Greenberg SD: The lungs and their response to disease. *Resident and Staff Physician* 1983; 29:28.

Gregory GA, et al: Treatment of the idiopathic respiratory distress syndrome with continuous positive airway pressure. *N Engl J Med* 1971; 284:1333.

Grimby G: Aspects of lung expansion in pulmonary physiotherapy. *Am Rev Resp Dis* 1974; 110(Suppl 1):149.

Gross D, King M: High frequency chest wall compression: A new noninvasive method of chest physiotherapy for mucociliary clearance. *Physiother Can* 1984; 36:137.

Haas F, et al: Time-related posturally induced changes in pulmonary function in spinal cord injured man (abstract). *Am Rev Resp Dis* 1978; 117:344.

Hedenstierna G, et al: Regional differences in lung function during anaesthesia and intensive care: Clinical implications. *Acta Anaesthesiol Scand* 1982; 26:429.

Hedstrand U, et al: Effect of respiratory physiotherapy on arterial oxygen tension. *Acta Anaesthesiol Scand* 1978; 22:349.

Hietpas BG, Roth RD, Jensen WM: Huff coughing and airway patency. *Respiratory Care* 1979; 24:710.

Holody B, Goldberg HS: The effect of mechanical vibration physiotherapy on arterial oxygenation in acutely ill patients with atelectasis or pneumonia. *Am Rev Resp Dis* 1981; 124:372.

Holten K: Training effect in patients with severe ventilatory failure. *Scand J Resp Dis* 1972; 53:65.

Hoskins TA, Habasevich RA: Cardiac rehabilitation. An overview. *Phys Ther* 1978; 58:1183.

Howell S, Hill JD: Acute respiratory care in the open heart surgery patient. *Phys Ther* 1972; 52:253.

Huszczuk A, Pokorski M, Casaco A: Respiratory responses following lifting the legs in normal man. *Am J Med Sci* 1982; 283:64.

Jardin F, et al: Influence of positive end-expiratory pressure on left ventricular performance. *N Eng J Med* 1981; 304:387.

Kigin CM: Chest physical therapy for the postoperative or traumatic injury patient. *Phys Ther* 1981; 61:1724.

Kottke FJ: The effects of limitation of activity upon the human body. *JAMA* 1966; 196:825.

Kumar A, et al: Pulmonary barotrauma during mechanical ventilation. *Crit Care Med* 1973; 1:181.

Lambert RL, Willauer G, Dasch FW: Postoperative status of dependent lung. *J Thorac Cardiovasc Surg* 1955; 30:713.

Leblanc P, Ruff F, Milic-Emili J: Effects of age and body position on airway closure in man. *J Appl Physiol* 1970; 38:448.

Light KE: Review of the aged respiratory system. *Physical and Occupational Therapy in Geriatrics* 1983; 3:4.

Lyager S: Ventilation/perfusion ratio during intermittent positive pressure ventilation: Importance of no-flow interval during the insufflation. *Acta Anesthesiol Scand* 1970; 14:211.

Mackenzie CF, Shin B: Evaluation of respiratory physical therapy. *N Engl J Med* 1979; 301:665.

Mackenzie CF, Shin B, Hadi F, et al: Changes in total lung/thorax compliance following chest physiotherapy. *Anesth Analg* 1980; 59:207.

Mackenzie CF, Shin B, McAslan TC: Chest physiotherapy: The effect on arterial oxygenation. *Anesth Analg* 1978; 57:28.

Macklem PT, Roussos CS: Respiratory muscle fatigue: A cause of respiratory failure. *Clin Sci Molec Med* 1977; 53:419.

Marini JJ: Postoperative atelectasis: Pathophysiology, clinical importance and principles of management. *Respiratory Care* 1984; 29:516.

May DB, Munt PW: Physiologic effects of chest percussion and postural drainage in patients with stable chronic bronchitis. *Chest* 1979; 75:29.

McAslan MT, Cowley RA: The preventive use of PEEP in major trauma. *Am Surg* 1979; 45:159.

Meyers JR, et al: Changes in functional residual capacity of the lungs after operation. *Arch Surg* 1975; 110:576.

Milic-Emili J: Recent advances in clinical assessment of control of breathing. *Lung* 1982; 160:1.

Mithoefer JC, Bossman OG, Thibeault DW, et al: The clinical assessment of alveolar ventilation. *Am Rev Respir Dis* 1968; 98:868.

Mueller RE, Petty TL, Filley GF: Ventilation and arterial blood gas changes induced by pursed lips breathing. *J Appl Physiol* 1971; 28:784.

Murray A: Cardiac survival and rehabilitation. *Physiotherapy* 1973; 59:383.

Nunn JF, et al: Hypoxaemia and atelectasis produced by forced expiration. *Br J Anaesthesiol* 1965; 37:3.

Oldenburg FA, Dolovich MB, Montgomery JM, et al: Effects of postural drainage, exercise, and cough on mucus clearance in chronic bronchitis. *Am Rev Resp Dis* 1979; 120:739.

Pardee NE, Winterbauer JD, Allen JD: Bedside evaluation of respiratory distress. *Chest* 1984; 85:203.

Pardy RL, Leith DE: Ventilatory muscle training. *Respiratory Care* 1984; 29:298.

Piehl MA, Brown RD: Use of extreme position changes in acute respiratory failure. *Crit Care Med* 1976; 4:13.

Pierson DJ, Lakshminarayan S: Postoperative ventilatory management. *Respiratory Care* 1984; 29:603.

Pryor JA, Webber BA: An evaluation of the forced expiration technique as an adjunct to postural drainage. *Physiotherapy* 1979; 65:304.

Ray JF, III, et al: Immobility, hypoxemia, and pulmonary arteriovenous shunting. *Arch Surg* 1974; 109:537.

Rochester DF, Aurora NS: Respiratory muscle failure. *Med Clin North Am* 1983; 67:573.

Rochester DF, Esau SA: Malnutrition and the respiratory system. *Chest* 1984; 85:411.

Schutz H, Taylor FA: Intracranial pressure and cerebral blood flow monitoring in head injuries. *Can Med Assoc J* 1977; 116:609.

Shearer MO, Banks JM, Silva G, et al: Lung ventilation during diaphragmatic breathing. *Phys Ther* 1972; 52:139.

Smoot EC: Fluid management of the surgical patient. *Resident and Staff Physician* 1983; 29:76.

Stremel RW, et al: Cardiorespiratory deconditioning with static and dynamic leg exercise during bed rest. *J Appl Physiol* 1976; 41:905.

Sutton PP, et al: Assessment of the forced expiration technique, postural drainage, and directed coughing in chest physiotherapy. *Eur J Resp Dis* 1983; 64:62.

Svanberg L: Influence of posture on the lung volumes, ventilation, and circulation in normals. *Scand J Clin Lab Invest* 1957; 25(*Suppl*):7.

Turino GM, Golding RM, Hememann HO: Water, electrolytes, and acid base relationships in chronic cor pulmonale. *Prog Cardiovasc Dis* 1970; 12:467.

Tyler ML: The respiratory effects of body position and immobilization. *Respiratory Care* 1984; 29:472.

Vraciu JK, Vraciu RA: Effectiveness of breathing exercises in preventing pulmonary complications following open heart surgery. *Phys Ther* 1977; 57:1367.

Webber BA: Current trends in the treatment of asthma. *Physiotherapy* 1973; 59:388.

West JB: Ventilation perfusion relationships. *Am Rev Resp Dis* 1977; 116:919.

Wolff RK, Dolovich MB, Obminski G, et al: Effects of exercise and eucapnic hyperventilation on bronchial clearance in man. *J Appl Physiol* 1977; 43:46.

Wright PC: Fundamentals of acute burn care and physical therapy management. *Phys Ther* 1984; 64:1217.

Zadai CC: Physical therapy for the acutely ill medical patient. *Phys Ther* 1981; 61:1746.

Zikria BA, Spencer JL, Kinney JM, et al: Alterations in ventilatory function and breathing patterns following surgical trauma. *Ann Surg* 1974; 179:1.

Books

Gaskell DV, Webber BA: *The Brompton Hospital Guide to Chest Physiotherapy*, ed 4. London, Blackwell Scientific Publications, 1981.

Haas A, et al: *Pulmonary Therapy and Rehabilitation: Principles and Practice*. Baltimore, Williams & Wilkins Co, 1979.

Mackenzie CF, et al: *Chest Physiotherapy in the Intensive Care Unit*. Baltimore, Williams & Wilkins Co, 1981.

Petty TL: *Intensive and Rehabilitative Respiratory Care*, ed 3. Philadelphia, Lea & Febiger, 1982.

Shoemaker WC (ed): *Critical Care: State of the Art*. Fullerton, California, Society of Critical Care Medicine, 1984.

Miscellaneous

Cabot R, Riley E: A program of resistive breathing for quadriplegics. Paper presentation, Annual Congress of the Professional Corporation of Physiotherapists of Quebec. Translation by S. Hornstein, 1980.

Hornstein S: Ventilatory muscle training. A clinical guide for physiotherapists. Unpublished manual, Spinal Cord Injury Unit, Shaughnessy Hospital, Vancouver, BC, 1984.

Hornstein S, Ledsome J, Dollfuss RE: Respiratory muscle training in kyphoscoliosis. Paper presentation, Canadian Lung Association, Edmonton, Alberta, 1984.

Riley E: Resistive breathing. Paper presentation, Annual Congress of the American Academy of Physical Medicine and Rehabilitation, 1978.

18

Cardiovascular and Thoracic Surgery

Maureen Fogel Perlstein, M.P.H., P.T., C.R.T.T.

Mary Mathews, B.S., R.N., C.C.R.N., R.R.T.

The chest physical therapist is a member of an extensive team of health care professionals. He should bear in mind the collective goal of this team, which is to help the patient attain the best possible state of health. This means a complete recovery from illness for most patients or, in the case of chronic illness, teaching the patient to live with his disease. Patient education is the means by which this goal can be attained. The clinical practice of chest physical therapy involves much teaching in addition to the application of technical skills. For example, therapists teach patients breathing exercises, effective coughing, relaxation techniques, posture correction, basic anatomy and simple pathophysiology. Therapists also teach skills to other health professionals and to patients' families. Although educational psychology is not the topic of this book, a few points about teaching and the therapist-patient relationship are appropriate.

Patients are exposed to a hospital environment presenting unfamiliar sights and sounds which are often frightening and painful. The therapist's clinical approach must be one not only of technical skill, but also of consideration for the patient's needs. A calm and quiet mood should be maintained to facilitate the patient's ability to relax and concentrate while information and instructions are explained to him. An unprepared therapist who repeatedly interrupts the treatment to look up information or gather equipment will lose both the patient's attention and confidence.

Learning may be defined as "any relatively permanent change in behavior which occurs as a result of experience or practice." Effective communication is the key to the "experience or practice" necessary for learning. Communication relies on sensory cues which include visual cues to lead movement, contact with the patient's skin for tactile stimulus, and appropriately timed verbal commands to coordinate the effort.

Tone of voice has a great influence on the quality of a patient's response. Soft tones should be used during breathing exercises to promote relaxation and enable the patient to turn his attention inward toward his pattern of breathing. Verbal instructions are given in a moderate tone of voice and are accompanied by demonstration of the desired exercise. Louder, sharp commands encourage quick, strong responses such as coughing.

The greatest impairments to learning in a therapy session are the patient's pain, fatigue and anxiety. Treatment sessions should be coordinated with pain medication schedules. Sessions should be kept brief enough to avoid overly fatiguing the patient. Patients' anxieties stem mainly from a lack of information about what will happen to them during therapy sessions. For example, a patient who will undergo a sternotomy for coronary artery bypass surgery must receive preoperative instruction about proper coughing technique and should be reassured that this coughing effort, while painful, should not damage the incision.

One brief note on patient cooperation is offered here. Patients are, for the most part, passive recipients of hospital services. They are targets for needles, receptacles for pills and the subjects of endless diagnostic tests. This is in great contrast to their role in chest physical therapy sessions, where patients (unless they are comatose) take an active part in treatment. Once patients understand that they are able to do something to help themselves, they will be more motivated to cooperate with the therapist.

The purpose of this section is to pull together knowledge of anatomy and pathophysiology with the specific skills of chest physical therapy and to apply them in a practical way. There are two ways of approaching this task. One is by listing disease entities and their treatments in separate categories. This would seem to be a convenient form of organization. As therapists, however, we are treating individual people, not diseases. In treating patients, one soon finds that there are few hard and fast rules which can be universally applied. Therefore, in addition to general guidelines, a second approach geared toward problem solving will be adopted to study clinical examples (see Chapter 33).

GENERAL GUIDELINES FOR THORACIC SURGERY PATIENTS

Patients undergoing extensive heart or lung surgery commonly experience respiratory complications. Atelectasis and retained secretions in the lung frequently develop after the surgery. The causes of pulmonary pathology in patients undergoing open heart surgery have been summarized in Table 18–1. These pre- and postoperative factors apply to patients who have had surgery on lung parenchyma, pleural cavity and chest wall.

The value of a comprehensive program of acute respiratory care to prevent and treat these complications has been firmly established. Although the value of intermittent positive pressure breathing remains a controversial issue, IPPB along with modalities of oxygenation, humidification and chest physical therapy comprises the primary treatment for these patients.

A complete discussion of thoracic surgical procedures is beyond the scope of this book but may be found in general surgical texts. A description of coronary artery bypass surgery and the chest physical therapist's treatment program will be presented. This will serve as a model which may be adapted by the therapist in his approach to other patients undergoing various other thoracic surgical procedures.

CARDIAC SURGERY

Coronary artery disease is one of the major causes of death in Americans today. Coronary atherosclerosis is a progressive disease process caused by deposits of plaques in the intima of the vessels. The plaque contains cholesterol lipoid material and lipophages. The left anterior descending coronary artery is most frequently involved, followed by the following arteries: right coronary, circumflex, left main and right posterior descending arteries. One or more of these arteries may be occluded, to varying degrees, resulting in tissue hypoxia, which leads to angina and myocardial infarction.

Percutaneous transluminal coronary angioplasty (PTCA) is an invasive nonsurgical approach to open narrowed coronary arteries. PTCA is safe and effective in the treatment of selected patients with

TABLE 18–1.

Causes of Pulmonary Pathology in the Patient Undergoing
Open Heart Surgery*

I. Preoperative factors.
   A. Pulmonary vascular congestion.
   B. Previous thoracic surgery.
   C. Premorbid activities.
   D. Underlying pulmonary disease such as emphysema.
   E. Prior exposure to severe air pollution.
   F. Cigarette smoking.
   G. Preoperative pulmonary trauma.
II. Factors during extracorporeal circulation.
   A. Pulmonary hypoxia.
      1. The lungs (pulmonary arteries) are not perfused normally during bypass.
      2. Moderately desaturated blood may be perfusing the bronchial arteries.
   B. Pulmonary collapse during extracorporeal circulation.
   C. Direct trauma from retraction and manipulation of the lungs.
   D. Microemboli in the pulmonary vasculature.
      1. Transfused blood contains minute fat emboli and particulate matter.
      2. Coronary suction during open heart surgery produces particulate matter of platelet, fibrous, and red cell aggregates.
      3. Coronary suction blood includes loose matter and debris from the wound.
      4. Extracorporeal circulation causes hemolysis.
   E. Phrenic nerve injury.
   F. Damage to the mucous membrane of the lung.
      1. Poor humidification of anesthetic gases.
      2. Allergic reactive inflammation to anesthetic gases.
      3. Chemical toxicity from anesthetic gases.
   G. Drying of the pleura from exposure.
III. Postoperative factors.
   A. Atelectasis.
      1. Narcotics for pain suppress the respiratory center.
      2. Incisional pain causes shallow breathing.
      3. Inactivity can cause shallow breathing.
      4. Endotracheal tube may be mistakenly placed in the right main-stem bronchus.
   B. Inability to clear secretions by coughing.
      1. Incisional pain.
      2. Weakness.
      3. Irritated throat from intubation.
      4. Presence of nasogastric tube.
   C. Surgical.
      1. Hemothorax.
      2. Pneumothorax.
   D. Second operation for bleeding.

*Adapted from Howard S, Hill J: Acute respiratory care in the open heart surgery patient. *Phys Ther* 1972; 52:254.

isolated coronary artery stenosis of the left anterior descending artery or right coronary artery. The technique employs a guiding catheter through which a dilation catheter is advanced which enters the diseased branch of the arterial system. The dilation catheter then traverses the stenotic segment under pressure inflation, leading to a circumferential compression of the plaque, resulting in the enlargement of the vessel lumen. A short anginal history increases the expectation of a successful angioplasty. A small percentage of angioplasty patients has abrupt reclosure of the dilated segment, requiring emergency coronary artery bypass graft; therefore, coronary artery surgery standby is mandatory.

The purpose of coronary artery bypass surgery is just to restore blood flow to the myocardium. Preoperative diagnostic tests include cardiac catherization, echocardiogram, electrocardiogram, and chest x-ray. Pulmonary function testing is of value in predicting pulmonary complications. Once identified, the high-risk patients may have surgery postponed in order to improve their pulmonary status. Surgical approach may be by mediastinum or thoracic incisions. Preoperative teaching should include coughing with splinting, breathing techniques including diaphragmatic breathing and huffing techniques.

A saphenous vein graft or internal mammary artery is usually used for an autogenous graft. Extracorporeal circulation through the bypass pump oxygenates and filters the blood during surgery. When pump runs are greater than two hours, incidence of ARDS rises. Hypothermia through cardioplegia may also be used to reduce contractility and oxygen demands of the myocardium. The cold injury to the phrenic nerve from the cardioplegia in the pericardium could probably be the cause of commonly found left lower lobe atelectasis in postoperative coronary artery bypass graft patients.

After the graft has been completed, direct current is used to defibrillate the heart. Once normal contractility is restored, extracorporeal circulation is removed. In cases of cardiogenic shock when it is impossible to remove the patient from the bypass pump, an intra-aortic balloon or left heart bypass may provide an artificial means of supporting the circulation. The intra-aortic balloon pump may be inserted transthoracic or through the femoral artery. If insertion is through the femoral artery, care must be taken to maintain the leg in an extended position so that the pressure controls inflating and deflating the balloon are not interrupted.

Following surgery, which may take up to two to four hours, the patient is brought to the surgical intensive care unit. An endotracheal tube remains in place and the patient is mechanically ventilated for approximately 24 hours. Due to the popularity of narcotic anesthesia, ventilatory support is necessary until the narcotic effect of anesthesia wears off. Ventilator support, which gives assistance to the heart as well as lungs, is utilized and, by so doing the work of breathing, reduces tissue oxygen demand and the level of required cardiac output. Vital signs including pulmonary artery pressures and central venous pressures are closely monitored. Chest tubes (pleural or mediastinal) are usually removed on the second postoperative day. Patients remain in the intensive care area, after which they are transferred to a cardiovascular surgical floor (Zone II).

Cardiac surgical patients have multiple causes for increased alveolar collapse and shunting, such as increase in capillary permeability or an increased pulmonary capillary pressure due to left ventricular failure or of infusion of inappropriately large amounts of fluid, decrease in colloid osmotic pressure with hemodilution and also with fall in lung volume due to decrease in lung compliance, or alteration in chest wall mechanics. Increase in the intestinal fluid also decreases the lung compliance. Immobilization in supine position decreases end expiratory volume by the diaphragm being pushed up. The higher the diaphragm, the higher the chance of lower lobe collapse.

PREOPERATIVE CHEST PHYSICAL THERAPY

Preoperative treatment consists of patient evaluation (see Chapter 6) and patient education. Many studies have been made to support the practice of preoperative patient education to minimize the incidence of postoperative pulmonary complications. Such sessions provide an excellent opportunity to develop rapport between the patient and therapist.

For the first one or two postoperative days, the patient receives small doses of morphine sulphate for pain relief and feels drowsy. Patients who have had preoperative instructions will be able to perform previously learned exercises with little difficulty. During preoperative evaluation, individual instruction should include a general discussion of the surgery and location of the incision. The patient should also be told that when he/she awakes after surgery, he/she will discover a tube in his/her throat which is helping the breathing function. He should understand that he will be unable to speak and should not try to speak while intubated, and that his voice will return when the tube is removed the day after surgery. The patients who are uninformed of this procedure could be awakened to a frightening and confusing experience.

The therapist should next explain that following open heart surgery, the patient may have a small amount of congestion in the lungs. Procedures of chest percussion and vibrations are explained and demonstrated. Patients with preexisting lung disease should receive chest physical therapy before surgery. Pulmonary function screening will be helpful for prescribing the type of breathing exercises for the patients. All patients should learn and practice breathing exercises, coughing with splinting, and general arm and leg exercises. Patients should be encouraged to ask questions during the teaching session.

Adaptation of Patients Undergoing Open Heart Surgery: Postural Drainage

Positions are modified to minimize stress on the cardiovascular system and sternotomy or thoracic incisions. Bed-flat position could be used until the chest tube is discontinued and the patient is stabilized. Trendelenburg positions could be used after removal of the chest tube for postural drainage of the lower lobes and when the patient is able to tolerate Trendelenburg. Log-rolling technique is used to turn patients to a side-lung position with pillows to support the uppermost leg and sternal incisions. When these patients are turned, meticulous care must be taken to ensure integrity of IVS Swan Ganz catheters, arterial lines, or intra-aortic balloon pumps.

Chest Percussion and Vibration

These techniques are applied posterolaterally on the thorax using a sidelying postural drainage position with rhythmic gentle clapping with cupped hands for three to five minutes per area. Chest physical therapy sessions should be coordinated with the pain medication schedule to increase the tolerance to treatment. It should also be done followed by respiratory care treatments such as ultrasonic nebulizer or bronchodilators when patients are receiving them in conjunction with chest PT. ECG monitors should be carefully watched for changes in rhythm. Treatment should be stopped if heart rate increases more than 10% to 20% above the resting level. If the patient's condition is stable, ectopic beats are not a contraindication for chest PT. However, if the number of ectopic beats increases significantly or a new foci appears, treatment should be stopped immediately.

Breathing Exercises

The interacting effect of increase of lung fluid, reduction of lung volume, immobility and failure to cough allow progressive collapse of alveoli over a few postoperative days. These plus probable cold injury to the phrenic nerve are the commonly found causes of atelectasis in postoperative open heart patients. Added risk of patients with degenerative diseases, patients who had valve replacement with elevated left heart filling pressures have stiffer lungs and therefore are more prone to microatelectasis. For these patients, lateral costal breathing exercises are stressed to expand the atelectatic areas. Inspiratory manuevers should be emphasized. Incentive spirometers should be used.

Cough

Cough usually is performed most effectively with the patients sitting or high sidelying splinting the incision with a pillow. Huff technique is effective on patients with low cough effort.

Arm and Leg Exercises

Passive range of motion exercises that are done on the first day following surgery are progressed to active assistive on the second and third day. Early ambulation is advisable as in any other surgeries. But the guidelines may vary from hospitals and surgeons. By the third postoperative day, most arm and leg exercises are done actively. These include:

1. Hand grasping, wrist flexion and extension, forearm flexion and extension, pronation and supination.

2. Shoulder shrugging motions.

3. Shoulder rotation: with the arms held extended at the side of the body, rotate from a neutral position to internal rotation and back.

4. Bilateral shoulder flexion: raising the arms overhead reinforces deep breathing patterns and prevents the frozen shoulder syndrome. Bilateral rather than unilateral movements are used to maintain incisional stability. External rotation and abduction are contraindicated with a sternotomy and should be avoided for 6–8 weeks.

5. Ankle: flexion and extension, circular motions.

6. Mass flexion and extension of the hip and knee are done to patient tolerance. Hip abduction and rotation may be done with both lower extremities if an intra-aortic balloon is not present. Patients *must* be reminded not to cross their legs because of the danger of developing deep vein thrombosis.

7. When the chest tubes are removed on about the second postoperative day, patients are permitted to dangle their legs at the bedside and then sit in a chair. Ambulation usually begins on the second or third day. These guidelines may vary among hospitals and among surgeons within the same hospital.

Treatment Schedule

As previously mentioned, treatments are recommended after pain medication and also preferably after aerosol treatment. A small number of patients may develop postpump psychosis from sleep deprivation and general fatigue. Also, patients are awakened day and night for a variety of diagnostic and therapeutic procedures in the intensive care area. Therefore, whenever possible, naps should not be interrupted for treatments. Therapists must keep in mind the contribution that sleep deprivation may make to postperfusion psychosis and to a patient's general fatigue.

Sveinsson has suggested factors that contribute to postperfusion psychosis:

1. A history of preoperative psychiatric illness.

2. Advanced age.

3. Severity of preoperative and postoperative illness.

4. Length of time spent in the intensive care unit with its monotony and absence of time orientation.

5. Sleep deprivation—the author's study found that sleep deprivation superimposed on the first four factors was the common precipitating factor in his subjects.

ANEURYSM AND VALVE DISEASES

Pre- and postoperative regimens for patients undergoing coronary artery bypass sugery are also followed for patients undergoing aneurysm repair and valve repair or replacement.

An aneurysm is an outpouching of an artery, vein, or cardiac chamber. Ventricular aneurysms are usually the result of dilatation of the myocardium weakened by infarction. The left ventricle is most commonly involved. Aneurysms of the thoracic aorta occur due to a variety of causes including atherosclerosis, syphilis, trauma, and congenital defect. The common surgical approach for resection of these aneurysms is by median sternotomy. These patients must remain at rest prior to surgery to prevent a potentially fatal rupture. Breathing exercises may be taught but coughing should be avoided preoperatively. The postoperative physical therapy management is the same as that for coronary artery bypass.

Valve Repair and Replacement

Diseases of the aortic, mitral, and tricuspid valves are usually the result of rheumatic fever. The acute process causing edema, inflammation, and scarring may result in either valvular stenosis or insufficiency. Bacterial endocarditis, syphilis, and trauma are other causes of valvular disease. Stenosis of the pulmonary valve is usually associated with other congenital heart defects such as transposition of the great vessels or tetralogy of Fallot.

Diseased valves may be repaired or replaced with various prosthetic devices. Median sternotomy is again used for valve replacement procedures with maintenance of extracorporeal circulation. Mitral valve stenosis may be treated by closed mitral commissurotomy. In this procedure, adherent cusps of the stenosed valve are separated. A left thoracotomy incision is used. Postoperative chest PT must emphasize range of motion exercises with special attention to the surgical side to prevent development of a frozen shoulder. Some patients undergoing surgery to correct rheumatic valvular disease have a special psychological problem. Many have been considered invalids from childhood by concerned but overly protective parents. These patients are especially anxious and resist exercises which they fear may place too great a strain on their heart. Extra patience and encouragement are necessary under these circumstances.

Thoracic Surgery

The number of operations involving lung parenchyma has increased in recent years due to the greater incidence of bronchogenic carcinoma. Cigarette smoking, the major cause of bronchogenic carcinoma, appears to be on the rise among young people. Resection of lung tissue is also used to treat tuberculosis, bronchiectasis, benign tumors, and fungal infections.

The procedures are named for the extent of lung tissue removed. Wedge resections are performed on small localized lesions. Segmentectomy is the excision of a bronchopulmonary segment. Lobectomy, the removal of a lobe, is indicated for large peripheral lesions not involving the lobar bronchi. Sleeve resection involves removal of the lobe and part of the mainstem bronchus. Then, as the name implies, the lower lobe is pulled up as with a "sleeve" and anastomosed to the proximal bronchus. Pneumonectomy, the removal of an entire lung, is indicated for lesions that originate in the mainstem and lobar bronchi.

A standard posterolateral thoracotomy incision is used to enter the chest. With the patient in a lateral decubitus position, the uppermost arm (on the involved side) is fully flexed anteriorly. The incision is made through an intercostal space corresponding to the location of the lesion to be excised. The incision divides muscle fibers of latissimus dorsi, serratus anterior, external and internal intercostals laterally, and trapezius and rhomboid muscles posteriorly. Chest tubes are placed at the conclusion of the procedure to evacuate accumulated fluid and air from the pleural space. In this manner, the pneumothorax created by entering the pleural space is resolved, and the remaining atelectatic lung tissue is reinflated.

Postoperative complaints of pain are both musculoskeletal and pleural in origin. The large number of muscles incised combined with the operative position contribute to the patient's complaints of severe shoulder soreness. Deep breathing and coughing are exceptionally painful following surgery. Therefore, treatments must be coordinated with pain medication schedules to be beneficial.

Underwater Chest Tube Drainage

Chest tube drainage is used to restore normal function to the chest. Normally, the thoracic cavity is a closed structure, but the trachea and esophagus are open to the atmosphere. Air enters and leaves the lungs through the trachea and bronchi. Surrounding the lungs are the pleura. The pulmonary pleura directly covers the lung surface. There is a potential space between the pulmonary and parietal pleura. The pressure in the pleural space is negative. This force is what keeps the lungs inflated. Air will flow from greater pressure to lesser pressure. During inspiration, as greater negative pressure is generated by the diaphragm, air flows into the lungs. At the end of inspiration when pressures are higher in the lungs, passive exhalation takes place.

Underwater chest tube drainage is used when the negative pressure in the pleural space has been altered. One example of this is following thoracotomy incision for removal of a lung segment (i.e., right middle lobe segmentectomy). The incision has opened the pleural space, and consequently, positive pressure will be present in the pleural space. This will allow the lung to collapse (pneumothorax). In order to resolve the pneumothorax, a chest tube will be placed to recreate the negative pressure in the pleural space. Following thoracic surgery, usually two chest tubes are placed. One is at the apex of the lung to drain air out (as air rises). The second tube is placed at the base of the lung to drain serous fluid (blood collecting secondary to the surgical procedure) since fluid will be subject to gravity and go to the bases of the lungs. When doing chest PT with a patient with chest tubes, the therapist should watch for any air bubbling through the tubes. This will note if there is an air leak. Initially, there will be some bubbling. But later, as it seals off, there will be less. If there seems to be an increase in bubbling, the service should be notified. There are many types of drainage systems currently available. Each practitioner should learn the particular systems in his hospital.

There is no problem in having the patient lie on his chest tubes. Patients of course do not *choose* to lie on the chest tube/incision. Consequently, they only will choose to lie on the unoperative side. They will thus develop atelectasis on the "good" lung; frequently, the surgical side will be clear of secretions as the patient is doing frequent drainage of the surgical lung. It is important to insist the patient turn to both sides for positioning and chest PT and to emphasize lying on the side opposite the incision.

Preoperative Chest Physical Therapy

Preoperative treatment includes patient evaluation and patient education. These procedures have been discussed earlier in this chapter.

Postoperative Treatment

Chest physical therapy following lung surgery closely follows that for coronary surgery, with certain modifications:

1. Postural drainage positions must be modified to allow for chest drainage tubes.

2. Chest percussion and vibration are performed in conjunction with postural drainage to remove retained secretions. The therapist

may use one hand to brace the incision while percussing with the other hand.

3. Breathing exercises should emphasize expansion of remaining lung tissue to fill the space left by removed lung tissue. In the case of pneumonectomy, fluid and air fill this space. Diaphragmatic, unilateral, and apical breathing exercises should be included on the remaining lung. Bilateral chest movement will be used to maintain chest mobility.

4. Coughing should be performed with the incision well supported by a pillow hugged closely about the axilla. Huffing or a series of progressively larger coughs may be tolerated better and therefore is more effective for some patients.

5. In addition to the usual arm and leg exercises, special consideration must be given to the upper extremity *on* the thoracotomy side. Patients tend to hold this arm still and splint it from pain. Unless range of motion exercises are repeated frequently, a frozen shoulder syndrome may result. Diagonal patterns used in PNF have been found to be an excellent method of range of motion exercise.

The lifting pattern is especially helpful in regaining the full range of motion on the involved side. Other suggested upper extremity exercises include:

1. Grasp a towel in both hands, raise it overhead, and return. The patient should inhale deeply as he reaches up and exhale as he lowers his arms. This exercise may be done in semireclining, sitting, or standing positions. Eventually the towel may be placed behind the head.

2. Use a towel to dry the back, using both hands alternatively in the uppermost position.

3. Use a towel or strap to emphasize unilateral and bilateral costal expansion.

4. Do push-ups against the wall. (Avoid breath holding.)

5. Perform functional tasks such as brushing hair, dressing, and reaching for objects.

6. Sit in a chair on the first or second day after surgery. Ambulation is begun as soon as possible, according to physician's order. If chest tubes remain in place due to a persistent air leak, the physician will usually want the patient to continue walking short distances. The

tubes should never be clamped; instead the pleurovac or other portable drainage system should simply be carried along.

Careful observation and palpation for subcutaneous emphysema should be done prior to percussion or vibration.

Vascular Surgery

Arterial and venous surgeries could be included in vascular surgery. Arterial surgeries include endarterectomies or carotid aneurysm repairs (abdominal, thoracic), dacron grafts like iliofemoral, femoral to femoral, or femoral-popliteal bypass grafts. Venous surgeries include caval ligations and institution of caval filtering devices.

RISK FACTORS IN VASCULAR SURGERY

Smoking

Tracheobronchial ciliary action is diminished by smoking; subsequently, clearance of secretions is diminished. Small airway clearance function is impaired which leads to obstructive problems and airway closure.

Obesity

Obesity decreases the lung volume which leads to hypoxemia. Lung volume is further decreased in supine position. Thoracic compliance is also decreased and work of breathing is increased.

Advanced Age

Age is associated with fall in vital capacity and diffusing capacity, and also in end expiration, the volume in basilar portions of the lungs of smokers and elderly individuals is lower than the critical closing volume.

Site of Operation

Vital capacity is decreased 70% after upper abdominal incisions and 50% after lower abdominal incisions. Functional residual capacity is also decreased. Decreased vital capacity may be the result of splinting to avoid pain.

Malnutrition

Malnutrition results in muscle wasting which is aggravated in postoperative days when ventilatory requirements and work of breathing is increased. Preexisting lung disease increases the risk of complications with ventilation and perfusion.

Chest Physical Therapy Treatment

Chest PT could be initiated preoperatively in patients who have a history of pulmonary disease. All evaluation should be followed postoperatively with chest PT techniques to prevent pulmonary complications.

PREOPERATIVE EVALUATION AND TREATMENT

Regardless of the surgical procedure, incision of the chest wall or abdomen will cause respiratory embarrassment. The vital capacity of patients undergoing thoracic or upper abdominal surgery has been seen to decrease 50%–75% of normal during the first 24 hours after surgery. It may take a week to 10 days or more before the normal vital capacity returns. Consequently, in high-risk patients—the elderly, the very young, smokers, the obese, those with abdominal or thoracic surgeries, those with preexisting lung disease—preop evaluation and treatment as well as postoperative therapy is extremely important to prevent respiratory complications.

The goals of chest PT for the surgical patient are to: (1) improve bronchial hygiene; (2) restore ROM, strength, and endurance; (3) prevent venous stasis and susceptibility to pulmonary emboli; (4) provide information/promote education of patient; (5) decrease anxiety; (6) facilitate breathing.

In the preoperative visit, the therapist or nurse can explain the postop regimen. The importance of deep breathing and coughing (even though it hurts) can be relieved by pain medication. Frequent position changes are important so secretions don't pool in the lung that is dependent. Explain how postural drainage with percussion and vibration will be done and demonstrate the technique. Reassure the patient that every effort will be made for his comfort (i.e., pain medication prior to CPT treatment). If the patient will be on a ventilator for 12–24 hours, explain that he may wake up with the endotracheal tube in place. He won't be able to talk and shouldn't try to talk. He may be hoarse when the tube is removed, but soon his voice will return even though he may have a sore throat for a short time.

Arm and leg exercises are important to promote good circulation and avoid venous stasis in the lower extremities. If the patient is having major surgery, even just ankle dorsiflexion, plantar flexion, and ankle "circles" are helpful.

The patient should be instructed in the use of the incentive spirometer and cough splinting techniques prior to surgery. The incision can be supported with the patient's hands, a blanket, or pillow. The pillow offers excellent support, especially if it is positioned across the full chest or abdomen with the arms over the pillow pressing down. This method gives the most support rather than just holding the pillow and pressing down.

REFERENCES

Periodicals

Bartlett R, et al: Respiratory maneuvers to prevent postoperative pulmonary complications: A critical review. *JAMA* 1973; 224:7.

Baxter W, Levine RS: An evaluation of intermittent positive pressure breathing in the prevention of postoperative pulmonary complications. *Arch Surg* 1969; 98:795.

Egbert L, Bendixen H: The effect of morphine on breathing pattern: A possible factor in atelectasis. *JAMA* 1964; 188:6.

Egbert L, et al: Reduction of postoperative pain by encouragement and instruction of patients. *N Engl J Med* 1964; 270:825.

Egbert L, et al: Value of the preoperative visit by an anesthetist: A study of doctor-patient rapport. *JAMA* 1963; 185:553.

Estanfanous F: Respiratory care following open heart surgery. *Surg Clin North Am* 1975; 55(5):1229.

Forthman J, Shepard A: Postoperative pulmonary complications. *South Med J* 1969; 62:1198.

Foss G: A method for augmenting ventilation during ambulation. *Phys Ther* 1972; 52:5.

Garzon A, Karson K: Hyperventilatory hypoxemia: A common pattern of respiratory insufficiency in surgical patients. *Ann Thorac Surg* 1970; 10:4.

Gormezano J, Branthwaite M: Pulmonary physiotherapy with assisted ventilation: Arterial blood gas changes following pulmonary physiotherapy with IPPB. *Anesthesia* 1972; 27:3.

Grimby G: Aspects of lung expansion in relation to pulmonary physiotherapy. *Am Rev Respir Dis* 1974; 110:145.

Guthrie A, Petty T: Improved exercise tolerance in patients with chronic airway obstruction. *Phys Ther* 1970; 50:9.

Howard S, Hill J: Acute respiratory care in the open heart surgery patient. *Phys Ther* 1972; 52:254.

Jones N: Conference on the scientific basis of respiratory therapy. Physical therapy—present state of the art. *Am Rev Respir Dis* 1974; 110:32.

Latimer R, et al: Ventilatory patterns and pulmonary complications after upper abdominal surgery determined by preoperative and postoperative computerized spirometry and blood gas analysis. *Ann J Surg* 1971; 122:622.

Martin C, et al: Chest physiotherapy and the distribution of ventilation. *Chest* 1976; 69:2.

McConnell D, et al: Postoperative intermittent positive pressure breathing treatments: Physiological considerations. *J Thorac Cardiovasc Surg* 1974; 68:6.

Millins R: Pulmonary physiotherapy in the pediatric age group. *Am Rev Respir Dis* 1974; 110:6.

Petty T: Conference on the scientific basis of respiratory therapy. Physical therapy. Introduction. *Am Rev Respir Dis* 1974; 110:29.

Ravin M: Value of deep breaths in reversing postoperative hypoxemia. *NY State J Med* 1966; 66:244.

Sharp J, et al: Respiratory muscle function in patients with chronic obstructive pulmonary disease: Its relationship to disability and to respiratory therapy. *Am Rev Respir Dis* 1974; 110:154.

Stein M, Cassara E: Preoperative pulmonary evaluation and therapy for surgical patients. *JAMA* 1970; 211:787.

Sveinsson I: Postoperative psychosis after heart surgery. *J Thorac Cardiovasc Surg* 1975; 70:4.

Thoren L: Postoperative pulmonary complications: Observations on their prevention by means of physiotherapy. *Acta Chir Scand* 1954; 107:193.

Van de Water J, et al: Prevention of postoperative pulmonary complications. *Surg Gynecol Obstet* 1972; 135:229.

Ward R, et al: An evaluation of postoperative respiratory maneuvers. *Surg Gynecol Obstet* 1966; 123:51.

Books

Basmajian JV: *Grant's Method of Anatomy*, ed 9. Baltimore, Williams & Wilkins Co, 1975.

Behrendt DM, Austen GW: *Patient Care in Cardiac Surgery*. Boston, Little, Brown & Co, 1985.

Bendixen H, et al: *Respiratory Care*, ed 2. St Louis, CV Mosby Co, 1965.

Bernhard VM, Towne JB: *Complications in Vascular Surgery*. Orlando, Florida, Grune & Stratton, 1985.

Buford TH, Ferguson TB: *Cardiovascular Surgery Current Practice*. St Louis, CV Mosby Co, 1969.

Cash E: *Chest, Heart and Vascular Disorders for Physiotherapist*. Philadelphia, JB Lippincott Co, 1975.

Gless Williams WL, Bare A, et al: *Thoracic and Cardiovascular Surgery*, ed 4. New York, Appleton-Century-Crofts, 1983.

Holden MP: *A Practice of Cardiothoracic Surgery*. Boston, John Wright-PSG, 1982.

Horwath PT: *Care of Cardiac Surgery Patient*. New York, John Wiley & Sons, 1984.

Kester RC, Leveson SC: *Practice of Vascular Surgery*. Pitman, Marshfield, Massachusetts, 1981.

King R: *Introduction to Psychology*. New York, McGraw-Hill Book Co, 1966.

Knott M, Voss D: *Proprioceptive Neuromuscular Facilitation*, ed 2. New York, Harper & Row, 1968.

Litwak RS, Jurado RA: *Care of Cardiac Surgical Patient*. New York, Appleton-Century-Crofts, 1982.

Mason DT, Collins JJ: *Myocardial Revascularization: Medical and Surgical Advances in Coronary Artery Disease*. New York, York Medical Books, 1981.

Moore WS, Baker DJ, et al: *Vascular Surgery: A Comprehensive Review*. Orlando, Florida, Grune & Stratton, 1983.

Peters RM, et al: *Scientific Management of Surgical Patients*. Boston, Little, Brown & Co, 1983.

Rahimtoola Shabbudin H: *Coronary Bypass Surgery*. Philadelphia, FA Davis Co, 1977.

Roberts AJ: *Coronary Artery Surgery: Application of New Technologies*. Chicago, Year Book Medical Publishers, 1983.

Roberts AJ: *Difficult Problems in Adult Cardiac Surgery*. Chicago, Year Book Medical Publishers, 1985.

Roe BB: *Perioperative Management of Cardiothoracic Surgery*. Boston, Little, Brown & Co, 1981.

Sawyer PN, Kaplitt MJ: *Vascular Graft Symposium: Vascular Graft*. New York, Appleton-Century-Crofts, 1978.

Sebistan D: *Davis-Christopher Textbook of Surgery*, vols 1 and 2. Philadelphia, WB Saunders Co, 1972.

Shapiro B, Harrison R, Trout C: *Clinical Application of Respiratory Care*. Chicago, Year Book Medical Publishers, 1975.

Unger F, Affeld K, et al: *Assisted Circulation*. New York, Springer-Verlag New York, 1984.

Wilson ES, Owens ML: *Vascular Access Surgery*. Chicago, Year Book Medical Publishers, 1980.

Zollinger R, Zollinger R, Jr: *Atlas of Surgical Operations*, ed 4. New York, Macmillan Publishing Co, 1975.

19

Neurology and Neurosurgery

Anne R. Smith, P.T., R.R.T.

The nervous system, a complex yet remarkably integrated network of nervous tissue encompassing brain, spinal cord, cranial nerves, spinal nerves, autonomic ganglia, and ganglionated trunks and nerves, is the control center of an individual's motor and sensory, voluntary and involuntary, and intellectual behavior.

Its structural components (Fig 19–1) include the neuron, highly specialized and characteristically excitable or irritable tissue, and the neuroglia, interstitial or supportive tissue which plays a role in the reaction of the nervous system to injury, in defense mechanisms, in the formation of myelin and perhaps in the conduction of impulses. A neuron is composed of a central portion or cell body, which contains the nucleus necessary to maintain the life of the cell, and peripheral processes: dendrites, which are usually multiple branchings that conduct impulses toward the cell body, and the single axon, a long extension ending in multiple terminal buttons or telodendria which conducts impulses away from the cell body. Shortly after its emergence from the cell body, an axon is surrounded by a membranous sheath containing Schwann cells. It may or may not be surrounded by myelin, an insulating shiny white substance that is formed by many layers of Schwann cell membrane coiled around the axon, except at its ending or at periodic intervals or constrictions known as nodes of Ranvier.

The neuron is also the functional unit of the nervous system and as such can receive stimuli, transmit nervous impulses and evoke responses. Stimuli, changes in the body's internal or external environment, originate in receptors (sense organs); responses, muscular con-

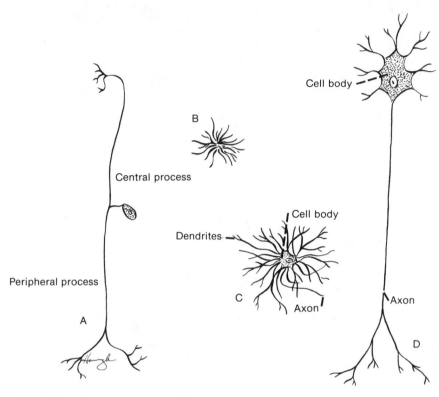

FIG 19–1.
Cells of the nervous system. **A,** sensory neuron. **B,** neuroglial cell. **C,** ventral (anterior) horn cell of the spinal cord. **D,** motor neuron.

traction and glandular activity are elicited in effectors (smooth and skeletal muscles and glands). Stimuli are conducted from receptors to a central integrating station by afferent or sensory neurons and from the central integrating station to effectors by efferent or motor neurons. It is this circuit that constitutes the reflex arc described by Ganong as "the basic unit of integrated neural activity." At the synapse, the junction of two neurons in a neural pathway, the axon of one neuron (presynaptic) comes in contact with the dendrites and cell body of another neuron (postsynaptic). Here the transmission of nervous impulses is mediated by a neurochemical transmitter, and the passage of the impulse is unidirectional from the first neuron to the next.

DIVISIONS OF THE NERVOUS SYSTEM

The nervous system can be divided into two parts. The central nervous system composed of the brain and spinal cord regulates and integrates sensory, motor and intellectual activity, whereas the peripheral nervous system including cranial and spinal nerves transports nervous impulses toward and away from the central compact portion. The autonomic nervous system, which controls the activity of smooth and cardiac muscles, blood vessels, glands and visceral organs, is considered to be a division of the peripheral nervous system.

Central Nervous System

Brain

The brain, which is surrounded by membranes or meninges (dura mater, arachnoid, pia mater) and protected by the bony skull and cerebrospinal fluid, is composed of three basic parts: the cerebral hemispheres, the brain stem and the cerebellum (Fig 19–2).

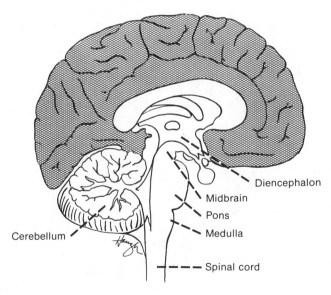

FIG 19–2.
Midsagittal section of the brain.

The paired *cerebral hemispheres,* which constitute the largest part of the brain, are composed of an outer gray portion (cortex or cerebrum) containing millions of cells, an underlying area of white matter containing vast numbers of nerve fibers (internal capsule), and deeply seated nuclear masses, the basal ganglia (Fig 19–3). The surface of the cerebrum is marked by numerous convolutions or folds (gyri) which are delineated by shallow grooves or sulci. Deeper grooves, the fissures, separate either the two hemispheres or the various lobes (frontal, parietal, temporal, occipital) of the hemispheres. When viewed laterally, the longitudinal fissure lies between the two hemispheres, the central fissure of Rolando divides the frontal from the parietal lobe, and the lateral fissure of Sylvius separates the frontal and parietal lobes from the temporal region. The cerebrum is the area where sensation is perceived, voluntary motion is initiated and intellectual activity probably occurs. The precentral gyrus of the frontal lobe constitutes the area of cortical representation of motor function; the postcentral gyrus of the parietal lobe is the area of cortical representation for reception of sensation from various body parts; and the remaining zones or association areas are concerned with activities such as vision, hearing, speech, perception, memory, learning, emotion and intelligence. The white matter

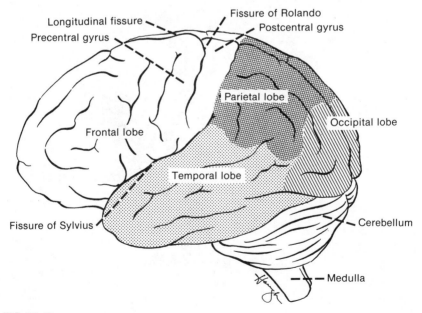

FIG 19–3.
Lateral view of left cerebral hemisphere, cerebellum, and lower brain stem.

of the cerebral hemispheres is primarily composed of three large groups of medullated fibers. Commissural fibers connect corresponding portions of cortex in the two hemispheres, association fibers interconnect cortical regions of the same hemisphere and projection fibers connect cortical regions with distant structures (i.e., brain stem, cerebellum, spinal cord) or more distant structures with the cortex. The basal ganglia, cellular masses of gray matter found at the base of the cerebrum, comprise a component of integrated motor function serving as relay stations for nervous impulses traveling to and from the cerebral cortex.

The *brain stem*, which somewhat resembles the stalk of a mushroom, is surrounded laterally by the cerebral hemispheres and posteriorly by the cerebellum. Its four components—diencephalon, midbrain (mesencephalon), pons and medulla—contain both gray nuclear masses and white matter. Structures within the diencephalon and midbrain comprise components contributing to integrated sensorimotor function, one of the most important of which is the thalamus of the diencephalon. For not only does it provide the relay stations for information from basal ganglia and cerebellum coursing to the cerebral motor cortex, but it also regulates and distributes most of the information traveling to the sensory cerebral cortex. The pons and medulla contain vital centers controlling both respiration and circulation. Finally, the brain stem is the area in which both the deep and superficial origin of the majority of the cranial nerves are found.

The *cerebellum* lies over the posterior surface of the pons and medulla and is partially surrounded by the occipital lobes of the cerebral hemispheres. It is composed of two lateral lobes—the cerebellar hemispheres, containing folds or folia, and a medial portion, the cerebellar vermis. An outer portion, the gray cortex, surrounds an inner core of white matter in which four pairs of nuclei are embedded. The cerebellum plays a monumental role in the coordination and synergy of somatic motor function, the regulation of muscle tone and the maintenance of equilibrium. By virtue of its connections with the midbrain, pons and medulla, it provides both a direct and an indirect influence on the activities of the brain stem, spinal cord and higher cortical centers.

The blood supply of the brain is provided by two pairs of arteries—the vertebrals and internal carotids (Fig 19–4). The vertebral arteries, which arise from the subclavian vessels, ascend through the foramina transversaria of the upper cervical vertebrae, pierce the spinal cord coverings in the region of atlas and base of skull and enter the posterior fossa through the foramen magnum. Here they course toward the

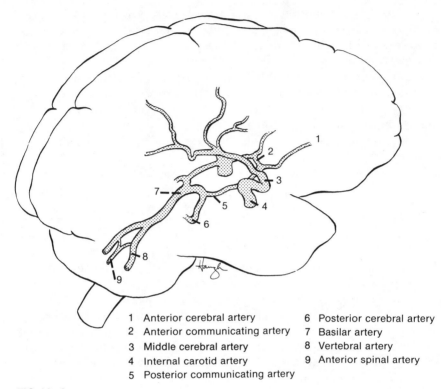

1 Anterior cerebral artery	6 Posterior cerebral artery
2 Anterior communicating artery	7 Basilar artery
3 Middle cerebral artery	8 Vertebral artery
4 Internal carotid artery	9 Anterior spinal artery
5 Posterior communicating artery	

FIG 19–4.
Arterial vessels of the brain.

ventral surface of the brain stem and subsequently join to form the singular basilar artery, which extends over the ventral surface of the pons, terminating in the region of its superior surface as two posterior cerebral arteries. The vertebral and basilar arteries send branches to supply areas of the pons, medulla and cerebellum, while the posterior cerebral arteries supply structures within the posterior region of the cerebral hemispheres. The internal carotids, which originate at the bifurcation of the common carotid arteries, enter the skull via the carotid canal in the region of the temporal bone and emerge in the middle cranial fossa lateral to the optic chiasm. Here they send off two main branches—the anterior cerebral arteries, which supply structures within the anterior cerebral regions, and the larger middle cerebral arteries, which course along the lateral fissures of the hemispheres to supply an area encompassing the precentral and postcentral gyri, basal ganglia, internal capsule and structures within the diencephalon. The arterial circle of Willis, via its paired posterior communicating and single anterior communicating arteries, provides the passageways through which the anatomically separate vertebral and internal carotid systems are connected. The anterior communicating artery joins the two anterior cerebral arteries while the posterior communicating arteries connect the posterior cerebral arteries with the internal carotids. Although these communications can preserve the integrity of blood flow to all areas of the brain in the event that one of its major vessels is interrupted, often this is not sufficient to prevent some damage from occurring. The superficial cortical and deeper penetrating branches of the major cerebral vessels do not generally anastomose. Also, variations in the structure of the circle as well as the absence of some of its parts may prevent this ideal communication from being realized. In contrast, cortical and deeper central cerebellar arteries anastomose freely.

Spinal Cord (Fig 19–5)

The spinal cord, which like the brain is surrounded by meninges and is afforded protection by the bony spine and cerebrospinal fluid,

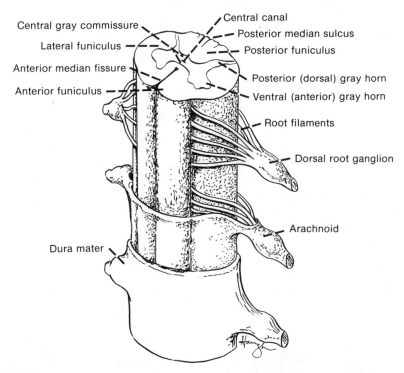

FIG 19–5.
Spinal cord, nerve roots, and meninges.

is an elongated cylindrical mass extending from the foramen magnum of the skull, where it is continuous with the medulla oblongata, to the upper border of the second lumbar vertebra beyond which it terminates in a cone-shaped structure, the conus medullaris. It is divided into symmetrical halves by a deep groove, the anterior median fissure, and a more shallow groove, the posterior median sulcus. On cross section, the cord is composed of a central gray substance, H- or butterfly-shaped, containing paired dorsal (posterior) and ventral (anterior) horns connected by a central gray commissure. This gray matter, consisting of groups of cell bodies and their processes, is surrounded anteriorly, posteriorly and laterally by columns of white matter (funiculi) containing bundles of myelinated or nonmyelinated fibers (axons) which ascend or descend to connect different areas of the cord or to connect the spinal cord and brain. The spinal cord is the area of attachment of the spinal nerves and the seat of action of the spinal reflexes.

The spinal cord receives its blood supply from the single anterior and paired posterior spinal arteries and the spinal branches of arteries supplying its adjacent structures (Fig 19–6). The anterior spinal arteries arise as two medial roots from the vertebral arteries and unite between the medullary pyramids before continuing to descend in the ventral median fissure. Branches of the artery supply the anterolateral gray and white regions of the cord as well as the anterior gray region of the posterior horn. The posterior spinal arteries arise as two branches from either the vertebral or posterior inferior cerebellar arteries and descend along the posterior surface of the cord medial to the dorsal roots to supply the posterior gray and white columns. The blood supply provided by the major longitudinal vessels is augmented by spinal or radicular branches of the vertebral, cervical, intercostal, lumbar and sacral blood vessels which enter the cord via the intervertebral foramina and whose anterior and posterior branches freely anastomose with the major vessels of the cord.

Peripheral Nervous System

Nerves, groups of neuron processes or fibers, course outward from the brain and spinal cord and serve to conduct impulses toward or away from the central nervous system. Their cell bodies are located in the brain, spinal cord or ganglia.

Cranial Nerves (Table 19–1)

The 12 pairs of cranial nerves, identified by number, are generally associated with structures located on or within the head and are sen-

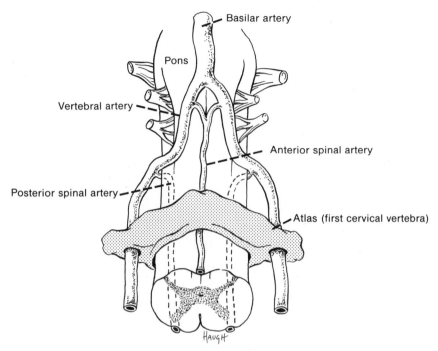

FIG 19–6.
Arterial supply of the spinal cord.

sory in function, motor in function, or a combination of the two (Fig 19–7). The nuclei of those nerves having a motor function originate within the brain stem, whereas those serving a sensory function generally originate from collections of cells in ganglia exterior to the latter. The first two cranial nerves are not true nerves but fiber tracts of the brain, and the 11th nerve (spinal-accessory) arises in part from the upper cervical segments of the spinal cord.

Spinal Nerves (Fig 19–8)

The 31 pairs of spinal nerves emerging laterally from the intervertebral foramina of the bony spine are named and numbered according to the vertebrae corresponding to the area of the cord from which they originate. Twenty-three pairs of nerves—twelve thoracic, five lumbar, five sacral, and one coccygeal—exit below the vertebrae for which they are named, while in the cervical region, one finds eight pairs of nerves and seven vertebrae. The first cervical nerves exit between the skull and atlas (C1) so that the first seven pairs of nerves exit above their

TABLE 19–1.

Function and Distribution of Cranial Nerves

NO.	NAME	FUNCTION	DISTRIBUTION
I	Olfactory	Special sense of smell	Nasal mucous membranes, olfactory region
II	Optic	Special sense of sight	Retina of eye
III	Oculomotor	Motor	Muscles of eye
IV	Trochlear	Motor	Muscles of eye
V	Trigeminal	Mixed	Muscles of mastication, skin of face, tongue, teeth
VI	Abducens	Motor	Muscles of eye
VII	Facial	Mixed	Muscles of expression, salivary glands, lacrimal glands
VIII	Acoustic		
	Vestibular	Special sense of equilibrium	Semicircular canals
	Cochlear	Special sense of hearing	Organ of Corti
IX	Glossopharyngeal	Mixed	Muscles of pharynx, larynx, posterior third of tongue, pharynx, parotid glands
X	Vagus	Mixed	Muscles of pharynx, larynx, thoracic and abdominal viscera
XI	Accessory	Mixed	
	Cranial		Joins branches of vagus
	Spinal		Sternomastoid, trapezius muscles
XII	Hypoglossal	Motor	Intrinsic muscles of tongue

vertebrae, while the eighth cervical nerves emerge below the body of C7 and above the body of T1. The spinal nerves are attached to the cord by two roots—the dorsal or posterior root, which contains a swelling or ganglion and is continuous with the dorsal gray column of the spinal cord, and the ventral or anterior motor root, which is continuous with the anterior gray column of the same. Lateral to the dorsal ganglion, these roots unite to form a short, mixed spinal nerve which emerges from the intervertebral foramen and subsequently divides into four branches—the recurrent or meningeal branch returns through the foramen to supply the coverings of the cord, the rami communicantes provide connections between the spinal nerve and sympathetic trunk, the posterior primary division or ramus innervates the skin and axial muscles of the back, and the anterior primary division or ramus innervates muscles of the lateral and anterior part of the body as well as skeletal muscles of the extremities. In the cervical, lumbar and sacral

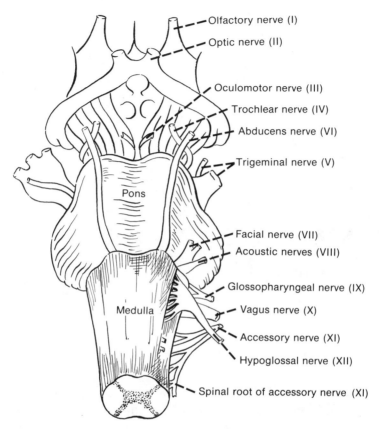

FIG 19–7.
Exit of cranial nerves from the brain.

regions, these anterior primary divisions intertwine to form plexuses whose terminal branches form the peripheral nerves which supply the individual muscles of the upper and lower limbs, while anterior primary divisions of the thoracic spinal nerves retain their segmental distribution and continue as the intercostal nerves found between the ribs. The function of spinal nerves is to carry impulses to and from the central nervous system. According to the Bell-Magendie law, the dorsal roots contain sensory or afferent fibers carrying impulses to the spinal cord, and the ventral roots contain motor or efferent fibers carrying impulses away from the cord. While the cell bodies of the afferent fibers lie in ganglia of the posterior roots, those of efferent fibers are found in the ventral horn cells of the anterior gray columns.

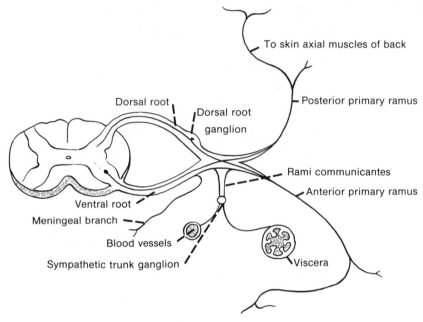

FIG 19–8.
Schematic representation of a spinal nerve.

Autonomic Nervous System

The autonomic nervous system is functionally defined as a motor (efferent) system which innervates the smooth muscles and glands of the body. Its characteristic components, the autonomic nerves, are composed of preganglionic neurons with cell bodies located within the gray matter of the brain stem or lateral gray horns of the spinal cord and axons which terminate in ganglia outside the central nervous system. These ganglia also contain cell bodies of postganglionic neurons and represent the location from which the postganglionic axons course to their destination. The divisions of the autonomic nervous system—sympathetic and parasympathetic—are anatomically determined by the location of cell bodies of the preganglionic fibers. The sympathetic portion (thoracolumbar), with preganglionic fibers originating in the lateral gray columns of the spinal cord, is characterized by chains of ganglia found along the sides of the vertebral column from the first thoracic to the second lumbar vertebrae (sympathetic chain). It innervates smooth muscles, vessels and glands and is closely interrelated with the roots of spinal motor nerves innervating skeletal muscle. The parasympathetic division (craniosacral), which is composed of preganglionic fibers originating in the gray matter of the brain stem and lateral gray columns of the second, third, and fourth sacral cord segments, supplies visceral organs of the head, thorax and pelvis. To summarize, generally the sympathetic nervous system contains short preganglionic and long postganglionic fibers, whereas the parasympathetic system contains long preganglionic and short postganglionic fibers with cell bodies that are located in ganglia close to the organ innervated. The autonomic nervous system is both automatic and involuntary since the majority of its functions are not consciously appreciated. It receives information concerning the body's internal environment and mediates responses which promote homeostasis.

MANIFESTATIONS OF DISORDERED NEURAL FUNCTION

Normal nervous system activity is dependent upon the integrity of the reflex arc, the basic neural components of which include an afferent and an efferent neuron. In a simple monosynaptic stretch reflex, for example, tapping the tendon of the biceps muscle causes involuntary contraction of the same. The stimulus generated by activating stretch receptors in the biceps tendon is transmitted to the spinal cord via the axon of the afferent neuron of the dorsal root. At the synapse within the cord the impulse passes from the afferent neuron to the anterior horn cell of the efferent neuron, then travels via its axon of the ventral root to terminate in the motor end plate of the skeletal muscle. Irritation of the posterior pharyngeal wall (afferent impulse, cranial nerve IX) stimulates the gag reflex or the swallowing reflex (efferent impulse, cranial nerve X). The stimulation of pressure in the baroreceptors of the carotid sinus (afferent impulse, cranial nerve IX) may cause initial tachycardia followed by reflex bradycardia and lowering of blood pressure (efferent impulse, cranial nerve X), which if severe can lead to cardiac arrest. Damage or interruption of the afferent or efferent component of the reflex arc will cause diminution or loss of the expected response.

The functional concept of the reflex arc, and its afferent and efferent neuron, can also be applied in more complex neural systems where, instead of the simple two-neuron complex, chains of neurons form afferent (sensory) and efferent (motor) pathways or tracts from brain to spinal cord, spinal cord to brain, and between structures within the brain. As examples, the lateral spinothalamic tract (Fig 19–9) carries the

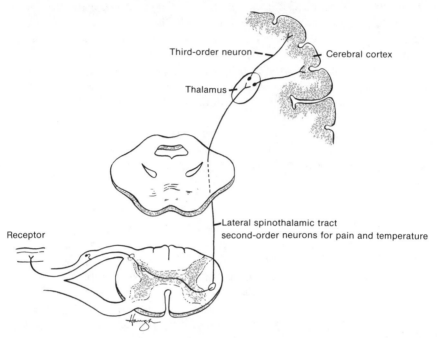

FIG 19–9.
Afferent pathway for pain and temperature sensations via the lateral spinothalamic tract.

sensations of pain and temperature from receptors in the skin to the spinal cord from which they ascend to the thalamus of the diencephalon (second-order neuron) and are finally projected to the cerebral sensory cortex (third-order neuron); the corticospinal tract (Fig 19–10) transmits impulses initiated in the cells of the cerebral motor cortex to the level of spinal cord containing the motor cells (ventral gray horn) of peripheral nerves innervating skeletal muscle. The corticobulbar tract also transmits impulses originating in the cerebral motor cortex, but these course to nuclei of the brain stem containing the cell bodies of cranial motor nerves; the pontocerebellar tract carries information about the coordination of movements from cell bodies within the pons to the cerebellar cortex; and the spinocerebellar tract transmits information regarding the tension within muscles and the position of joints to the cerebellum. The integrated and coordinated action of numerous neural pathways effects normal sensation, movement, postural and muscle tone, and the function of visceral organs so that lesions of any portion of the constituent neurons, in cell bodies or fiber processes, result in other than normal function.

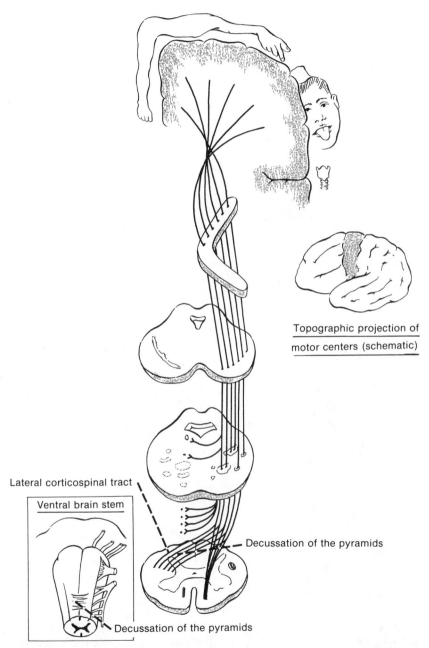

Topographic projection of
motor centers (schematic)

Lateral corticospinal tract

Ventral brain stem

Decussation of the pyramids

Decussation of the pyramids

FIG 19–10.
Efferent motor pathway of the pyramidal system.

Motor Function

Nervous impulses causing reflex (involuntary) as well as voluntary motion are channeled to the motor end plates of skeletal muscle by peripheral motor nerves, the cell bodies of which are located in the anterior gray horns of the spinal cord or in nuclei within the brain stem. These *lower motor neurons,* which comprise the final common path through which muscular activity is effected, receive information that may either initiate or modify muscular contraction from more than ten neural pathways. Impulses causing voluntary motion arise in cells of the cerebral sensorimotor cortex, from whence they are transmitted via the corticospinal and corticobulbar tracts to synapse with lower motor neurons. The neurons of corticospinal and corticobulbar paths constitute the *upper motor neurons.*

Paralysis and Muscle Tone

Lesions of lower motor neurons produce paralysis of the involved muscles, flaccidity (loss of muscle tone), atrophy (loss of muscle bulk) and absent or diminished reflexes. The final common path becomes disconnected, so to speak, from the influences of pathways from higher brain centers, the motor nerve degenerates and once contractile and elastic muscle is eventually replaced by fibrous tissue. The most striking example of this type of lesion is that of poliomyelitis, in which ventral horn cells of the spinal cord are destroyed. The axons of lower motor neurons may be the seat of lesions also. With severance of a peripheral spinal nerve as a result of trauma, the affected muscle becomes paralyzed and atrophied and varied degrees of sensory disturbance occur.

Upper motor neuron lesions produce complete or partial paralysis of the involved muscles, usually spasticity or rigidity (increased muscle tone), increased deep tendon reflexes and the appearance of pathologic reflexes. Although the final common path remains intact, the influences from higher brain centers become distorted. The impulses of facilitatory and inhibitory mechanisms, feedback circuits interconnecting pathways within brain structures (i.e., cerebellum and brain stem) either directly or indirectly with corticospinal and corticobulbar pathways, are no longer delicately balanced with the forces effecting skilled voluntary movement so that the overall quality of motion is the product of the interrelated influence of both the pyramidal (corticospinal and corticobulbar pathways) and extrapyramidal (all other contributing motor pathways) systems acting on the final common path. Hypertonicity and hyperreflexia are believed to occur because the lower motor neuron receives impulses lacking the inhibitory control of higher brain centers. When *spasticity* is present, there is increased resistance to sudden passive stretch of the involved muscles, often followed by relaxation of the latter. The simultaneous contraction of both flexor and extensor musculature present in *rigidity* prevents rapid passive motion in any direction but does not exhibit this type of release. While lesions of pyramidal pathways usually characterized by spastic paralysis cause alteration of skilled voluntary movement, lesions of extrapyramidal pathways, especially those involving the basal ganglia, are typified by rigidity, an increase or lack of gross movements or a lack of associated movements. Interruption of the blood supply of one half of the cerebral motor cortex resulting from hemorrhage of a middle cerebral artery, for example, may produce eventual spastic paralysis of one or both limbs of the opposite side of the body (contralateral monoplegia or hemiplegia) since the majority of the descending fibers of the corticospinal tracts cross in the medulla (decussation of the pyramids) and then continue their descent in the lateral funiculus of the spinal cord. If a lesion is in the region of cell bodies or fibers of corticobulbar pathways, cranial nerve impairment may occur. Disease of basal ganglia may result in the excess movements of athetosis, chorea or hemiballismus, or in the poverty of movement, resting tremor, masked facies and loss of armswing during walking seen in Parkinson's disease.

Posture (Fig 19–11)

Posture, the attitude or position of the body, which is dependent upon the integration of a variety of reflexes from spinal cord to cerebral cortical levels and which is primarily mediated through extrapyramidal pathways, comprises a component of normal motor function. In humans, it provides the means by which we are able to maintain an upright balanced position and also maintains and continuously adjusts this underlying stability so that voluntary motion may be performed. Static (tonic) postural reflexes, those characterized by the constant state of contraction found in certain portions of the body musculature, are seen in antigravity muscles of the head, spine, hips and extremities; whereas phasic postural reflexes are dynamic, allowing movement.

Abnormal postures that may be encountered in patients suffering from central nervous system dysfunction are: decerebrate rigidity, in which the limbs are extended and internally rotated and the static or tonic postural reflexes that normally offer resistance to gravity are markedly increased; and more commonly decorticate rigidity, in which the upper extremities are held in an attitude of flexion and the lower extremities are extended. Lesions of the cerebral cortex, in which brain stem function is generally preserved, may produce decorticate postur-

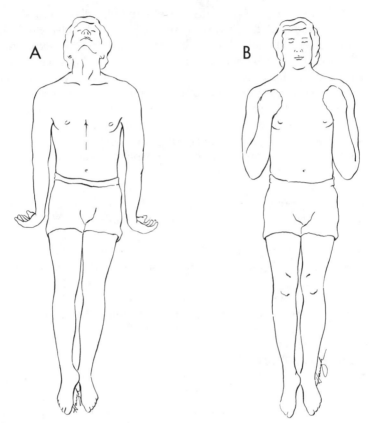

FIG 19–11.
A, decerebrate posture. **B,** decorticate posture.

ing, whereas involvement of brain stem structures may be associated with decerebrate posturing. Opisthotonos, posturing typified by severe hyperextension so that in the supine position the back is so arched that the body rests on the head and the feet, may be seen in patients suffering from tetanus, strychnine poisoning or meningitis.

Coordination

Although the cerebellum does not exert direct control over the muscular contraction necessary for voluntary movement, loss of appropriate influence from this vitally important region of the brain causes movement to become abnormal. Coordinated and especially rapidly performed movements (i.e., talking or running) are affected by cerebellar disease because its synergistic and quickly reactive function is impaired. Lesions of the cerebellum producing clinical signs characteristic of a lack of coordination between muscle groups may be manifested by ataxia (clumsy, wide-based staggering gait), dysmetria (inaccurate direction of motion or pointing past an intended target), dysdiadochokinesia (lack of smooth progression of motor activity, inability to perform rapid alternating movements), dysarthria (unintelligible uncoordinated speech), rebound (inability to halt motion in a limb contracting against resistance when that resistance is removed) and intention tremor (jerky movements upon voluntary motion). In addition, an altered state of muscle tension characterized by hypotonia may be present.

Brain Stem Function

Disordered or altered function of structures within the lower brain stem, certain cranial nerves and those nerves innervating the muscles of respiration is frequently encountered in the neurologic surgery patient.

Swallowing (Fig 19–12)

The swallowing reflex is a complex mechanism which is dependent upon a normally functioning swallowing center (located in the medulla in the floor of the fourth ventricle close to but separate from the respiratory center) and intact afferent and efferent neural pathways. It is considered to consist of three stages—oral or voluntary, pharyngeal and esophageal. After food has been prepared by the muscles of mastication (nerve supply, mandibular portion of cranial nerve V), it is propelled backward by the intrinsic muscles of the tongue (nerve supply, cranial nerve XII), where it comes into contact with swallowing receptor areas of the posterior pharyngeal wall, base of tongue, soft palate and pillars of the tonsils. At this point, the completely involuntary pharyngeal and then the esophageal stages are initiated. Impulses from the receptor area are transmitted to the swallowing center by sensory branches of the fifth and ninth cranial nerves and then there is a series of automatic responses that serve to propel food or fluid from the pharynx to the esophagus (pharyngeal reflex) and to protect the airway above and below the oropharynx (pharyngeal and laryngeal reflexes). The soft palate elevates to close off the nasopharynx; the palatopharyngeal folds constrict to pass the food into the posterior pharynx; the vocal cords close and the epiglottis swings over the laryngeal opening; and, as the pharynx is elevated to receive the food, the larynx is moved upward and forward, the pharyngoesophageal sphincter is relaxed and

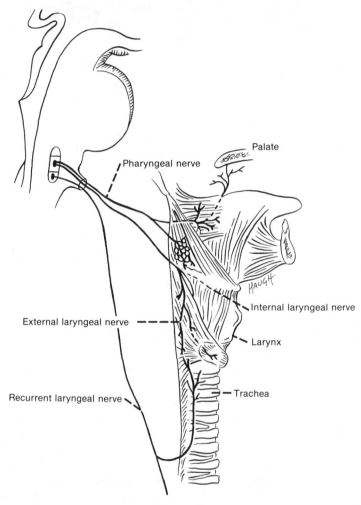

FIG 19–12.
Innervation of muscles of the pharynx, larynx and trachea (branches of the vagus nerve).

the pharyngeal constrictor muscles are contracted to initiate peristaltic waves that propel food into the esophagus. During this pharyngeal stage of swallowing, the respiratory center of the medulla is inhibited by the swallowing center of the same so that respiration ceases during any phase of its cycle for the 1–2 seconds in which the process of swallowing takes place.

The efferent impulses to muscles involved in swallowing are transmitted by branches of the fifth, ninth, tenth and twelfth cranial nerves, but the majority of these are mediated through motor branches of the vagi (cranial nerve X). The muscles that elevate the soft palate and constrict the posterior pharynx (levator, veli palatini, glossopalatine, pharyngopalatine, superior and middle pharyngeal constrictors) are supplied by rostral or pharyngeal divisions of the vagi. The stylopharyngeus muscles that elevate and expand the pharynx to receive a bolus of food are innervated by motor divisions of the glossopharyngeal nerves. The laryngeal musculature, which receives its innervation from the laryngeal branches of the vagi, plays an important role in opening and closing the glottis (the true vocal cords and their intervening space) and in protecting the airway from aspiration of secretions or foreign material. The cricothyroid muscles which tighten the vocal cords are innervated by the superior laryngeal nerves, and the remaining laryngeal muscles are supplied by branches of the recurrent laryngeal nerves.

Paralysis of the elevators of the soft palate causes regurgitation of food and liquids through the nose, may result in a nasal type of speech due to lack of closure of the nasopharynx from the oropharynx, and may be manifested by an absent gag reflex (Fig 19–13). Paralysis of pharyngeal constrictor muscles causes difficult swallowing (dysphagia) and inability to propel food from pharynx to esophagus, and paralysis of laryngeal sphincters may allow aspiration of food, liquids and secretions into the tracheobronchial tree. In addition, lesions of the swallowing center (i.e., polio, tumor invasion) as well as primary diseases of muscle (myasthenia gravis, muscular dystrophy) create disturbances in normal swallowing activity. The peristaltic activity propelling food and fluids from the esophagus to the stomach constitutes the esophageal phase of swallowing and is entirely mediated by afferent and efferent branches of the vagus nerves. Accumulation of food and liquids in the upper esophagus and pharynx as a result of esophageal paralysis may cause suffocation or aspiration.

Coughing

Coughing, which can be voluntarily initiated or reflexly activated in response to irritation or the presence of foreign matter in the larynx, trachea or carina, is, in addition to mucociliary transport, one of the vitally important functions that keeps the respiratory passageways free from foreign material. The cough reflex is initiated in centers within the medulla, its afferent and efferent components being transmitted by the vagus nerves. Following stimulation, a large volume of air is inspired and the epiglottis and vocal cords close to hold the air within

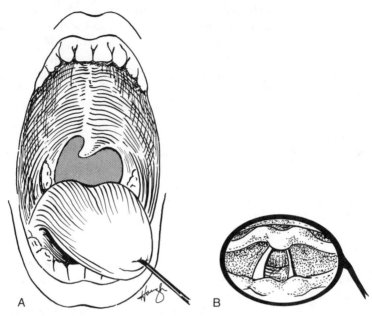

FIG 19–13.
A, sagging of left palate and pharyngeal wall with deviation of uvula to the right that might occur with damage of the left vagus nerve. **B,** paralysis of left vocal fold that might occur with damage of left recurrent laryngeal nerve.

the lungs. Then forceful contraction of abdominal muscles pushes the lungs against the diaphragm to increase the pressure of air within the thoracic cavity. At this time, while the cords and epiglottis are open, air that is forcefully expelled from compressed lung tissue and compressed airways propels foreign material to the pharynx where it can be expectorated or swallowed.

Cough effectiveness is compromised when inspiratory muscles are weakened or paralyzed (i.e., polio, neuromuscular disease, quadriparesis), if vocal cord paralysis prevents adequate closure of the cords, when strength of the abdominal musculature is impaired, or if protective airway reflexes (pharyngeal, laryngeal and tracheal) are depressed (i.e., comatose patients, postoperative neurologic surgery patients). Some or all of these factors, which may cause not only retention or inadequate mobilization of secretions but also pooling of secretions in the pharynx and aspiration of secretions into the tracheobronchial tree, may necessitate the passage of an artificial airway, oxygen administration and the institution of mechanical assistance of ventilation.

Vomiting

Vomiting, a reflex activity occurring generally in response to irritation or overdistention of the upper gastrointestinal tract, psychogenic stimuli (i.e., unpleasant odors or sights) or rapid changes of motion, allows the contents of the upper gastrointestinal tract to be forcefully expelled. Following stimulation, impulses are transmitted by sympathetic and vagal afferents to the vomiting center lying in the dorsal part of the lateral reticular formation of the medulla. A series of motor responses mediated through both cranial nerves (V, VII, IX, X, and XII) and spinal nerves of the diaphragm and abdominal musculature occurs. A deep breath is taken, the sphincter of the esophagus is opened, the glottis and posterior nasal passages are closed and the stomach is squeezed by the simultaneous contraction of the diaphragm and abdominal muscles (Valsalva maneuver) to evacuate its contents upward through the esophagus.

Direct irritation or lesions of the vomiting center associated with tumor invasion, meningeal irritation, increased intracranial pressure and head injury may cause central or "projectile vomiting" in which the vomitus is very forcefully ejected but in which there is little of the nausea or forceful action of the skeletal muscles usually associated with the vomiting act.

Circulation

The flow of blood toward and away from the various tissues of the body passes through the arteries and veins of the circulatory system and provides the means by which nutrients are carried to the tissues and the waste products of tissue metabolism are removed. It is dependent upon a number of factors: the pumping action of the heart, the volume of blood circulating within the system, appropriate tone or resistance of the circulatory vessels and a generated pressure which allows adequate flow of blood from the periphery to the heart (venous return). Although circulation for the most part is regulated locally by the metabolic demands of individual organs (i.e., liver, kidneys and brain receive a greater proportion of the total blood flow or cardiac output than resting muscle), it is controlled, especially during periods of stress, by structures within the nervous system as well as factors within the blood.

The vasomotor center found within the reticular portion of the brain stem in the lower one third of the pons and upper two thirds of the medulla contains excitatory and inhibitory portions. The excitatory vasoconstrictor system sends continuous impulses to almost all vessels via the sympathetic nerves to promote vasomotor tone, whereas the vasodilator system causes vasodilatation by inhibiting the activity of the vasoconstrictor portion. In addition, the sympathetic nervous system exerts either an excitatory or an inhibitory effect on the heart so that its rate and force of contraction are altered. The parasympathetic nervous system, however, plays only a minor role in the regulation of circulation; it exerts a small influence in reducing the contractile force of the heart so that secondary reduction of the heart rate occurs.

Especially during periods of stress, rapid response to stimuli and simultaneous control of large portions of the circulation, which override local regulation by the tissues, characterize the nervous control of circulation. Baroreceptors, stretch or pressure receptors found in large systemic vessels, but especially those of the carotid and aortic bodies, detect changes in blood pressure and serve to keep average systemic pressure within the circulatory vessels constant. If mean arterial pressure falls, the baroreceptors are stimulated so that vasoconstriction occurs, the force and rate of heart contraction increase and blood pressure rises. Conversely, if an increase in blood pressure is sensed, vasodilatation accompanied by decreased rate and force of heart contraction causes blood pressure to fall. If cardiac output falls or a severe loss of blood volume occurs, as in circulatory or hemorrhagic shock, the blood vessels constrict to raise blood pressure in order to increase the amount of blood flow to vital organs. When neurogenic shock occurs, blood volume is adequate but there is marked loss of generalized vasomotor tone, resulting in greatly decreased blood pressure. At a mean arterial pressure of 50 mm Hg or less, decreased blood flow to the vasomotor center initiates a very powerful sympathetic vasoconstrictor response (central nervous system ischemic response) in which blood pressure is increased, peripheral vessels may be occluded and an abdominal compression reflex may be activated in order to preferentially direct blood flow to the brain. Neurogenic shock may occur secondary to depression of the vasomotor center in deep general anesthesia, when sympathetic outflow to the vessels is depressed by spinal anesthesia, when there is direct damage of the brain stem (i.e., basilar skull fractures, concussion) or if increased cerebrospinal fluid pressure occludes blood flow within the brain. It is counteracted by placing the patient in the Trendelenburg position or in the supine position with the legs elevated to increase venous return to the heart and direct blood flow to the brain or with pharmacologic agents. If unreversed, it results in death of cells within the vasomotor center within 3–10 minutes.

Respiration

The respiratory center containing large numbers of neurons which are found bilaterally in the reticular portion of the pons and medulla is that region of the brain where ventilation (the movement of air into and out of the lungs) is controlled. Of its three major portions—the pneumotaxic center of upper pons, the apneustic center of lower pons and the medullary center of medulla oblongata—the last controls the basic rhythmicity of respiration and is probably the most important. This medullary rhythmicity area receives regulatory impulses from pneumotaxic and apneustic centers, other brain regions, vagus and glossopharyngeal nerves (chemoreceptors and baroreceptors of aortic and carotid bodies, pulmonary stretch receptors) as well as facilitatory impulses mediated through the spinal cord from not only the proprioceptors of muscle spindles within the respiratory muscles, but probably also from other sensory receptors throughout the body. The product of the information integrated within the respiratory center of the brain stem is effected through the final common path of the lower motor neurons governing the force of contraction of the respiratory muscles. The leaves of the diaphragm, the major muscle of respiration, are supplied by the phrenic nerves generally formed by the paired third, fourth and fifth cervical roots. A mnemonic to remember is "three, four, and five keep us alive." The 11 pairs of intercostal muscles are innervated by their respective intercostal nerves formed by the ventral rami of the upper 11 pairs of thoracic nerves. Disturbance of central respiratory regulation and respiratory muscle function can cause alveolar hypoventilation, alveolar hyperventilation and abnormal patterns of breathing.

Hypoventilation. The effectiveness of alveolar ventilation (the volume of ventilation found in the gas-exchanging portions of the lungs), which is determined by measuring the pressure exerted by CO_2 in the arterial blood, determines the amount of oxygen that is added to alveolar gas as well as the amount of carbon dioxide removed from the same. If alveolar ventilation falls, Pa_{CO_2} rises (hypercapnia) and Pa_{O_2} decrease (hypoxemia).

Hypoventilation can occur when the respiratory center is depressed by anesthesia, morphine and barbiturates or in the presence of central nervous system embarrassment resulting from brain swelling (cerebral edema) secondary to head injury, inflammation, hemorrhagic lesions, tumors, increased intracranial pressure and lesions within the medulla. Frequently, impairment of the cough and swallowing reflexes occurs in conjunction with respiratory center depression, so that in addition to the alveolar hypoventilation that may be produced, inadequate mobilization and pooling of secretions can contribute to the development of aspiration pneumonia. Placement of an artificial airway, administration of oxygen and mechanical assistance of ventilation may be required.

The weakness of respiratory muscles found in peripheral neuromuscular disease (i.e., myasthenia gravis, Guillain-Barré, quadriparesis, polio) is another important factor producing hypoventilation. Failure of these muscles (especially the diaphragm) to generate adequate tidal volumes during inspiration, as well as impaired action of the abdominal musculature during the compressive phase of coughing, can lead to the development of pulmonary infection. Although a person with normal respiratory muscle strength can increase his ventilation and cough effectively to meet the stress imposed by pulmonary infection, the patient afflicted with neuromuscular weakness may be unable to adequately increase his ventilation. Because of his reduced vital capacity and limited ventilatory reserve, he must expend so much energy to increase ventilation that extreme fatigue and respiratory failure occur. Administration of oxygen, intubation and mechanical assistance of ventilation may be required. In addition, ventilation-perfusion inequality frequently contributes to or hastens the development of the hypoxemia and hypercapnia (increased P_{CO_2} in arterial blood) that ultimately result in respiratory failure.

Finally, the alveolar hypoventilation seen in central nervous system and peripheral neuromuscular disease occurs secondary to neurologic dysfunction and can be present even if the lungs are normal. If, however, the patient suffers from neurologic and primary respiratory disease, the stress placed upon the respiratory system is compounded. Although the treatment of respiratory failure in this group of neurologically impaired patients is the same as that for respiratory failure due to any other cause (see Chapter 26), it is important to appreciate that disease of this seemingly unrelated system, even in the presence of normal lungs, can significantly impair pulmonary function.

Hyperventilation. Hyperventilation (decreased P_{CO_2} in arterial blood) may occur when lesions are present within the central nervous system or when coma produced by metabolic abnormalities (i.e., ketoacidosis, lactic acidosis, metabolic acidosis of uremia) stimulates the respiratory center. Localized lesions of midbrain and upper pontine structures may cause central neurogenic hyperventilation characterized by rapid shallow respirations that are not altered by the administration of oxygen, a Pa_{CO_2} less than 30 mm Hg and an ineffective pattern of ventilation that serves primarily to ventilate the anatomical dead space.

Abnormal Patterns of Ventilation. Damage or depression of the brain at nearly all of its levels can affect the pattern of ventilation. Cheyne-Stokes respiration, a type of periodic breathing characterized by alternating periods of apnea and hyperpnea, is believed to be caused by a delayed response of the medullary chemoreceptors to blood gas changes within the lungs (especially changes in Pa_{CO_2}). It may be present when there is damage, hemorrhage or chronic hypoxia of the brain, in the presence of diffuse cortical involvement and in isolated lesions of the diencephalon. In addition, it is frequently seen in patients suffering from congestive heart failure. Biot's breathing, another type of periodic breathing typified by periods of apnea separated by short bursts of irregular breaths, may also be associated with brain damage and is often a serious clinical sign. Finally, severely compromised function of the medullary region of the respiratory center may cause permanent apnea or the loss of automaticity of breathing seen in Ondine's curse.

Altered Levels of Consciousness

Although alteration in the level of consciousness may be encountered in a large variety of disease states, it is a manifestation of neurophysiologic dysfunction of structures within the brain which may occur as a result of intracranial processes (i.e., head injury, brain infection, cerebrovascular insult, seizure disorders, increased intracranial pressure and herniation or displacement of structures within the brain) or extracranial processes (i.e., serious systemic infection; serious metabolic disturbances such as diabetic acidosis, hepatic dysfunction and uremia; drug overdose and alcohol intoxication; carbon dioxide and metal poisoning and systemic shock secondary to hemorrhage or compromised vascular function). Some mechanisms involved in its development include direct destruction of cortical and diencephalic tissues by space-occupying lesions, interference with the metabolic activity of their neuronal structures and alteration of their blood flow as a result of circulatory dysfunction or mechanical obstruction.

The classification of normal and altered levels of consciousness is variable and the terminology used may be interpreted differently by several observers. Coma may be characterized by a profound loss of consciousness, absent reflexes, lack of response to verbal or noxious stimuli, and primitive posturing or withdrawal in response to noxious stimuli. In lesser degrees of coma, the reactions of the patient as well as his level of orientation may be described by terms such as semicomatose, stuporous, confused, disoriented and lethargic. However, description of the actual state in which one finds a patient may provide more meaningful information for determining whether there is improvement or deterioration and should include items regarding the patient's orientation to place, time, and person; his ability to follow commands; if he is restless or irritable; if he can answer questions; and whether he can be aroused easily, not at all, or only in response to noxious stimuli.

Seizures

Convulsive seizures, which are characterized by the sudden yet involuntary onset of increased contraction and relaxation of all or some of the body musculature, may occur if neuronal activity within brain tissue is increased (epilepsy) or when there are brain lesions resulting from infectious disease (meningitis, viral encephalitis, brain abscess), tumor invasion, head trauma, asphyxia at birth, prematurity, postcardiopulmonary arrest, lead poisoning, subdural and epidural hematoma, subarachnoid hemorrhage, metabolic disturbances (electrolyte imbalance, hypoglycemia, diabetes) and vitamin deficiency (B_6). Consciousness may be lost as in grand mal seizures; the patient may be conscious, experiencing seizure activity in a limb, for example, due to localized irritation of the area of cortex supplying that extremity; or the seizures may be severe and almost constant as in status epilepticus.

Increased Intracranial Pressure

Because the intracranial space is surrounded by a rigid casing of bone and occupied by brain tissue and fluid that is relatively noncompressible, an increase in the volume of its contents can seriously compromise neural function, reduce cerebral blood flow, impair neural tissue metabolism and ultimately cause destruction of neural tissue. Although the integrity of blood flow to the brain is preserved despite small increases in intracranial pressure by autoregulatory mechanisms that allow for displacement of the cerebrospinal fluid, as intracranial pressure approaches mean systemic pressure, these compensatory mechanisms are spent and there are symptoms of papilledema (inflammation of the optic nerve where it enters the eyeball) and possibly headache (pain produced as a result of traction on vessels and dura), vomiting and deterioration in the level of consciousness.

Brain swelling or cerebral edema is closely interrelated with and often difficult to distinguish from increased intracranial pressure. Retention of salt and water within the tissues and vessels of the brain frequently occurs as a sequel of craniocerebral trauma and in response to tumor invasion (especially metastatic lesions), acute brain abscess, intracranial or subarachnoid hemorrhage, toxic or metabolic disturbances and ischemia caused by spasm of vessels or a limited supply of oxygen within the tissues. The increase in intracranial pressure occurring with mass lesions (hemorrhage, abscess, tumor) may cause herniation or distortion of structures within the cerebral regions or displacement and compression of the brain stem. This may be accompanied by abnormal breathing patterns, abnormal postures and disturbances of consciousness. Increased carbon dioxide and reduced oxygen concentrations in the arterial blood will cause dilatation of cerebral vessels with a consequent increase in blood flow and blood volume. In a brain that is already edematous, hypercapnia and hypoxemia, which may be present with ineffective patterns of ventilation, suppression of the respiratory center and shunting of pulmonary blood because of retained secretions, produce even more edema and consequently a greater increase in intracranial pressure. If the process is not reversed, death occurs from anoxia and destruction of brain tissue. Finally, hydrocephalus is characterized by enlargement of the ventricular system in which there is an accumulation of cerebrospinal fluid within or outside of the brain. It can occur as a result of ventricular obstruction or obstruction to the flow of venous blood and be of the high-pressure, low-pressure, normal-pressure, communicating and noncommunicating types. Treatment of the condition generally includes the placement of shunts to remove excess cerebrospinal fluid. If left untreated, it causes atrophy and destruction of brain tissue.

ACUTE TREATMENT OF THE NEUROLOGICALLY IMPAIRED PATIENT

As a review of the material presented thus far, several predisposing factors may be associated with the development of respiratory complications in the presence of neurologic impairment: decreased level of activity especially as a result of an acute process or decreased motor function, decreased strength of the respiratory muscles which reduces the ability of the patient to increase ventilation or cough effectively, disturbances of the swallowing mechanism and mechanisms of airway protection which may permit aspiration and/or development of pulmonary infection, disordered or depressed control of respiration associated with ineffective patterns of ventilation, and alterations in the level of consciousness which impair the patient's ability to actively promote his own bronchial hygiene.

Techniques of chest physical therapy are administered in order to prevent the development of respiratory infection, atelectasis, or retained secretions; to treat these problems if they occur; and to promote not only maximum strength but also maximum efficiency of the respiratory muscular apparatus and cough mechanism. The importance of instructing the patient and his family, as well as developing home programs when indicated, cannot be overlooked.

Neuromuscular Disorders (Fig 19–14)

Several disorders of the neuromuscular system are associated with respiratory muscle weakness or paralysis. In many instances, although the neuropathology of disease is understood, the cause is unknown. The course of the specific diseases varies, and in many the symptoms of bulbar involvement occur. Also, acute phases of these disease processes frequently require intensive supportive care until the neurologic symptoms subside. When the acute and recovery phases of polio are complete, the patient is left with residual paralysis, flaccidity and atrophy of the involved muscles resulting from the destruction of anterior horn cells of the spinal cord. Guillain-Barré syndrome is characterized by ascending paralysis that progresses generally in a distal to proximal direction, often including respiratory and bulbar musculature. Gradual, though almost complete recovery of motor function usually occurs as the myelin of nerve roots and peripheral nerves regenerates. A similar pattern of neurologic dysfunction may be seen in acute intermittent porphyria, a derangement of porphyrin metabolism. Recurrence of the two previously mentioned diseases sometimes occurs. Amyotrophic lateral sclerosis, on the other hand, is a devastating disease in which paralysis is progressive, irreversible and rapidly fatal. The rationale for institution of supportive measures, and especially those of assisted ventilation, when these patients become completely helpless poses philosophical questions for some and remains a controversial issue. The lesions of multiple sclerosis are characterized by demyelination and subsequent degeneration and scarring of white matter of the brain and spinal cord. Symptoms and manifestations are variable; the disease is chronic, slowly or rapidly progressive and typified by exacerbations and

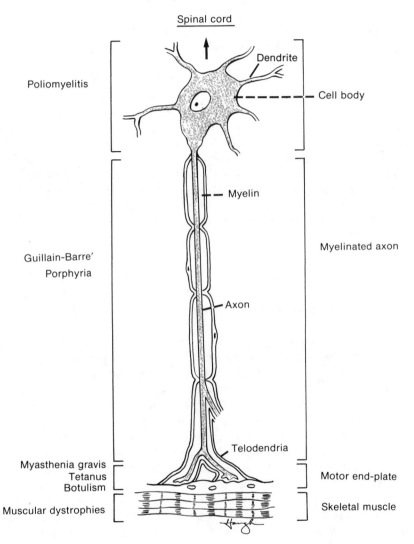

Multiple sclerosis

Amyotrophic lateral sclerosis

Spinal cord

Poliomyelitis

Dendrite

Cell body

Myelin

Guillain-Barre'
Porphyria

Myelinated axon

Axon

Telodendria

Myasthenia gravis
Tetanus
Botulism

Motor end-plate

Muscular dystrophies

Skeletal muscle

FIG 19–14.

Diagram of motor neuron indicating the site of involvement in some diseases affecting the
neuromuscular system.

remissions. Motor dysfunction, sensory disturbances and symptoms of bulbar involvement are common. The rigidity of muscles and poverty of movement seen in Parkinson's disease occur as a result of degeneration of brain structures. Myasthenia gravis, which is believed to be caused by some disturbance of transmission of nervous impulses at the motor end plate, is characterized by extreme fatigability of muscles, especially those of the eyelids, jaws, face, neck and trunk. Involvement of respiratory and bulbar muscles as a result of either myasthenic or cholinergic crises often causes respiratory failure requiring mechanical support of ventilation. Tetanus and botulism are caused by toxic agents which may also interfere with the transmission of impulses at the myoneural junction. Whereas botulism poisoning can cause generalized flaccid paralysis, tetanus is characterized by generalized rigidity and severe spasms of the body musculature. Finally, paralysis resulting from the primary degeneration and subsequent fatty infiltration of muscle typical of the muscular dystrophies may be rapidly or slowly progressive; the central nervous system and peripheral nerves, however, remain intact.

Clinical Considerations

It is not unusual for the patient suffering from neuromuscular weakness to be admitted to the hospital because the development of an upper respiratory infection, which to us may pose only the discomforts of the common cold, causes serious respiratory distress, difficulty mobilizing secretions and the possible development of pneumonia. An aggressive program of postural drainage, percussion and vibration preceded by aerosol therapy, given in conjunction with or following intermittent positive pressure breathing, might prevent the development of respiratory failure. The aerosol will help to liquefy secretions. Breathing exercises may be performed while the patient is positioned for postural drainage. Although this method might seem somewhat complicated, a variety of techniques are integrated rather than administered one by one in an attempt to effectively mobilize secretions without causing unnecessary fatigue in an already tired patient. Manual pressure applied over the abdomen or sternum and upper abdomen may also help to improve the effectiveness of the cough in a patient with weak abdominal muscles. As the patient's condition improves, the focus of attention might be redirected to emphasize strengthening and more effective use of the respiratory musculature and improvement of the cough. Finally, as soon as possible before discharge, a home program of exercise and bronchial hygiene may be taught to both patient and family in order to prevent the development of recurrent pulmonary infection.

Chest physical therapy treatment of the patient requiring mechanical ventilation (see Chapter 26) should at the very least include positional rotations to prevent microatelectasis and accumulation of secretions resulting from constant volume ventilation, as well as from interference with the normal mucus clearance mechanism, upper airway and cough. Postural drainage, percussion and vibration may be administered prophylactically or therapeutically. These patients are often managed in intensive care units where unified care requiring the cooperative effort of nurses and therapists is essential. Coordination of treatment with nursing activities (i.e., while the patient is on his side, sheets are changed and treatment is given) is sometimes helpful. Breathing exercises for strengthening respiratory musculature as the patient is nearing discontinuance from the ventilator, as well as ambulation with a hand ventilator when possible, may be utilized to improve general and respiratory muscle strength during appropriate phases of weaning (see Chapter 26).

Cervical Spinal Cord Injury
Patients suffering from traumatic section of the cervical spinal cord require aggressive supportive care during the initial period following injury. During this phase of spinal shock, all reflex, motor, sensory and autonomic function is lost below the level of the lesion. Often the loss of intercostal muscle action even if the diaphragm and accessory muscles are functioning, combined with the loss of abdominal muscle power necessary for effective coughing, causes severe respiratory embarrassment. Even if the patient is immobilized on a special bed or frame and/or cervical traction is in place, postural drainage, percussion and vibration can be administered. Many of these devices can be placed in head-up and head-down positions. If the patient is in traction and treatment is to be administered in a head-down position, countertraction may be applied to the lower extremities. Care should be taken to prevent sudden jarring of the weights or resting of the weights on the floor. The patient who has undergone decompressive laminectomy, anterior spinal fusion or posterior spinal fusion should be log rolled—care being taken to avoid the neck and shoulders during the application of percussion techniques, or vigorous tugging on the upper rib cage during vibration. In addition, after decompressive laminectomy or posterior cervical fusion, treatment should not be administered in the head-down position. Breathing exercises should be initiated early and are often best performed in a flat or head-down position as this places

the diaphragm at a mechanical advantage during inspiration if the abdominal muscles lack tone and allows the weight of the abdominal contents to push against the diaphragm during expiration. Early and progressive cough instruction is important in order to teach the patient how to effectively clear his secretions. Many patients fear that they will choke and need our instruction and encouragement. Deep breathing and breath holding followed by huffing may help to optimize high-velocity airflow during expiration in order to compensate for a weak cough. When the patient is up in a chair, application of an abdominal binder can partially compensate for a loss of abdominal tone, place the diaphragm in a more normal resting position and facilitate the return of venous blood to the heart. It is important that the binder remain beneath the lower margins of the ribs so that chest expansion is not restricted.

The primary goal of comprehensive treatment of the quadriparetic patient is to restore him to an optimal level of function. It is a long process, often requiring admission to a rehabilitation facility, which in many instances takes anywhere from 6 to 12 months. Patients who are left with marked residual paralysis of respiratory muscles may require intermittent or continuous support of ventilation using positive pressure breathing devices, cuirasses or electrophrenic stimulators. If they continue to experience difficulty mobilizing secretions, their families should be taught home programs of bronchial hygiene designed to meet the individual needs of the patient.

Central Nervous System Depression

In contrast to the patient who may be alert yet unable to deep breathe and cough effectively because of neuromuscular weakness, the patient who exhibits central nervous system depression may possess normal strength of respiratory muscles but disordered function of their controls. In further contrast, while the patient after abdominal or thoracic surgery may deep breathe and cough poorly because he is splinting due to pain or is depressed by pain medication (especially narcotics), the patient suffering from brain tumor, brain infection, cerebrovascular or hemorrhagic insult (thrombosis, embolus, subarachnoid hemorrhage, subdural or epidural hematoma) or recent neurologic surgery (craniotomy) usually experiences no pain but is depressed as a result of the intracranial process.

Clinical Considerations

The period coinciding with and following intracranial insult as well as that following neurologic surgery is one in which patency of the airway, adequate oxygenation of the brain, protection of the airway and mobilization and removal of secretions are essential. Many of these patients are unconscious or obtunded, exhibiting depressed protective airway reflexes, depressed cough and ineffective patterns of ventilation. Some patients will cough spontaneously but fail to do so on command, many require suction for removal of secretions, others require intubation or tracheostomy and suction until they can protect their airways, and still others require ventilatory support. Positional rotations as well as postural drainage, percussion and vibration can usually be administered in modified positions (flat bed), except after craniotomy surgery when the patient's head is elevated in order to reduce cerebral edema by increasing the venous return of blood to the heart. Stretch applied to the rib cage immediately preceding inspiration may facilitate deep inspiration even in the comatose patient, perhaps as a result of increased sensory input or increased reflex activity. The patient who is arousable but lethargic may respond more appropriately to the stimulation of firm pressure applied to the chest than to verbal commands; manual sensory stimulation timed with simple commands or the therapist's sounds of deep breathing are sometimes helpful. If a patient becomes agitated when percussion is being administered, a slower rate of percussion may be better tolerated; if not, percussion should be discontinued. The patient who is having a seizure should not be treated until seizure activity is controlled. Also, during the administration of treatment to the patient with hydrocephalus, care should be taken to avoid applying pressure to areas where shunt tubing is located. Finally, whenever there are questions concerning contraindications or precautions to be taken during the administration of treatment, therapists should not hesitate to consult with the physician in order to provide the most appropriate therapy for each individual patient.

SUMMARY

The various techniques of chest physical therapy utilized during the acute phase in the treatment of the neurologically impaired patient are no different from those that other types of patients receive. An understanding, however, of the causes and effects of neurologic dysfunction should help us to become more aware of the respiratory problems that these people so frequently exhibit. Prophylactic, therapeutic and rehabilitative programs based on evaluation results and utilizing appropriate respiratory therapy modalities when indicated will enable us to administer comprehensive therapy contributing to the needs of the total patient.

REFERENCES

Periodicals

Alvarez SE, Peterson M, Lansford BR: Respiratory treatment of the adult patient with spinal cord injury. *Phys Ther* 1981; 61(12)1737–1745.

Bellamy D, et al: A case of primary alveolar hypoventilation associated with mild proximal myopathy. *Am Rev Respir Dis* 1975; 112:867.

Bethune DA: Neurophysiological facilitation of respiration in the unconscious adult patient. *Physiotherapy (Canada)* 1975; 27:241.

Campbell RL: Electrophrenic respiration. *Respir Care* 1976; 21:846.

Chopra SK, Taplin GV, Simmons DH, et al: Effects of hydration and physical therapy on tracheal transport velocity. *Am Rev Respir Dis* 1977; 115(6)1009–1014.

Christensen MS, Kristensen HS, Hansen EL: Artificial hyperventilation during 21 years in three cases of complete respiratory paralysis. *Acta Med Scand* 1975; 198:409.

Dail CW: Respiratory aspects of rehabilitation in neuromuscular conditions. *Arch Phys Med Rehabil* 1965; 46:655.

Elam JO, et al: Impairment of pulmonary function in poliomyelitis. *Arch Intern Med* 1948; 81:649.

Greene W, L'Heureux P, Hunt C: Paralysis of the diaphragm. *Am J Dis Child* 1975; 129:1402.

Haas A, et al: Respiratory function in hemiplegic patients. *Arch Phys Med Rehabil* 1967; 48:174.

Lane DJ, Hazelman B, Nichols PJR: Late onset respiratory failure in patients with previous poliomyelitis. *Q J Med* 1974; 172:551.

North JB, Jennett S: Abnormal breathing patterns associated with acute brain damage. *Arch Neurol* 1974; 31:338.

Radecki LL, Tomatis LA: Continuous bilateral electrophrenic pacing in an infant with total diaphragmatic paralysis. *J Pediatr* 1976; 88:969.

Trout CA: Preventing the need for mechanical ventilation. *Respir Care* 1976; 21:526.

Watson CA, Ross JE, Ramsey M: Identification of neurosurgical patients susceptible to pulmonary infection. *J Neurosurg Nurs* 1984; 16(3):123–127.

Books

Adams RD: *Diseases of Muscle, A Study in Pathology*, ed 2. New York, Harper & Row, 1975.

Applebaum EL, Bruce DL: *Tracheal Intubation*. Philadelphia, WB Saunders Co, 1976.

Bendixen HH, et al: *Respiratory Care*. St Louis, CV Mosby Co, 1965.

Blackwood W, Corsellis JAN (eds): *Greenfield's Neuropathology*, ed 3. London, Edward Arnold Publishers, Ltd, 1976.

Bushnell SS, et al: *Respiratory Intensive Care Nursing*. Boston, Little, Brown & Co, 1973.

Carpenter MC: *Core Text of Neuroanatomy.* Baltimore, Williams & Wilkins Co, 1972.

Cash JE (ed): *Chest, Heart and Vascular Disorders for Physiotherapists.* London, Faber and Faber, 1975.

Cherniack RM, et al: *Respiration in Health and Disease,* ed 2. Philadelphia, WB Saunders Co, 1972.

Chusid JG: *Correlative Neuroanatomy and Functional Neurology,* ed 16. Los Altos, California, Lange Medical Publications, 1976.

Comroe JH, Jr, et al: *The Lung,* ed 2. Chicago, Year Book Medical Publishers, 1962.

Cooper JS: *Living With Chronic Neurologic Disease.* New York, WW Norton and Co, 1976.

Elliott FA: *Clinical Neurology,* ed 2. Philadelphia, WB Saunders Co, 1971.

Epstein BS: *The Spine: A Ratiological Text and Atlas,* ed 4. Philadelphia, Lea & Febiger, 1976.

Ganong WF: *Review of Medical Physiology,* ed 7. Los Altos, California, Lange Medical Publications, 1975.

Gilroy JSM: *Medical Neurology,* ed 2. New York, Macmillan Publishing Co, 1975.

Grant JCB: *Atlas of Anatomy,* ed 5. Baltimore, Williams & Wilkins Co, 1962.

Grinker RR, Sahs AL: *Neurology* ed 6. Springfield, Illinois, Charles C Thomas, Publisher, 1966.

Guttman L: *Spinal Cord Injuries,* ed 3. Oxford, Blackwell Scientific Publications, 1976.

Guyton AC: *Textbook of Medical Physiology,* ed 5. Philadelphia, WB Saunders Co, 1976.

Hedley-Whyte J, et al: *Applied Physiology of Respiratory Care.* Boston, Little, Brown & Co, 1976.

Hightower NC, Janowitz HD (eds): Digestion, in Brobeck JR (ed): *Best and Taylors Physiological Basis of Medical Practice,* ed 9. Baltimore, Williams & Wilkins Co, 1973.

Hirschberg GG, Lewis L, Thomas D: *Rehabilitation.* Philadelphia, JB Lippincott Co, 1964.

Hislop HJ, Sanger JO (eds): *Chest Disorders in Children.* Washington DC, American Physical Therapy Association, 1968.

Hutchinson EC, Acheson EJ: *Strokes, Natural History, Pathology, and Surgical Treatment.* London, WB Saunders Co, 1975.

Lockhart RD, Hamilton GF, Fyfe FW: *Anatomy of the Human Body.* Philadelphia, JB Lippincott Co, 1959.

Matzke HA, Foltz FM: *Synopsis of Neuroanatomy,* ed 2. New York, Oxford University Press, 1972.

Merritt HH: *Textbook of Neurology,* ed 5. Philadelphia, Lea & Febiger, 1973.

Murray JF: *The Normal Lung.* Philadelphia, WB Saunders Co, 1976.

Needham CW: *Neurosurgical Syndromes of the Brain.* Springfield, Illinois, Charles C Thomas, Publisher, 1973.

Petty TL, et al: *Intensive and Rehabilitative Respiratory Care,* ed 2. Philadelphia, Lea & Febiger, 1974.

Rothman RH, Simeone FA (eds): *The Spine,* vols I and II. Philadelphia, WB Saunders Co, 1975.

Shapiro BA, Harrison RA, Trout CA: *Clinical Application of Respiratory Care.* Chicago, Year Book Medical Publishers, 1975.

Shapiro BA, Harrison RA, Walton JR: *Clinical Application of Blood Gases,* ed 2. Chicago, Year Book Medical Publishers, 1977.

Slager VT: *Basic Neuropathology.* Baltimore, Williams & Wilkins Co, 1970.

Thorn GW, et al (eds): *Principles of Internal Medicine,* ed 8. New York, McGraw-Hill Book Co, 1977.

Vick NA: *Grinker's Neurology,* ed 7. Springfield, Illinois, Charles C Thomas, Publisher, 1976.

Wechsler IS: *Clinical Neurology,* ed 9. Philadelphia, WB Saunders Co, 1963.

West JB; *Respiratory Physiology—The Essentials.* Baltimore, Williams & Wilkins Co, 1974.

Whisler WW: The neurosurgical patient, in Goldin MD (ed): *Intensive Care of the Surgical Patient.* Chicago, Year Book Medical Publishers, 1971.

Youmans WB, Siebens AA (eds): Respiration, in Brobeck JR (ed): *Best and Taylors Physiological Basis of Medical Practice,* ed 9. Baltimore, Williams & Wilkins Co, 1973.

Youmans JR (ed): *Neurological Surgery,* vols 1–3. Philadelphia, WB Saunders Co, 1973.

Young JA, Crocker D (eds): *Principles and Practice of Respiratory Therapy,* ed 2. Chicago, Year Book Medical Publishers, 1976.

20

Respiratory Rehabilitation Secondary to Neurological Deficits: Understanding the Deficits

Mary Massery, P.T.

It is often observed in a rehabilitation setting that patients with neurological deficits continue to acquire respiratory problems long after their acute phase has subsided. Research has repeatedly documented a decrease in pulmonary function for the chronic neurologically impaired patient, yet many therapists do not appear to fully comprehend why this occurs. This section will try to elaborate the causes of respiratory complications secondary to neurological deficits (Chapter 20) and what clinicians can do to minimize or eliminate these complications (Chapters 21 and 22). The focus of this treatment approach is primarily aimed at the physical therapist. Every effort was made to explain specific physical therapy (PT) concepts so that all clinicians, respiratory therapists (RRT), and nurses (RN) included could benefit from the ideas presented.

DIAGNOSES ADDRESSED

The following primary diagnoses will be covered in this section: spinal cord injuries (SCI), head traumas, cerebral vascular accidents (CVA), multiple sclerosis (MS), amyotrophic lateral sclerosis (ALS), Parkinson's, cerebral palsy (CP), muscular dystrophy (MD), poliomyelitis (polio), spina bifida, and neuropathies. However, it is by no means an exhaustive list. The primary consideration for application of these treatment techniques is the residual physical deficits left by a neurological insult. Therefore, a patient presenting with hemiplegia will be treated with hemiplegic techniques, regardless of how the original deficit was acquired (from a CVA, head trauma, or CP, etc.). Likewise, quadriplegia or paraplegia not only refers to patients that have suffered from SCIs, but any patient that presents with quadriplegic or paraplegic deficits.

However, three aspects of neurological disorders must be clarified here, to assist the therapist in discerning which techniques, described later, are appropriate for his or her particular patient. They are (1) progressive vs. nonprogressive injuries, (2) cerebral vs. noncerebral injuries, and (3) rehabilitation vs. habilitation. Single insult injuries, such as SCIs, head traumas, CVAs, or CPs, are nonprogressive. The damage was only once inflicted and does not repeat itself. Progressive diseases, on the other hand, such as MS, ALS, Parkinson's, or MD, show increasing neurological deficits over time. Goals for these groups will be different, with maximal respiratory functioning stressed for the single insult diagnoses, and comfort and ease of respiration stressed for progressive diagnoses. Similar treatment consideration is given for patients with detrimentally affected cerebral functioning, such as with head traumas, CVAs, and Parkinson's, versus those whose deficits are at the spinal level, such as with SCIs, neuropathies, myopathies, and polio. Patients with only spinal involvement may respond favorably to complex techniques and demonstrate better conscious carryover, whereas those with impaired cerebral functioning may respond better to techniques that act primarily upon the subconscious and require little cognitive participation. Finally, the difference between rehabilitation and habilitation must be understood. Rehabilitation involves restoring function, habilitation teaches functioning for the first time. Children with acquired deficits in utero or shortly after birth have never experienced normal movement patterns. Therefore, they cannot depend on the memory of past experiences to help correct abnormal patterns as the adults going through rehabilitation can. This important difference must be accounted for when developing their treatment programs.

PLANES OF RESPIRATION

Before specific treatment techniques and progressions can be discussed, an understanding of what affects the chest walls, thereby affecting respiratory functioning, is critical. This treatment approach is based on the premise that respiration does not take place in a one-dimensional plane, but rather as a three-dimensional activity. It expands in an anterior-posterior plane, an inferior-superior plane, and a lateral plane (Fig 20–1). Too often, therapists treat patients with neurologic dysfunctions with apparent disregard for this extremely important fact. This one-dimensional fallacy has been perpetrated by techniques documented and taught to new therapists that limit the patient's breathing program to one or two postures (supine and sitting). Few approaches were found in the literature that deals with the chest as a three-dimensional object (other than for postural drainage). We must therefore change our perspective of the chest and lungs when determining treatment protocol in order to become more effective. The forces that act upon the chest walls will be detailed first.

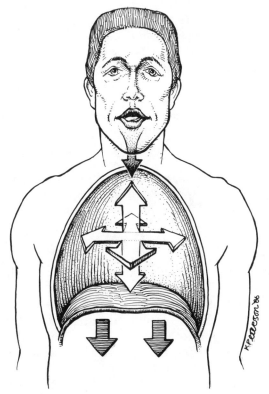

FIG 20–1.
Planes of respiration (anterior-posterior, inferior-superior, and lateral).

EFFECTS OF GRAVITY

If chest expansion takes place in three planes, the effect of gravity upon these planes must be considered. Physical therapists would not exercise a weak muscle without taking into account the effect of gravitational pull on that muscle, thereby making the positioning of the limb in space an important consideration in treatment planning. How many times is the same consideration given for the weakened respiratory muscles? Gravity can assist, resist, or have no effect on the movement of the chest wall, according to the chest's position in space. Consider weakened intercostal muscles. Placing a patient with this deficit in a supine position for initial treatment in his rehabilitation program and then asking the patient to "breathe up into your hands" is asking the patient to attempt the most difficult gravitational posture first (breathing into the anterior plane with gravity resisting the movement). It would seem more appropriate to start retraining techniques in a gravity-eliminated posture, such as sidelying, or a gravity-assisted posture such as hands-knees, and then progress to gravity-resisted postures such as supine. In view of this, we will examine the planes of respiration and the effects of gravity upon these planes in all treatment techniques discussed in this section.

Gravity will also affect the positioning of the intestines under the diaphragm. In the "normal," neurologically intact person, this seems to have a minor effect on respiratory functioning. However, for many neurologically impaired persons with a marked loss in abdominal tone (many SCIs or Guillian Barré), intestinal positioning becomes an important factor in their respiratory functioning.

The abdominal wall acts as the anterior support for the intestines, causing the intestines to sit high in the abdominal cavity. This forces the diaphragm to rest high, at approximately the level of the fifth rib in an erect posture (Fig 20–2). The diaphragm contracts, drawing its origins toward its insertion (concentric contraction). These muscle fibers, which originate down as low as the 10th rib, must rise up superiorly and then medially toward the central tendon (see Chapter 1—bucket-handle effect). This movement pattern provides anterior and lateral expansion of the lower chest. This is generally of about 2–4 inches when measured around the chest at the xiphoid process during maximal inspiration. Without abdominal wall support, the intestines shift inferiorly and anteriorly, the "beer-belly" effect, allowing gravity to position the diaphragm lower in the abdominal cavity (see Fig 20–2). This puts the diaphragm at an extreme mechanical disadvantage.

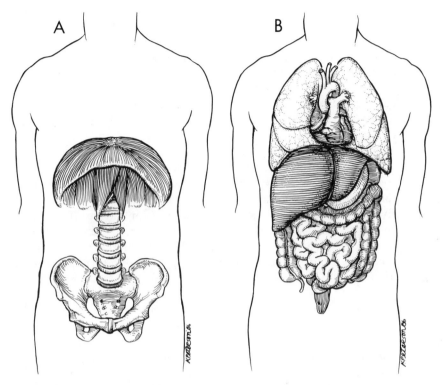

FIG 20–2.
Proper mechanical positioning of the diaphragm relative to the abdominal viscera. Note the high dome shape of the diaphragm.

Instead of having to rise up and over the intestines, the lateral fibers of the diaphragm can now move more horizontally to reach the central tendon, thereby significantly reducing excursion in both the lower anterior and lateral planes of expansion. This adverse positioning may be so significant as to cause a negative lower chest expansion upon inspiration for patients with quadriplegia. Quantitatively, this may be seen as a ½- to 1-inch decrease in lower chest expansion, again measured at the xiphoid process, when the patient proceeds from maximal expiration to maximal inspiration. Thus, the net difference in chest expansion pre- and postneurological injury could potentially be up to 4–5 inches.

Since gravity causes the intestines to shift, the effect on the diaphragm will be most dramatic in a gravity-dependent position such as sitting or standing, rather than in a gravity-eliminated position such as supine. Thus, the importance of providing the patient with an external abdominal wall support in these upright postures should be undeniably clear. Although not as effective as the abdominal muscles themselves, abdominal supports help restore the natural mechanical advantage of the diaphragm. Specific types and placements of abdominal supports will be covered in Chapter 21.

In addition to changing muscle effectiveness, gravity will also affect bony structures. Obviously, this will affect a growing child more so than a fully developed adult, but both will be affected. Since bones grow according to stress laid upon them, abnormal stresses will produce abnormal bony developments. This is the case for the person with severe neurological deficits. Gravity becomes the main force acting upon the bones and joints, unopposed by normal muscle action. This can result in many skeletal deformities such as, flattening or flaring of the anterior rib cage, narrowing of the upper chest, loss of normal spinal curves, and chest cavus deformities. Prevention of these deformities, rather than their cure, must be the aim of a good long-term respiratory program for the neurologically impaired.

GRAVITY: EFFECTS ON DEVELOPING CHESTS

Thus far, the effects of gravity on the planes of respiration, muscles, performance, and bony changes in the adult have been discussed. This same force, gravity, plays an extremely crucial role in the skeletal development of the chest in the newborn. "Normal," neurologically intact infants move freely in and out of postures, such as prone, hands-knees, standing, etc., as they progress developmentally, allowing gravity to alternately assist or resist the movements. Through this, the infant begins to strengthen and develop muscle groups and learn to interact with the gravitational force in his environment.

This combination of normal movement patterns in a gravity field accounts for the normal development of the bones, muscles, and joints that comprise the chest wall. Conversely, infants with severe neurological impairments do not have that same freedom of movement within their environments. This applies to children with congenital deficits, such as CP, MD, or spina bifida, or for children who acquire deficits at an early developmental age, such as some CVAs, head traumas, or SCIs. These children become subjugated to the effects of gravity upon their growing and developing bodies because they are unable to independently counteract its constant presence. A variety of reasons may account for their inability to change their own positions in space: (1)

muscle weakness, (2) tonal problems (e.g., spasticity, flaccidity), (3) reflex dominance, (4) incoordination, or a combination of the above. Typically, these children spend significantly more time in supine than in any other posture, which can lead to undesirable changes in the thorax.

Understanding the basic steps and principles in normal chest development is essential for accurately assessing abnormal chest deformities often seen in this handicapped population. Initially, the newborn's chest is triangular in shape, narrow and flat in the upper portion, and wider and more rounded in the lower portion (Fig 20–3). The neck accessory muscles are too weak and unable to assume the necessary position to assist in respiration, and the infant's arms are held in flexion across the chest, significantly hampering movement of the upper chest. This all points to underdevelopment of the upper chest region in the newborn. The infant, being a diaphragmatic breather, shows greater development of the lower chest; hence, the triangular shape of the rib cage.

As children develop, they begin to reach out into their environment with their upper extremities, which begins the development of

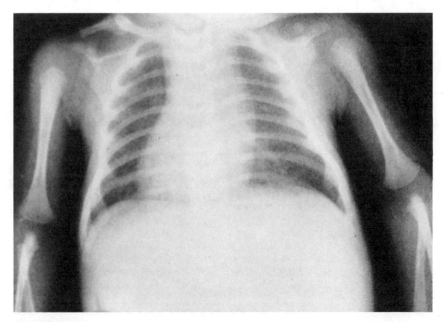

FIG 20–3.
Newborn chest configuration. Note triangular shape.

the pectoralis region of the upper chest. This constant stretching on the anterior upper chest helps to expand the chest laterally. An increase in intercostal and pectoralis muscle strength improves the infant's ability to counteract the force of gravity upon the anterior upper chest in supine, leading to the development of a slight convex configuration of the area. In addition, the development of the child's neck musculature provides the upper chest with a stable base in which to operate the upper chest accessory muscles (primarily the sternocleidomastoid, scalenes, and trapezius muscles) to aid the development of a more rectangular shape of the chest.

The next significant development occurs when the child begins to assume erect postures (e.g., sitting, kneeling, standing). Until this time, the ribs are aligned fairly horizontally, with narrow intercostal spacing. In fact, the newborn's chest only comprises approximately one third of the total trunk cavity. As the child begins to move up against the pull of gravity, the ribs rotate downward (primarily the lower ribs), creating the sharper angle of the ribs as seen in the adult (Fig 20–4). This markedly elongates the rib cage until it eventually occupies more than half of the trunk cavity (Table 20–1). A comparison of chest x-rays of the newborn and adult clearly show these developmental trends (see Figs 20–3 through 20–5).

Children with severe neurological deficits often show a very different picture of their chest development. Frequently, they do not develop adequate upper extremity and neck muscle control (e.g., weak muscles, tone problems, reflex dominance, or incoordination), causing their up-

TABLE 20–1.

Comparison of Infant and Adult Chests

CHEST	INFANT	ADULT
Size	Occupies one third of trunk cavity	Occupies half of trunk cavity
Shape	Triangular	Rectangular
Ribs	Evenly horizontal	Progressively more diagonal inferiorly
Intercostal spacing	Narrow	Wider
Upper chest	Narrow apex, flattened anterior	Squarer apex, rounded anterior
Lower chest	Very round, wide	Flatter than infant, width consistent with upper chest
Diaphragm	Adequate, less domed	Adequate, domed
Accessory muscles	Inadequate	Adequate

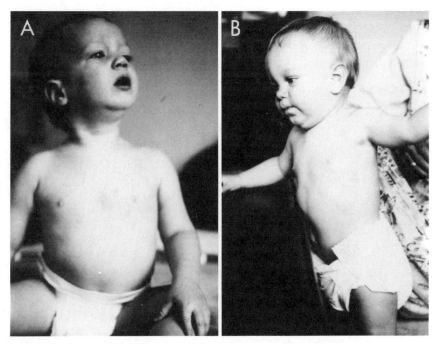

FIG 20–4.
A and **B,** ten-month-old infant chest configuration. Note shape of chest changes and angle of ribs.

per chests to retain the more primitive triangular, flattened shape. Inadequate muscle control also renders their accessory muscles less able to assist if needed in respiration. In some cases, the child's diaphragm remains so strong and unbalanced by other accessory muscles that it creates a cavus deformity at the sternum (Fig 20–6). This occurs when the intercostal muscles are incapable of maintaining the anterior chest wall's position against gravity and the abdominal muscles are weak or flaccid. This may also eventually cause an anterior flaring of the lower ribs.

Most of these children with severe impairments require significant assistance to maintain an upright posture; therefore, they are often left in a recumbent position. Thus, the rib cage shows less downward rotation and elongation than that of the normally developing child. In some cases of prolonged supine posturing, the chest will become flattened anteriorly and the lower ribs will flare laterally (Fig 20–7). These changes occur in response to the child's primary breathing pattern in his primary posture (here being supine). These children breathe into

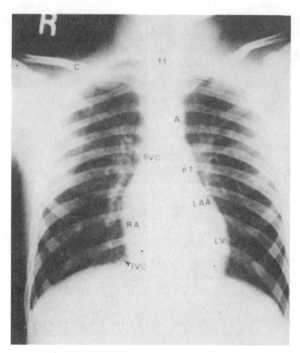

FIG 20–5.
Normal adult chest x-ray. Chest shape is rectangular, ribs angled downward, upper and lower chest equally developed.

the lateral plane of respiration because gravity's force is eliminated, whereas breathing into the anterior plane would require antigravity muscle strength.

As long as the neurological deficits are present, these children will never develop normally. However, frequent position changes, inhibition of abnormal tone, facilitation of their weakened chest muscles, and promotion of coordinated breathing patterns are important factors in stimulating "normal" chest development. Optimum respiratory function cannot be expected from a severely underdeveloped chest.

MUSCULAR AND TONAL INFLUENCES ON THE CHEST

Adverse effects of gravity are counteracted by functioning musculature. Recall that inspiration/expiration occurs due to pressure gradients between the air outside the lungs and the air inside. These gradients

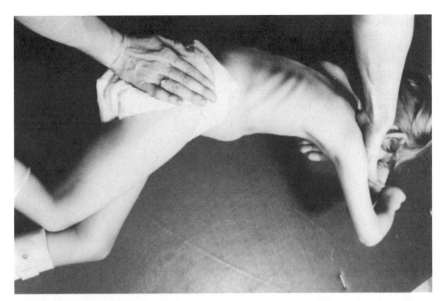

FIG 20–11.
Intercostal retraction.

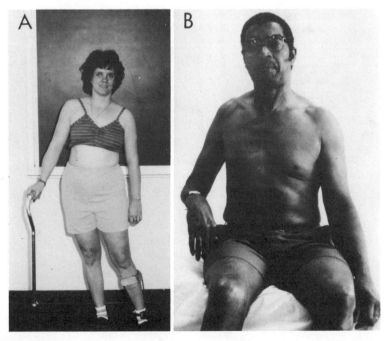

FIG 20–12.
A and **B,** patients with hemiplegia. Note asymmetry of trunk.

are achieved through movements in the chest walls. Muscle contractions provide the "power" to move these walls. If these muscles do not overcome the effect of gravity because of weakness, paralysis, abnormal tone, or inadequate muscle control, the chest will be unable to expand in all three planes of respiration, thus limiting pulmonary function. Because of this important fact, all muscles originating or inserting into the chest wall become "respiratory muscles." Table 20–2 lists these muscles with how they affect chest expansion and other specific respiratory function. They are listed from the lowest neurologic level of

TABLE 20–2.

Specific Function of Respiratory Muscles

Abdominal muscles
1. Innervation T_5–T_{12}
2. Builds up intrathoracic pressure
3. Needed for efficient cough
4. Needed for proper viscera placement under diaphragm
Intercostal muscles
1. Innervation T_{1-12}
2. Provides anterior and lateral expansion of upper and lower chest
Pectoralis muscles
1. Innervation C_5–T_1
2. Provides upper chest anterior expansion
3. Assists in development of rectangular shape of chest from early triangular proportions
Serratus muscle
1. Innervation C_5–C_7
2. Provides posterior expansion when upper extremities are fixated
Scalenes muscles
1. Innervation C_3–C_8
2. Provides superior expansion
Diaphragm muscle
1. Innervation C_3–C_5
2. Provides inferior, lateral and anterior expansion
3. Major muscle of
    a. Passive respiration
    b. Effective coughing
4. Concentric contractions increase chest cavity size
5. Good eccentric control needed for
    a. Forced expiration
    b. Elongated phonation
Sternocleidomastoid (SCM) and trapezius muscles
1. Innervation CN XI and C_1–C_4
2. Provides superior expansion
Erector spinal muscles
1. Innervation C_1 and down
2. Provides spinal stability required for rib cage mobility

innervation (thoracic) to the highest (cervical). Impairment to any of these muscles may therefore result in respiratory deficits.

Another factor that will determine a muscle's effectiveness as a chest wall mover is neurologic tone in the muscle. Rigidity, or constant isometric contractions, as seen in some head traumas and Parkinson's, will render the chest immobile, severely limiting its ability to expand in any plane. Spasticity, more often to a lesser degree than rigidity, can render the chest immobile. Spasticity (e.g., SCI, CP, head trauma), is frequently activated by quick movement of the affected muscle area either actively or passively. A quick activity like coughing may activate this abnormal tone and work against the patient as he tries to produce an effective cough. The other extreme of abnormal muscle tone is flaccidity or lack of any tone. In this case, the muscle is entirely unable to move the chest walls or to counteract the effects of gravity (may be seen in SCI, CVA, MD, CP, head trauma, and advanced stages of ALS, MD, MS). Of the three types of abnormal tone, flaccidity is the most severely influenced by the effects of gravity.

At the same time, postural reflexes and their effect on muscle tone must be considered. For instance, the tonic Labrinthyne reflex (TLR) increases extensor tone when the person is supine and, conversely, increases flexor tone when the person is prone. For the neurologically intact person, these reflexes are integrated into all their movement patterns through childhood. This allows the child to freely move in and out of flexion or extension in either posture. This primitive reflex only shows its influence in physically stressful situations like lifting weights on a bar bell from a supine position. This is not the case with many persons with neurological impairments, especially those who have not yet gone through this integrative process (CP or any congenitally acquired deficits). For these patients, the primitive TLR stays a dominant force, interfering with their ability to move freely in supine and prone positions. Because of this, a child with CP with increased extensor tone will see an even greater increase in that abnormal tone if placed supine (TLR in supine increases extension). That will make it more difficult for the child to attempt any flexion phase of a breathing pattern in supine (coughing or exhalation). How often are these children left supine as the therapist teaches them altered breathing patterns? Abnormal muscle tone can significantly affect a neurologically impaired person's performance in a respiratory rehabilitation program. As the Bobaths (originators of the neurodevelopmental treatment philosophy) repeatedly state, you cannot superimpose normal movement on abnormal tone. Therefore, positioning of the patient, as well as tonal inhibitory or facilatory techniques, become of vital importance when developing a treatment plan for respiratory restoration.

SPECIFIC RESPIRATORY IMPAIRMENTS

The first half of this chapter discusses the forces that influence the functioning of the neurologically impaired chest. Understanding these forces will allow one to discern the impairments that will appear as a direct or indirect result of those neurological deficits. Decreased chest expansion, abnormal or inefficient breathing patterns, abnormal bony changes, decreased cough effectiveness, decreased coordination of breathing with functional activities, decreased ability to phonate, and decreased ability to self-maintain bronchial hygiene can all be direct results of severe neurological deficits. These specific impairments will be addressed now in detail.

DECREASED CHEST EXPANSION

Muscle weakness or abnormal tone, combined with the effects of gravity that were previously discussed, will serve to decrease the ability of the chest to expand in one or all three planes of respiration. Quantitatively, chest expansion can be measured by taking vital capacities readings and comparing them to the norms, or it can be measured by taking a lower chest measurement with a tape measure. Although both methods will give an objective measurement, neither technique can assess which planes of respiration are being compromised. Subjective assessments skills are needed to determine limiting factors. Table 20–3 gives detailed summaries of such assessments for persons with all levels of SCIs. These characteristics can be extrapolated to subjective chest assessments of other neurological disorders, especially where true neuromuscular weakness is present.

ABNORMAL BREATHING PATTERNS

Limitations in chest expansion will inevitably lead to changes in breathing patterns. Severely involved CVAs, head traumas, or end-stage MS, ALS, MD, or Parkinson's, may show severe abnormalities in their breathing patterns. This is most often due to changes in their CO_2 levels or insults to the respiratory center in the medulla causing patterns like Cheyne-Stokes to evolve. This chapter focuses on the neurologically involved persons that are capable of actively changing their breathing patterns rather than those that are so severely impaired that they are incapable of change (Table 20–4).

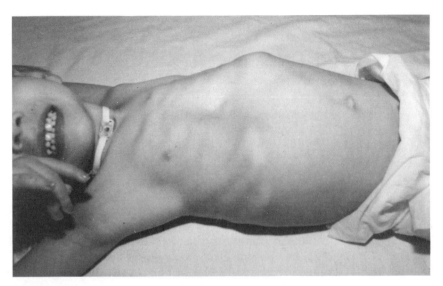

FIG 20–6.
Sternal cavus deformity (see text for explanation).

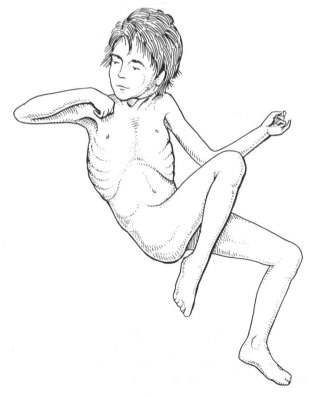

FIG 20–7.
Musculoskeletal changes secondary to static positioning and neurological deficit.

TABLE 20–4.
Common Abnormal Breathing Patterns

1. Paradoxical breathing patterns.
2. Diaphragmatic and upper accessory muscles breathing patterns.
3. Asymmetrical breathing patterns.
4. Lateral breathing patterns.
5. Shallow or asynchronous breathing patterns.

Most therapists have heard of paradoxical breathing, although many may not be aware that there are two types. The first is caused by a strong diaphragm in the absence of the intercostal muscles and other accessory muscles (polio, paraplegics, etc.). The diaphragm contracts causing the abdomen to rise, while the upper chest collapses without the assistance of the intercostal muscles (Fig 20–8). This type of paradoxical breathing, or see-saw breathing, is generally more pronounced in those persons with abdominal weakness or paralysis and in children. Without abdominal muscles, the patient will be unable to stop the strong descent of the diaphragm, thus exaggerating the see-saw action.

The second type of paradoxical breathing occurs when there is isolated diaphragm paralysis while the supportive accessory muscles are still intact. The see-saw action here is the opposite motion of that described above (Fig 20–9). In this case, the intercostal muscles contract, expanding the rib cage anteriorly, laterally, and primarily in the superior chest, while the abdominal muscles push up on the flaccid diaphragm to assist the intercostal muscles in achieving maximal chest expansion. There, the abdomen draws in during inspiration while the upper chest expands, instead of the lower abdomen expanding and the upper chest collapsing, as we saw in the intercostal paralysis. Unlike with intercostal paralysis, diaphragmatic paralysis will require some kind of assisted ventilation for at least some part of the day. This is because the diaphragm normally supplies 75%–80% of the total expansion necessary to provide adequate alveolar ventilation. Total accessory muscle breathing is inefficient and generally incapable of providing adequate long-term ventilation. The risk of respiratory muscle fatigue is greater in this pattern. Assisted ventilation is assuredly needed during sleep since conscious use of the accessory muscles is not possible.

Patients with intact diaphragms, absent intercostal and abdominal muscles, but intact upper accessory muscles, like paraplegics and spina bifida patients, try to counteract the strength of the diaphragmatic pull by using their sternocleidomastoid muscles in conjunction with the sca-

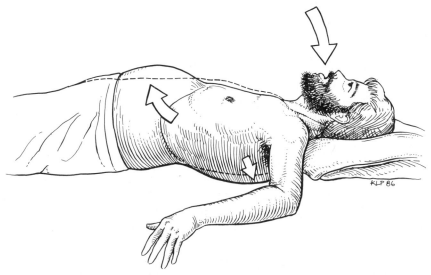

FIG 20–8.
Paradoxical breathing, strong diaphragm, absent accessory muscles.

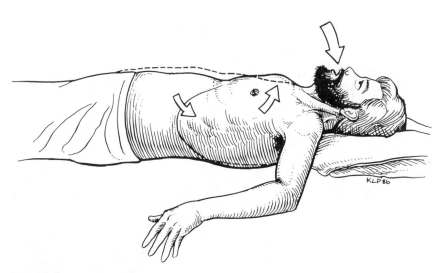

FIG 20–9.
Paradoxical breathing, diaphragm paralysis.

lenes and trapezius muscles (Fig 20–10). This allows superior expansion of their chest, thereby retaining some upper chest expansion. This must be cognitively coordinated with the inspiratory phase. On subjective breathing assessment, these patients present with shortened neck muscles, active and observable contractions of the accessory muscles during inspiration, and sometimes actual lifting of the head to provide a better mechanical advantage for the overworked neck muscles during inspiration. Intercostal retractions, or the collapsing of the intercostal spaces upon inspiration, will be seen here (Fig 20–11). The paralyzed intercostal muscle tissue will be sucked in toward the lungs during the creation of negative pressure within the chest, thus the observance of the retractions. This may be the most accurate way of assessing intercostal paralysis without an EMG test.

Neurological insults that affect the chest asymmetrically, such as CVAs and some head traumas, will show another type of breathing pattern abnormality. These patients can still actively expand their unaffected side in all three planes of respiration. Often, they accentuate this asymmetry to achieve more expansion on their unaffected side, by sidebending toward their involved side (Fig 20–12). This leads to in-

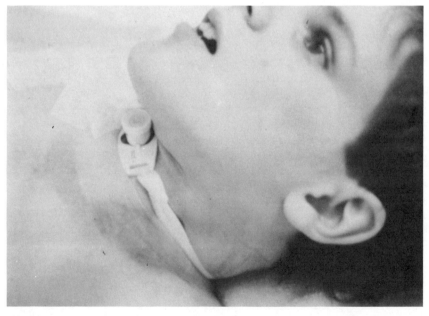

FIG 20–10.
Shortened neck musculature secondary to accessory muscle breathing pattern.

TABLE 20–3.

Spinal Cord Injured: Neuromuscular Effects on the Respiratory System

Paraplegics: as low as T$_{12}$
1. Weakened and/or absent abdominal, intercostal, and erector spinal muscles
2. Planes of respiration limited:
    a. Slight decrease in anterior expansion
    b. Slight decrease in lateral expansion
3. Will see:
    a. Decrease chest expansion
    b. Decrease vital capacity (VC)
    c. Decrease ability to build up intrathoracic pressure
    d. Decrease cough effectiveness
    e. May have paradoxical breathing pattern

Quadriplegic C$_5$–C$_8$
1. Missing aforementioned muscles and weakened:
    a. Pectoralis
    b. Serratus
    c. Scalenes
2. Planes of respiration limited:
    a. Marked decrease in anterior expansion, both upper and lower chest
    b. Marked decrease in lateral expansion
    c. Slight decrease in posterior expansion
3. Will see:
    a. Significant decrease in chest expansion with resulting decrease in VC
    b. Significant decrease in forced expiratory volume (FEV)
    c. Significant decrease in cough effectiveness
    d. Paradoxical breathing pattern in acute phase

Quadriplegics: C$_3$–C$_4$
1. Missing aforementioned muscles and show weakness in:
    a. Scalenes
    b. Diaphragm
2. Planes of respiration limited:
    a. Marked decrease in anterior expansion
    b. Marked decrease in lateral expansion
    c. Some cases: slight decrease in inferior expansion
3. Will see:
    a. As mentioned above
    b. Plus may have decrease in tidal volume (TV)

Quadriplegics: C$_1$–C$_2$
1. Missing aforementioned muscles and show weakness in last of accessory muscles available:
    a. SCM
    b. Trapezius
2. Planes of respiration limited:
    a. All limited severely
    b. Now show severe decrease in inferior and superior expansion
3. Will see:
    a. As mentioned above
    b. Plus significant decrease in TV
    c. Decrease in ability to maintain bronchial hygiene
    d. Lack of coordination of breathing with functional activities

adequate ventilation on the affected side which puts them at a higher risk of developing respiratory complications secondary to inadequate ventilation. In addition, the adverse effects on their posture can lead to undesired musculoskeletal changes over a prolonged period of time. Abnormal breathing patterns will take a greater toll on children than on adults because of their changing skeletons (see bony changes). Prevention of these secondary changes is of utmost importance.

Patients with generalized weakness, such as Guillain-Barré, some myopathies or neuropathies, or incomplete SCIs, may show a tendency toward "lateral breathing." That is, in supine, their weakened diaphragms and intercostal muscles cannot effectively oppose the force of gravity in the anterior plane, causing the chest to expand primarily in the lateral plane where gravity is eliminated. The plane of respiration used during breathing for these patients will vary according to posture, e.g., in sitting it would be inferior expansion, and in sidelying it would be anterior expansion. Overall, these patients have the best prognosis for effective breathing retraining methods because most of their neuromuscular system has at least partial innervation.

The last breathing pattern to be discussed involves patients with central nervous system deficits such as MS, Parkinson's, and some head traumas. Their breathing pattern is altered not so much by muscle weakness as it is by (1) chest immobility due to abnormally high neuromuscular tone (spasticity, rigidity, tremors) which severely limits chest expansion in any plane, (2) cerebellar incoordination, or (3) improper sequencing due to lesions in the brain, most commonly seen with medullary lesions. Breathing is usually symmetrical, shallow, sometimes asynchronous, and frequently tachypneic (respiratory rates over 25 breaths/minute). Initiation and follow-through of a volitional maximal inspiration becomes extremely difficult for these patients in the later stages of the progressive diseases. This will markedly curtail their ability to produce an effective cough and to maintain bronchial hygiene.

The patients described in this chapter frequently need to use their accessory muscles cognitively, to arrive at a work efficient, ventilation efficient, breathing pattern. Because of this, they should be considered for night-time ventilatory assistance. Muscle weakness or breathing inefficiency may cause a state of chronic hypoventilation during sleep. Drowsiness, lack of concentration, disturbed sleep, and/or irritability are common complaints of this state. In the clinical setting, we see many quadriplegic patients and other severely involved neurological patients who are lethargic after awakening. Hospital staff may incorrectly label these patients as lazy or uncooperative. It should be assessed whether this behavior is volitional or whether it is due to a state of hypoventilation and hypoxemia which may have developed overnight. Assessments can be made by taking blood gases during sleep or by screening high-risk patients for this disorder with an ear oximeter during sleep. Patients showing deficiencies should use night-time ventilatory assistance or be given adequate time upon awakening to cognitively restore proper O_2 saturation levels with altered breathing techniques. Rigorous exercising or ADL (activities of daily living) training may not be appropriately scheduled first thing in the morning for these patients.

CHANGES IN PULMONARY FUNCTIONS

The abnormal breathing patterns discussed above develop secondary to the patient's neurological deficits. However, those new patterns then change the patient's pulmonary function, which in turn affects their functional respiratory status. Specifically, changes in RR, TV, and VC will be addressed here.

Alveolar minute ventilation is the product of TV times RR. The optimal relationship between these two parameters is those values that result in minimizing the mechanical work that the lungs must perform in a particular breathing pattern. In other words, it is the combination of RR and TV that requires the body to put out the least muscular effort per breath. Because most of the abnormal breathing patterns that have been discussed here thus far reduce the patient's TV, the only recourse is to increase RR. Normal RR is between 12–20 breaths/minute; however, for this neurological population, it is not uncommon to see RRs at least twice that figure.

Although adjusting RR does bring the patient's respiratory system back to a state of equilibrium, it may not produce the most efficient pattern in the long run. The idea of the oxygen "cost" of breathing in that pattern must be considered in its long-term functional use. Ideally, TV at rest should be about 10% of one's actual VC. At this level, the "normal" person needs less than 5% of the total oxygen available to the body to operate the respiratory mechanisms. When performing a physical task or exercising, this oxygen consumption rate increases slowly, never quite reaching a point where the oxygen "cost" of operating the respiratory system outweighs the "cost" of performing the activity. However, for patients with impaired chest function, such as in this population, the total oxygen consumption level of the respiratory muscles at rest can be as much as 4–10 times that amount. These patients may have TV/VC ratios that are already in the 33%–67% range at rest, indicating inefficient breathing patterns, inadequate VCs, or both. When they attempt a mild exercise, they become quickly short of breath. They do not have adequate oxygen reserves to supply the respiratory and the nonrespiratory muscles simultaneously, thus severely limiting their exercise tolerance. Therefore, although these patients may show adequate maintenance of alveolar minute ventilation at rest, a mild increase in their activity level may magnify their respiratory insufficiencies.

An adequate VC is imperative in restoring a patient's functional status. Without the ability to expand the chest maximally under his own muscle power, VC will initially decrease. For example, studies show that quadriplegia resulting from SCIs may reduce the patient's VC to 33% of the predicted value, increasing the TV/VC ratio to 30%. For SCIs, an adequate VC is generally considered to be 66% of the expected value. This would restore the TV/VC ratio to approximately 15%, thus decreasing the work of breathing. If VC remains less than 60% of the predicted value, most research indicates that these patients will demonstrate inadequate coughs. Similarly, a FEV_1 less than 60% indicates lack of sufficient power behind the cough. When VC remains or decreases to only 25%–30% of the predicted norm, then ventilation assistance usually becomes necessary.

ABNORMAL BONY CHANGES

A change in breathing patterns may cause bony skeletal changes over a prolonged period of time. Earlier, discussion revolved around the adverse effects that gravity can play on the skeleton if the body is unable to counteract that force or is unable to contract the muscles that could balance that effect on the body. Pronounced deformities are more prevalent in children, of course, because of their cartilaginous state; however, both children and adults can show undesired musculoskeletal changes. Specifically, what changes do occur? A flattened anterior chest is perhaps the most common change in both the adult and child. Most frequently, this is due to prolonged supine positioning in conjunction with weakened or absent intercostal muscles, such as with quadriplegia (see Fig 20–7). In the presence of a strong, unopposed diaphragm, a cavus deformity of the sternum may also accompany the flattened chest. A variation may show the cavus deformity with anterior flaring of the lower rib cage due to the direct relationship between the ribs and diaphragmatic contractions (see Fig 20–6).

Upper chest abnormal bony changes occur when the intercostal and/or other accessory muscles that normally supply upper chest expansion are impaired. The diaphragm is not positioned to assist in expansion of this area. Therefore, without those accessory muscles, the anterior wall of the upper chest will become flattened and appear more narrow than that of the normal upper chest. Good shoulder, scapular, and pectoralis muscle functioning appears clinically to help maintain the stretch needed on the upper chest for maintenance of lateral expansion of that area. For adults, this means that their chests may revert back toward the more primitive triangular shape of the infant's chest, although never as markedly as in the child (Fig 20–13).

Spinal curves are not spared deformities. In a weakened, low tone patient, the common change is scoliosis since the patient cannot adequately maintain himself upright against gravity. Slowly, the spine collapses upon itself, seeking stability with the resultant scoliosis. All types of neurological diagnoses discussed in this chapter are at risk for developing this unwanted scoliosis. The second change, lumbar and thoracic kyphosis, is again due to the force of gravity upon a mobile supine. Secondary to the kyphoses, many patients develop a cervical lordosis. In sitting, the patient hunches over his trunk making eye con-

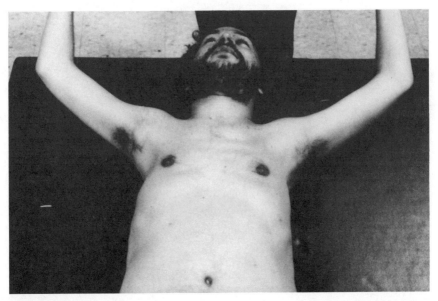

FIG 20–13.
Musculoskeletal changes in adult chest secondary to spinal cord injury (SCI). Note flattening of the anterior wall, and narrowing of the upper chest.

tact and head righting difficult (Fig 20–14). To compensate, they exaggerate the cervical lordosis with head protraction, thus regaining head posturing for establishing eye contact.

These spinal changes affect the functioning of the respiratory system adversely. With a kyphotic thorax in an upright posture, expansion of the chest in all three planes of respiration will be impaired. The ribs require a stable base from which to become properly mobilized. A kyphotic, weak spine does not provide the necessary stability for optimal rib functioning. Therefore, proper elevation and angulation of the ribs becomes impossible. This limits overall chest expansion.

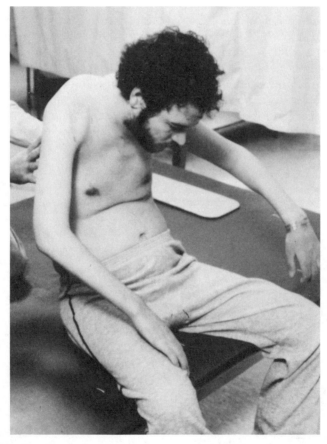

FIG 20–14.
Independent upright posturing. Adult patient with quadriplegia. Kyphosis restricts chest movement for respiration.

Musculoskeletal changes in children must be addressed. They are in a state of habilitation rather than rehabilitation. Because of this, the neurological deficit affects their chest formation more severely. Their rib cages remain more triangular in shape since the muscles of the upper chest never develop fully or normally. The ribs also remain more horizontal than in the normal adult, probably due to less upright posturing and lack of intercostal and abdominal muscle contractions upon their rib frames. Their necks and shoulders do not mature developmentally, often due to overuse of the neck acccessory muscles. This leads to a permanent shortening of the strap muscles, making the child appear to be without a "neck" (see Fig 20–7). Proper elongation of the cervical spine then cannot occur, resulting in skeletal changes to that area. Scoliosis, along with thoracic kyphosis, tend to be more pronounced here than in the adult. In very low toned children with a strong diaphragm but absent abdominal muscles, the intestines may not be positioned under the rib cage—the "beer belly" effect. These children have large protruding abdomens and a collapsed lower rib cage. It is most noticeable in sitting where the ribs appear to be cutting into the abdominal cavity, rather than resting over its contents (Fig 20–15). Breathing in this posture is severely impaired. To reiterate a common theme, prevention of these devastating deformities must be a top priority.

DECREASED COUGH EFFECTIVENESS

With decreased chest expansion, the presence of abnormal breathing patterns, and undesired bony changes, the patient's ability to cough effectively will be drastically reduced. Vital capacities will be impaired as will the ability to build up sufficient intra-abdominal pressure, especially for those patients with weakened, flaccid, or incoordinated abdominal musculature. Particularly for many head traumas, Parkinson's, CP, and CVA patients, their inability to coordinate an effective cough will be significant.

This inability may be due to cerebellar damage or to high neuromuscular tone (spasticity, rigidity, tremors). Frequently, the quick action required to produce an effective cough will be the same action that will trigger a sudden increase in the abnormal neuromuscular tone. Objectively, when the patient can not expel at least 60% of his actual vital capacity in one second (FEV_1), he will be incapable of producing an effective cough without some assistance or retraining.

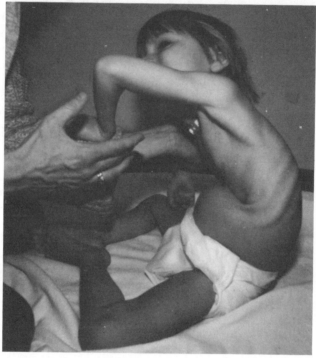

FIG 20–15.
Independent upright posturing in a patient with congenital quadriplegia. Note relationship of rib cage and abdominal viscera.

BREATHING COORDINATION IN ADL

Consistent with their inability to produce an effective cough, many patients with neurological deficits also demonstrate an inability to coordinate an altered breathing pattern with their everyday activities (ADL). Efficient breathing may be at a conscious level initially, impeding these patients from focusing on relearning other physical tasks. Clinically, this is seen when attempting to teach a patient a transfer technique or a new task that requires all of their effort and concentration. The patients may become extremely short of breath, not necessarily because the physical demands of the activity are too great, but rather their concentration on executing the new activity has reduced their ability to breathe at a conscious level. In this case, children, due to habilitation, have the definite advantage over adults, who must go through rehabilitation. The adult must unlearn patterns and then relearn the desired one before successfully integrating it into the subconscious. Children, however, have no ingrained cycles to break, making integration of more efficient breathing patterns into their ADL activities generally easier.

Consider the task of learning to ride a bicycle. Initially, it takes concentrated effort and physical work. Once the activity becomes a learned activity or integrated into the subconscious mind, riding becomes effortless, with most people even learning to converse while still pedaling or learning to ride "no-handed." Coordinating a new breathing pattern with ADL activities requires the same integrative process.

MAINTAINING BRONCHIAL HYGIENE

All these changes in respiratory functioning lead to a decreased ability of the neurologically impaired to independently maintain bronchial hygiene. Complete expansion of the chest in all three planes of respiration and in all postures is impaired, so their ability to properly aerate all portions freely, into and out of gravity, impairs their ability to perform independent bronchial drainage. Inefficient breathing patterns may cause them to remain in a state of chronic hypoventilation. Inability to produce an effective cough impairs their ability to clear their own lungs of secretions. Therefore, most of these patients will require some assistance, either physically or through verbal instruction, in order to maintain proper bronchial hygiene.

IMPAIRED PHONATION

Aphasia, as a secondary impairment to neurological deficits, is generally recognized by all members of the medical team as a serious problem that requires active treatment. However, many persons with neurological impairments display serious deficits in communication that remain untreated and their deficits remain unacknowledged. Primarily, that deficit is inadequate breath support for phonation; in other words, the patient's inability to control the force and duration of exhalation for the purpose of phonation. Duration of phonation and voice intensity are regulated by a delicate balance between airway resistance, provided by the laryngeal muscles, and the force of exhalation, provided by the muscles of respiration (Fig 20–16). They work in concert as a team. When the respiratory muscles are malfunctioning as in the neurological diseases discussed here, the patient's ability to regulate the

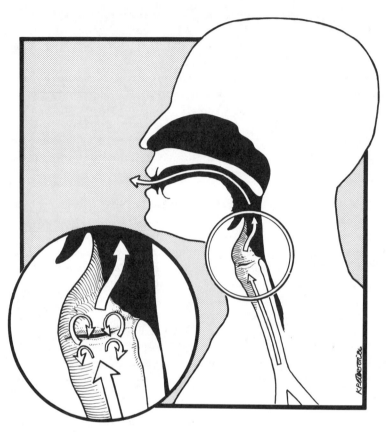

FIG 20–16.
Relationship of air flow and vocal folds.

flow of air out of the lungs may be impaired. Good eccentric control of
the diaphragm, the ability to slowly release the muscle during exhalation, is needed to produce normal lengths of phonation. Otherwise, the
risk is that the air will be expelled from the lungs too quickly because
of the natural elastic recoil of the diaphragm, rendering that volume
of air useless for phonation. Therefore, both a decrease in tidal volume
and a decrease in eccentric control of the respiratory muscles, will lead
to impairments in speech production.

The average adult breathes at a ratio of 1:1 or 2:1 (exhalation
time: inhalation time) during quiet breathing. The average ratio during phonation becomes (E:I) 5:1, with 8–10 syllables per breath being
a comfortable speaking length. Clinically, many patients are seen to

struggle with two- to three-syllable phrases because of inadequate breath support. How often are these same patients not referred to speech therapy for training because they are not diagnosed as having a "speech problem" (e.g., many SCIs, MDs, polio, or spina bifida)? Optimally, these patients should be able to phonate (an "ah" or "oh" sound) for at least 10–12 seconds during a controlled expired vital capacity. Again, how many of their voices fade away after 4–5 seconds? Without the ability to communicate with normal speaking lengths and normal voice intensities, these patients' successful reentry into society's mainstream becomes significantly more difficult.

Another misconception about these patients is that they are mentally slow or retarded because they do not use all the proper figures of speech. In reality, these patients may exclude such things as prepositions or verbs because of the extended time it takes them to communicate. For them, it is more expedient to forego their enclosure.

A marked example of this was seen in our clinic. A 3-year-old girl who sustained a complete C_{4-5} spinal cord lesion at birth and had not received prior rehabilitation was seen. Upon initial examination, her speech was choppy, brief, and grammatically incorrect. She rarely initiated conversation and her voice intensity was very low. It was suspected that she perhaps suffered some anoxic brain damage to account for her developmentally delayed speech. After an intense breathing retraining program in conjunction with a physical rehabilitation program, her speech changed drastically. She spoke fluently, with 8–10 syllables/breath, correct grammar, and louder and more varied voice intensities. Instead of being quiet and more reserved as she had been prior to treatment, the mother reported that the child was a "regular chatterbox." Her new communication skills appeared to improve her self esteem. At that point, it became understood that her cognitive skills were well underestimated upon initial screening.

Because of all this, air flow out of the lungs should be just as important to clinicians as air flow into the lungs. An evaluation of diaphragmatic eccentric control becomes necessary for all patients who demonstrate respiratory impairments. Optimum head and neck positioning, also crucial to maximizing the patient's ability to phonate, must be evaluated. High neuromuscular tone may impair the patient's ability to regulate the outgoing air flow in addition to inhibiting the inflowing air, and therefore may need to be inhibited through positioning or handling techniques. All concerned disciplines should incorporate a phonation facilitation program into their rehabilitation program, especially for those patients who would otherwise not receive any speech training.

TABLE 20–5.
Respiratory Rehabilitation Goals

↑ or maintain chest expansion
↑ VC and TV where indicated
Improve cough effectiveness
Alter RR and breathing patterns where indicated
↑ coordination and eccentric control of the diaphragm
↑ coordination of breathing with functional activities
↑ ability of patient to maintain good bronchial hygiene

GOALS OF A NEUROLOGIC RESPIRATORY PROGRAM

The combination of secondary effects to a neurological insult, such as decreased chest expansion, abnormal breathing patterns, impaired phonation, etc., are responsible for leaving the person with chronic neurological deficits at greater risk for developing respiratory complications, even long after their acute phases have subsided. The long-term goal of any respiratory rehabilitation program for these patients is obvious; reduce their risk for developing these complications. First and foremost is the need to increase or maintain chest expansion in all three planes of respiration. Second, the patient's vital capacity and tidal volume, where indicated, must be increased toward normal values. Respiratory rates and breathing patterns may need to be altered, which could mean increasing or decreasing the use of accessory muscles to achieve maximal breathing efficiency. With this, a goal to improve the coordination and eccentric control of the diaphragm for improved phonation must be included. Improving cough effectiveness and therefore improving FEV_1, is needed. These goals lead us finally to a need for increased coordination of breathing with functional activities and increased ability of the patient or family to maintain good bronchial hygiene for prophylactic care. These goals are summarized in Table 20–5. When implementing this program, it is imperative to recall that the patient's respiratory needs do not exist in a vacuum. They must be able to apply what they learn from this program into all phases of their lives. Thus, incorporation of these goals into ADL or multipurpose activities will yield the most successful results.

21

Respiratory Rehabilitation Secondary to Neurological Deficits: Treatment Techniques

Mary Massery, P.T.

Attaining the respiratory goals stated at the end of Chapter 20 requires the employment of a variety of techniques. Some will be passive in nature, such as passive positioning of the patient, or application of an abdominal binder for better diaphragmatic positioning. Some will require very active participation on the therapist's and/or patient's part, such as in assistive cough techniques or in glossopharyngeal breathing instruction. Other techniques will be subtly incorporated into the patient's total physical rehabilitation program, requiring little overt attention to the patient's respiratory performance. All these diverse aspects of treatment techniques play an important role in the total development of a successful respiratory rehabilitation program for the severely neurologically impaired. No single technique is appropriate in all cases. Sound clinical judgment and experience must be exercised when applying these ideas on each patient. It is this author's hope that the techniques itemized in this chapter will stimulate the clinician's creative talents, to extrapolate and improve upon these techniques according to specific patient population needs.

PASSIVE TECHNIQUES

Passive respiratory techniques are those that require no active participation from the patient and very little participation from the therapist.
These techniques will be discussed first. Critical acute care techniques
are discussed specifically in Chapters 16 and 17.

All patients spend some portion of their day in a horizontal position for rest or sleep. Using this opportunity to assist the patient in
passive drainage of lung secretions would appear to be a natural beginning in the development of a patient's long-term respiratory program.
Specific postural drainage positions have been covered extensively in
this book (see Chapter 12). Using a combination of these positions in
your patient's bed position rotation, in the hospital, or at home can
help to achieve multiple goals. First, it can assist the patients in clearing
secretions passively that they may have difficulty doing actively. Second, these position changes provide for skin relief and better circulation. Finally, they assist in retarding the development of joint contractures or bony changes. A four-position rotation (supine, prone, side-to-
side) is usually an effective and reasonable means of incorporating
these goals into a long-term prophylactic program. Specific positions
may be altered as an acute need arises. See Chapter 12 to determine
which positions are best suited to your patients. Instruction in positioning to the family and patient is necessary for maintaining long-term
bronchial hygiene. Observation of all precautions and contraindications
to passive positioning is still warranted.

Just as passive positioning of the patient in bed helps to maintain
bronchial hygiene, passive positioning of the patient's skeletal frame in
antigravity postures (sitting, standing), helps to maximize the patient's
mechanical advantage of breathing. For example, patients with SCIs
resulting in quadriparesis will be unable to align their intestinal contents properly under the diaphragm to allow for maximal expansion of
the chest in all three planes of respiration (see Chapter 20). Use of an
abdominal support, from the iliac crest to the base of the xiphoid process, helps to restore this vital intestinal positioning in an upright position (Fig 21–1). Research has well documented significant improvements in vital capacity, inspiratory capacity, and tidal volume in sitting
with use of a strong abdominal support. These binders have long been
used in nursing to provide for better circulation and in the prevention
of hypotension.

The abdominal binder's value in cosmesis may be underrated.
Many of these neurological patients were once "normal," healthy indi-

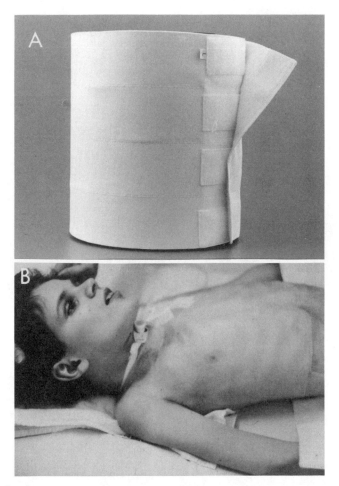

FIG 21–1.
A, abdominal binder—Velcro fastener. **B,** placement of abdominal binder.

viduals with high self-esteem who took great pride in their appearance. They now present with a "beer belly" (the anterior and inferior shift of the intestines due to flaccid abdominal muscles), which may be psychologically disturbing to them. Thus, the use of a binder here may greatly aid in the restoration of that person's self-esteem which should be a high priority goal in *any* rehabilitation program.

In the past few years, another type of abdominal support has evolved, which aids the severely neurologically impaired person more adequately. This is usually known as a body jacket (Fig 21–2). It is a

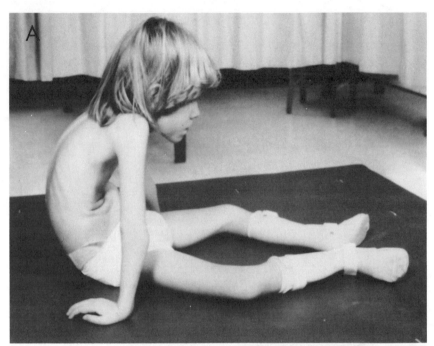

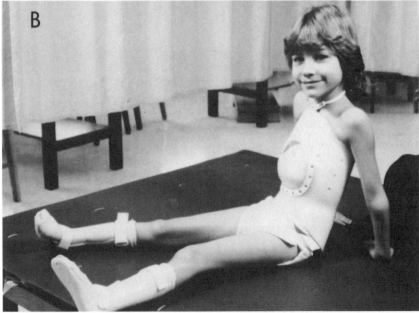

FIG 21–2.
A, patient with C5 congenital quadriplegia independent long sitting. **B,** long sitting with body jacket support. Note changes in head position and eye contact.

rigid trunk support molded individually to the shape of the patient's entire trunk from the axilla down to the pubis. It is made up of two separate front and back pieces, with an anterior cutout in the abdomen to allow for better diaphragmatic movement. Many of these jackets also use a strong elastic support across the cutout to allow for diaphragmatic motion while minimizing unwanted displacement of the abdominal contents. This extreme type of abdominal support is very appropriate for the growing child who needs more spinal stability, along with intestinal positioning, to breathe adequately in sitting, or the completely flaccid quadriplegic patient, who may also require the same support. Because head and neck positioning are so interdependent on trunk positioning, a body jacket may be the difference to these patients between being bedridden or being able to get up in a wheelchair. It allows for significantly better head control, eye contact, longer phonation, and possibly better articulation (if inadequate breath support caused phonation impairments, see "phonation," Chapter 20) than a simple elastic abdominal support could. However, because it limits trunk movements, its usefulness for each patient must be assessed carefully.

Logically, the next consideration under passive respiratory techniques, is proper wheelchair positioning. Optimal performance in respiratory functioning, as well as many other areas of rehabilitation, depends on good alignment of the body against the forces of gravity. Symmetry must be strived for, through the use of a body jacket, lateral trunk supports in the wheelchair, abdominal binders, or some other means (Fig 21–3). This is especially important for patients with hemiplegia where habitual asymmetrical posturing leads to musculoskeletal problems later on. Symmetrical breathing patterns and uniform aeration of all lung segments is augmented by careful daily positioning. Therefore, everything from the type of neck support to the height and width of the arm rests to the length and type of the foot supports must be carefully analyzed for each chronically impaired patient.

ALTERING BREATHING PATTERNS

Inhibition of the Diaphragm

Only after all passive positioning techniques have been employed should active respiratory techniques in those postures begin. Specific techniques are discussed here in detail. Progressions for use of these techniques in different therapeutic postures are addressed in the next chapter.

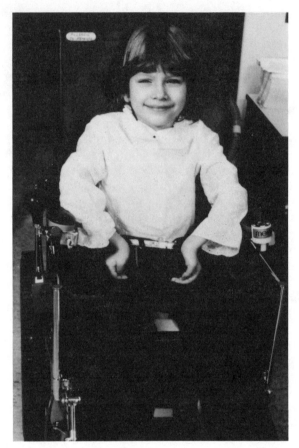

FIG 21–3.
Wheelchair alignment considerations.

Because the diaphragm normally supplies 75%–80% of the inspired air during quiet breathing, diaphragmatic breathing is the preferred pattern of breathing. Chapter 10 demonstrates many facilitation techniques to encourage this type of breathing and therefore will not be reiterated here. However, following some neurological insults, strictly diaphragmatic breathing may not be possible or even preferred. Unlike pulmonary rehabilitation programs for chronic lung patients, where diaphragmatic breathing is always encouraged and use of accessory muscles discouraged, restoration of independent, efficient breathing patterns for the neurologically impaired patient may require the regular use of accessory muscles. Two techniques are described to inhibit the sole use of the diaphragm during inspiration, in order to facilitate the use of accessory muscles, especially the intercostal muscles, sternocleidomastoid, scalenes, and trapezius muscles. These techniques are not ends in themselves, but rather they allow for a search of the most effective breathing pattern for that patient.

Inhibiting the diaphragm is often necessary during breathing retraining for patients with high level SCI, polio, spina bifida, head trauma and CP deficits. All share in common some malfunction of the diaphragm. With the high level quadriplegic in the first three diagnostic categories, the diaphragm may be too weak to produce an adequate tidal volume or vital capacity without the assistance of some accessory muscles. In these cases, the diaphragm inhibiting technique is used to encourage the use of supportive muscles so the patients learn to use their weakened diaphragms in consort with intact accessory muscles. Not only does this allow for an increased tidal volume and vital capacity, but it also provides better aeration of all the lung segments and better mobilization of the entire thorax.

In contrast to the first reason that this technique may be used, an unusually strong diaphragm, acting without constraints from surrounding musculature, may also need to be inhibited. For example, a paraplegic or lower level quadriplegic patient with an intact diaphragm but absent abdominal and intercostal muscles may demonstrate a paradoxical breathing pattern (see abnormal breathing patterns, Chapter 20). Unaltered, over a prolonged period of time, this pattern tends to cause an elongation and narrowing of the lower chest with a flattening of the anterior rib cage and collapsing of the upper chest. In this case, the accessory muscles must be encouraged to keep the diaphragm in check, hopefully avoiding the undesirable changes that its use alone can cause. The goal of this breathing retraining method is to stop the paradoxical movements of the chest during respiration by balancing the use of the upper and lower chest inspiratory muscles. Spastic intercostal muscles, like in many chronic stage SCIs, may intercede to prevent this paradoxical movement by maintaining the upper chest's position during inspiration. Balancing the chest's movements should produce an increased tidal volume and vital capacity potential, while mobilizing a greater portion of the chest, just as the technique does in the first case presented. Patients with CP or head traumas that display paradoxical breathing may also benefit from this technique.

To perform the diaphragm inhibiting technique, the patient is positioned supine with arms resting comfortably at his side. The heel of the therapist's hand is placed lightly on the patient's abdomen, slightly below the base of the xiphoid process. No instructions are given to the patient at this point. As the patient begins to exhale a normal breath of air, the therapist gently allows the heel of his hand to move up and in toward the central tendon, following the patient's diaphragmatic recoil (Fig 21–4). When expiration for that breath is completed, the therapist strictly maintains hand position. During the following inspiratory phase, the diaphragm will experience some gentle resistance to its movement. Upon the next expiration, the technique is repeated with the therapist carefully pushing the heel of his hand further up and in, maintaining each new gain during the following inspiratory phase. Usually, after two or three breath cycles, the patients begin to unconsciously alter their breathing patterns to accommodate the diaphragm's inability to produce enough chest expansion in the lower rib cage for an adequate tidal volume. The therapist should carefully observe which accessory muscles the patient spontaneously chooses. Are they used symmetrically? What is the general quality of their movement? Do they appear fatigued or uncoordinated?

It is not until this point that the therapist should acknowledge ver-

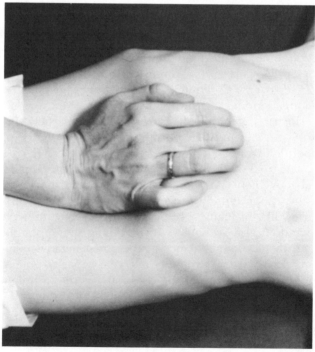

FIG 21–4.
Hand position for diaphragm inhibiting technique in supine.

bally any alteration of the patient's breathing pattern. Without changing his hand position, the therapist tells the patient what it is that they like about his altered breathing pattern (balance between upper and lower chest expansion, less cavus motion of the sternum, less paradoxical motion, etc.). Then the patient is asked if he notices any difference from before, to bring this breathing pattern to a conscious level. Only after some orientation to this pattern, usually no more than 4–6 breathing cycles in the full inhibiting pattern, should the therapist begin to gradually reverse the pressure.

While slowly releasing pressure with each cycle of inspiration, the therapist asks the patient to attempt cognitively to reproduce the desired pattern. It should take the same number of cycles to release the pressure as it did to apply it. This technique easily allows for gradations of inhibition, from full inhibition, where the patient is forced to use upper accessory muscles or risk becoming short of breath, to barely a proprioceptive reminder to change his breathing pattern. It also allows for gradation of inhibition while the patient is learning to assume control over the new breathing pattern. If during the releasing phase of this technique the patient begins to lose control over the new pattern, the therapist can gently reapply some pressure during the next exhalatory phase to help the patient regain that control. After that point, the therapist can release or reapply pressure as necessary until the desired pattern is obtained and full release of pressure is completed.

This technique is particularly effective with patients who are having difficulty cognitively altering their own breathing pattern, such as with small children, brain-damaged patients, or slow motor learners, because it requires no cognitive effort on their part until success has already been achieved. Extra care must be taken not to initiate any applied pressure quickly, due to the likelihood of then eliciting unwanted abdominal or diaphragmatic spasticity or eliciting a stronger diaphragmatic contraction due to the quick stretch reflex. The technique, used properly, should never be painful. The therapist must keep his hand on the abdomen, not the rib cage.

The second technique is for the more advanced patient and simply presents a physical block to diaphragmatic excursion. The patient is positioned in a prone on elbows position (Fig 21–5). With most severely neurologically impaired patients, the lower chest will be in direct contact with the surface, so anterior expansion is inhibited and lateral costal expansion is severely limited. The upper chest is in extension and the upper extremities are fixated, making facilitation of the accessory muscles very natural. Now, through the use of head and neck patterns, such as in PNF (proprioceptive neuromuscular facilitation) diagonals,

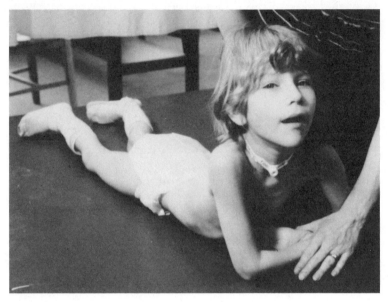

FIG 21–5.
Diaphragm inhibiting in prone on elbows position.

or static-dynamic activities, such as in weight shifting to one supporting limb while reaching out with the other extremity, the therapist can facilitate a preferred breathing pattern for that patient (Fig 21–6). These are the same patterns the therapist can use to achieve such goals as increased head and neck control, increased shoulder stability, or increased upper body balance. Therefore, the therapist is helping the patients to coordinate movement goals with alternative breathing patterns. It becomes all the more likely that the patients will incorporate these patterns functionally into their daily activities—the ultimate goal.

A word of caution: The supine diaphragmatic inhibiting technique is more passive and less threatening to the patient than the prone on elbows technique. Prone on elbows itself can inhibit the diaphragm so completely for this patient population that they become extremely short of breath. Consequently, do not position the patients in this more demanding posture until success appears likely.

Segmental Breathing

Patients having difficulty coordinating the use of accessory muscles with their diaphragms may require specific segmental breathing in-

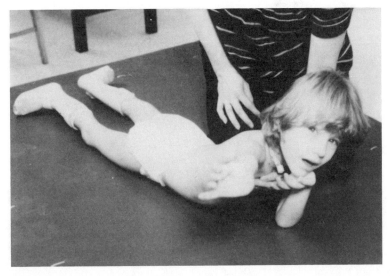

FIG 21–6.
Static-dynamic upper extremity activities in prone on elbows to encourage upper chest accessory muscle participation.

struction first. Chapter 10 goes into detail about many such techniques that will not be reiterated here. However, other techniques found to be particularly effective with this neurological population are presented.

Proper proprioceptive input is very important while facilitating a specific muscle or muscle group for segmental breathing. For example, to increase the use of the pectoralis muscle in upper chest expansion, the therapist should place his hand in the same direction as the contracting muscle fibers. The heel of the hand should be near the sternum while the fingers are aligned up and out toward the shoulder. Then the patient is asked to breathe up and into the therapist's hands, while the therapist applies a quick manual stretch to the muscle fibers (down and in toward the sternum) (Fig 21–7). This elicits the quick stretch reflex of the muscle while simultaneously providing added sensory input, all of which facilitates a stronger and more specific muscle contraction. This same principle can be applied to any muscle or muscle group during segmental breathing exercises (e.g., to facilitate the trapezius or sternocleiodmastoid muscles for increased superior expansion or to facilitate the intercostal muscles for increased lateral expansion).

Asymmetrical segmental breathing is often needed for hemiplegic

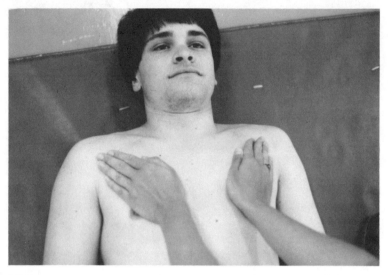

FIG 21–7.
Hand placement for segmental facilitation of pectoralis.

patients (CVAs, head traumas, some CPs, etc.). This is most effectively accomplished by inhibiting the uninvolved side. Frequently, the best posture in which to achieve this is in sidelying. When the patient lies on his uninvolved side, lateral chest expansion into that side becomes inhibited due to the physical barrier. This forces the patient to then expand the involved side of the chest instead. The therapist can supply sensory and motor input through the hands to the patient's upper, mid, or lower chest on their involved side to work on isolated segmental breathing (Fig 21–8). Early in the rehabilitation process, the patient may have difficulty performing lateral chest expansion against gravity in sidelying (gravity-resisted movement). If so, take the patient down to a ¾ supine position to lessen the work load imposed by gravity. Gradually, work them back up to a full sidelying posture to achieve the greatest strengthening benefits.

Another posture for performing segmental breathing techniques is prone on elbows, which can facilitate segmental expansion of the posterior or anterior (see the second diaphragm inhibiting technique) upper chest. This is significant because for the first time, gravity is assisting anterior excursion of the chest while resisting posterior excursion. To emphasize posterior expansion, the patient performs an upper body push-up, with or without the therapist's assistance. This requires the use of the serratus anterior muscle which provides lateral scapular

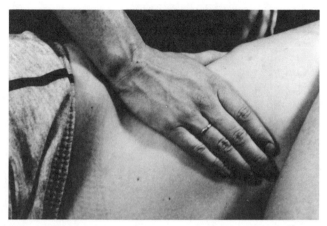

FIG 21–8.
Hand placement for lower chest facilitation in sidelying.

movement and thereby allows for maximal posterior excursion of the thorax. The patient is instructed to take a deep breath in during the push-up, and to exhale the air (passively or forcefully) when returning to the starting position. Forceful exhalation in this activity can be used as a forerunner to effective cough retraining. To emphasize anterior expansion, the patient can be instructed in head and neck patterns (i.e., PNF patterns) to encourage neck extension. The patient is instructed to inhale during the extension component to facilitate accessory muscle participation.

Varying Respiratory Rates

In addition to altering breathing patterns through segmental breathing techniques, changing respiratory rates (RR) may also be necessary before arriving at an efficient breathing pattern for each patient. Neurological patients subconsciously increase their RR to compensate for a decrease in their tidal volumes (TV). Attempting to restore the status quo involves increasing TV while concurrently decreasing RR. The segmental breathing techniques described previously in depth will help to increase the patients' TV and VC. The counterrotation technique to be discussed now is particularly useful in controlling the RR and is perhaps, in this author's view, the most useful manual technique for this type of rehabilitation program. It is extremely valuable for patients who have decreased cognitive functioning, or for very young children because the therapist's hands direct the results rather than relying on the patient's cognizance of verbal commands. It is also an inhibitor of high neuromuscular tone, such as spasticity or rigidity (which may be a desired end in itself). Finally, as described in the next section, it can be adapted easily as a very effective assisted cough technique. One significant contraindication is bony instability of the spine.

In bed or on a mat, the patient is placed sidelying with knees bent and arms resting comfortably out in front of his head or shoulders (the higher the better). Relaxed positioning of the patient is essential to the success of this technique because normalizing neuromuscular tone is the first step in attempting to decrease a high RR. Patient discomfort is likely to do the opposite, increase tone, and increase RR.

The therapist's own position is equally as important because it directs the force that is applied to the patient's chest. Standing behind the patient near the hips, the therapist turns diagonally to the patient until facing the patient's head at roughly a 45-degree angle. The therapist then positions his hands lightly on the patient. If the patient is sidelying on his left, the therapist's left hand is placed on the patient's right pectoralis region with care being taken not to unintentionally use the thumb or fingertips. The heel of the right hand is placed solidly in the patient's right gluteal fossa (the hollow of the buttocks) (Fig 21–9,A). The therapist leaves his hands in place and follows the patient's respiratory cycle, noting its rate, rhythm, and the patient's overall neuromuscular tone. Only after this assessment should the clinician begin the active phase of the technique.

Phase 2 of the technique involves learning the proper stretching procedure. Waiting for the patient to complete an expiratory phase, the therapist then skillfully pulls the left hand down and back, stretching quickly along the grain of the pectoralis muscle, toward the therapist's stomach, while at the same time pushing the other hand up and forward along the grain of the gluteus maximus, away from the stomach. If the therapist is on a true diagonal to the patient's body, the hands will be counterrotating the trunk on a diagonal plane. This is decisive to the technique's success. Only then is the chest cavity closed off in all three planes of respiration. When the technique is performed as a quick stretch technique, it will facilitate a larger and stronger inhalation, thus increasing TV.

When the patient inspires, the therapist switches hand placement to capitalize on the improved chest expansion. The left hand slides back to the patient's left scapula, while the right hand slides forward just anterior to the patient's left iliac crest (Fig 21–9,B). The therapist is encouraged to use the flat or heel of the hand whenever possible to minimize unintended patient discomfort and to maximize the facili-

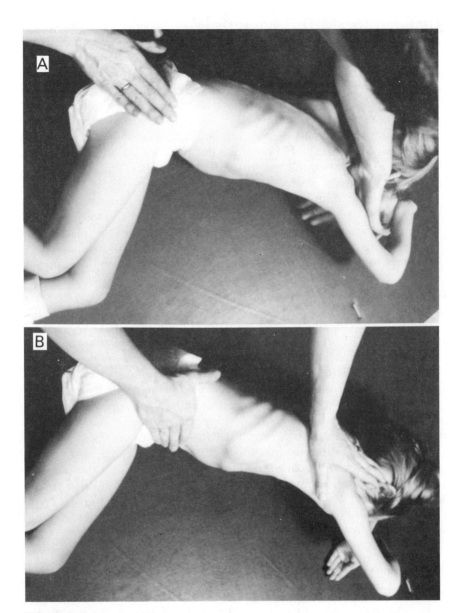

FIG 21–9.
A and **B,** hand placement for decreasing respiratory rates technique in sidelying.

tated area. The clinician slowly stretches on the new grain during inspiration to expand the chest three dimensionally. At the end of inspiration, the patient is given a quick stretch further into that same diagonal pattern to facilitate the reciprocal muscles for the flexion or expiratory phase of the technique. Just as for inspiration, the therapist then quickly reverts back to the other hand positions to utilize expiration fully. The whole sequence is repeated at the end of exhalation.

Initially, the therapist begins and ends the respiratory cycle according to the patient's RR. However, as the patient's tone is relaxed and increased TVs are promoted through the effects of counterrotation, the therapist gradually slows the rate of rotation down. The patient will usually accommodate to the new respiratory rate as the clinician gains more control over the patient's breathing pattern. With many patients, the results can be marked. If the patient can cognitively follow commands, he is alerted to this change and assisted in independently breathing at the slower rate by decreasing the manual input from the therapist. As with the diaphragm-inhibiting technique, the therapist can reestablish control quickly if needed by simply reapplying stronger facilitation.

For some extremely rigid patients (i.e., Parkinson's, some head traumas, or CP), this technique may be appropriately preceded by a PNF technique called rhythmic initiation. The patient is gently logrolled in a small ROM in sidelying. Then the rolling is progressively increased achieving more of a roll from sidelying toward prone. This progression of movement inhibits high tone more slowly and for these patients may be necessary before attempting tone inhibition through the counterrotation of the decreased RR technique.

It should be apparent that this technique need not be used exclusively for respiratory goals, but rather incorporated into the patient's total rehabilitation program. It is a natural precursor to active rolling or it can be used as a vestibular stimulator. Intertwining goals, respiratory, mobility, strengthening, etc., should be the therapist's true long-term goal.

Glossopharyngeal Breathing

For a small population of neurological patients, worthwhile altering of breathing patterns requires more than just promoting the use of different accessory muscles or changing RR. In the last decade, more high level SCIs (above C_2) have survived the initial trauma because of advances in medical technology. However, the rehabilitation therapist is then faced with the difficult task of restoring "quality of life." For these patients, as well as many old polio patients, mastery of the glossopharyngeal breathing (GPB) technique has provided just such a means. This breathing pattern allows patients to regain some control over their lives and to regain control over their respiration which was lost as a result of the high neurological insult.

GPB is a technique for breathing that was developed in the 1950s by polio patients looking for a way to reduce their dependence on the "iron lung" for respiration. They found that by using their lips, soft palates, mouths, tongues, pharynx, and larynx, they could actually swallow air into their lungs. Only intact cranial nerves were required. This method is sometimes referred to as "frog breathing" because it uses the principles of inspiration common to the frog. The patient learns to create a pocket of negative pressure within the buccal (mouth) cavity by maximizing that internal space, thereby causing the outside air to rush in. At that point, the patient closes off the entrance (his lips) and proceeds to force the air back and down his throat with a stroking maneuver of the tongue, pharynx, and larynx. Research has consistently shown that use of this technique with severely impaired neurological patients has increased pulmonary functions significantly, especially for TV and VC. If GPB is their only means of respiration off of a ventilator or phrenic nerve stimulator, mastery of this technique is critical to their survival in case of mechanical failure. All attempts should be made to successfully teach GPB to this patient population.

A clinical example may help to illustrate its usefulness. A 14-year-old male sustained a C_1 complete SCI while trying to race in front of a train on a minibike. After he was medically stable, two phrenic nerve stimulators were implanted in his chest to supply artificial respiration. The patient had no nonmechanical means of respiration. Neuromuscularly, the patient had limited use of one trapezius, sternocleidomastoid, and intrinsic neck muscles. The patient and family feared that long-term nursing home placement would be inevitable because of the danger of his phrenic nerve stimulator malfunctioning or a battery wearing out, causing immediate respiratory distress. The family believed it could not bear the psychological burden placed on them. GPB instruction was suggested and began slowly, as the patient stated that he was always a slow physical activity learner. After a painstaking two-month period, the patient learned to breathe without the use of his phrenic nerve stimulator for 3–5 minutes before hypoventilating. Within the next 1–2 months, this same patient learned to breathe for up to two hours off of his stimulator, using GPB only. To the staff's surprise, he even learned to talk and operate his "sip and puff" wheelchair while using GPB.

It was only after this accomplishment that the rehabilitation staff and the family decided that living at home was a possibility. The patient was comfortable with the idea of being alone in his room or house for up to two hours because he could breathe on his own and operate his wheelchair into another room to get assistance, or he could get to a telephone and call for help. The patient's family felt much less anxious about the risk of finding their son compromised at home due to a stimulator malfunction because he could now breathe independently with GPB. The patient was then successfully discharged to his home. This does not imply that this was the only factor considered in his discharge planning, but it was perhaps the most significant.

Instruction in GPB takes time and concentration. It is best to start off in small time blocks of 10–15 minutes because it can be very fatiguing at first. However, it is important to successful learning of the technique that the patient get consistent, preferably daily training. Once the patient has mastered the technique, practice sessions can be lengthened considerably, and the patient can be taught self-monitoring techniques. Specific goals of GPB training must be explained to the patient prior to the beginning of treatment in order to gain his support and cooperation. In addition to providing the ventilator or stimulator-dependent patient with a TV necessary for gaining independence from mechanical assists, GPB has many other benefits. For the quadriplegic patient who has a partially intact diaphragm (C_{3-4}) or the loss of essential accessory muscles (C_{5-8}), GPB can help to (1) increase VC to produce a more effective cough, (2) assist in a longer and stronger phonation, and (3) act as an internal mobilizer of the chest wall.

The muscles used in this technique do not have the same internal proprioceptive, sensory, or visual feedback mechanisms that the trunk and limb muscles have, making corrections in performance of the method more difficult. The patient cannot "see" his tongue pushing the air back or truly "feel" the pharynx swallowing the air into the lungs, so the therapist's external feedback system is very influential. Use of a mirror can greatly enhance the visual component of feedback. Small changes like adjustment in posture or a suggestion of another sound to imitate may be all that is needed for the patient to learn the stroking maneuver correctly. Success in GPB can be assessed objectively with a spirometer. For those patients incapable of breathing on their own, any TV reading will indicate successful intake of air. For patients who are not ventilator dependent, a VC reading that is greater than 5% over the base line, indicates successful use of GPB. Lower level quadriplegics, C_5–C_8, have demonstrated increases in VC by as much as 70%–100%.

Therapists can monitor their own success with this technique by taking VC readings with and without GPB or by subjective analysis. Maximal inhalation, followed by three or four successful GPB strokes, will provide a feeling that their chest will burst if they attempt to inhale more air. Instead, a feeling of indigestion is usually indicative of swallowed air in the stomach.

During the initial treatment session, the therapist demonstrates to the patient what a stroking maneuver looks like several times, to give him an idea of the motion required. The therapist continues to mimic the pattern as the patient attempts to duplicate it initially. This gives the patient an active model and decreases feelings of uneasiness surrounding the necessary facial grimaces. If the patient is able to breathe on his own, his ability to hold his breath and to close off his nasal passageway should be checked because air leakage is a common cause of failure. The patient is then instructed to take in a maximal inspiration before attempting the stroking to eliminate the possibility of using other necessary muscles during the technique.

The patients are instructed to bring their jaws down and then forward as if reaching their lips up for a carrot dangling just above their upper lip (without tilting the head back) (Fig 21–10,A). Their lips should be shaped as if they were to make the sound "oop." Then the patients are told to close their mouths, reaching the bottom lip up to the top lip (Fig 21–10,B). The tongue and jaw are drawn back toward the throat, with the mouth and tongue formation of the word "up" or the sound "L" (Fig 21–10,C). Most patients learn the stroking maneuvers by making the sounds at first, but as they become more proficient, the sounds and excessive head and neck motions become diminished. In most cases, the student (patient) outperforms the teacher (therapist) in time, because through consistent use, they learn all of its finer subtleties.

Although this technique can be broken down into several stages like it has been here for the purpose of description, most of the literature cautions the therapist against it. Simple, minimal instructions seem to accomplish more, perhaps because the continuity of movement is so essential to the success of the inhalation. Specific instructions such as the ones here can be given later if necessary.

Common problems encountered with GPB instruction are as follows: (1) an open nasal passage or glottis that allows the air to escape; (2) a feeling of indigestion indicating that the air is being swallowed into the esophagus rather than the trachea; (3) incorrect shape of the mouth as the air is being drawn in, usually not puckered enough; (4) incoordinated backward movement of the tongue; or (5) incorrect

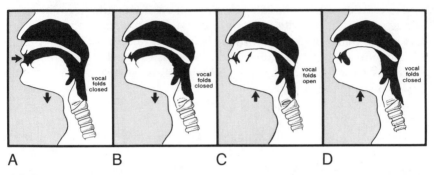

FIG 21–10.
Glossopharyngeal breathing. (See text for details.) **A,** mouth opened to draw in air; **B,** jaw closed to entrap the air; **C,** air pushed back with tongue into trachea; **D,** vocal folds closed to prevent passive air leaks. Entire maneuver then repeated.

sounds while performing the technique, such as the word "gulp" or an "M"·sound. Tolerance to GPB can be increased when mastery of a single stroke becomes consistent. For patients using it as an assist to their own voluntary respiration, 3–4 strokes on top of a maximal inspiration is usually sufficient. Ventilator- or stimulator-dependent patients may need to use as many as 10–14 strokes per breath. These figures should be used only as rough guidelines. Each patient will use a slightly different technique with a different number of strokes, with the only important factor being a method that works for them.

Any or all of the altered breathing techniques described here, (1) use of passive techniques, (2) inhibition of the diaphragm, (3) segmental breathing, (4) changing RRs, or (5) GPB can be used for patients with chronic neurological impairments. Accurate assessment of each patient's pulmonary deficits (see Chapters 6 and 7: Specific Respiratory Impairments) will determine which procedures will be the most beneficial.

ASSISTIVE COUGH TECHNIQUES

Producing effective coughs is important to any respiratory program. With the wide range of physical and cognitive capabilities that the neurologically impaired population has, having only one assistive cough technique in their program does not appear to be adequate. Yet the current literature makes no reference to more than a few techniques for these patients, and describes them in only two developmental postures. Some of these patients may respond to those techniques with increased tone, thus rendering the cough ineffective. For others, muscle weakness may make coughing effectively improbable in gravity-resisted postures. Still other patients may demonstrate isolated paralysis or incoordination deficits which would require yet other assistive cough approaches. Because of these patients' diverse neurological deficits and respiratory needs, 10 different assistive cough techniques will be detailed here in five different developmental postures (Table 21–1). Hopefully, this wide variety of techniques will enable therapists to more readily find a suitable approach for each of their neurological patients. GPB may be used in conjunction with any of these techniques if needed, but will not be discussed again under each new technique. For cough techniques more applicable to the acute care patient, such as the postsurgical patient, see Chapter 11.

Supine

Three techniques work well in this posture. One is adapted from the diaphragmatic breathing technique described in Chapter 10, and is a common technique seen in the literature for these patients. The second has limited benefits and should only be used when all others fail. The third incorporates both upper and lower chest participation. Accurate assessment of each patient's tone, strength, and mobility level is necessary before deciding which posture and technique to use.

TABLE 21–1.
Assistive Cough Techniques

POSITION	TECHNIQUE
Supine	Costophrenic assist Heimlich-type assist Anterior chest compression assist
Sidelying	Costophrenic assist Heimlich-type assist Combination of Heimlich-type assist and costophrenic assist Massery counterrotation assist
Prone on elbows	Head flexion assist
Sitting	Para-long-sitting self-assist Quad-long-sitting self-assist Short-sitting self-assist
Hands-knees	Rocking

To perform the first assistive cough technique in supine, the therapist places his hands on the costophrenic angles of the rib cage (Fig 21–11,C). At the end of the patient's expiratory phase, the therapist applies a quick manual stretch down and in on the lower chest walls, facilitating a stronger diaphragmatic and intercostal muscle contraction. As the patient then inspires air, the therapist applies a series of three repeated contractions, down and in, (as in the PNF approach) to encourage maximal inhalation. The patient is then asked to "hold it" (to hold the air in). Just prior to instructing the patient to actively cough out, the therapist applies strong pressure through his hands, up and in toward the central tendon of the diaphragm. In this manner, the patient is not only assisted with forced expiration but also with increased intrathoracic pressure, both of which are necessary for an effective cough.

This technique's obvious use would be for SCIs, spina bifida, MDs, neuropathies, and myopathies. The therapist must remember to evaluate the effect of gravity in this posture for each patient. Depending on the patient's neuromuscular tone, costophrenic assistance may also be appropriate for head traumas, MS, ALS, Parkinson's, and CPs. Finally, because it facilitates a symmetrical cough, it may be beneficial for CVAs or any other hemiplegic deficit. In most cases, this technique can be used from the acute phase through the patient's rehabilitation phase, thus accounting for its popularity.

The second technique, called the Heimlich-type assist, requires the therapist to place the heel of his hand just inferior to the patient's xiphoid process, taking care to avoid direct placement on the lower ribs (see Fig 21–4). The patient is instructed to "take in a deep breath and hold it." As the patient is instructed to cough, the therapist quickly pushes up and in under the diaphragm with the heel of his hand, like in a Heimlich choking maneuver. Technically, this procedure is very effective at forcefully expelling the air, as in a cough, but it can be extremely uncomfortable for the patient due to its concentrated area of contact. In addition, its abrupt nature combined with the sensory input that the therapist's manual contacts supply may elicit undesired high neuromuscular tone. Due to its limited usefulness, the Heimlich-type assist should only be used when the patient does not respond to other techniques and the need to produce an effective cough is imminent, or for home use by family members, owing to its ease of application and relatively effective results. Patients with low neuromuscular tone, or flaccid abdominal muscles fare best with this procedure.

The third assistive cough is called anterior chest compression assist, since it compresses both the upper and lower chest during the cough-

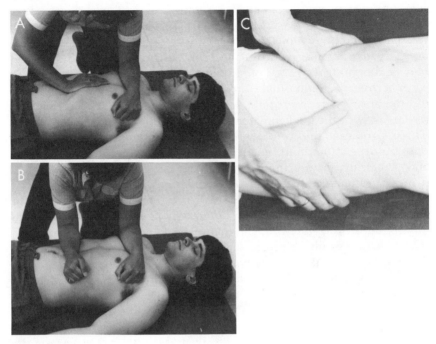

FIG 21–11.
Assistive cough techniques in supine position. **A** and **B,** variations of the anterior chest compression assist. **C,** costophrenic assist.

ing manuever. The therapist puts one arm across the patient's pectoralis region to stabilize or compress the upper chest while the other arm is either placed parallel on the lower chest (Fig 21–11,B) or placed like in the Heimlich-type manuever under the xiphoid process (Fig 21–11,A). The commands are the same as in the other techniques. The therapist applies the greatest force through the lower chest during the expulsion phase. This technique is indicated for patients with very low toned chests where maintenance or compression of the upper anterior chest wall during coughing cannot be achieved independently.

Sidelying

For assistive coughs, this is the most versatile of all the developmental postures. It allows for substantial mobility of the upper side while stabilizing the chest and trunk with the lower side. All three planes of respiration can be utilized except for lateral expansion on the lower side. Often it is used as a reflex inhibiting posture, becoming a very desirable posture for relax dominated patients such as children with CP. The inherent asymmetry of this posture can be viewed as a positive or a negative feature according to each patient's deficits, and should only be determined as such on an individual basis.

The first technique makes use of the costophrenic positioning of the therapist from the supine procedure. However, in sidelying, the technique is performed unilaterally to the upper side (see Fig 21–8). Three significant differences are present: (1) the patient is less supported in the trunk than in supine, and thus, better balance reactions and stabilizing factors in the trunk are necessary; (2) gravitational planes are changed. Lateral chest expansion becomes an antigravity movement rather than unaffected as in supine. Conversely, anterior chest excursion, which was in an antigravity plane in supine, becomes unaffected by it in sidelying; (3) finally, the cough is asymmetrical, primarily assisting only the lung segments of the upper side and could therefore be considered a segmental assistive cough.

Some of its benefits to patients should be apparent. First, sidelying, because of its increased balance demands, allows a natural progression from supine for the patient working on increasing trunk stability in functional activities. Second, lateral excursion is now resisted, making this posture the next step in a cough strengthening program where the intercostal muscles are being encouraged to play a more active role. Many paraplegics, who already have a strong diaphragm but still demonstrate a weak intercostal contraction, use this sequencing. Conversely, patients who require diaphragmatic strengthening may be taught assistive coughing techniques in this posture first, since anterior excursion is in a gravity-eliminated plane. When successfully taught here, the patient could then be progressed to supine, where the motion becomes gravity resisted, thus more challenging. Finally, this position encourages hemiplegic patients to also use their involved side of the chest when coughing. The patient lies on his uninvolved side. Clearing of secretions from the weak side is then assisted from gravity, while active chest expansion on that side is resisted by gravity. Simultaneously, the patient is required to use more balance reactions on the weaker side.

The second assistive cough in sidelying is the Heimlich-type assist. The procedure is identical to that in supine with all stated precautions still prevailing. The significant difference is this posture's effect on neuromuscular tone. With the patient's knees flexed, and with assuming a reflex inhibiting posture such as sidelying, the chances of increasing a patient's tone are significantly reduced. For this reason, patients who would benefit from this procedure usually tolerate it better in this position. For the therapist, it is slightly more difficult to execute than in supine because the patient's trunk must be stabilized.

Combining the two previous techniques, one gets the third side-lying assistive cough. Using both hands, the therapist assists lateral compression of the chest with one hand (costophrenic assist) while the other assists inferior chest compression during the forceful expulsion (Heimlich-type assist). In this manner, more planes of respiration are being utilized, thus becoming more effective at clearing secretions than either technique alone. Unfortunately, family teaching is often more difficult to accomplish than the Heimlich-type assist alone, but the extra component to this technique makes it that much more effective. It may be an excellent beginning for an immobile hemiplegic assistive cough program, since the Heimlich aspect of the technique provides the necessary force, while the lateral component provides the desired facilitation to the involved side.

The most effective assistive cough for the widest cross-section of neurological patients, in this author's clinical experience, is the fourth and final method described in sidelying, the Massery counterrotation assist. The positioning and procedures required for the counterrotation technique described in altering breathing patterns still apply for both the patient and the therapist (see Fig 21–9). It is important for the therapist to recall that spinal stability is a prerequisite for this procedure.

The therapist begins by following the patient's breathing cycle with his hands positioned over the patient's pectoralis and gluteal areas (compression, or flexion, position). Once the pattern is established, the therapist uses slight facilitation, a quick manual stretch on the diagonal, to maximize the next few inhalations. This is accomplished by pulling the upper chest down and back diagonally with the hand positioned over the pectoralis region, while the hand in the gluteal fossa pushes the lower chest wall up and forward diagonally at the very end of an exhalation. Immediately after this inspiratory facilitation, the therapist slides his hands to their expansion, or extension, positions (upper hand over the scapula, lower hand over the iliac crest) to physically assist the patient in chest expansion, thus maximizing inspiratory potential. This sequence is generally repeated for 3–5 cycles, or until the patient appears to have achieved good ventilation to all lung segments.

At this point, the patient is ready to begin the coughing phase of the procedure. With an accentuated quick compression of the chest at the end of exhalation (hands in flexion positions), the patient is asked to take in as deep a breath as possible. Sliding his hands immediately back to the extension positions, the therapist assists the patient in chest expansion, and then instructs the patient to "hold it" at the end of that inspiration. The patient is then commanded to cough out as hard as possible while the therapist quickly and forcefully compresses the chest with his hands in their flexion positions.

The importance of following a true diagonal plane of facilitation during both the flexion and extension phases of this technique cannot be overemphasized. Failure to do so will result in shifting of the air within the chest cavity rather than the desired forcing out. This air shifting can occur to varying degrees, when the upper and lower chest are not utilized together, as in all the other assistive cough techniques. When done properly, the Massery counterrotation assist is the only one to rapidly close off the chest cavity in all three planes of respiration in all areas of the chest. Unless the patient volitionally closes his glottis, it is impossible to withhold the air from being forcefully expelled.

Other effects of counterrotation make this procedure particularly beneficial to patients with low levels of cognitive functioning. (1) The rotation component is a natural high tone inhibitor. Thus, this is the least likely of all techniques discussed so far to elicit an increase in abnormal tone during the coughing phase. In fact, the opposite usually prevails. Gentle rotation prior to passively coughing in a comatose patient can reduce high tone and frequently reduce a high RR. Both of these will reduce the possibility of the patient keeping his glottis closed during the expulsion phase. Almost eliminated is the possibility of increasing abnormal tone which could prevent the patient's chest from being compressed maximally. (2) Counterrotation is an excellent mobilizer for a tight chest, which in itself can facilitate spontaneous deeper breaths. TVs can therefore be increased for many patients by mobilizing the chest walls. (3) Finally, rotation can be a vestibular stimulator, and may assist to arousing the patient cognitively, allowing him to take a more active role in the procedure.

But the true beauty of the technique is the fact that no active participation on the part of the patient is required for success. Incoherent or unresponsive patients, such as those with low functioning head traumas, CVAs, or CPs, will still demonstrate good secretion clearance with this technique. The mechanics of the procedure dictate that the air within the lungs be rapidly and forcefully expelled regardless of the patient's level of active participation. Obviously, patient participation is desirable to clear secretions even more effectively and for teaching the patient to eventually clear his own secretions, but it is not critical.

With extremely tenacious secretions, use of vibration instead of quick chest compression during the cough itself may be more effective.

This prolongs the cough phase and gives the secretions time to be moved along the bronchi for successful expulsion. These patients may also require a series of three or four cough cycles before clearing most of their secretions. In general, patients from all the diagnostic groups discussed thus far with or without good cognitive functioning are appropriate for this procedure. The majority of them find it to be the most comfortable and effective assistive means of producing secretions.

When to suction these patients will be addressed here. Since suctioning is preferable after successful mobilization of secretions, the cognitive low functioning patients should be suctioned after chest mobilization and assistive coughing. However, realistic coordination of a patient's schedule in a large setting to allow for suctioning by another discipline to occur immediately after chest mobilization may be impossible or improbable. In addition, optimally, the patient's position should not be changed after secretions have been adequately mobilized, or they may recede back to a level where they cannot be suctioned effectively. Suctioning should be an integral part of these patients' chest mobilization programs, and should be performed by the clinician doing the mobilizing, be that the PT, the RT, or the nurse. If properly incorporated into the patient's program, the end result should be a decreased need for suctioning with more successful clearance of secretions per necessary suctioning.

Prone

A prone on elbows assistive cough, head flexion assist, is used when participation of the accessory muscles during forceful expulsion is desired. As previously discussed, the position itself inhibits full use of the diaphragm by preventing lower anterior chest excursion. This forces the patient to use an alternate breathing pattern that facilitates accessory muscle use. Because this change in breathing patterns often occurs spontaneously, prone on elbows is a good posture for promoting spontaneous use of the accessory muscles in a more difficult activity (coughing). However, without the full use of the diaphragm, the resultant cough will assuredly be weaker than in other postures, and should not be the exclusive means of assisting a cough for patients who have productive secretions present. After mastering the timing of the procedure, most patients move back to another posture and technique to capitalize on their functional increase in chest expansion and compression abilities. For a small population of patients who can assume a prone on elbows posture independently (i.e., some patients with quadriplegia), this technique may be used functionally. Here, they can assist their own cough when the need arises, rather than wait for someone to assist them in a position change.

The head flexion assist requires good use of head and neck musculature, seen in patients sustaining a spinal level injury below C_4 (i.e., SCIs, spina bifida, etc.). It can be utilized either as a self-assisted or therapist-assisted procedure, using the principles of extension activities to facilitate inspiration and flexion activities to facilitate expiration. With the patients prone on their elbows, the therapist instructs them to extend their heads and necks up and back as far as possible, breathing in maximally as they do so (Fig 21–12,A). The patients are then instructed to cough out as hard as they can while throwing their heads forward and down (Fig 21–12,B). This head and neck pattern can be

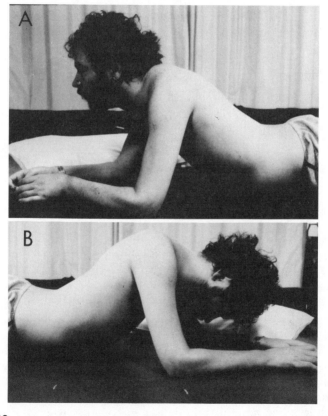

FIG 21–12.
Head flexion assistive cough in prone on elbows. **A,** extension and inspiratory phase; **B,** flexion and coughing phase.

initially assisted by the therapist to establish the desired movement pattern, and gradually progressed to a resisted pattern to promote increased accessory muscle participation and to strengthen those muscle groups.

Sitting

The coughing techniques discussed in this posture are intended to be used as self-assisted procedures, thus usually taught later in a patient's rehabilitation process. The first procedure, long sitting self-assist, was developed at the Rehabilitation Institute of Chicago by a patient for his own use (an SCI quadriplegia patient). The patient is positioned on a mat in a long sitting posture (legs straight out in front of the patient), with upper extremity support. The therapist instructs the patient to extend his body backward while inhaling maximally. The therapist then tells the patient to cough as the patient throws his upper body forward into a completely flexed posture (Fig 21–13,B). Once again, the extension aspect of the procedure is used to maximize inhalation while the flexion aspect is used to maximize expiration. The self-directed chest compression occurs mainly on the superior-inferior plane of respiration only.

The second assistive cough, the para-long-sit assist, employs the same principles as the techniques described for the quad-long-sit assist. This technique was developed by an SCI patient with a low thoracic insult. These patients have active spinal extension and can achieve greater trunk extension and flexion safely, achieving greater chest expansion prior to the cough and greater chest compression on a superior-inferior plane during the cough. The patient positions his upper extremities in a butterfly position or uses elbow retraction depending on the level of injury (Fig 21–13,C). During the flexion phase, the patient throws himself onto his legs, thereby involving both the upper and lower chest (Fig 21–13,D). This can be taught very successfully to patients with paraplegia, provided they do not have any interfering tone problems.

The third assistive cough, short-sitting self-assist, is performed in a short-sitting posture, such as in a wheelchair or over the edge of a bed. The patient is instructed to place one hand over the other at the wrist and place them in his lap. As in the previous technique, the patient is then asked to extend his trunk backward while inhaling maximally, followed by a strong voluntary cough. During the cough, the patient pulls his hands up and under the diaphragm, resembling the motion of a Heimlich maneuver (Fig 21–14). The hands mimic the abdominal mus-

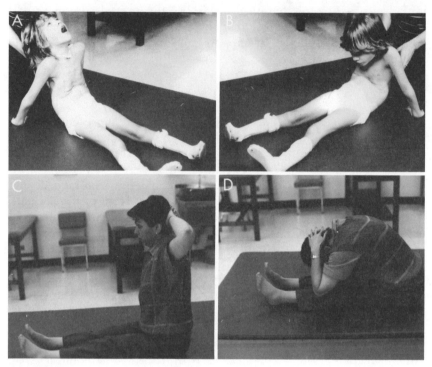

FIG 21–13.
A and **B,** assisted cough in long sitting (quadriplegic). **C** and **D,** paraplegic.

cles which would ordinarily contract to push the intestinal contents up and under the diaphragm to aid its recoil ability. This short-sitting technique employs more substantial use of the diaphragm than the long-sitting procedure and is therefore generally more effective as an assistive cough. Both techniques can be combined with improving functional balance goals. It is an effective self-assisted method for patients who have weak diaphragms or abdominal musculature. Most SCI or spina bifida patients, C_5 or below, can successfully learn this technique. Quadriplegics usually require trunk support from their wheelchairs to perform it independently and safely, whereas most paraplegics can perform it from an unsupported short-sitting position. Patients who lack good upper extremity coordination, such as many Parkinson's and MS patients, cannot perform the procedure quickly or forcefully enough to make it effective, and usually require assistance from another person.

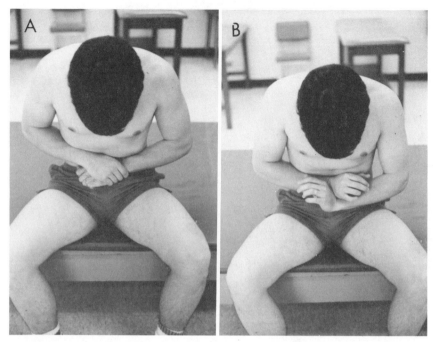

FIG 21–14.
Assisted cough in short sitting. **A,** hand position for patient with good hand function; **B,** hand position for patients with only wrist function.

Hands-Knees

The last assistive cough to be discussed is performed most frequently as a multipurpose activity, working on increasing the patient's balance, strength, coordination, and functional use of breathing patterns (including quiet breathing and coughing), simultaneously. The patient assumes an all-fours position (hands-knees). He is then instructed to rock forward, looking up and breathing in as he moves to a fully extended posture (Fig 21–15,A). After this, the patient is told to cough out as he quickly rocks backward to his heels with a flexed head (Fig 21–15,B). Once again, the importance of flexion and extension components of a cough are noted. The rocking can be done with or without a therapist's assistance. For patients with generalized or spotty weakness throughout (some SCI, head traumas, Parkinson's, MS, CP, or spina bifida patients), this method is perfect for incorporating many functional goals into a single activity. It can help prepare them for more challenging

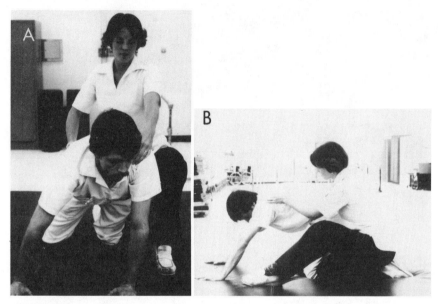

FIG 21–15.
Assisted cough in hands-knees position. **A,** extension or inspiratory phase; **B,** flexion or coughing phase.

respiratory activities that they will undoubtedly meet after their discharge from a rehabilitation center.

PHONATION

In contrast to the above procedures that assist the patient in swift expulsion of the air, procedures intended to restore a patient's vocalizing skills must prolong rather than abbreviate expiration. Coughing can be considered a gross motor skill that relies more on the force than the fine control of the muscles, for its effectiveness. Conversely, phonation requires precise, fine motor control of the diaphragm and vocal cords to provide a consistent air flow through the larynx. Both are expiration activities that depend on the preceding inspiration for their performance. Because of these differences, procedures to achieve both goals of improved coughing and improved phonation will be different in their emphasis.

Because of the patient's tidal volume and total inspiratory capacity are the "power source" for phonation, they become important concerns in a rehabilitation program. Generally, a normal tidal volume is adequate for conversational speech. However, larger quantities of air, thus greater inspiratory capacities, are required for singing or professional speaking. Therefore, breathing exercises described in Chapter 10 for improving inspiration should be taught prior to instructing the patient in better expiration control. Diaphragmatic and/or segmental breathing techniques, along with the use of quick stretches or repeated contractions, will facilitate the desired deeper inhalation.

Several simple techniques can be employed to improve eccentric control of the diaphragm and intercostal muscles in preparation for speech. Vibration to the lower chest during expiration assists in a slower, more controlled recoil of the diaphragm. Why this occurs is not fully understood. It may be that the sensory and proprioceptive stimulation that the vibration provides augments the patient's concentration on those muscles. Regardless, clinically we see that it results in longer phonation for many neurologically impaired patients. The patient is instructed to phonate an "ah" or "oh" sound for as long as possible. The therapist simultaneously vibrates the patient's chest with an even and gentle force throughout and slightly beyond the full expiration phase, using the hand placement of the Heimlich-type assist or costophrenic assistive cough technique. This is very different from the rapid, forceful pressure that was applied to the patient's chest when promoting a deep cough. As clinicians, be certain that the patients understand this important difference. The therapist must stress to the patient that they should not let air escape prior to vocalization, and that they should try to keep the voice intensity consistent throughout the procedure. This will promote equal eccentric contractions of the diaphragm during the entire course of their phonation. Progress can be readily monitored by timing the patient's vocalization, before, during, and after this technique. Ten to twelve seconds of vocalization is generally considered adequate for functional use in speech.

For children, this technique can be modified. The child is asked to say "ah" or "oh" for as long as possible while the therapist percusses his or her hands alternately on the child's upper or lower chest in supine or sidelying, so as to produce a series of staccato sounds. Most children enjoy the new sound that this makes and will try repeatedly to phonate longer and louder to accentuate the different intensities. Therapeutically, this requires them to take a deeper inhalation prior to vocalizing, followed by an elongated expiratory phase, both of which are necessary for functional speech. As the child becomes more adept at it, the therapist can apply more pronounced clapping over the chest, accomplishing a wider range of voice intensities and doubling as a means of percussion for postural drainage.

Speech activities that do not require a therapist's physical assistance can be done in a group or individual setting. Singing, for instance, promotes strong and prolonged vocalization with maximal inspiration, which is a main goal in a phonation program for this patient population. Similarly, whistling promotes long, even expirations, but without vocalization. Both are easily incorporated into a group activity on the nursing floor or in therapy. Along recreational lines, games that promote controlled blowing further the refinement of motor control over the respiratory muscles. This can be accomplished by blowing bubbles, especially large ones, blowing out candles, especially trick candles, blowing a ping-pong ball through a maze, or by blowing air hockey discs across the table rather than pushing them. Obviously, the possibilities for recreational use are endless, and simply require imagination on the part of the therapist.

Further refinement of breath control for speech can be promoted by interrupting the outgoing air flow. Functional speech is a series of vocal stops and starts. This procedure is geared toward improving functional communication skills. The therapist tells the patient to take a deep breath and then to count out to 10. After a few numbers, the patient is commanded to "hold it." He is then told to start up where he left off, with the therapist periodically interrupting as he proceeds. Because this activity requires the patient to stop and start diaphragmatic recoil at will, it is more advanced and should be used only after some control of the diaphragm has been mastered.

SUMMARY

Numerous ideas, techniques, and procedures were presented to diversify the neurological patients' respiratory rehabilitation program, which better accommodates their variety of respiratory deficits. Several passive positioning and equipment considerations were noted as well as five different methods for altering breathing patterns and 10 different ways to assist a patient in producing a more effective cough. Finally, several activities to improve communication skills were discussed. In the next chapter, integration of these techniques into the patient's total rehabilitation program will be presented in detail.

22

Respiratory Rehabilitation Secondary to Neurological Deficits: Treatment Progressions

Mary Massery, P.T.

TREATMENT PROGRESSIONS BY THERAPEUTIC POSTURES

In the previous two chapters, much attention has been paid to specific respiratory rehabilitation techniques, such as positioning considerations, altering breathing patterns, assistive cough techniques, and improving phonation. Coordination of all these procedures into an effective respiratory rehabilitation program requires skillful application according to the underlying principles laid down in Chapter 20. How are the three planes of respiration and the patient's skeletal system affected by the forces of gravity in different postures, and how is the patient's tone and muscle control affected by each posture? In each position discussed in this chapter, supine, sidelying, prone, sitting, standing and hands-knees, the specific effects of gravity on that posture, plus reflex influence, tone considerations, postural or skeletal considerations, and a therapeutic exercise progression will be presented. These exercise progressions are an expression of this author's philosophy and clinical experience with respiratory rehabilitation for the neurologically impaired, and are not intended to rule out the use of other traditional modes. Rather, they will hopefully inspire other clinicians to expand upon their own repertoire of treatment techniques.

Supine

The effects of gravity on each plane of respiration must be the first aspect of any posture analyzed. Only after that can the therapist determine which techniques will be the most beneficial in that position. In supine, anterior chest expansion is gravity resisted or in an antigravity plane; lateral and superior-inferior expansion is unaffected by gravitational forces or in a gravity-eliminated plane; and posterior expansion is posturally limited.

The influence of neurological reflexes can be felt in all postures and is usually a significant factor for children with CP and many patients with head trauma. Supine offers strong posturing for the tonic labyrinthine reflex (TLR), which increases extensor tone, and for the asymmetrical tonic neck reflex (ATNR), which promotes asymmetry in the chest by increasing extensor tone when the head is turned toward that side of the body, and increasing flexion tone on the other side. Spasticity of the abdominal muscles tends to be high in this posture, for many patients with SCIs. When dominant reflexes and marked spasticity are present, the chest becomes significantly immobile, rendering supine a poor starting point for many of these patients. Patients who are low toned with generalized or spotty weakness may be the most appropriate ones to begin in this position.

Early traditional treatments in this posture will be addressed first. Airshifting, a procedure in which the patient takes in a deep breath of air and shifts it from the lower to the upper chest and back again, has frequently been the patient's introduction into a neurological respiratory rehabilitation program. While it may help to improve the patients' cognitive awareness of their chests and their ability to control its movement, its significance as a chest mobilizer has not been satisfactorily proven. These patients typically have pronounced deficits in vital capacities. Thus, it would appear unlikely that they could maximally mobilize their own chests through this internal stretching method.

The second common technique used in this posture is diaphragmatic strengthening using weights on the abdomen. Caution is expressed for its indiscriminate use until the therapist has determined whether the applied resistance is actually strengthening the diaphragm or whether it is instead inhibiting it like the diaphragm-inhibiting technique described in Chapter 21. If the resistance of the weights plus the effect of gravity on anterior expansion in supine is too strong, or the patient's endurance too weak, this method will force the patient to alter his breathing pattern to an upper chest accessory muscle pattern rather than achieving the original goal of strengthening diaphragmatic breathing. Individual responses to this technique must therefore be carefully assessed before including or excluding it from the patient's respiratory program.

For new treatment procedures presented in Chapter 21, supine offers a fairly wide range of usage. Patients restricted to supine early in their rehabilitation can have diaphragmatic and intercostal breathing promoted through segmental breathing techniques. In addition to facilitating a preferred breathing pattern, segmental techniques also strengthen the diaphragm and mobilize the lower chest. Upper chest expansion can be promoted in this posture over the pectoralis region with segmental breathing techniques and diaphragm inhibition.

These procedures are antigravity for anterior excursion and should be used in this posture only if the patient is restricted to supine or demonstrates adequate strength to resist gravity. Conversely, encouragement of lateral chest expansion is begun in this posture because it is in a gravity-eliminated plane. Emphasis to one side of the chest is easily accomplished through manual input, which may make supine the preferred starting position for patients with hemiplegia that can breathe into an antigravity plane. When paradoxical breathing is present as with many patients with SCI, the diaphragmatic inhibiting technique is appropriate to encourage the use of accessory muscles. After instruction in desired breathing patterns has been initiated, use of either assistive cough (costophrenic or Heimlich-type) or phonation activities may be employed. Both cough procedures are antigravity activities and require more strength of the patient than in sidelying. On the other hand, the communication procedures work well in this posture because expiration is readily controlled by the therapist.

In summary, supine is an excellent beginning posture for CVAs or other diagnoses where asymmetry of the chest is the major concern. Supine is a more advanced posture for patients whose major deficit is symmetrical muscle weakness or paralysis, below a "fair" or "C" muscle grade, as in SCIs or other neuromuscular disorders.

Sidelying

This versatile posture readily lends itself to functional incorporation of respiratory goals within the patient's total rehabilitation program. In this posture, the effects of gravity have changed. Lateral expansion becomes an antigravity movement on one side and posturally limited on the other, while the rest of the chest, anterior-posterior and superior-inferior expansion, is in a gravity-eliminated plane.

Posturally, the diaphragm shifts downward to the dependent side, along with the intestines, allowing for freer movement of the chest on the uppermost side. Abnormal dominant reflexes, such as the ATNR, or the TLR, are less influential here because of the posture itself. Meanwhile, head and eye righting reactions, which are significant to upright posture functioning, can now be elicited in a sidelying on elbows position. Functionally, the posture promotes lateral trunk flexion of the uppermost side which can naturally lead into trunk rotation and movements such as rolling or coming to sitting. All these properties can be used advantageously when planning the patient's respiratory functioning progression. However, sidelying, by its nature, will always be asymmetrical. Both adverse and desired effects from this must be assessed prior to treatment for each individual patient.

As in supine, the sidelying progression begins with segmental breathing which leads to altered breathing patterns. Lower chest expansion, primarily the diaphragm's anterior excursion, can be either facilitated or inhibited here without the direct influence of gravity. Decreased resistance from gravity, combined with reduced reflex and spasticity influence in this posture, will usually successfully elicit more voluntary responses here than in supine. The patients learn control of the movement without contending with the added resistance from gravity and a possible increase in tone. Thus, sidelying is ideal for the more acute patient with SCI or any other patient whose primary problem is muscle weakness or paralysis.

Upper chest anterior excursion and/or upper chest superior excursion can be promoted through the diaphragm-inhibiting technique or through segmental facilitation over the pectoralis region. Balancing the use of the diaphragm and accessory muscles should be started in this posture when possible.

In contrast to the progression for upper and lower chest expansion, lateral chest expansion of the uppermost side becomes more difficult in sidelying, providing a natural progression for any hemiplegic patients from supine. After encouraging bilateral expansion of the lower chest in supine, the patient can be upgraded to sidelying with the uninvolved side dependent (against the surface). In order to breathe into his involved side, the patient must counteract gravity. At the same time, the patient surrenders neurological overflow support from the musculature on the uninvolved side because lateral excursion is posturally inhibited in this position. This is frequently the most difficult breathing activity for a patient with hemiplegia (from any diagnosis) to master because the therapist removes two support systems at once. Thus, it should not be attempted until some success in supine has been achieved. However, once successful here, most patients with hemiplegia will demonstrate better bilateral symmetrical breathing patterns in all other postures.

A patient's high RRs can often be altered in this posture through the use of the counterrotation technique. At the same time, this technique serves as an excellent external chest mobilizer. The Massery counterrotative assistive cough naturally follows and is definitely the preferred coughing procedure in this posture. The Heimlich-type assist, or the combination of these two, can be used successfully if counterrotation is not possible for medical or orthopedic reasons (unstable spine). Recall that the Massery counterrotative technique is the only assistive cough that closes off all three planes of respiration during forceful expulsion, which significantly improves on the two planes of respiration (in only the lower chest region) that the Heimlich-type or costophrenic techniques compress.

Phonation is usually more challenging in sidelying because the chest is asymmetrical. The same techniques, vibration, songs, interrupted air flow, etc., are used to increase breath support here, but only after the patient has first learned them in supine. For patients with hemiplegic deficits, placing them on their uninvolved sides while performing these procedures forces them to develop better breath control with their involved musculature, thus roundaboutly promoting more symmetrical use of the chest in other postures.

For patients who are developmentally delayed, such as children with CP, this posture offers a wonderful opportunity to combine improving their respiratory functioning simultaneously with promoting normal movement patterns. The therapist should begin by facilitating head righting reactions through assumption of sidelying on elbow posture, typically the sidelying posture one would assume while watching television. Through the use of PNF or NDT therapeutic exercises in this posture, it can accomplish six different goals: (1) elongates the weight-bearing side, allowing for better passive aeration of the dependent side while promoting lateral trunk flexion on the uppermost side; (2) facilitates asymmetrical posturing, thus inhibiting a dominant STNR which frequently locks these patients into symmetrical patterns of the extremities and trunk; (3) encourages the patient to maintain a head righting posture with the help of their own extremities, thereby promoting an internal feedback system for maintaining posture, essential for purposeful upright posturing; (4) begins work on better balance reactions of the upper body, which also is needed in upright posturing; (5) develops better head and neck control, thus assisting in breath control and optimal laryngeal position for vocalizing, which leads finally to (6) promotes vocalization. As a point of interest, how many neurologically intact persons ever converse from a sidelying position without first righting their heads and assuming this described posture? Do likewise for the patients before working on phonation activities in sidelying (Fig 22–1). All six of the above items combined are needed to help the patient successfully carry over a new breathing pattern into the next more challenging posture, sitting. Without the development of good voluntary trunk and head control, which this posture supports, the patient will be unable to control and isolate the movements of his chest for maximal respiratory functioning or phonation skills. This is a perfect illustration of the importance of combining goals in rehabilitation programs.

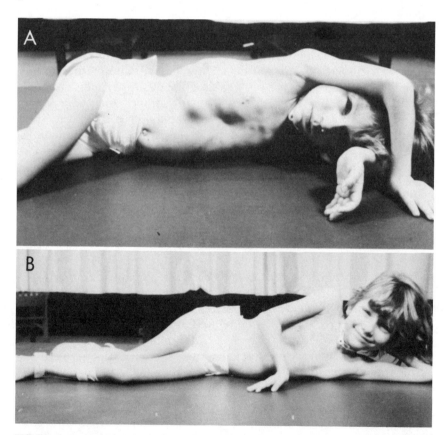

FIG 22–1.
A, sidelying without head righting. **B,** sidelying with head righting. Note changes in trunk and eye contact potential.

Progressing to rolling and assumption of sitting from sidelying, the patient learns to incorporate new breathing patterns into more functional activities. These two activities work well for all types of patients, especially those with symptoms like Parkinson's, using either PNF or NDT facilitation techniques. When rolling from supine to sidelying, facilitation can be given to promote either flexion or extension patterns, allowing for greater flexibility for breathing retraining techniques here. Rolling with the leading upper extremity in an extension pattern encourages the patient to inhale, while rolling with the leading upper extremity in a flexion pattern encourages exhalation (Fig 22–2). The clinician's evaluation of each patient's needs best determines which rolling pattern would be beneficial.

From a sidelying on one elbow posture, the patient can be facilitated up into a long-sitting position or on through to a side-sitting posture, emphasizing expiration on the way up (flexion phase) and inspiration on the way back down (extension phase) (Fig 22–3). Early on, the activity can be broken down into smaller ranges of motion to stress either better breathing control or better quality of movement of the patient's entire body. Eventually, some patients can be resisted through the movement to strengthen the muscles and breathing patterns as well as to challenge the patients' ability to control their own quality of movement. Due to the strong rotation components, this activity is also good for chest mobilization.

In summary, sidelying appears to have the most options for the severely involved patient, those with high neuromuscular tone, excessive reflex domination, and abnormally strong symmetrical posturing (some CP, Parkinson's, head trauma). For hemiplegic patients where asymmetry is the primary dysfunction, sidelying can encourage active use of the weak or involved side of the chest by inhibiting the uninvolved side. This is generally considered a more advanced posture for these patients because of the increased demands from gravity on lateral expansion. On the other hand, patients with spinal level weakness (SCI, spina bifida, polio) find the effects of gravity favorable upon their weakest plane of expansion, anterior expansion. Thus, it is often used as an early posture in their breathing retraining programs. Likewise, patients suffering from progressive diseases (MS, ALS, MD) find sidelying a particularly comfortable breathing posture in the latter stage of their diseases, most likely due to the decreased effect of gravity on their diaphragms. The versatility of this posture should be obvious from the above statements.

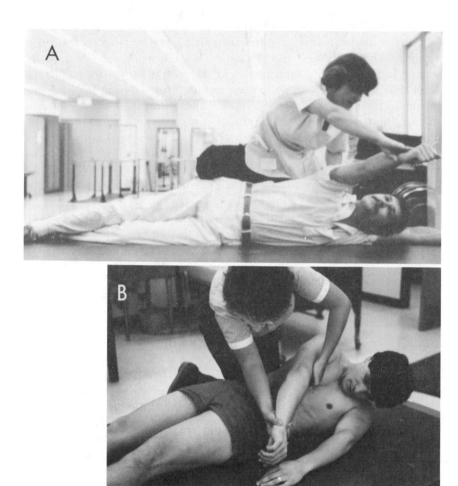

FIG 22–2.
A, rolling with extension: facilitating inhalation while rolling from supine to sidelying. **B,** rolling with flexion: facilitating exhalation while rolling to sidelying.

Prone

This posture posturally inhibits anterior chest excursion, thereby severely curtailing the ability of the diaphragm to function in the anterior plane. Posterior chest expansion now becomes antigravity for the first time, while superior-inferior and lateral expansion are in gravity eliminated planes. Abnormal reflexes become more dominant in this pos-

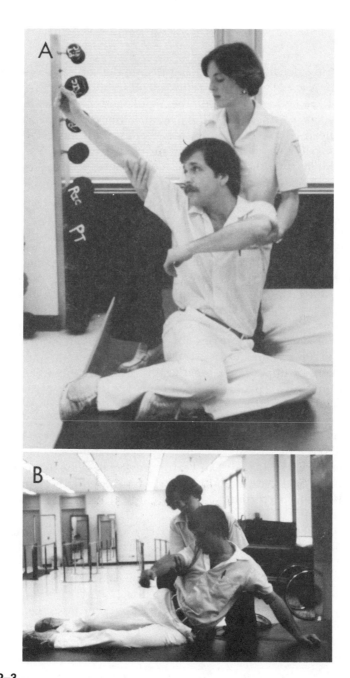

FIG 22–3.
A, a sidesitting flexion phase encourages exhalation. **B,** returning to prone: extension phase to encourage inspiration.

ture than in sidelying, often making assumption of flat prone unfeasible and impractical. The TLR reflex increases flexor tone here, as can the STNR reflex, especially in the trunk and proximal joints. The ATNR becomes difficult to inhibit because the position itself requires that the head be turned to one side, feeding into this reflex pattern, unless the patient is up in a prone on elbows position. Patients with abnormal high tone show similar results. Because of these strong tonal influences, managing a reflex dominated patient's breath control in prone or prone on elbows is the most challenging position for the therapist.

However, this posture can be used effectively for the patient with low tone and nonreflex domination (SCI, neuropathy, etc.) when stressing incorporation of new breathing patterns into functional activities. All therapeutic exercises here are performed in a prone on elbows position, creating ripe conditions for accessory muscle facilitation. The diaphragm is inhibited, yet the anterior upper chest is gravity assisted. In addition, the fixated upper extremities allow the patient to use his pectoralis and serratus muscles for respiration along with the more common accessory muscles (SCM, trapezius, scalenes, intercostals). Encouragement of upper chest breathing is nicely accomplished through head and neck PNF patterns, which concurrently work to (1) improve head control and righting reactions, (2) promote active movement out of synergy patterns, and (3) assist in reflex integration via inhibition of total body response to head positioning. These exercises can be progressed from active-assisted through resisted to independent activities.

From here, the patient can be progressed to static-dynamic activities. This requires the patient to support his upper body on one upper extremity while performing a nonweight-bearing task with the other upper extremity (see Fig 21–6). Greater trunk and shoulder control is necessary to perform this type of acitvity, which can be an excellent means of reestablishing chest stability. Throughout both, PNF head and neck patterns and static-dynamic activities, the upper chest is mobilized, thus reducing the risk of developing chest rigidity and its resultant impairments on respiratory function.

Without the significant use of the diaphragm, assistive coughing here is not nearly as effective as in any other posture. Primarily, the head flexion assist is used to strengthen the use of accessory muscles in a functional activity for intended use with the diaphragm in other postures.

This posture may be frightening to patients who are strictly diaphragmatic breathers. In the clinical setting, therapists often rush their patients with quadriplegia into a prone on elbows position with the intent of strengthening and stabilizing the shoulder girdle. However, if those patients have not developed an alternative breathing pattern, inhibition of the diaphragm may cause them extreme shortness of breath, understandably frightening them and usually negating any desired results in the posture.

In summary, a prone on elbows progression is most appropriate for the patient with lower toned, neuromuscular weakness. Use of reflex integration activities with breathing retraining exercises here is most appropriate for the patient already resolving any reflex domination. Lastly, prone on elbows is the best posture mechanically for facilitation of upper accessory muscles; however, the posture itself may cause anxiety for strong diaphragmatic breathers.

Sitting

This posture is the first antigravity (upright) posture that patients assume. Habits developed here carry over to other upright postures such as kneeling or standing. Therefore, integrating good breathing habits in sitting is vital before progressing the patient to more difficult antigravity postures.

For the first time, superior chest expansion is in a gravity-resisted plane of respiration and inferior expansion is in a gravity-assisted plane. Also for the first time, no planes of respiration are posturally inhibited, with all others being in a gravity-eliminated plane. The diaphragm and abdominal contents have shifted inferiorly because of gravity, being most pronounced in those patients with flaccid abdominal tone and no external supports, such as a binder. Because of this, concentric contractions of the diaphragm become easier, while eccentric contractions become more difficult, such as in coughing, forced VCs, or phonation activities. This makes it easier to understand why patients with SCIs show substantially higher residual lung volumes and lower VCs in sitting than in supine. Research has confirmed this, showing that for patients with SCIs, the highest VC reading is obtained in a slightly head-down supine position, where eccentric control of the diaphragm and intestinal positioning can be assisted by gravity. Flat supine positioning will show a slightly lower VC. Clearly then, the two assistive coughs performed in sitting are less likely to be as effective as the techniques described in supine or sidelying. For these reasons, they remain more advanced techniques.

Abnormal reflex dominance likewise changes here. The TLR reflex, which was so significant in supine and prone, becomes inactive while the ATNR and STNR become more significant. Although the effects of these reflexes are usually more apparent in children, their subtle influence must be watched for in the adult population as well, especially in CVAs and head traumas. These patients may use the asymmetry of the ATNR reflex to strengthen the muscular response of their weaker side. Therefore, the therapist should check closely to determine if a patient is relying on reflex support to produce a preferred breathing pattern. Uncurtailed, the breathing pattern may not be reproducible in other postures, thus not functional for them. Sitting is rarely the posture in which instruction in breathing retraining or coughing is begun; rather it is the posture that tests its functional use.

Concurrently, in sitting, the spine becomes unsupported for the first time, requiring active back extension or external supports. Notably then, good postural alignment is the initial concern in this position. For patients who cannot assume or maintain an upright posture without support, correct wheelchair alignment must be accomplished. These considerations were discussed in depth earlier. For those patients who can actively maintain the posture without support briefly before fatiguing, manual therapeutic assistance is appropriate. One such technique involves providing the patient with manual assistance for proper lumbar positioning, thus enabling the patient to work on thoracic and cervical extension more efficiently. This assists the patient in learning to balance the stability needs of the spine with the mobility needs of the rib cage. Once mastered, the manual support for the lumbar spine can be gradually withdrawn, presenting the patient with a greater challenge.

To perform the technique, the patient is seated over the edge of a firm surface such as a mat table. The therapist places her thumbs into the patient's sacroiliac joints (the dimples just above the buttocks) and aligns the rest of the hand along the posterior lateral border of the pelvis. As the patient is commanded to "sit up as straight as possible," the therapist presses her thumbs forward to produce an anterior, or forward, tilting of the pelvis (Fig 22–4). By properly aligning the lumbar spine, increasing its lordotic configuration, the thoracic and cervical spines become better aligned, which makes the paraspinal muscles' active participation in back extension more feasible. Only after this alignment is achieved should breathing or phonation exercises begin. Then ironically, improving spinal strength, improving sitting balance, and realigning head and neck positions can be considered respiratory rehabilitation goals here instead of just physical rehabilitation goals.

For the patient who is severely neurologically impaired and has difficulty learning accessory muscle breathing, a rocking chair may be the answer. Rocking the chair can be accomplished solely by move-

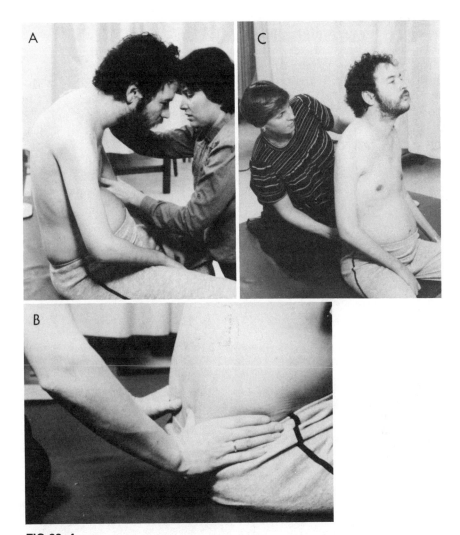

FIG 22–4.
Facilitating back extension. **A,** independent sitting posture of a patient with quadriplegia. Note trunk and head posture. **B,** hand placement to facilitate better spinal posture. **C,** sitting posture with facilitation. Note changes in thorax and head alignment.

ments of the head and neck, which is ideal for patients with high levels of quadriplegia. For safety reasons, the therapist must securely strap the patient in the rocking chair with straps of lateral supports prior to the activity. The patient is then instructed to bring the head forward to start the rocking motion, inhaling as he does so, and to exhale as he returns back (Fig 22–5). This coordinates the active contraction of the accessory muscles with inspiration, while promoting expiration during their relaxed phase. It serves as an important activity for strengthening these muscles and increasing their endurance, while performing a functional activity. It demands quick recruitment and activation of the appropriate muscle fibers to accommodate the precise timing of the rocking motion. But perhaps its most important attribute is that the rocking chair allows these severely limited patients to initiate their own movement, which may be all but lost in any other position. This is especially significant for children who have never known the feeling of self-initiated movement, adding to improved feelings of self-esteem and control over their bodies. Clinically, most young children respond enthusiastically to this new freedom, as a "normal" child would to a swing. Most are willing to do "less desirable therapeutic exercises" if it "buys" them more time in the rocking chair. Similar home use is strongly recommended.

For the less neurologically involved patient, therapeutic exercise progressions in sitting are open ended. No planes of respiration are posturally inhibited, allowing more freedom of trunk rotation, and thus chest mobilization, than did the previous three postures. Func-

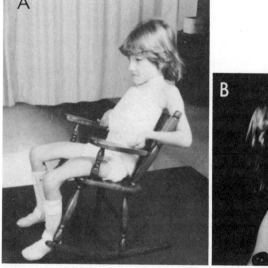
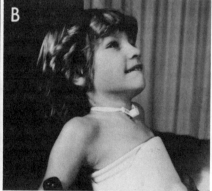

FIG 22–5.
Rocking chair activity. **A,** rocking movement performed by a patient with C5 quadriplegia. Note active participation of neck muscles. **B,** close-up of accessory muscle action during initiation of rocking movement.

tional incorporation of breathing patterns, rather than their beginning instruction, is the primary goal in this posture. While working on any number of balance or strengthening activities, breathing styles can be promoted or inhibited, such as with many bilateral upper extremity patterns in PNF. Another technique, called the butterfly procedure, promotes increased symmetrical participation of the whole chest during maximal inhalations and maximal exhalations.

While sitting over the edge of a firm surface, the patient, with or without the therapist's assistance, places his hands behind his head, making "wings" of his elbows (external rotation of the shoulder). The patient is instructed to inhale maximally while extending his back and upper extremities (increased external rotation of the shoulder), maximizing anterior chest expansion (Fig 22–6,A). After full extension, the patient pulls his elbows down and toward his lap into a flexed posture, which compresses the anterior chest, thus maximizing exhalation, exhaling as he proceeds (Fig 22–6,B). The upper extremity portion of the technique can be performed independently, assisted or resisted, depending on each patient's needs. This technique not only promotes symmetrical use of the chest, which is ideal for hemiplegic deficits, but it also promotes both deeper inhalations *and* exhalations. For patients with high residual volumes in their lungs, this technique is particularly useful.

Improved ventilation on one side of the patient's chest can be accomplished by adding a component of rotation to the above procedure. The patients inhale as they twist and look over their shoulder on the side to be emphasized (Fig 22–6,C). Likewise, to improve exhalation, the patients bring their elbow from that side down and across to their opposite knee during the expiration phase (Fig 22–6,D). Both aspects provide a better stretch to the intercostal muscles, promoting their active participation in both inspiration and expiration.

A variation of the sitting posture, side-sitting, facilitates significant reduction in high abnormal tone due to its strong rotational components. Although this position is seldom used functionally by adults, it does achieve maximal chest mobilization in all three planes of respiration and can be used for that purpose. Children generally assume and function in this posture more readily due to their greater flexibility. Therefore, it is more commonly seen in their exercise programs than in the adults' program. Again inspiration is encouraged during the extension phase and expiration during flexion.

The use of therapeutic exercise equipment in this posture must not be forgotten or excluded because it allows the patients to work independently on their long-term goals. The more advanced patients can

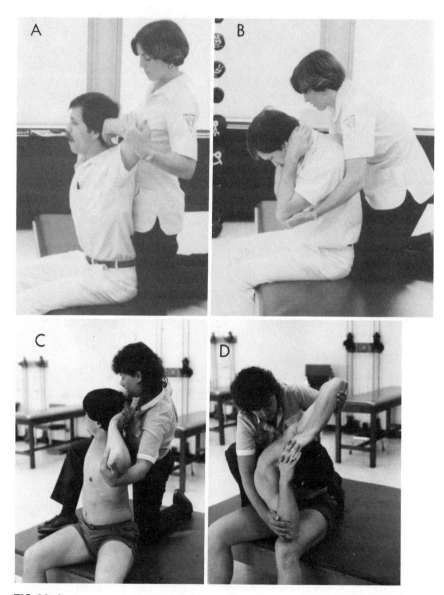

FIG 22–6.
A, butterfly technique facilitating inspiration. **B,** butterfly technique facilitating exhalation. **C,** butterfly with trunk rotation facilitating inspiration. All 3 planes of respiration are stretched on the patient's right side. **D,** butterfly with trunk rotation facilitating exhalation. All planes compressed on the right side.

use pulleys to strengthen their trunks and upper extremities while challenging their ability to use a proper breathing technique. A variety of PNF bilateral upper extremity patterns can be employed to encourage inspiration during trunk extension and expiration during trunk flexion, with either component of the activity being set up for resistance or assistance from the weights (Fig 22–7). Since all PNF patterns are performed on a diagonal, the chest will be stretched in all three planes. However, these activities must be performed bilaterally to ensure the participation of the trunk muscles which then ensures active chest participation. The same results could be accomplished through the use of slings, springs, balls, etc. The individual therapist's creative talents remain the only limit to the number of different techniques that can be used in this posture to promote better respiratory functioning.

In summary, sitting is the first upright posture in these patients' respiratory rehabilitation programs and is generally considered more advanced. One exception is for strict diaphragmatic breathing retraining. Those patients capable of maintaining intestinal positioning can use gravity for the first time to aid concentric contractions of the diaphragm. This is the only breathing pattern retraining begun in this

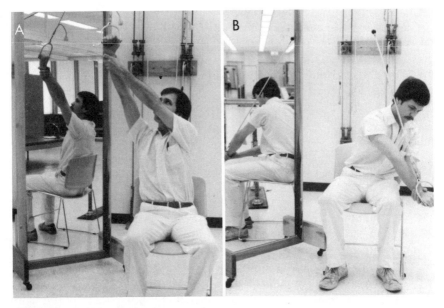

FIG 22–7.
Use of pulleys in a respiratory program. **A,** bilateral upper extremity PNF pattern (chopping). **B,** note trunk flexion and rotation.

posture. The increased balance, strength and postural endurance requirements of this posture make functional incorporation of other breathing patterns more challenging and thus more difficult. In addition, coughing, or forceful eccentric contraction of the diaphragm, is gravity resisted for the first time. On the other hand, these same attributes mean an increased potential for mobility that was not possible in the lower postures. This opens more options such as the use of equipment (i.e., pulleys, canes, or rocking chairs) or modifications of the posture (i.e., side-sitting, long-sitting, supported or unsupported short-sitting) for incorporating the patients' breathing patterns into their other physical rehabilitation goals.

Standing

All the principles for treatment progressions in sitting apply to standing as well. The only significant difference is that standing requires better balance reactions and wheelchair considerations are no longer needed. However, good posturing remains important in all positions.

Hands-Knees

In contrast to the vertical alignment of sitting and standing, the hand-knees posture is horizontally aligned. All are without posturally inhibited planes of respiration. Posterior expansion again becomes antigravity as it was in prone; but now, anterior expansion, rather than being prevented, is assisted.

All others are in a gravity-eliminated plane. Dominant reflexes present in prone will also be influential here with some minor differences. The TLR reflex will be less active because the body is no longer in contact with the surface. The most active reflex becomes the STNR because the active involvement of the extremities in the maintenance of this posture reinforces its actions. Thus, patients dominated by this reflex should be found an alternative posture in which to work.

Assuming an all-fours position causes the distal components of the extremities to become fixated, or stabilized, while the proximal components are moved, or mobile. This is in opposition to the actions in sitting or standing. The patients can then reverse the action of the proximal muscles, causing them to pull the chest out toward their arms, assisting in chest expansion. In addition, diaphragmatic breathing is in a gravity-assisted plane, providing a golden opportunity to combine the action of the diaphragm with all the accessory muscles to improve maximal inhalation and vital capacity. This posture is most appropriate for individuals with incomplete SCIs or other diagnoses that result in spotty weakness, because it can improve respiratory functioning while promoting balance, strength, and range of motion. Specifically, one such technique is rocking.

The patient rocks forward onto the upper extremities while inhaling and looking up (extension phase), and then exhales while pushing back onto the heels with head bowed (flexion phase) (see Fig 21–15). As in other posturally uninhibited postures, rotational components may be added to stretch the chest three dimensionally or to stress one side or the other. This technique can also be easily modified to accommodate any special deficits such as limitations in range or lack of proximal stability with the therapist's assistance.

The self-assistive cough is a natural progression for patients who have developed some control with this slower paced motion. The patient's ability to combine the necessary speed and force of movement required to produce an effective cough in this posture indicates a patient who has nearly completed his respiratory rehabilitation.

In summary, this posture is used in the more advanced stages of the patient's respiratory rehabilitation program with the emphasis on achieving multiple goals with each activity (i.e., improving pulmonary function, improving balance, improving coordination, etc.). This is also a good posture for teaching independent home programs for maintenance of bronchial hygiene and independent assistive coughs.

OTHER CONSIDERATIONS

Ideas that can be used in different postures for many types of patients will be presented. The first such item is the use of a oxygen nasal cannula during the initial phase of ADL or other new activity training. Patients with SCIs, for example, who use their accessory muscles to increase their tidal volumes, commonly find that they become short of breath when learning new activities such as transfer techniques. Concentrating on performing a new task reduces the ability to simultaneously control a new breathing pattern; thus, they "forget" to breathe adequately during the activity. Or, this shortness of breath can be due to increased oxygen demand without adequate reserve volume. Tidal volumes should be approximately 10% of the patient's vital capacity, but clinically many patients with quadriplegia show tidal volumes in the range of 33%–67% of their vital capacities, which leaves little reserve to fall back on when oxygen demands increase, resulting in shortness of breath. If these patients are provided with supplemental oxygen through a simple nasal cannula at a rate of 1–2 L O_2/min or 24%–28% F_{IO_2} (see Chapter 29), they can concentrate on learning the new task without also having to think about getting adequate ventilation. As the activity becomes learned and requires less conscious effort, the cannula can be weaned and the patient can learn to coordinate both activities.

The second item involves recreational integration of respiratory goals. Some patients do not feel comfortable performing breathing exercises per se but when these exercises are incorporated into a fun or competitive situation, they may suddenly excel. Countless creative ideas have been used. In a class or group setting of patients with high levels of quadriplegia (in PT, recreational therapy, or on the nursing floor), games involving sipping or sucking will help to promote maximal inspiration and better ventilation. One such idea that this author has used successfully is the "longest draw through the longest straw" game. Slits are cut at both ends of many straws and then loosely fit onto one another to make longer straws. Sipping fluid through these makeshift straws becomes progressively more difficult as the distance the fluid must travel increases and the suction leakage becomes more marked. In our facility, a contest was set up to determine who could sip through the longest straw. The group's low VC average led the staff to project that no patient would succeed further than through 4–5 straws. However, all patients easily passed that mark. The winner, in fact (a male patient with C_5 quadriplegia from a SCI), sipped through 37 straws before the game was called due to time. Interestingly enough, this was the same patient who cooperated minimally with routine VC and breathing exercises. When the procedures were made competitive, this patient clearly rallied, showing a significant improvement in his respiratory capabilities.

Other game ideas include modified ping-pong, blowing the ball across the table instead of using a paddle, or ice hockey using the same method. A maze can be made requiring the patient to blow the ball through the correct channels and monitoring their progress by timing each effort or counting how many breaths were needed per trial. Blowing out candles, especially for the younger population, continues to use the same idea. Singing and whistling, as detailed earlier in this chapter, helps to facilitate longer phonation.

Contests to see who can hold their breath the longest maintains airway openings longer, which some researchers think may prevent microatelectasis and facilitates collateral ventilation. Incentive spirometry may also be used for this purpose. For younger children, a modified version of the popular "red light, green light" game encourages fine tuning of the respiratory muscles. The leader rapidly changes commands to sip in, blow out, or hold it, with the child most closely following the commands becoming the winner, and getting a chance to become the new leader. These few ideas just begin to explore the realm of possibilities.

CONCLUSION

Obviously the main goal throughout the exercise progression presented in this chapter is to prevent the harmful effects of prolonged bed rest or prolonged singular positioning on the patient's pulmonary function. The literature repeatedly shows decreased TV and minute volumes, less frequent deep inspirations, poorer bronchial hygiene, and less active cough reflexes for patients confined to bed, even without any neurological impairments. Thus, the patient population that presents with significant neurological deficits to the external mechanisms of the chest is at even greater risk for showing decreased pulmonary functions. Their chances of developing respiratory complications such as pneumonia or atelectasis, secondary to these deficits, are of course elevated. It is thus the clinician's responsibility to get these patients mobile as soon as possible, using as many different postures as possible. It is also their responsibility to stress to the patient and family the importance of following through on a long-term prophylactic program. Carrying out a judicious respiratory rehabilitation program while simultaneously keeping these patients mobilized should markedly reduce these risks, thereby improving the quality of these patient's lives.

REFERENCES

Aberion G, Alba A, Lee MH et al: Pulmonary care of duchene type of muscular dystrophy. *NY State J Med* 1973; 73:1206–1207.

Alexandre H, Colombo F, Curri D, et al: Breathing alterations in head injured patients. *J Neurosurg Sci* 1982; 51:209–218.

Alexander MA, Johnson EW, Petty J, et al: Mechanical ventilation of patients with late stage duchene muscular dystrophy: Management in the home. *Arch Phys Med Rehabil* 1979; 60:289–292.

Alvarez SE, Peterson M, Lunsford BR: Respiratory treatment of the adult patient with spinal cord injury. *Phys Ther* 1981; 61:1737–1745.

Ashworth B, Hunter AR: Respiratory failure in myasthenia gravis. *Proc R Soc Lond (Biol)* 1971; 64:489–490.

Axen K, Pineda H, Shunfenthal I, et al: Diaphragmatic function following cervical cord injury: Neurally mediated improvement. *Arch Phys Med Rehabil* 1985; 66:219–222.

Axen K: Ventilatory responses to mechanical loads in cervical cord-injured humans. *J Appl Physiol* 1982; 52:748–756.

Bobath K, Bobath B: Neuro-developmental treatment of cerebral palsy. *Am J Phys Ther* 1967; 11:1039–1041.

Bonner CD: Rehabilitation instead of bed rest? *Geriatrics* 1969; 24:109–118.

Braun SR, Giovannoni R, Levin HB, et al: Oxygen saturation during sleep in patients with spinal cord injuries. *Am J Phys Med* 1982; 61:302–309.

Braun SR, Giovannoni BA, O'Connor M: Improving the cough in patients with spinal cord injury. *Am J Phys Med* 1984; 63:1–10.

Brown JC, Swank SM, Matta J, et al: Late spinal deformity in quadriplegic children and adolescents. *J Pediatr Orthop* 1984; 4:456–461.

Bryan AC: Conference on the scientific basis of respiratory therapy: Pulmonary physiotherapy in the pediatric age group. Comments of a devil's advocate. *Am Rev Respir Dis* 1974; 110:143–144.

Cahill JL, Okamoto GA, Higgins T, et al: Experience with phrenic nerve pacing in children. *J Pediatr Surg* 1983; 18:851–854.

Carter RE: Experiences with high tetraplegics. *Paraplegia* 1979; 17:140–146.

Carter RE: Medical management of pulmonary complications of spinal cord injury. *Adv Neurol* 1979; 22:261–269.

Carter RE: Unilateral diaphragmatic paralysis in spinal cord injured patients. *Paraplegia* 1980; 18:267–274.

Cherniack RM, Cherniack L, Naimark A: Respiration in health and disease, ed 2. Philadelphia, WB Saunders Co, 1972.

Cherniack NS, Fishman AP: Abnormal breathing patterns. *Med Clin North Am* 1975; 59:1–45.

Cherniack NS: Abnormal breathing patterns: Their mechanisms and clinical significance. *JAMA* 1974; 230:57–58.

Cheshire DJ, Flack WJ: The use of operant conditioning techniques in the respiratory rehabilitation of the tetraplegic. *Paraplegia* 1979; 16:162–174.

Clough P: Glossopharyngeal breathing: Its application with a traumatic quadriplegic patient. *Arch Phys Med Rehabil* 1983; 64:384–385.

Collier CR, Dail CW, Affeldt JE: Mechanics of glossopharyngeal breathing. *J Appl Physiol* 1956; 8:580–584.

Conomy JP, Braatz JH: Guillain-Barré syndrome: The physical therapist and patient care. *Phys Ther* 1971; 51:517–523.

Cooper CB, Trend PS, Wiles CM: Severe diaphragm weakness in multiple sclerosis. *Thorax* 1985; 40:631–632.

Curran FJ: Night ventilation by body respirators for patients in chronic respiratory failure due to late stage muscular dystrophy. *Arch Phys Med Rehabil* 1981; 62:270–274.

Dail CW, Affeldt JE, Collier CR: Clinical aspects of glossopharyngeal breathing. *JAMA* 1955; 158:445–449.

Dail CW: Respiratory aspects of rehabilitation in neuromuscular conditions. *Arch Phys Med Rehabil* 1965; 46:655–675.

Davis LF: Continuing education class: Developmental disorders. Sponsored by: National Institute of Continuing Education in Developmental Disabilities. 1978; 10:14–15.

Davis LF: Continuing education class: Speech-motor dysfunction. Sponsored by: National Institute of Continuing Education in Developmental Disabilities. 1979; 4:28–29.

DeReuck AV, Porter R: Ciba Foundation Symposium: Development of the Lung. Boston, Little, Brown & Co, 1967.

De Troyer A, Deisser P: The effects of intermittent positive pressure breathing on patients with respiratory muscle weakness. *Am Rev Resp Dis* 1981; 124:132–137.

Donovan WH, Taylor N: Ventilatory assistance in quadriplegia. *Arch Phys Med Rehabil* 1973; 54:485–488.

Dowell AR, Buckley CE, Cohen R, et al: Cheyne-Stokes respiration: A review of clinical manifestations and critique of physiologic mechanisms. *Arch Intern Med* 1971; 127:712–726.

Fisher HB: Improving voice and articulation. Boston, Houghton-Mifflin Co, 1975.

Foldstad H, Blom S, Linderholm H: Artificial respiration by phrenic nerve stimulation (diaphragm pacing) in patients with cervical cord and brain stem lesions. *Scand J Rehabil Med* 1983; 15:173–181.

Fugl-Meyer AR: A model for treatment of impaired ventilatory function in tetraplegic patients. *Scand J Rehabil Med* 1971; 3:168–177.

Fugl-Meyer AR, Grimby G: Respiration in tetraplegia and in hemiplegia: A review. *Int Rehabil Med* 1984; 6:186–190.

Fulford FE, Brown JK: Position as a cause of deformity in children with cerebral palsy. *Dev Med Child Neurol* 1976; 18:305–314.

Gordon E: Respiratory control after acute head injury. *Lancet* 1973; 1:483.

Greenberg M, Edmonds J: Chronic respiratory problems in neuromyopathic disorders: Their nature and management. *Pediatr Clin North Am* 1974; 21:927–934.

Griggs RC, Donohoe KM: Recognition and management of respiratory insufficiency in neuromuscular disease. *J Chronic Dis* 1982; 35:497–500.

Griggs RC, Donohoe KM, Utell MJ, et al: Evaluation of pulmonary function in neuromuscular disease. *Arch Neurol* 1981; 38:9–12.

Grimby G, Hook O: Physical training of different patient groups: A review. *Scand J Rehabil Med* 1971; 3:15–25.

Gross D, Ladd HW, Riley EJ, et al: The effect of training on strength and endurance of the diaphragm in quadriplegia. *Am J Med* 1980; 68:27–35.

Haas F, Axen K, Pineda H, et al: Temporal pulmonary function changes in cervical cord injury. *Arch Phys Med Rehabil* 1985; 66:139–144.

Hamilton EA, Nichols PJ, Tait GB: Late onset of respiratory insufficiency after polio. *Am Phys Med* 1970; 10:223–229.

Harrison BD, Collins JV, Brown KG, et al: Respiratory failure in neuromuscular diseases. *Thorax* 1971; 26:579–584.

Hixon TJ: Dynamics of the chest wall during speech production: Function of the thorax, rib cage, diaphragm, and abdomen. *J Speech Hear Res* 1976; 19:297–357.

Hixon TJ, Putman AH, Sharp JT: Speech production with flaccid paralysis of the rib cage, diaphragm, and abdomen. *J Speech Hear Disord* 1983; 48:315–327.

Homma I, Nagai T, Sakai T, et al: Effect of chest wall vibration on ventilation in patients with spinal cord lesion. *J Appl Physiol* 1981; 50:107–111.

Hornstein S, Ledsome JR: Ventilatory muscle training in acute quadriplegia. Accepted for publication by *Physiother Can* 1986.

Houser CR: Breathing exercises for children with pseudohypertrophic muscular dystrophy. *Phys Ther* 1971; 51:751–759.

Huang CT, Kuhlemeier KV, Ratanaubol U, et al: Cardiopulmonary response in spinal cord injury patients: effect of pneumatic compressive devices. *Arch Phys Med Rehabil* 1983; 64:101–106.

Huldtgren AC: Ventilatory dysfunction and respiratory rehabilitation in post traumatic quadriplegia. *Eur J Respir Dis* 1980; 61:347–356.

Keesee PD: Abnormal reflex activity and voice usage deviations in cerebral palsy. *Phys Ther* 1976; 56:1358–1360.

Kendall HO, Kendall FP, Wadsworth GE: *Muscles: Testing and Function*, ed 2. Baltimore, Williams & Wilkins Co, 1971.

Kim R: The chronic residual respiratory disorder in postencephalitis parkinsonism. *J Neurol Neurosurg Psychiatry* 1968; 31:393–398.

Kirby NA, Barnerias MJ, Siebens AA: An evaluation of assisted cough in quadriparetic patients. *Arch Phys Med Rehabil* 1966; 47:705–710.

Knott M, Voss DE: Proprioceptive neuromuscular facilitation, ed 2. New York, Harper & Row, 1968.

Lavigne JM: Respiratory care of patients with neuromuscular disease. *Nurs Clin North Am* 1979; 14:133–143.

Le CT, Price M: Survival from spinal cord injuries. *J Chronic Dis* 1982; 35:487–492.

Ledsome JR, Sharp JM: Pulmonary function in acute cervical cord injury. *Am Rev Respir Dis* 1981; 124:41–44.

Levitt S, Miller C: The interrelationship of speech therapy and physiotherapy in children with neurodevelopmental disorders. *Dev Med Child Neurol* 1973; 15:188–193.

Maclean IC, Mattioni TA: Phrenic nerve conduction studies: A new technique and its application in quadriplegic patients. *Arch Phys Med Rehabil* 1981; 62:70–73.

Maloney FP: Pulmonary function in quadriplegia: Effects of a corset. *Arch Phys Med Rehabil* 1979; 60:261–265.

Mazza FG, DiMarco AF, Altose MD, et al: The flow-volume loop during glossopharyngeal breathing. *Chest* 1984; 85:638–640.

Metcalf VA: Vital capacity and glossopharyngeal breathing in traumatic quadriplegia. *Phys Ther* 1966; 46:835–838.

Micheli J: The use of the modified Boston orthosis system for back pain: Clinical indications. *J Orth Pros* 1985; 39:41–46.

Montero JC, Feldman DJ, Montero D: Effects of glossopharyngeal breathing on respiratory function after cervical cord transection. *Arch Phys Med Rehabil* 1967; 48:650–653.

Mortola JP, Sant'ambrogic G: Mechanics of breathing in tetraplegics. *Am Rev Resp Dis* 1979; 119:131–134.

Newsom DJ: The diaphragm and neuromuscular disease. *Am Rev Respir Dis* 1979; 119:115–117.

Nixon V: *Spinal Cord Injury: A Guide to Functional Outcomes in Physical Therapy Management.* Rockville, Maryland, Aspen Systems Corp, 1985.

North JB, Jennett S: Abnormal breathing patterns associated with acute brain damage. *Arch Neurol* 1974; 31:338–344.

Oakes DD, Wilmot CB, Halverson D, et al: Neurogenic respiratory failure: A five-year experience using implantable phrenic nerve stimulators. *Ann Thorac Surg* 1980; 30:118–121.

Payton OD, Hirt S, Newton R: *Bases for Neurophysiologic Approaches to Therapeutic Exercise: An Anthology.* Philadelphia, FA Davis Co, 1977.

Popova LM, Nicolajenko EM, Bobrovskaja AN: The influence of acid-base balance on the respiratory center function and cerebral blood flow in patients with respiratory muscle paralysis during long-term artificial ventilation. *Eur Neurol* 1972; 8:161–163.

Porter R (ed): *Breathing: Hering-Breuer Centenary Symposium* London, Churchill, 1970.

Rankin J, Dempsey JA: Respiratory muscles and the mechanisms of breathing. *Am J Phys Med* 1967; 46:198–244.

Rothman, JG: Effects of respiratory exercises on the vital capacity and forced expiratory volumes in children with cerebral palsy. *Phys Ther* 1978; 58:421–425.

Roussos C, Macklem PT: The respiratory muscles. *N Engl J Med* 1982; 307:786–797.

Sandham JD, Shaw DT, Guenter CA: Acute supine respiratory failure due to bilateral diaphragmatic paralysis. *Chest* 1977; 72:96–98.

Semans S: The bobath concept in treatment of neurological disorders: A neurodevelopmental treatment. *Am J Phys Med* 1967; 46:732–785.

Shaffer TH, Wolfson MR, Bhutani VK: Respiratory muscle function, assessment, and training. *Phys Ther* 1981; 61:1711–1723.

Siegel I: Management of muscular dystrophy: A clinical review. *Muscle Nerve* 1978; 1:453–460.

Siegel IM: Pulmonary problems in duchene muscular dystrophy: Diagnosis, prophylaxis, and treatment. *Phys Ther* 1975; 55:160–162.

Silver JR, Moulton A: The physiological and pathological sequelae of paralysis of the intercostal and abdominal muscles in tetraplegic patients. *Paraplegia* 1969; 7:131–141.

Sivak ED, Streib EW: Management of hypoventilation in motor neuron disease presenting with respiratory insufficiency. *Ann Neurol* 1980; 7:188–191.

Sivak ED, Gipson WT, Hanson MR: Long-term management of respiratory failure in amyotrophic lateral sclerosis. *Ann Neurol* 1982; 12:18–23.

Stanley WG: Follow-up care of the spinal cord injured patient. *Am Fam Physician* 1981; 24:105–111.

Sullivan CE, Berthon JM, Issa FG: Remission of severe obesity—Hypoventilation syndrome after short-term treatment during sleep with nasal continuous positive airway pressure. *Am Rev Resp Dis* 1983; 128:177–181.

Taylor N, Glenn WW: Respiratory training for quadriplegics. *N Engl J Med* 1972; 286:1267–1268.

Tecklin JS: Physical therapy for children with chronic lung disease. *Phys Ther* 1981; 61:1774–1781.

Tobin MJ, Cohn MH, Sackner MA: Breathing abnormalities during sleep. *Arch Intern Med* 1983; 143:122–228.

Van Hanswyk E, Yuan H: Orthotic management of thoracolumbar fractures with a total contact TLSO. *J Orthop Pros* 1979; 33:10–19.

Van SH: Treatment of a patient with a complete C1 quadriplegia. *Phys Ther* 1975; 55:35–38.

Vella LM, Hewitt PB, Jones RM, et al: Sleep apnea following cervical cord surgery. *Anaesthesia* 1984; 39:108–112.

Wehner R: Respiratory care for patients with amyotrophic lateral sclerosis. *J Pract Nurs* 1981; 31:24–25.

Weinberg B, Bosma JF: Similarities between glossopharyngeal breathing and injection methods of air intake for esophageal speech. *J Speech Hear Disord* 1970; 35:25–32.

23

Surgery of the Alimentary Tract, Abdomen, Head, and Neck

Lyn Hobson, P.T., R.R.T.

Robert Berry, R.N.

Cynthia Webster, B.S.R.

As we develop in our roles as professional health care workers, we begin to appreciate the variety of medical problems that the human body is capable of developing and enduring. The human body is an incredibly complex system capable of withstanding an incredible amount of anatomical and physiological insult. There are various disease entities that can be treated without surgical intervention and there are those that require corrective surgery in order to return to a predisease state of life or at least to one of reasonable comfort.

This chapter provides the therapist with a synopsis of the more common surgical procedures involving the alimentary tract, abdomen, head, and neck. The pathophysiology of pulmonary complications does not differ with each surgery. We encourage the reader to investigate the references presented at the end of this chapter for further study.

SURGERY OF THE ESOPHAGUS

Some of the more common pathologies requiring surgery of the esophagus include congenital disorders, injuries, achalasia, hiatal hernias, neoplastic growths, and esophageal varices.

Congenital Disorders

The two most common congenital disorders requiring surgery are atresia (a localized stenosis of the esophagus which if unrepaired leads to death from aspiration) and tracheoesophageal fistula (occurs when the two pathways fail to be completely divided by the partition during embryologic development). These disorders are repaired by having the esophagus reconstructed surgically through a right thoracotomy or sternal split.

Injuries

The types of injuries to the esophagus are varied and include knife wounds, swallowing of corrosive fluids, rupture of the esophagus and lodging of foreign objects in the esophagus. Knife wounds to the esophagus are rare and usually occur in the cervical region. They are treated by immediate surgical repair, with the type of approach varying with the area affected.

Swallowing of corrosive fluids occurs accidentally with children and deliberately with adult suicides. It results in a chemical burn and subsequent ulceration of the esophagus and stomach. The extent of the injury depends on the solution and amount ingested. Acids and solutions of mercuric chloride and phenol affect the stomach more than the esophagus. Strong alkalis cause extensive erosion and damage of the esophagus with severe fibrotic strictures remaining after the esophagus has healed. Healing after ingestion of corrosive fluids always results in scarring and stricture of the esophagus, requiring frequent dilatations. Esophagectomies may be done at the time of injury, or later if the strictures and scarring of the esophagus are severe. A new esophagus is then fashioned from the jejunum or colon and passed up through the diaphragm and chest into the neck.

Rupture of the esophagus is rare and is usually seen in alcoholics. It occurs when the patient vomits after eating excessively heavy meals, as a result of the sudden distention of the esophagus. A longitudinal tear appears in the esophagus, with the vomitus spilling into the pleural space (usually on the left) and ultimately causing a pyopneumothorax. Immediate transthoracic repair and irrigation must be performed.

Lodging of foreign bodies (dental plates in adults; marbles, whistles and coins in children) causes local mucosal edema, which may completely occlude the esophagus, tear the wall of the esophagus if large or sharp enough, or cause fatal mediastinitis. Treatment is extraction of the object with special forceps, with the patient under general anesthesia, or transthoracic surgical repair of tears.

Achalasia

This is caused by spasm of the lower end of the esophagus and is most frequently seen in young women in their twenties. The spasm is caused by contraction of the smooth muscle of the esophagus and results in the part above the stricture becoming grossly dilated with decomposing food. Correction of the problem is surgical with the Heller procedure (the smooth muscle is divided through a thoracotomy or upper abdominal incision).

Esophageal Varices

Esophageal varices occur when portal hypertension from cirrhosis of the liver causes the veins at the lower end of the esophagus to become dilated and tortuous. It occurs when anastomoses form between the portal and systemic circulation. Bleeding is frequently severe and is treated with transfusion and insertion of a special tube with two balloons; the small one is fed into the stomach and inflated to prevent dislodgment, and the large one fits inside the esophagus and is inflated to control bleeding. Surgical procedures to correct the problem include portacaval shunts, removal of part or all of the esophagus and feeding gastrostomy.

Hiatal Hernias

In this condition the stomach protrudes into the thorax through the opening for the esophagus in the diaphragm (esophageal hiatus). It is a common condition seen frequently in women past middle age. Regurgitation of acid from the stomach into the esophagus causes heartburn and is a result of the weakened diaphragm muscle in this area. The problem is accentuated with obesity, pregnancy, ascites or any other form of abdominal distention. The constant regurgitation of acid into the esophagus can lead to chronic inflammation, ulceration, fibrosis and obstruction. Various surgical procedures can be used to correct the problem. A thoracic incision, abdominal incision or both are made. A fundal plication involves wrapping the fundus of the stomach around the lower end of the esophagus. In Boeremia's procedure the stomach is stitched to the anterior abdominal wall. All procedures are designed to reduce the stomach to its correct anatomical location and re-form the angle between the esophagus and stomach.

Neoplastic Growths

Cancer of the esophagus will be discussed in Chapter 24. Suffice it to say that the malignancy is usually quite advanced when the patient begins to experience difficulty with swallowing. The condition is treated with either radiation (to relieve symptoms) or surgery. Radical excision involves removing the affected esophagus, as well as a considerable length above and below. In a second operation the cervical stump is connected to the stomach with a piece of the jejunum or colon (colon upswing). A bypass procedure, again using the colon or jejunum, is used when the esophagus cannot be safely removed. This procedure relieves the obstruction and allows the patient to continue to eat. In either of these procedures a gastrostomy or feeding jejunostomy may be performed in order to feed the patient. (A tube is placed directly into the stomach or jejunum to allow nutritionally balanced fluids and solutions to be inserted.) Frequently when surgery is not feasible, a plastic tube can be passed through the stricture to relieve the obstruction for several months (although occlusion of the tube by tumor does eventually occur).

Chest Physical Therapy

Treatment of the patient following esophageal surgery depends on the site of the incision. Essentially all procedures use either a thoracic incision, in which case the patient is treated as a thoracotomy patient, or an abdominal incision is used and the patient is treated the same as after abdominal surgery (to be covered later in this chapter).

Treatment of patients who have had colon upswing surgery must be mentioned. Special consideration in positioning must be made. In order to prevent the possibility of putting a "stretch" on the anastomosed section of the colon, these patients should be log rolled with the head kept in a neutral position or flexed (do not hyperextend the neck). The head of the bed should remain elevated 30 degrees at all times. Physicians do not like these patients positioned bed flat unless their respiratory status becomes compromised. In these cases the aggressiveness of positioning must depend on the physician's wishes. When the patient's bronchial hygiene becomes a priority, the physician may instruct the therapist to place the patient in postural drainage positions.

These patients should not be nasotracheally or orally suctioned, as there is a possibility of traumatizing the cervical anastomosis. Other than those two exceptions, these patients should be evaluated and treated as any other patients, with the appropriate respiratory therapy modalities, percussion, vibration, breathing exercises and cough instruction. These patients will frequently have difficulty with diaphragmatic breathing since the diaphragm is split during surgery. Occasionally the phrenic nerve is cut and the affected half of the diaphragm will be paralyzed. Therapists can obtain this information from the surgeon, if it is not mentioned in the chart. The therapist often is the one to assess the diaphragmatic dysfunction by his assessment and therapy.

SURGERY OF THE ABDOMEN

When an organ or organ system within the body begins to malfunction, the body has unique ways of communicating this to us. Each of us has a specific set of activities that we follow every day. When the body sends out a signal that causes an interruption in our daily routine, the health-conscious individual seeks out medical attention to discover what is causing this deviation from the norm. Specific symptoms of abdominal distress could include a loss of appetite followed by a gradual weight loss, nausea and vomiting, a fever of undetermined origin, or a change in bowel habits.

When the patient presents with the symptoms mentioned, immediate attention is given to an examination of the abdomen. A systematic assessment of the abdomen is done by utilizing the techniques of inspection, auscultation, percussion, and palpation. Inspection should include observation of rashes, lesions, dilated veins, and distention. Auscultation of the abdomen is performed in a systematic manner, listening to each of the four quadrants of the abdomen. The examiner should listen first for the presence or absence of bowel sounds. He should then listen for bruits (vascular sounds) in each of the four quadrants. Percussion is done to determine resonance, tympany, and dullness. Palpation of the abdomen is used as the final assessment technique since it usually causes the most discomfort of the four to a tender abdomen. Light palpation and deep palpation can be performed in all four quadrants of the abdomen in order to determine abdominal tenderness or the presence of masses. The patient is observed at all times when utilizing all four of these techniques for signs of tenderness or pain. This exam is usually followed by a series of diagnostic tests to determine the etiology of the patient's complaint. Depending on the diagnosis made, the patient may be treated either conservatively or through surgical intervention. At this point, some of the more common surgical procedures of the abdomen will be discussed.

Surgery performed on the internal organs of the abdomen can present special problems to the patient in need of postoperative pulmonary hygiene. *The closer the surgical incision is to the diaphragm, the more difficulty the patient will have with techniques such as cough effort, diaphragmatic breathing, and use of the incentive spirometry.* These problems are addressed at the end of this section. Here we discuss some of the more common disease entities requiring surgical intervention of the abdomen. Therapists desiring more information in a particular area may utilize the references offered at the end of this chapter.

ALTERATIONS IN THE DIGESTIVE PROCESS

Gastrectomy

The gastrectomy, or removal of the stomach, can be either partial or total. The partial gastrectomy is indicated when duodenal or gastric ulcers have not responded to medical treatment and in some carcinomas of the stomach. There are several other surgical techniques for the treatment of the unresolved ulcer, but the goal of all these surgical procedures is to reduce acid. With a partial gastrectomy, 70% to 80% of the stomach is removed. An anastomosis is then made to either the duodenum (Billroth I) or to the jejunum (Billroth II). This will reduce acid secretion and divert it from the ulcerative area. Total gastrectomy is the removal of the entire stomach. This is usually indicated for carcinoma of the stomach with no metastatic involvement. Again there is an anastomosis, but here the small intestine is joined to the proximal portion of the esophagus. Possible postoperative complications include shock, infection, hemorrhage, and pulmonary complications. Intraoperatively, a nasogastric tube is put in place and is maintained for several days with the patient receiving nothing by mouth.

Exploratory Laparotomy

The exploratory laparotomy is performed by the surgeon when the patient presents with specific acute complaints for which an etiology cannot be determined. Frequently the cause for the specific complaints is determined intraoperatively, but at times the patient is closed with a conclusive diagnosis still pending.

Cholecystectomy

Cholecystitis is an inflammation of the gallbladder. The patient may present with either chronic or acute symptoms that can be accompanied by the presence of calculi or gallstones (cholelithiasis). The precise etiological factor for precipitating the inflammatory process is not exact. The obstruction of the cystic duct or bacterial invasion are two factors that are considered. The most common precipitating factor is the presence of calculi. If a conservative treatment of dietary management is not effective and the symptoms persist and increase, surgical intervention is indicated. The surgical procedure is referred to as a cholecystectomy (removal of the gallbladder) accompanied by a choledochotomy (exploration and drainage of the common bile duct). If an emergent situation occurs or if the patient is assessed as a poor surgical risk, a cholecystotomy (removal of calculi from the gallbladder) may be performed. This is only a temporary measure, and the likelihood of calculi recurring is great. As a part of the surgical procedure, a rubber T tube may be placed in the common bile duct to maintain the patency of the duct after surgery and to allow for the drainage of bile.

Pancreatectomy

This surgical procedure is also refered to as the Whipple's procedure and is the surgical treatment of choice for carcinoma of the pancreas. The head of the pancreas is most commonly involved and carcinoma rarely occurs before the age of 40. Its highest incidence is in males between the ages of 50 and 60. Surgery is performed in the hope of treating pancreatic cancer but does not seem to improve the extremely poor prognosis. The surgical procedure consists of the excision of the head, body, and tail of the pancreas. The duodenum, pylorus, and approximately 40% of the stomach are removed; the jejunum is anastomosed to the stomach. The main bile duct is removed and the gallbladder is anastomosed to the jejunum. Patients with carcinoma of the pancreas usually die within one year of the onset of the initial symptoms. Approximately one-half of the deaths occur within three months. Metastasis is rapid and includes the regional lymph nodes, liver, lungs, intestines, adrenals, and bone.

Portacaval Shunt

The patient with a diseased liver is always at risk of it becoming increasingly cirrhotic. When this happens, its microvasculature is interrupted and portal hypertension increases. Collateral circulation develops and flows along certain vessels that are weaker than normal vessels. As the pressure in the collateral circulation increases, the vessels become overdistended and esophageal varices result. The main concern here is rupture of the vessels and hemorrhage. If hemorrhage occurs, the patient's life is in jeopardy and emergency surgery is indicated. A portacaval shunt is created to divert the blood flow from the high pressure venous system to the low pressure systemic veins in order to relieve the pressure in the esophageal varices. These patients' postoperative course is critical since their underlying liver disease is extensive.

Bowel Resection

Interference with elimination from the gastrointestinal tract can be due to an obstruction anywhere along the bowel. The obstruction can be partial, allowing certain amounts of intestinal contents to pass, or complete, causing a total stoppage of all intestinal contents. Elimination can also be interrupted by polyps or intestinal neoplasms. Most mechanical obstructions require surgical intervention. The diseased portion of the bowel may be removed with the healthy segments anastomosed.

Colostomy

This surgical procedure involves a portion of the colon that is brought outside of the abdominal cavity. Colostomies can be temporary or permanent. The colostomy is often performed concomitantly with the bowel resection to relieve obstruction. The temporary colostomy is used when there is a possibility that the bowel will heal and can be reanastomosed while retaining rectal sphincter control. It may also be utilized to rest the distal portion of the intestine following trauma to the abdomen or severe diverticulitis. The permanent colostomy is most often done for colorectal cancer when the tumor is too close to the rectal sphincter to allow resection of the tumor and still retain sphincter function.

Ileostomy

Debilitating diarrhea with cramping, a toxic megacolon, obstructions, and the increased risk of cancer in persons with long standing ulcerative colitis are all indications for an ileostomy. An ileostomy brings a portion of the ileum out to the external environment. This procedure brings the terminal portion of the ileum through the abdominal wall which creates an opening for intestinal elimination. The colon and rectum are removed. While the ileostomy can be temporary, when done for ulcerative colitis, it is usually permanent.

Jejunoileal Shunts

In some severely or morbidly obese patients, surgical intervention may be necessary when conservative treatment has failed. Jejunoileal shunts are the most common and most successful type of treatment. These shunts create a surgically induced malabsorption syndrome. The procedure involves a resection of 20 feet of the ileum and jejunum, with an end-to-end anastomosis of the remaining 15 inches of the proximal jejunum and 4 to 8 inches of the distal ileum. The desired goal is a weight loss that brings the patient within 50 pounds of the ideal weight.

Endorectal Ileal Pullthrough

Over the past seven years the UCLA Medical Center has been performing an endorectal ileal pullthrough procedure with an isoperistaltic ileal reservoir for patients with ulcerative colitis and colonic polyps. This is a technically difficult operation, but the long-term results indicate that the pullthrough operation is a good alternative to a proctocolectomy with an ileostomy.

Patients have indicated that they were minimally limited in their athletic and social activities, compared to the period between operations when they had an ileostomy. The surgical procedure is the second phase of surgical repair. Reports also indicate that patients experience no bladder dysfunction or abnormal sexual function.

Complications From Abdominal Surgery

Postoperative complications are frequent and include perforation, peritonitis, obstruction, hemorrhage, pain, pneumoperitoneum, ileus retention of urine, subphrenic and pelvic abscess, portal pyelophlebitis, ascites, renal failure, respiratory failure and pneumonia. The first four conditions have been discussed earlier in the chapter. The other complications will be mentioned briefly.

Pain at the site of the surgery is normal and is due to the incision, internal sutures, swelling and inflammation. The patient reacts to the pain by breathing rapidly and shallowly and moving around in bed as little as possible. Respiratory excursions frequently stretch the incision, causing further pain.. The patient begins to splint that area and hypoventilate on that side of his chest. Coughing is painful as it stretches the incision and also causes the patient to fear evisceration of the incision. He begins to cough in a manner designed to put as little stress on the incision as possible. All these factors, plus the effects of the anesthetic and intraoperative medications (see the section on treatment of the surgical oncology patient in Chapter 24) and the site of the incision, may cause the patient recovering from abdominal surgery to develop pneumonia and atelectasis. The situation is complicated further when narcotics are given to relieve pain. As Bendixen showed, this causes patients to breathe shallowly and evenly, without sighing. Sighing or taking deep breaths prevents microatelectasis and is done by normal individuals 2–4 times a minute. Patients breathing in this manner develop diffuse areas of microatelectasis throughout both lungs. Severely compromised patients may then develop respiratory failure.

Pneumoperitoneum occurs when air is trapped in the peritoneal cavity at the time of surgery. It usually occurs in surgeries of the upper abdomen, with excess air collecting under the diaphragm. This excess air interferes with the normal function of the diaphragm by preventing or impeding its descent. The patient experiences severe pain in the area. Interference with the normal function of the diaphragm, in addition to the pain, further compromises the patient's ability to breathe and cough effectively. After several days the air is absorbed and all symptoms disappear. Until that time the patient is given pain medications.

Retention of urine following surgery is a common occurrence, seen mostly in elderly patients. It is treated by inserting a urinary catheter into the bladder and allowing urine to drain into a bag. It is removed when the problem is reversed. Ileus, or paralysis of the intestines, can occur normally after abdominal surgery. The bowel does in fact contract, but the movements are infrequent and uncoordinated and are therefore ineffective. The entire bowel, or only a portion, may be involved. It is detected by listening to the abdomen with a stethoscope. Lack of bowel sounds indicates ileus. The patient has an NG tube in place to drain fluids from the stomach and is not allowed food or fluids until bowel sounds are heard. Normal bowel sounds are rarely heard for 24 hours after surgery but usually occur soon after that time. Transcutaneous nerve stimulators (TNS) have been found to be extremely effective in treating ileus. The reason for this is unknown.

Subphrenic and pelvic abscesses are collections of pus and are usually located under the diaphragm. In this case hiccups and localized pain are seen. In the pelvic cavity localized pain usually reveals the location of abscesses. They are treated with antibiotics or surgical

drainage. When located subphrenically, respiratory infections and atelectasis occur frequently. Portal pyelophlebitis occurs usually in conjunction with peritonitis or ascites and is due to pressure or invasion of
the infection into the mesenteric veins. They in turn send clots to the
portal veins. It occurs infrequently now as patients are treated prophylactically following surgery with antibiotics to prevent infection.

Ascites is the excess production of serous fluid within the abdominal cavity. It is commonly seen in right-sided heart failure due to back
pressure in the systemic venous system, renal failure also due to back
pressure, malignancies, chronic inflammation and portal hypertension
again due to back pressure. Treatment involves removal of the underlying cause, which is frequently impossible, or paracentesis, which is
done as a palliative measure to relieve pressure. The excess fluid prevents effective descent of the diaphragm and may even compress the
lower lobes of the lungs, causing a restrictive disease.

Renal failure occurs frequently following major surgery and is usually a transient phenomenon. Generally it is treated with hemodialysis
or peritoneal dialysis. Hemodialysis is used when failure does not appear to be resolving. It involves connecting one of the patient's arteries
and veins to a mechanical pump which circulates blood through a tube.
This tube is immersed in a fluid, whose composition is altered in order
to cause substances like urea to diffuse through the wall of the tube
into the fluid. Peritoneal dialysis involves the placement of one or two
cannulae into the abdominal cavity. Fluids with special compositions
are then put into the abdominal cavity. Their properties cause urea
and other blood substances to diffuse into the peritoneum. These fluids
are then drained out into a bag. Generally 24 exchanges are done, with
one hour for infusion and one hour for drainage. The excess fluids
produce a restrictive factor on the lungs, much like ascites. Therapists
with patients receiving this form of dialysis should arrange for their
treatments to occur during the last 15 minutes of drainage.

Postoperative Pain Management

One of the greatest hindrances to postoperative pulmonary hygiene is
the lack of effective pain management prior to therapy. Executing
good pulmonary hygiene for the patient in pain can be challenging.
The first line of defense for someone in pain is usually self-imposed
immobility. Fortunately, a variety of pain-relieving modalities can be
employed that will make the patient more comfortable, thus ensuring
greater participation.

The patient's postoperative orders will always include pain medications to be given every three to four hours as needed for relief. Intramuscular injections such as Demerol, morphine sulphate, and codeine are given in the immediate postoperative period in specific dosages as ordered by the physician. In the days to follow, as the surgical incision heals, the physician may elect to change the medication to an oral form. It is important for the therapist to determine if the patient will require premedication prior to therapy. After the medication is given, it is suggested that approximately 30 minutes elapse before therapy is begun. By this time, the patient should be experiencing the pain-relieving effects of the drug, thus allowing therapy to begin. Those therapists carrying a consistent daily case load may elect to call the patient care unit to request premedication if it has already been determined that effective pain relief will be necessary prior to therapy.

Several electronic devices for pain control are capable of stimulating peripheral nerves, either directly (through implantation) or percutaneously. Two of the most effective devices are the TNS (transcutaneous nerve stimulator) and the epidural morphine infusion. Both of these methods have become widely accepted and have gained popularity as a valid clinical tool for pain relief. The TNS is the application of an electric current through the skin to a peripheral nerve or nerves for the control of episodes of acute pain; in each instance, the nerve impulses carrying pain from the peripheral areas are blocked. With the continuous morphine sulfate infusion, a catheter is implanted into the epidural space intraoperatively by the anesthesiologist or nurse anesthetist. A prescribed amount of this drug is usually mixed in a 100-cc bag of dextrose and water. After surgery, the intravenous medication is placed in a drip control pump. Its rate of infusion is regulated by the department of anesthesia until the catheter is removed. The length of time the catheter remains in the patient is usually determined by the progress the patient achieves in the first few days following surgery. Respiratory depression has always been the major side effect of morphine sulfate. When it is given as a continuous infusion, epidurally, this risk is significantly reduced.

The therapist should not hesitate to request that the patient be premedicated. It is only through effective postoperative pain relief that the patient will derive the maximum benefit of attempts to assist in pulmonary hygiene.

Chest Physical Therapy Treatment

Treatment of a patient before and after abdominal surgery has been discussed at length in the chapter on oncology, and so will not be dealt with here. Therapists should remember that pneumonia and atelectasis occurrence in these patients is more than 60%. Therefore, treatment of these patients is essential. First, abdominal incisions are large and painful. Therapists would be wise to concentrate on lateral-costal breathing exercises, rather than diaphragmatic exercises which draw the patient's attention to the incision. (Remember, lateral-costal expansion is mostly due to contraction of the lateral diaphragmatic fibers. This exercise will therefore cause the patient to use his diaphragm without realizing it.)

Second, abdominal distention is a common occurrence following surgery and acts to restrict breathing. Patients with large amounts of distention may find it uncomfortable to assume postural drainage positions and become dyspneic when in the Trendelenburg position. These patients should be treated in modified positions (bed flat) when possible. In turning these patients, make sure that the drainage tubes have enough length to prevent pulling them out, stretching or kinking the lines. Coughing may also be a problem with these patients since their abdominal muscles have been cut. (Abdominal muscles are the most important muscles in coughing.) Special techniques used to assist the patients with these maneuvers have been discussed in Chapter 11 on coughing.

Other than these modifications, treatment of abdominal surgical patients should be no different than that of other patients. Respiratory therapy equipment should be ordered as needed. Percussion and vibration should be done in postural drainage positions (when possible). Breathing exercises and cough instruction are especially important due to the diaphragm being compromised and the respiratory muscles cut. The patient should perform these exercises independently in the therapist's absence. The patient may need to be nasotracheally or orally suctioned if the cough is ineffective and the patient has many retained secretions. Positional rotation should be coordinated with the nursing staff.

SURGERY OF THE HEAD AND NECK

Most surgeries of the head and neck are done to treat malignancies. The incidence of these tumors is increasing. In 1975, 62,000 new cases of cancer of the head and neck were diagnosed. (Of these, 29,000 were primary cancers and the other 33,000 involved circulatory and lymphatic tumors with cervical lymph node adenopathy, thyroid tumors and tumors of the central nervous system.) These tumors have been briefly discussed in Chapter 24 on oncology. The most common types of head and neck cancers treated surgically are epidermoid cancers of the intraoral region, including tongue, pharynx, larynx and salivary glands.

Radical Neck Dissection

Radical neck dissection always involves removal of certain structures including lymph nodes, vessels, fat and fascia; various nerves including the spinal accessory (makes the patient unable to elevate his shoulders or shrug), ansa hypoglossi, sensory branches of the cervical plexus, and cervical branch of the facial nerve; internal and external jugular veins, and branches of the subclavian and external carotid arteries; the sternocleidomastoid and omohyoid muscles; and the submaxillary salivary gland and a portion of the parotid gland. If the tumor is extensive, further structures may be excised, including external or internal carotid; thoracic or right jugular lymph duct; platysma, digastric and mylohyoid muscles; and the thyroid gland. The radical neck dissection may be done on one side or bilaterally. It is frequently done in conjunction with other procedures including hemimandibulectomies or laryngectomies. Postoperative complications are frequent and will be discussed at the end of this section. Some surgical complications include injury of the lingular nerve, the superior or recurrent laryngeal branches of the vagus nerve (causing vocal cord paralysis), the phrenic nerve (causing paralysis of half of the diaphragm) or the bronchial plexus (causing paralysis of the arm); injury to the external, internal or common carotid arteries; and puncture of the apex of the pleura, causing a pneumothorax.

Radical Laryngectomy

Radical laryngectomy involves removal of the larynx and associated lymph nodes in conjunction with a radical neck dissection. A permanent tracheostomy is performed at the same time, with the trachea being externalized. A laryngectomy tube is used to maintain patency of the airway immediately after surgery. This is removed before the patient goes home, and a clean cloth is tied around the neck over the opening or stoma. This cloth filters air, prevents aspiration of particles or foreign objects into the lungs and is esthetically more acceptable than an exposed tube to the patient. There are obvious precautions and complications to having an open access to the lungs. Three important functions of the larynx are lost with laryngectomy: the ability to speak, the ability to bear down, as in the Valsalva maneuver, and the ability to cough. Laryngectomy patients need to have speech therapy to learn new ways of speaking. They need stool softeners and should be well hydrated to facilitate bowel regularity. They need to learn cough facilitation techniques or self suctioning to clean their secretions.

Radical Thyroidectomy

Radical thyroidectomies include removal of all of the thyroid and the surrounding lymph nodes. They are done to treat diffuse malignancies of the thyroid. These patients must receive thyroid extract daily for the rest of their lives. They are closely followed to ensure proper levels of the drug in their blood.

Maxillectomy

Maxillectomies involve removal of the maxilla and are usually done to treat cancers on the roof of the mouth that have extended into the maxilla. The gap created by removal of the bone is replaced with a split-thickness skin graft. These surgeries are rare and can be devastating as they destroy the bony boundaries of the eye, oral cavity and nasal cavity. This causes many of the postoperative complications.

Hemimandibulectomy

Removal of half of the mandible is usually done in conjunction with a radical neck dissection when the tumor has invaded the mandible as well as the neck. These surgeries are frequently referred to as *monobloch dissections*. These patients have temporary tracheostomies in place to prevent collapse of the airways from swelling, and feeding gastrostomies to maintain nutrition.

Postoperative Complications

Due to the extensive nature of this type of surgery, complications are common and include respiratory complications, postoperative hemorrhage, infection, rejection or necrosis of skin flaps, gastric complications and oral cutaneous fistulas. These various complications will be discussed briefly. Therapists desiring further knowledge should refer to one of the books in the reference section at the end of the chapter.

Aspiration pneumonia is one of the most common respiratory problems faced by the patient with head and neck surgery. For this reason, most of these patients have a temporary tracheostomy performed at the time of surgery. Protection of the lower airways will always be a problem because of the extensive surgeries, especially when the cords become paralyzed as a result of nerve damage. The aspirated substances cause inflammatory reactions and provide a good medium for bacterial growth. Aspiration pneumonia is responsible for about 90% of the deaths in these patients. Even when aspiration does not occur, pneumonia and atelectasis are frequently seen. Trauma to the tissues of the neck causes an inflammatory reaction in the lungs with hyperactivity of the glands that produce mucus. The patient's cough is ineffective due to the tracheostomy (the patient cannot build up pressure as the tracheostomy bypasses the cords). Ciliary activity is sluggish due to medications given during surgery, and the patient's ability to take a deep breath is impaired. This is a result of postoperative vital capacities being one fourth of their normal values in most patients. To compound the problem, the artificial airways also bypass the normal filtering systems of the upper airway, making contamination of the lower airways by bacteria more of a probability.

To summarize, there is an increase in the amount of secretions, while the normal clearance mechanisms of the airways are bypassed or rendered ineffective by surgery. Secretions begin to accumulate in dependent lung segments, causing atelectasis or pneumonia. Phrenic nerve injury with a resultant paralysis of half of the diaphragm, and pneumothorax from puncture of the pleura also occur in these patients. Paralysis of the diaphragm will affect the patient's ability to take a deep breath.

Hemorrhage occurs in 9% of all patients undergoing head and neck surgery. If it occurs immediately after surgery it is referred to as *primary* hemorrhage and is treated with transfusions or surgery. It occurs in 2%–3% of these surgeries. Ten days to three weeks later a carotid blowout may occur as a result of infection and necrosis. It occurs in 6% of head and neck surgeries and is an emergency, treated by local pressure, infusion of IVs and blood, and surgical repair once the patient is stable. The mortality from this *secondary* hemorrhage is high.

Massive infection of head and neck wounds is rare, and when it occurs is usually due to staphylococcal or streptococcal organisms. Small areas of infection are not unusual and do not often cause problems. The infection is treated with antibiotics and drainage of the area. Rejection or necrosis of the skin flaps is a serious complication. It is caused by infection or retardation and failure of a new blood supply to develop. Gastrointestinal hemorrhaging is the most common gastric complication and is usually due to the development of peptic or gastric ulcers from stress. Finally oral-cutaneous fistulas with drainage occur in about half of the cases. They are treated with pressure dressings and usually close within a few days.

Chest Physical Therapy Treatments

Treatments of the patient following head and neck surgery requires empathy on the part of the therapist. These patients often have a grotesque appearance with huge bloated faces and long incisions that run in several different directions with drains protruding from them. Their eyes are usually swollen shut, and their skin is shiny, inflamed and bruised in appearance. Therapists must be careful to treat these patients as they would any other. It is important that each procedure be explained to the patient in detail prior to its implementation. Therapists should encourage patient participation as much as possible. Instructions should be clear and concise and should include explanations of why they are being done.

Flaps are a major consideration when positioning the patient. The patient should be log-rolled to prevent torsion or twisting of neck and head areas. Flaps should be carefully checked after positioning to make sure that they lie flat with no puckers or air bubbles trapped beneath. The patient should be repositioned on his back if the flap begins to appear blanched or blue during treatment. Despite the high rate of respiratory complications, proper care of flaps remains a major priority. It takes several weeks after surgery for good revascularization to occur. Necrosis of the flap will greatly prolong the patient's hospitalization, increase the chance of infection and require several surgeries to transplant new skin flaps.

Patients with head and neck surgery have their heads elevated 30 degrees at all times to decrease the amount of edema seen in the head and neck. Most physicians will allow these patients to be positioned bed flat (though never in the Trendelenburg position) for the duration of the treatment. The head of their beds should then be returned to 30 degrees, although the patient should remain on his side for at least 30 minutes.

Evaluation and treatment of these patients are essentially the same as for other patients. It is important that they receive preventive treatments, even when chest assessment reveals clear lungs, throughout the course of their hospitalization. This is due to the high rate of respiratory complications and the fact that most deaths are caused by pneumonia. These patients should also receive a home program designed to maintain good bronchial hygiene for their lungs.

Respiratory therapy modalities are very important in these patients. The patient should have a heated aerosol device on at all times to ensure adequate humidity of the airway since the nose and mouth are bypassed by the tracheostomy. Ultrasonic nebulizers should be used to liquefy secretions. Positional rotation is essential due to the amount of secretions and the fact that the patient must have his head elevated at all times. Even with good rotation in modified positions, secretions will tend to accumulate in dependent segments.

Percussion should be done very gently. It should never be done on or close to skin flaps. Vibration is the most useful technique for mobilizing secretions in these patients. One therapist can create an artificial cough with the self-inflating bag while the other vibrates during exhalation.

The patient should be taught breathing exercises and how to "huff" to clear his airway of secretions. Therapists will find that these patients are very cooperative and eager to do as much as possible for themselves. These exercises enable the patient to take an active role in his therapeutic programs. Range of motion to the affected side should not be done until the flap is well healed. Therapists are advised to wait until the physicians are sure the revascularization of the flap has occurred.

Home programs should include a means of humidifying the airways. Inhalation of air in a steamy bathroom is a good way to liquefy secretions. Patients who do not have artificial airways should be taught to breathe the steam through their mouths as the nose filters out most water particles. Breathing exercises and coughing should be continued at home. By the time the patient goes home, he should be able to assume postural drainage positions. This should be done on a bed or on the floor over two or three pillows, with the lateral and posterior segments of both lower lobes being emphasized. Percussion and vibration should be taught to family members if the patient has more than the normal amount of secretions. Range of motion exercises to the affected shoulder and arms can be included since flaps will have been revascularized at the time of discharge. These range of motion exercises should not involve stretching contractures or tight joints as it may cause the flaps to tear.

SUMMARY

Some of the more common surgeries of the alimentary tract, head and neck have been discussed in this chapter. The information presented is very basic and is geared toward giving the therapist a cursory idea of the extent of the surgical procedures. Institutions vary in their approaches to the postoperative patient, and therapists are advised to consult individual physicians as to the aggressiveness of their treatment programs.

REFERENCES

Periodicals

Fonkalsrud EW: Endorectal ileal pullthrough with isoperistaltic ileal reservoir for colitis and polyposis. *Ann Surg,* 1985; 202:145-153.

Norwood SH, Civette JM, Kesler AFB: Abdominal CT scanning in critically ill surgical patients. *Ann Surg* 1985; 202:166-175.

Books

Bendixen HH, et al: *Respiratory Care.* St Louis, CV Mosby Co, 1965.

Goldin MD: *Intensive Care of the Surgical Patient.* Chicago, Year Book Medical Publishers, Inc, 1971.

Hardy JD: *Critical Surgical Illness.* Philadelphia, WB Saunders Co, 1971.

Hedley-White J, Burgess GE: *Applied Physiology of Respiratory Care,* ed 2. Boston, Little, Brown & Co, 1976.

Moroney J: *Surgery for Nurses,* ed 12. New York, Churchill Livingstone, Inc, 1971.

Nardi GL, Zuidema GD: *Surgery,* ed 3. Boston, Little, Brown & Co, 1972.

Nash DF: *Surgery for Nurses and Allied Professions,* ed 6. London, Edward Arnold Publishers, Ltd, 1976.

Stahl WM: *Supportive Care of the Surgical Patient.* New York, Grune & Stratton, 1972.

Stuart AG, Smith AN, Samuel E: *Applied Surgical Pathology.* London, Blackwell Scientific Publications, 1975.

Taylor S: *Harlow's Modern Surgery for Nurses,* ed 9. London, William Heinemann Medical Books Ltd, 1973.

Taylor S, Cotton L: *A Short Textbook of Surgery,* ed 3. Philadelphia, JB Lippincott Co, 1973.

24

Oncology

Lyn Hobson, P.T., R.R.T.

Cynthia Webster, B.S.R.

Cancer is a generic term used to encompass many diseases character-ized by an excessive proliferation of cells which serve no useful func-tion and in fact interfere with normal bodily and cellular functions. These cells are referred to as *neoplasms* (meaning new growth) or *tu-mors*. They can arise in any body tissue at any age, with deleterious effects on the host due to their invasive nature. They invade local tis-sues by direct extension, and the rest of the body by way of the lym-phatic and circulatory systems. The course of the disease is dependent on many factors, including the age and state of health of the host, the tissue from which the tumor arose (some cancers grow and invade vital organ centers more rapidly than others), the treatment the host re-ceives and the frequency and severity of secondary complications such as pneumonia and cachexia.

BENIGN TUMORS

Tumors are classified as either benign or malignant according to their effect on the body. Benign tumors generally do not cause death unless they are located in a vital, inoperable site (such as deep in the brain) but will, however, frequently cause the host discomfort. For instance, a benign neoplasm in a main-stem bronchus may cause severe respira-tory distress, while growth of tumor cells near nerve cells may cause pain.

Benign tumor cells closely resemble the normal tissue cells from which they arise. They have limited growth potential and tend to remain localized at the site of origin. Growth occurs by expansion rather than by infiltration. The tumors are encapsulated and thus easily removed surgically. Once removed, they rarely recur.

MALIGNANT TUMORS

Malignant neoplasms are much more destructive in nature than are benign cells; they proliferate rapidly and spread throughout the body. Their rapid growth causes them to develop many abnormal immature cells that have little resemblance to the normal cells from which they arose. Death frequently occurs as a result of these cells' effects on the host. Surgical removal, radiation and chemotherapy may temporarily destroy or slow the growth of these cells, but eventually most of them will recur. Malignant tumors have an irregular shape with ill-defined borders due to their invasion of surrounding cells and tissues. This local invasion makes them difficult to remove surgically and frequently causes necrosis of the invaded tissue as a result of tissue destruction.

Malignant tumors have a tendency to form secondary tumors at distant sites, known as *metastasis*. These metastases are transported by the lymphatic system, circulatory system, direct invasion or serosal spread. Lymphatic spread of cancer usually occurs by cancer cells splitting off to form emboli after they have invaded the lymphatic system. Occasionally tumor cells will not detach, and the cancer will proliferate as a continuous growth within the lymphatic vessel. The emboli of cancer cells lodge in a lymph node where they grow until the whole node is involved. Cells then once again detach and invade further lymph nodes. Invasion of lymph nodes is a sure sign that the cancer is spreading, and the sooner it occurs the more ominous the sign. Carcinomas are known to spread by this route; some, such as malignant melanomas and cancer of the tongue, invade the lymph system early, while others, such as squamous cell carcinomas of the skin or lips, invade the lymphatic system late in the disease. Lymphatic spread will frequently invade the circulatory system via the thoracic duct and continue to spread by that route.

Circulatory spread of cancer is similar to invasion and spread via the lymphatic system. Cancer cells invade blood vessels and either grow along the vessel or detach and are mechanically transported as emboli to a new location, where they lodge and grow. Growth at the new site can occur only if the cancer cells have infiltrated the vessel wall. Many blood-borne cancer cells do not survive. Circulatory metastases occur most frequently in the following organs—in order: liver, lungs, bone marrow, brain and adrenal glands. Sarcomas most frequently metastasize by this route, as well as carcinomas of the lung, breast, kidney, prostate and thyroid.

Direct invasion of surrounding tissues by cancer cells occurs along the lines of least resistance, usually along tissue planes. All tumors grow and directly invade local tissues as well as metastasizing to distant sites. Serosal spread occurs when cancer cells are detached from the surface of the tumor and spread by mechanical means. This occurs in the intraperitoneal cavity and the intrapleural cavity, with spread generally to the dependent portions of the cavities. Serosal spread also occurs through cerebrospinal fluid in certain brain tumors. It may occur when surgeons operate to remove tumors, with some cells inadvertently being carried deep into the operative site.

Systemic Effects of Malignant Tumors

Malignant tumors, by their destructive nature and uncontrolled growth patterns, produce many local and systemic effects. Locally, the rapid growth of the tumor encroaches on healthy tissue, causing destruction, necrosis, ulceration and hemorrhage. Pain may or may not occur depending on how close tumor cells, swelling or hemorrhage occurs to the nerve cells. This process also occurs locally at metastatic sites.

Systemically, the host frequently presents with a gradual or rapid weight loss, muscular weakness, anorexia, anemia and so on. Further spread of the cancer leads to obstruction of the gastrointestinal (GI) tract and vital organs (such as the brain, where pressure by tumor cells frequently causes partial paralysis and eventually coma, or compression of the ureters by tumor leading to uremia and coma). Hemorrhage caused by direct invasion or necrosis leads to further anemia or even death if the situation is severe. Terminal cancer patients become very cachexic as a result of tissue destruction and the body's nutrients being used by the malignant cells for further growth. Pain presents as a late symptom and is caused by infiltration, compression or destruction of nerves. Secondary infections frequently occur as a result of the host's decreased immunity, causing respiratory failure if located in the lungs or toxemia with acidosis if in the blood. Death can occur as a result of any of these processes.

Psychological Response of the Patient to a Malignancy

Patients usually respond to being told they have a tumor by asking: "Is it cancer?" At this time their physician will explain the meaning of the diagnosis and its consequences. The patient is never told more than he can intellectually and emotionally handle. The first response is usually denial. The patient looks and feels normal, and it is easy to convince himself that he does not have the disease. As the treatment program is planned and explained to the patient in detail, he finds it harder and harder to suppress the truth from himself. Each new treatment and explanation force the patient to confront the reality of the disease.

Patients respond differently to the various forms of treatment. Surgery, though disfiguring, is frequently the most accepted form of treatment as the patient considers the tumor physically removed and therefore no longer a threat. Radiotherapy (or radiation) is viewed as the most mysterious form of treatment as the patient cannot see, feel or hear anything happening during the treatment. This becomes a real problem when the side effects suddenly begin to occur. To compound the problem, it is frequently weeks or months before the effectiveness of the treatment can be evaluated. Chemotherapy is also stressful to the patient because of its various side effects. Gastrointestinal problems including nausea or vomiting will make the patient very anxious prior to each course of treatment. The patient continues to deny his disease as the first course of treatments ceases. He may try to convince himself that the disease has been eliminated.

Denial usually continues until recurrence or spread of the disease is discovered. At this time the patient becomes very angry and lashes out at all medical personnel. He will frequently blame recurrence of the disease on the individuals who planned and executed the initial treatment. It is at this time that the thought first occurs to the patient and family that the disease may not be cured. Understandably, they become skeptical of further treatment plans. It is not unusual for families to resort to wild, far-out treatment potions and programs made by people who are willing to capitalize on those looking for a miracle. This stage is called "the bargaining stage" by Dr. Kubler-Ross in her book, *On Death and Dying*. Patients will literally do anything in exchange for their lives.

As the disease continues to progress, the patient realizes that no form of bargaining will influence the course of the disease. He becomes very depressed as he views his inevitable impending death. Counseling with clergy, social workers and psychologists is frequently very helpful at this point. Finally the patient accepts what is occurring in his body. His greatest concern becomes that he be allowed to die with dignity. To some patients this means being allowed sufficient medication to relieve pain, while still being alert enough to interact with family members. For others, it means not having to take medication at all, and others may wish to be totally sedated. The goals of the medical staff at this point should be to make the patient as comfortable as possible.

Prognosis

The prognosis of a patient with cancer depends on many factors, including the type of cancer and the stage at which the cancer is found. The staging of a cancer is an attempt to define the extent of the cancer at a given moment and may not be related to prognosis. (Some cancers progress slowly from one stage to another, while others are considered stage IV at the time of diagnosis, such as Wilms' tumor.)

Stage I.   Examination reveals a mass limited to the organ of origin. The lesion is operable and there is no nodal or vascular spread. A cancer found at this stage has the best prognosis (70%–90% chance of survival).

Stage II.   Examination reveals local spread into surrounding tissues and lymph nodes. The lesion is operable but success of surgery is uncertain due to the greater local spread (about 50% chance of survival).

Stage III.   Examination reveals an extensive primary lesion with fixation to deeper structures. There is invasion of lymph nodes and surrounding bone. The lesion is operable in that some of it can be removed, offering temporary relief, but gross amounts of tumor remain (about 20% chance of survival).

Stage IV.   Examination reveals an extensive primary lesion, with lymphatic and bone invasion as well as evidence of distant metastasis. It is inoperable (less than 5% chance of survival).

Staging of cancers is imperfect since it is impossible to tell microscopically the advanced stage of the tumor. Doctors use staging to determine the mode of treatment. Generally, cancers are treated one stage beyond their classification. If a cancer is known to progress rapidly through the stages (such as lung cancer, which has a high conversion rate), then it is treated very aggressively.

Treatment of Cancer

The mode of treatment selected is the one that can best cure the patient with minimum functional and structural impairment. Generally, cancers that have a low chance of survival are treated more radically. Cancer can be treated by surgery, radiation or chemotherapy. Frequently, the standard treatment is a combination of the three methods.

Surgery

Surgery is the oldest way of treating cancer. Generally, the surgeon attempts to remove the cancer and the affected lymph nodes in one operation. The risks the patient incurs in these surgeries are the same as in any surgical procedure. Frequently, the physician will "prepare" a patient for surgery with preoperative chemotherapy or radiation if a tumor appears large or shows signs of inflammation. This helps stop the growth of the tumor temporarily, or may even shrink the tumor for better operative results. A major problem that occasionally occurs during surgery on a neoplasm is splintering off of malignant cells that seed deep within the operative site, forming new areas of malignant growth. (This occurs frequently with tumors of the head and neck.)

At times radical surgery is performed on patients with advanced cancer when it is the only chance of a cure, no matter how marginal that chance might be. The decision to operate is a mutual one arrived at by the physician and the patient. Patients feel that the inconvenience of the surgery is worth the chance to survive. These surgeries are frequently palliative in nature, designed for functional purposes or to prevent uncomfortable side effects and pain. Removal of tumors from upper airways, the buccal cavity, head and neck and the digestive tract, though disfiguring, saves the patient from a painful death of hemorrhage, asphyxia or malnutrition. Complex operations involving removal of several abdominal organs, large amounts of colon and stomach are done to relieve obstruction, to prevent erosion or hemorrhage and to treat cancer of the colon.

Following primary operative and histopathology reports, it is often possible to divide the results into two groups: (1) patients in whom the treatment was unsuccessful, resulting in residual neoplastic tissue; (2) patients in whom the treatment was judged successful and appear to be "free of disease." Amputation and disarticulation of limbs and pelvis are performed for functional purposes and for relief of pain when the possibility of a cure is slight. All of these surgeries are worth the operative complications and disfigurement if they make the patient more comfortable, functional, or hopeful for a cure. For these reasons, it is the responsibility of the physical therapist to deliver optimal rehabilitation and maintenance to each patient as required.

Radiation

Radiation has been used successfully since the late 19th century to treat malignancies. Decaying radioactive elements produce ionizing radiations. They are also produced when subatomic particles accelerated in a vacuum are permitted to "escape" or produce electromagnetic radiation by hitting a "target." These ionizing radiations are used to destroy malignant cells. Generally the dose required to destroy tumor cells is less than that required to destroy normal cells. The dose of radiation used is measured by the rad (the energy absorbed per unit weight of tissue). Several things are taken into consideration when discussing doses of radiation: (1) the size and numbers of fractions into which the dose is divided (larger fractions are more effective), (2) the length of time over which the dose will be administered, (3) the total amount of tissue to be irradiated and (4) the recovery time from the irradiation.

Radiation is used either externally (where a generator creates a beam of radiation or electrons that reaches the tumor and destroys it and its extensions) or internally (where radioactive elements are introduced into body cavities or tumors). Some tumors, such as Hodgkin's disease, are radiosensitive and radiocurable. Other tumors are radiosensitive but not radiocurable (i.e., they only temporarily disappear when irradiated, for example, Wilms' tumor). Some tumors are radioresistant (do not respond to radiation) and must be treated surgically (such as malignant melanomas and osteogenic sarcomas).

Radiotherapy can cause many side effects, including local erythema, desquamation, pigmentation, drying of the irradiated tissues (very irritating when this involves the mouth or pharynx), radiation sickness (this involves nausea and vomiting and is frequently psychological in origin), and a fall in the white and red blood cell counts. Late side effects include permanent skin changes characterized by atrophy, thinning, blanching, telangiectasis, subcutaneous fibrosis and ulceration. These changes are less frequently seen today due to better equipment and more skilled radiotherapists. Such side effects also occur in the lung and spinal cord when they are irradiated.

Radiation is used to treat many head and neck tumors, and of necessity the temporal bone is sometimes included in the paths of radiation. The pathological changes noted can include bony changes such as resorption, fibrosis, empty lecunae, and sequestration; soft tissue changes include thickening of the epithelium in the canal and in the tympanic membrane, and subepithelial fibrosis. These changes can be manifested clinically as persistent otitis externa, with otorrhea and otelgia. Radiotherapy has important late sequelae within the regions of the irradiation.

Chemotherapy

The treatment of cancer by drugs is a relatively new development dating back to 1945, when nitrogen mustard was first used to treat lymphomas. These drugs are nonspecific and attack all cells equally, especially those that are rapidly proliferating, such as gastrointestinal epithelia. (This is why so many patients being treated with chemotherapy suffer from severe nausea.) The drug of choice can be phase specific (killing cells during one phase of cell life), cycle specific (killing proliferating cells more effectively than resting cells) or noncycle specific (killing proliferating and resting cells equally). Chemotherapeutic agents are used most frequently in combination with surgery, radiotherapy or both. In advanced forms of cancer, chemotherapy is frequently the agent of choice. Because these drugs are so cytotoxic, the specific drug and dosage must be carefully calculated so as to be compatible with life. If at any given time a drug is not stopping the progression of the disease or is too destructive to the host, then dosage and drug adjustments must be made. The side effects of these drugs are severe, including anemia, leukopenia, thrombocytopenia, stomatitis, nausea, vomiting and diarrhea.

CHEST PHYSICAL THERAPY IN THE PATIENT WITH CANCER

Psychological Aspects

Patients with terminal disease are difficult to treat at any time, but the patient who is facing death from a malignancy presents special problems. Very few diseases have received as much publicity as cancer. From the time we are children, our parents, family, friends and the media (television, movies, newspapers) bombard us with tales of horribly painful deaths by cancer. This conditioning affects the patient and all who come in contact with him, whether they be family, therapists or nurses.

It is very important that medical personnel who come into contact with patients suffering from cancer recognize and resolve some of their feelings toward the disease. Therapists frequently react to the patient with empathy, compassion and even pity not only for what the patient is experiencing at the present but also for what the patient could experience in the future. Often these feelings are governed not by what the therapist has experienced clinically but by his preconceived notions of the disease. It is natural to feel helpless in changing the final outcome of the disease, but one must realize that these feelings are conveyed to the patient by one's actions, expressions and attitudes. These feelings will make it difficult for the therapist to be aggressive enough to be effective when encountering the cancer patient.

The goal of therapy in these patients is to improve the quality of life, not to effect a cure for the underlying disease. In dealing with cancer patients, one realizes that there will come a time when it is proper to withdraw supportive treatment, but until that decision is made by appropriate personnel, therapists must give aggressive or at least supportive care to these patients. Therapists who learn to evaluate and treat cancer patients according to their respiratory involvement, and not their underlying disease, will find that they approach patients with a more positive attitude. Patients respond to this positive attitude by becoming more cooperative and involved with their treatments. Even patients who are resistant to treatment may respond when told firmly by a therapist that the treatment is necessary to make them better or more comfortable.

Therapists treating cancer patients will frequently have to use their imagination in order to persuade or manipulate the patient into receiving treatment. These patients generally react in one of three ways to therapy. Some patients are cooperative and become actively involved in their respiratory care plan. Others are passive and will let the therapists do anything, as long as it requires a minimum of effort on the part of the patient. Lastly, some patients are very resistant to treatment. This may be due to an excessive amount of discomfort incurred by the treatment (although treatment plans can be modified to balance minimum discomfort with maximum results). If the patient's condition is terminal and all forms of treatment cause him excessive discomfort, then it is appropriate to discontinue treatment with the physician's approval. Many of these patients experience tremendous frustrations at having lost all control of their lives. They can no longer control their future by setting goals, and frequently they cannot control what is happening to them at the present in the hospital. They are forced into a passive role as a patient and sometimes the only thing they can actively control is their therapy. They try to convince the therapist not to treat them by crying, complaining of pain or fatigue or flatly refusing treatment.

Therapists often find that patients respond when the treatment program is presented as a joint effort on the part of the patient and the therapist. This allows the patient to become active in doing something therapeutic for himself. Of course one must realize that there will be times when the patient is too emotionally upset or physically ill from treatments or pain to be treated. At these times it would jeopardize the rapport between patient and therapist to insist on treatment.

Treatment

Treatment programs should be tailored to the needs of the patient and as such must depend heavily on the results of the initial evaluation of the patient by the therapist. These techniques have been discussed at length in Chapters 6–13. When treating persons with carcinomas, the physical therapist should have a clear idea of what he or she expects to find. A few things the therapist should note from the chart for the cancer patient are type of cancer, date of diagnosis, stage of the disease, metastatic sites, method of treatment, white blood cell count (low counts make the patient susceptible to secondary infections), platelet count (low counts make the patient susceptible to hemorrhage) and times that the patient receives pain medication (generally 45 minutes to one hour after medication is given is the best time to treat the patient).

A chest physical therapist is generally called in to see the cancer patient in one of three situations: before surgery when the patient is being prepared for radical surgery, after surgery and late in the disease when the patient has reached a fairly advanced compromised state and is bedridden (home health care). In any of these three situations the therapist may be consulted to prevent a possible problem (prophylactic) or to treat an existing problem (therapeutic). These patients should be treated no differently than any other patient. The aggressiveness of the treatment program should depend on the condition of the patient and the priorities set by the physician for that patient.

Preoperative Treatment

The preoperative evaluation of the chart and patient should reveal any potential postoperative problems. Many studies on patients undergoing surgery have revealed that certain factors seem to contribute to postoperative respiratory complications. Therapists should be familiar with these factors so that they can anticipate problem patients and work to prevent those patients from getting into trouble.

One of the most important factors is the site of the incision. Surgery of the extremities has a very low rate of postoperative respiratory complications (10%–30%). This is because the respiratory muscles are not cut; therefore breathing and coughing do not pull on the incision. The closer one gets to the thorax, the higher the incidence of postoperative respiratory complications. High abdominal incisions (cholecystectomies) result in a high rate of atelectasis, and of pneumonia following surgery (60%–90%). The incisions for these surgeries cut through the abdominal muscles, which play an important role in coughing. The incision is stretched every time the patient takes a deep breath, causing him pain and fear of evisceration of the incision. Consequently he splints the area. Thoracic incisions, interestingly enough, result in a lower rate of postoperative respiratory complications (70%). This is due to the thorax being fixed and moving little during respiratory excursions. Sternal incisions move little during breathing, whereas incisions between ribs are compressed during inspiration, lessening the pull on the incision. Patients with this type of incision find it much easier to cough and take deep breaths than those with abdominal incisions.

The condition of the patient prior to surgery must also be considered. The incidence of postoperative pneumonia is very high in older patients (3:1), overweight patients (2:1), those who smoke (4:1) and those with abnormal pulmonary function studies (23:1). Patients presenting with any of these factors should receive special attention. It is obvious that the more risk factors a patient has, the more likely he will be to have postoperative problems.

Surgery also has certain effects on the lungs regardless of the nature of the operation and the site of the incision. First of all, there is a trememdous drop in the patient's postoperative vital capacity (down to 25%–50% of normal). This makes it physiologically much harder for the patient to take deep breaths and therefore more difficult to produce an effective cough. The cough may be further compromised by swollen, sore vocal cords (a result of the endotracheal tube), which do not approximate well. Poor approximation of the cords limits the amount of intrathoracic pressure that can be created and thereby the velocity of expelled air and effectiveness of the cough (see Chapter 9).

Many patients are given medication during surgery designed to dry all body secretions (including oral and pulmonary secretions) and to prevent intraoperative aspiration. This dehydrates the mucous blanket of the lungs, making secretions tenacious and difficult for the ciliary escalator to mobilize. The ciliary escalator is itself affected by the medication and anesthesia. It reacts by moving much slower and less effectively, making it difficult to mobilize normal secretions (much less dehydrated secretions!).

After checking the patient's chart an initial chest assessment should be performed (see Chapter 6). Potential problem areas should be noted (such as ineffective cough, chronic production of secretions) and, if necessary, a therapeutic treatment program initiated to correct the problem. (This is covered in detail later in this chapter.) Therapists should explain to the patient the purpose of prophylactic bronchial hygiene, emphasizing that pulmonary congestion following surgery is common and that their physicians wish to prevent such problems by preoperative instruction. Explaining the pathophysiology of postoperative respiratory complications in basic terms frequently helps the patient understand the need for such a program.

Patients should be instructed in all chest physical therapy techniques that might be used with them after surgery. Therapists should explain to the patient that the combinations of postoperative techniques chosen will be those that will best help him at that moment. These combinations of techniques may well change from day to day as the patient's condition changes. Breathing exercises and cough instruction should be specific to the future incision. Patients should be taught to splint incisions with their hands or a pillow when coughing. They should practice this technique several times before surgery. Explain to them that taking deep breaths and coughing while painful, is very essential to their lungs following surgery.

Positional rotation to prevent pooling of secretions should be mentioned. Explain to the patient that turning will be painful and that nurses and therapists will assist him in this maneuver. Percussion and vibration should be performed on the patient, so that he can become familiar with the technique. Explain that these techniques will help dislodge tenacious secretions and make it easier for him to cough. Generally, therapists will find it helpful to present the program several days before surgery and review it again the day before surgery. It is helpful whenever possible to have the same therapist see the patient before and after surgery. This preoperative instruction will make the patient less anxious and better able to cooperate with his postoperative treatment.

Therapeutic chest physical therapy should be instituted when a potential problem is revealed in the therapist's initial evaluation of the chart (such as a long history of smoking, lung disease, recurrent pneumonias in a specific area) or chest assessment (such as decreased lateral expansion on one side—this is the first sign of lung pathology and frequently precedes auscultatory and radiographic changes). Decreased diaphragmatic excursion and a productive or ineffective cough are good reasons for further patient training. It is to the patient's advantage that his lungs be in the best possible condition prior to surgery!

Once the therapist has isolated the problem, he should determine the best methods by which the problem can be resolved. The need for respiratory therapy equipment must be assessed. Does he need an ultrasonic nebulizer to help liquefy thick secretions? The various techniques of chest physical therapy that can be applied have been discussed previously. The indications and contraindications for the various techniques remain applicable to these patients. Specifically percussion should not be performed over rib metastasis or an operable lung tumor. Postural drainage in the Trendelenburg position should not be performed if the patient has brain metastasis or a brain tumor or abdominal distention such as ascites. Generally if there are no contraindications, percussion and vibration to the involved area in the appropriate postural drainage positions are performed following USN. Breathing exercises and cough techniques should be taught to the patient and done by him during the treatment. Following postural drainage the patient should sit up, cough and then be repositioned on his side (bed flat in a modified postural drainage position). If the patient has an ineffective cough then the therapist or nurse should nasotracheally suction him to clear the trachea and pharynx of mobilized secretions. The patient is told to remain in this position for 20 minutes, performing his breathing exercises. (Physiologically it takes the cilia approximately 20 minutes to mobilize a particle from the base of the lung to the trachea. Positioning a patient facilitates the drainage of that segment and allows the patient to receive maximum benefit from the treatment.) Patients with ineffective coughs may need to be suctioned again at this time.

The patient is taught basic positional rotation (with emphasis on the area of his problem), breathing exercises and cough techniques. These are to be done by him throughout the time the therapist is absent. They allow him to become an active partner in the team, working to improve the condition of his body. The nurse should also be instructed in the program so she can reinforce the therapy in the therapist's absence. For a compromised patient, the nurse may need to assist or even perform the techniques. This program should continue until the time of surgery, with the therapist also giving the patient the necessary preoperative training.

Postoperative Treatment

Following surgery therapists are asked to see patients prophylactically or therapeutically. Prophylactic or preventive treatments are ordered if one or more of the risk factors mentioned in the previous section are present, if there were intraoperative respiratory complications (i.e., aspiration), or if the patient does not appear able to maintain his own bronchial hygiene following surgery (i.e., is lethargic, confused or unable to cough and take deep breaths). Assessment of the chart and patient is exactly the same as mentioned previously. Again, potential problem areas must be noted by the therapist. Generally, most patients have difficulty taking deep breaths and coughing effectively. This is due to the site of the incision, swelling or pain of the vocal cords, decreased vital capacity and medications given during and after surgery. (Narcotics cause the patient to breathe very regularly and shallowly. This results in hypoventilation and microatelectasis of various areas of the lung.) Fear of pain or evisceration of the incision may also cause the patient to breathe shallowly and cough poorly. Good communication between therapist and patient should allow these fears of the patient to be expressed.

Prophylactic treatment programs are planned according to the needs of the patient. Ultrasonic nebulizers to liquefy secretions may assist the therapist in maintaining good bronchial hygiene. Postoperative breathing exercises and cough instruction are essential, as these are the areas presenting the most difficulty. It is important that the therapist reinforce the patient positively in these instructions. Patients who are doing poorly respond when told, "You're not doing badly considering this is your first day after surgery. By tomorrow your cough should be much stronger." Therapists should carefully check the patient's posture and breathing patterns to ensure that he is ventilating well and not guarding a painful area. If this is detected, it should be pointed out to the patient, with specific breathing exercises given for the guarded area. Patients who continue to have trouble with breathing and coughing should receive extra instruction as mentioned in Chapters 8 and 9.

Following surgery most patients have difficulty concentrating on their breathing exercises and cough instruction, and they fatigue quickly. As a result we have found it helpful to do percussion and vibration to both lower lobes in modified postural drainage positions. This dislodges any dried, retained secretions and prevents further accumulation of secretions while the patient is inactive. It is helpful in preparing the patient for the treatment to explain that percussion is a massaging technique. Patients who are already anxious after surgery respond to this approach better than when told they are going to be "beaten." The percussion should be done slowly, rhythmically and gently, so that the patient relaxes during the treatment. This modality is very helpful in preventing a postoperative problem in a patient who is comatose, confused or too lethargic to cooperate. Following percussion and vibration the patient should sit up and be encouraged to cough. Patients unable to cough should be suctioned. Percussion and vibration should be continued until the patient becomes more active.

In recent years, the use of mechanical vibration as a treatment modality for acutely ill postoperative patients has received considerable attention. It has been suggested that mechanical vibration has the ability to dislodge retained secretions in those persons who are unable to tolerate percussion and vibration as techniques for clearing accumulated secretions. When vibration is applied to the muscles of the chest wall, a slow tonic contraction occurs followed by a reciprocal inhibition of the antagonists of the vibrated muscle. Further, the use of high-frequency vibration for mucociliary clearance is possible when the proper postural drainage position is not possible. Another feature of the noninvasive high-frequency vibration technique is that it has been demonstrated to be effective as a short-term desensitization procedure.

Positional rotation is of paramount importance in these patients and must be coordinated with the nursing staff. The burden of responsibility for positional rotation must fall on them, as nurses are with the patient throughout the day. Frequent turning of the bedridden patient will prevent accumulation of secretions, bedsores and venous stasis. The various positions have been discussed previously, but in general the therapist should make sure that the patient is being positioned in good side-lying positions, bed flat and sitting up.

Therapeutic treatment of the postoperative patient is exactly the same as preventive treatment, with the compromised area being emphasized. Respiratory therapy modalities should be ordered as needed. Breathing exercises should be specific to the area of involvement (i.e., teach the patient right lateral-costal breathing exercises if he has a right lower lobe pneumonia). Postural drainage with percussion and vibration should be done predominantly to the involved segment area. It is important, however, that uninvolved areas continue to be treated to prevent cross infection or accumulation of secretions within those areas. The treatment thus becomes partially preventive and partially therapeutic. Generally, the involved area should be treated two out of three times. Treatment should not cease when the involved area clears. It is important to realize that the previously involved area will remain "weaker" and more susceptible to infection than other areas of the lung. Thus it is important to continue treatment as long as the patient is bedridden.

The reasons for discontinuing chest physical therapy treatment in these patients are the same as those for other patients. Patients who are afebrile, ambulating and have clear lungs by auscultation and chest x-ray should be discontinued, even if they plan to remain in the hospital indefinitely. Patients who are chronically bedridden may be discontinued if they are motivated and able to assume responsibility for their bronchial hygiene. It is generally a good idea to continue treatment of patients who chronically produce a moderate amount of sputum, even if they are afebrile. The chronic production of sputum makes these patients retain secretions more readily than other patients and thus be more susceptible to infection. Therapists should check on patients periodically when they are uncertain about their ability to maintain bronchial hygiene.

Treatment of the Medical Cancer Patient

Treatment of the nonsurgical cancer patient is either preventive or therapeutic. Generally these patients remain fairly active and free of lung complications until late in their disease. As they become bedridden, the threat of lung infection becomes greater. These patients have a great deal of difficulty in fighting these infections as they are already compromised hosts. In fact pulmonary complications cause a large number of deaths in cancer patients. Consequently, physicians will frequently order prophylactic chest physical therapy to help prevent pulmonary infections. This is seen less with DRGs.

The therapist is frequently consulted when the patient becomes bedridden or is on reverse isolation as a result of a drop in the white blood count which causes him to have lowered resistance. Initial chart and patient evaluation remains the same as mentioned earlier in the chapter. Treatment must be tailored to the needs of the patient. Generally these patients are more difficult to work with as their bodies have suffered tremendous trauma and change. They are frequently in a great deal of pain and emotionally unstable. It is especially important to establish rapport between therapist and patient. The therapist should explain the purpose of the treatment and the possible modalities that might be involved. In general positional rotation, breathing exercises and cough instruction are sufficient to maintain bronchial hygiene in the alert patient. Bone metastasis can make it difficult for the therapist to position these patients. Coordination with pain medication may make it easier for the patient to tolerate treatment. Therapists should notify the physician when the treatment causes the patient undue pain and discomfort. At that time he is the one who must determine the aggressiveness of the treatment plan.

Confused, lethargic, and comatose patients usually need aggressive positional rotation. Therapists may also wish to do percussion and vibration (after ensuring that there are no rib metastases). Percussion over rib metastasis causes pain and possible rib fractures. These patients should be stimulated to cough following treatment (tracheal tickle or catheter) and suctioned as needed. Again the aggressiveness of the treatments must be determined by the physician and therapist.

Therapeutic treatment in the cancer patient is the same as in any other patient, with some special considerations. Chart and patient assessment will reveal the location of the respiratory problem. Respiratory therapy modalities should be implemented as needed. Selection of appropriate chest physical therapy modalities should be made according to the nature of the patient's pulmonary problem and the extent of his disease. Breathing exercises and cough instruction should be taught to the alert patient. Percussion and vibration to the involved area in a postural drainage position (if tolerated) should be implemented. Positional rotation should be coordinated with the nursing staff. Treatment plans must be geared to the needs of the patient.

Therapists will frequently encounter patients who have contraindications to every form of chest physical therapy treatment. In those cases the treatment must depend on the discretion of the therapist, after consultation with the physician. Generally the treatment in these cases must depend on the benefit to the patient. Patients with rib metastasis, who have copious amounts of thick secretions, may feel temporary relief after gentle percussion and vibration are performed around the metastasis. Therapists should use their imagination in an effort to modify treatments so that the patient may receive some benefit. For instance, vibration over the sternum in a sitting position may be sufficient to clear the larger airways and offer some relief.

Discontinuing chest physical therapy in these patients should occur when the respiratory problem is resolved or when the physician decides that it is no longer of benefit to the patient. Treatments that cause the patient undue anxiety or pain and discomfort may harm the patient more than help him. There may come a time when the patient or family requests that all supportive care be discontinued. Physicians may decide that death is imminent and discontinue the treatment. At times the therapist may feel that death is imminent and try to discontinue the treatment, only to discover that the physician wishes treatments continued. These situations are frequently very frustrating for therapists. They will find it helpful to discuss the case with the physician to determine what his goals are for that patient. Frequently he possesses information not written in the chart which makes continued or discontinued therapy more understandable. Physicians are usually willing to discuss the chest physical therapy program with concerned therapists who feel strongly about continued treatment. If these feelings interfere with treatment, then it may benefit both patient and therapist if another therapist takes over the case.

SPECIAL CASES

Listed below are some of the more common types of cancer that the therapist may encounter. Information on the specific cancers is designed to provide therapists with very basic knowledge. Specific forms of chest physical therapy treatment are not mentioned as they have been covered in depth in the previous section. Therapists wishing further 'knowledge on specific cancers should consult one of the excellent texts in the reference section at the end of the chapter.

Lung Cancer

Primary cancer of the lung is a very lethal disease, with only 5% of the patients surviving for five years, regardless of the type of cancer, the stage of diagnosis or the method by which the cancer was treated. Eighty percent of the patients diagnosed with lung cancer are dead within one year, with the average survival being 6–9 months after diagnosis. At the time of diagnosis 50% of the cancers are inoperable, while 50% of those undergoing surgery (25% of all lung cancers) are found to be unresectable. The incidence of lung cancer is four times higher in men than in women, with the average age of onset being 50–60 years. It is more frequently seen in patients with chronically diseased or scarred lungs.

Etiologic factors that may play a role in the development of lung cancer are cigarette smoking and exposure to coal tars, asbestos and radioactive dusts, such as uranium or radon. While the relationship between cigarette smoking and the development of lung cancer is still controversial, recent studies show that 80% of lung cancers are due to cigarette smoking. A combined study of lung cancer patients by the American Cancer Society, the National Cancer Institute and the U.S. Department of Health, Education and Welfare indicated that 80% of patients with lung cancer had a 20–30-year history of smoking two or three packs of cigarettes per day.

Bronchogenic carcinoma accounts for 95% of primary malignant lung tumors. Histologically bronchogenic carcinoma can be divided into the following types: squamous or epidermoid, polygonal or undifferentiated large cell, small round cell or oat cell, giant cell and adenocarcinoma. Squamous cell carcinomas account for 45% of all lung cancers, with prognosis being better in this type of tumor than with the others. They are usually centrally located and frequently cause bronchial obstruction with pneumonia, atelectasis, bronchiectasis or lung abscesses occurring distal to the tumor. The common route of spread is to regional lymph nodes. Polygonal carcinoma cells are large and polygonal in shape. Metastatic spread occurs early in this tumor via the lymphatic and circulatory systems.

Oat cell carcinoma is usually malignant. Though temporarily responsive to radiotherapy, patients rarely survive more than 3–4 months after diagnosis. Oat cell carcinoma accounts for 35%–40% of all lung cancers and is usually centrally located, with metastatic spread occurring early in the disease via the circulatory and lymphatic systems. It is the most rapidly spreading lung cancer. Giant cell carcinoma occurs in 1% of primary lung cancers. It is usually peripherally located and very malignant, with death occurring in 3–4 months. Adenocarcinoma occurs in 10%–15% of all lung tumors and is usually situated peripherally. It is an unusual tumor in that it is rarely diagnosed until after it has invaded the chest wall. It is also one of the rare lung cancers that is unrelated to cigarette smoking.

Metastatic spread of lung cancer occurs early in the disease, usually through the lymphatic and circulatory systems. The more common sites of secondary growth are the brain, adrenals, bones, liver and kidneys. The preferred therapy of lung cancers is surgery, if the tumor has not spread and is not of the oat cell variety. Radiation is frequently used before and after surgery to improve the results. The response to radiation without surgery depends on the type of cancer, with adenocarcinomas being unaffected while oat cell carcinomas virtually disappear for short periods of time. Generally radiation is used for symptomatic relief of cough, hemoptysis and compression of large airways by tumor. Chemotherapy is usually not very effective, producing intolerable side effects (nausea, weakness, vomiting) in a previously asymptomatic host, without prolonging life. As a result it is not used as frequently as other therapy in the treatment of lung cancer.

Bronchiolar carcinoma accounts for 3%–4% of all malignant lung tumors (in comparison to the bronchogenic carcinomas which account for 95% of primary lung tumors). Unlike bronchogenic carcinoma, men and women are equally affected. It is less malignant than bronchogenic carcinoma in that it rarely metastasizes. Death usually occurs as a result of respiratory insufficiency. The remaining 2% of malignant lung cancers are numerous and relatively rare and will not be discussed in this text. Therapists desiring further information should consult one of the references at the end of the chapter.

Metastatic tumors lodge to form secondary tumors in the lung more frequently than in any other organ but the liver. Metastatic spread usually occurs via the lymphatic and circulatory systems, with carcinomas of the kidney, breast, pancreas, colon, stomach and uterus being the most prone to metastasize to the lungs. The metastases are diffuse (lymphangitic), nodular or a combination of the two forms. The diffuse lymphangitic metastases present on x-ray as fine nodular densities spread throughout the lungs in a reticular pattern. This form of tumor frequently interferes with normal lung function, producing alveolar capillary block syndrome (i.e., the tumor serves as a barrier between alveoli and blood, preventing gas exchange). These patients generally present with dyspnea, rapid respirations, decreased tidal volumes and cyanosis. Patients with this form of metastatic spread usually die 2–4 months after lung involvement. Metastatic nodules occur in the lung as either solitary lesions or multiple diffuse lesions, with the latter occurring more frequently. The location of the nodules determines the symptoms of the patient, which usually include a productive cough, hemoptysis and wheezing. These nodules frequently obstruct bronchi, causing pneumonia, atelectasis or abscess distal to the tumor. Prognosis for nodular metastasis is poor though not as grave as for lymphangitic metastases.

Treatment of metastatic lung cancers is difficult and rarely successful. Solitary lesions respond the best, with surgery being the method of treatment. Unfortunately, treatment by chemotherapy or radiation is ineffective, as most of these tumors metastasize from adenocarcinomas, which do not respond to either form of therapy. As a result, treatment of lung metastases is usually done to relieve symptoms rather than to effect a cure.

Cancer of the Gastrointestinal Tract

Cancer of the GI tract carries a better prognosis as one descends from the esophagus to the colon. Cancers of the esophagus account for 2% of all cancers and have a very low survival rate (6% survival for five years). One reason for their high mortality is that they are not diagnosed until late. As such, treatment is usually palliative. Surgery and radiotherapy are the methods used to treat this cancer. Surgery is used less, as most cancers have invaded local areas extensively by the time of diagnosis. The surgery is usually radical and may include esophagectomy, splitting the diaphragm, and resection of the tail of the pancreas, spleen and celiac nodes. Second-stage surgeries are usually done to try to reconstruct an alimentary pathway for the patient by upswinging part of the colon between the mouth and stomach. Respiratory complications occur often following these surgeries (especially respiratory failure and secondary bacterial infections). Treatment by radiation is used to reduce the size of the tumor and therefore relieve symptoms caused by obstruction when surgery is not feasible. Chemotherapy has little effect on these tumors.

Cancer of the stomach is generally a disease of later life, occurring twice as often in men as in women. Adenocarcinomas comprise 97% of the malignancies that are sarcomas (most commonly lymphomas and leiomyosarcomas). These occur most frequently in the lower socioeconomic groups of Japan, Chile and Iceland. The prognosis depends on the stage of the disease at the time of diagnosis, with approximately 25%–30% of all patients with stomach cancer surviving for five years. The treatment of choice is surgery. Radiation and chemotherapy have proven ineffective in treating these malignancies. Surgery includes radical subtotal gastrectomy with removal of a large portion of the stomach, the lesser and greater omenta, and sometimes the spleen and distal pancreas. If the tumor has extended, the involved areas are also removed. Total gastrectomy is done only if absolutely necessary, as postoperative morbidity is very high.

Cancer of the colon and rectum causes more deaths in the United States than any other form of cancer, with men and women equally affected. The tumors are usually adenocarcinomas and are spread by the lymphatic and circulatory systems. The treatment of choice is either surgery or radiation. Surgical procedures involve removal of the cancer-containing bowel with intestinal anastomoses or abdominoperineal resections with permanent colostomies. Tumors of the colon are fairly radiosensitive, with clearance of the tumor occurring in 50%–75% of the cases. The five-year survival rate for this cancer is about 25%. Respiratory problems in patients with GI tract cancer occur fairly frequently as a result of abdominal pain which causes the patient to splint and makes it difficult for him to cough effectively. Secondary bacterial infections of the lung occur late in the disease when the patient is bedridden.

Cancer of the digestive organs is usually quite advanced when diagnosed and includes cancer of the pancreas, liver, extrahepatic bile ducts and gall bladder. Mortality is high, with death occurring in most cases in less than one year. Cancer of the pancreas comprises about 2%–3% of all tumors and is seen most frequently in men. The tumors are usually radioresistant and unresectable at the time of diagnosis. Temporary palliation of symptoms with chemotherapy is possible in 10%–20% of the cases. Primary cancer of the liver occurs in about 2% of all tumors, usually in men of Oriental extraction. It is treated with partial hepatectomies, when feasible, and chemotherapy (which may induce temporary remission). Death usually occurs within six months. (Metastases to the liver are treated much the same as primary tumors, and they have the same prognosis as liver cancer.) Cancer of the gall bladder comprises 4% of all cancers and is seen most frequently in women. The only treatment possible is surgical removal of the gall bladder with partial or subtotal hepatectomy. Cancer of the extrahepatic bile ducts is rare, with surgical treatment being the only effective therapy. Malignancies of the digestive glands have many respiratory complications due to their anatomical location. Pain from the area, with or without surgery, causes the patient to hypoventilate and splint the area. Secondary bacterial infections occur fairly early in the disease in the hypoventilated areas of the lung.

Cancer of the Head and Neck

Malignancies of the head and neck are grouped together by their anatomical location rather than histologically. They account for only 5% of all malignancies but are frequently the most difficult to treat. They occur most frequently in patients who smoke or have a high alcohol intake. Treatment involves radical, disfiguring surgery and irradiation. Most patients are managed by a multidisciplinary approach, including surgeons of otolaryngology, plastic surgeons, oral surgeons, radiation oncologists and medical oncologists. Lesions in the oral cavity are removed surgically in a block dissection, with neck dissections performed at the same time when lymph nodes are palpable. Elective neck dissection is also done at this time in certain forms of cancer that are known to spread quickly (cancer of the tongue, alveolar ridge, and the floor of the mouth). Pre- and postoperative radiation is frequently used to reduce the size of the tumor and effect better results. (These tumors are generally radiosensitive.) At times the radical neck dissections are done palliatively to prevent painful deaths by asphyxia, starvation, or hemorrhage. These patients are difficult to manage after surgery, having many respiratory, nutritional and emotional problems. The five-year survival rate is low (5%) with most deaths, occurring from nutritional or respiratory complications.

Lymphomas

The malignant lymphomas are a group of disorders characterized by malignant proliferation of the lymphoreticular tissue. They include Hodgkin's disease (40%), lymphosarcomas and reticulum cell sarcomas. They account for 5% of all cancers and usually present with lymph node enlargement. Treatment is by radiation and/or chemotherapy (a delicate combination to manage as extensive radiation reduces bone marrow tolerance to chemotherapy). Prognosis depends on the stage of the disease at diagnosis, with 75% of early-stage lymphomas having a five-year survival, whereas only 25% of late-stage lymphomas survive for five years. These patients rarely have lung involvement until late in their disease, when secondary bacterial pneumonias occur as a result of the patient's compromised condition.

Leukemias

The leukemias are a group of diseases involving hematopoietic cells or their precursors. The bone marrow is always involved. Leukemia accounts for 8% of all malignancies, with men affected 75% of the time. The different types are acute lymphocytic leukemia (ALL), a disease of childhood; chronic lymphocytic leukemia (CLL), a disease of the aged; acute myelogenous leukemia (AML), a disease occurring equally in all age groups; and chronic granulocytic (myelogenous) leukemia (CML), which occurs in middle and late life. The disease is frequently designated as acute or chronic, with acute referring to undifferentiation of proliferating cells and chronic referring to a fairly complete differentiation of cells. The proliferating cells invade all tissues and organs and are responsible for the clinical manifestations of the disease. The leukemias are treated by chemotherapy, with prognosis widely varied. Patients with acute leukemia have a very low survival rate—less than 1% survival for five years. The survival rate varies with the type of leukemia—from 13 months after diagnosis in patients with AML, to 3.5 years in patients with CML, while there is 50% survival for five years in patients with ALL, and seven years for patients with CLL. Death usually occurs as a result of secondary infections. Respiratory complications (e.g., pneumonia) occur late in the disease and are usually bacterial in origin.

Bone Tumors

Primary malignant tumors of the bone are rare. They are all sarcomas and are treated by all three forms of therapy. They differ from most malignancies in that they spread through the circulatory system. Death usually occurs from secondary growth of a metastatic tumor. The different types of bone cancer include: osteosarcoma (28% of all bone tumors), chondrosarcoma (13% of bone tumors), fibrosarcoma (4% of all bone tumors) and multiple myeloma. (Actually the cancer is a malignancy of the plasma cells but occurs most frequently in the marrow of bone, invading surrounding bone early in the disease. It compromises

35%–40% of all bone tumors.) Prognosis for five-year survival for a primary bone cancer depends on the type, varying from 5% for osteosarcoma and 10% for multiple myeloma to 20%–25% for chondrosarcomas and fibrosarcomas. Most malignant bone lesions (65%) are metastatic from a carcinoma located elsewhere in the body. They occur most frequently in the spine and pelvis. These lesions make it difficult to position the patients, thereby making them good hosts for secondary pulmonary involvement.

Central Nervous System

Tumors of the central nervous system comprise 2%–10% of all tumors. They occur more frequently among the white races and equally among women and men in all age groups. Eighty percent of these tumors involve the brain and 20% involve the spinal cord. Forty percent of central nervous system tumors are metastatic lesions from other primary cancers (especially from lung, breast, kidney, melanomas and GI tract). Primary tumors of the central nervous system are unusual in that they rarely metastasize beyond the central nervous system. Glial tumors account for 45%–50% of all central nervous system tumors and include astrocytomas (20%–30% of glial tumors), glioblastomas (50%–55% of all glial tumors and the most malignant) and medulloblastomas (5%–15% of all glial tumors). Tumors of the membranes include meningiomas (20% of central nervous system tumors) and schwannomas (tumor of the sheaths of Schwann occur in 8% of central nervous system tumors).

All tumors of the central nervous system are associated with high mortality. Initial treatment of these tumors involves surgical excision. Frequently, these tumors have invaded deep into the brain at the time of diagnosis and cannot be completely removed surgically. In such cases surgeons remove as much of the tumor as possible in order to relieve the pressure on the brain. Most malignant brain tumors are very radiosensitive and decrease in size rapidly with irradiation. Radiation is used when surgery cannot be performed, when total tumor excision is not possible surgically and when multiple sites of tumor are suspected. Respiratory complications occur when the patient becomes bedridden or when the tumor invades or applies pressure to the respiratory centers located in the pons and medulla. Patients with central nervous system damage frequently breathe shallowly with consistent tidal volumes, unlike the normal person who breathes with irregular tidal volumes. The consistent tidal volumes allow small areas of the lung to collapse (microatelectasis). Secondary bacterial infections of the lung occur late in the disease as a result of hypoventilation, immobility of the patient and decreased resistance of the host.

SUMMARY

Only the most basic information on cancer has been presented in this chapter. It was designed to acquaint the therapist with basic concepts on oncology. Therapists dealing frequently with this subject should utilize all available sources including nursing staff, attending physicians and textbooks to learn more about the subject.

REFERENCES

Periodicals

Barber LM: Occupational therapy for the treatment of reflex sympathetic dystrophy and posttraumatic hypersensitivity in the injured hand, in Fredericks S, Brody GS (eds): *Symposium on the Neurological Aspects of Plastic Surgery*. St Louis, CV Mosby Co, 1978, p 115.

Blitz B, Dinnerstein J, Lowenthal M: Attenuation of experimental pain by tactile stimulation: Effect of vibration at different levels of noxious stimulus intensity. *Percept Mot Skills* 1964; 19:311–316.

Boysen M, Natvig K, Winther FO, et al: Value of routine follow-up in patients treated for squamous cell carcinoma of the head and neck. *J Otololaryngol* 1985; 14:211–214.

Calverly PMA, Chang HK, Wight D, et al: High frequency chest wall compression (HFCWC) assists and improves gas exchange in normal man (abstract). *Am Rev Respir Dis* 1983; 127:283.

Gross D, O'Brien C, Wight D, et al: Enhanced peripheral mucus clearance with high frequency chest wall compression (abstract). *Physiologist* 1983; 26:35.

Harf A, Bertrand C, Chang HK: Ventilation by high frequency oscillation on the thorax or at the trachea in rats. *J Appl Physiol* 1985; 124–127.

King M, Phillips DM, Gross D, et al: Enhanced mucus clearance with high frequency chest wall compression (HFCWC). *Am Rev Respir Dis* 1983; 128:511–565.

Mosely JR: Alterations in comfort. *Nurs Clin North Am* 1985; June:427–430.

Pavia D, Thompson ML, Philipakos D: A preliminary study of the effect of a vibratory pad on bronchial clearance. *Am Rev Respir Dis* 1976; 113:92–96.

Saunders JM, McCorkle R: Models of care for persons with progressive cancer. *J Otolaryngol* 1985; 14:365–378.

Zidulka A, Gross D, Minami H, et al: Ventilation by high frequency chest wall compression in dogs with normal lungs. *Am Rev Respir Dis* 1983; 127:709–713.

Books

Ackerman LV, Regato JA: *Cancer,* ed 4. St Louis, CV Mosby Co, 1970.

Baum GL: *Textbook of Pulmonary Diseases,* ed 2. Boston, Little, Brown & Co, 1974.

Bendixen HH, et al: *Respiratory Care.* St Louis, CV Mosby Co, 1965.

Bouchard R, Owens NF: *Nursing Care of the Cancer Patient,* ed 3. St Louis, CV Mosby Co, 1976.

Committee on Professional Education of UICC International Union Against Cancer: *Clinical Oncology.* Berlin, Springer-Verlag, 1974.

Guenter CA, Welch MH: *Pulmonary Medicine.* Philadelphia, JB Lippincott Co, 1977.

Hardy RE, Cull JC: *Counseling and Rehabilitating the Cancer Patient.* Springfield, Illinois, Charles C Thomas, Publisher, 1975.

Hedley-White J, et al: *Applied Physiology of Respiratory Care.* Boston, Little, Brown & Co, 1976.

Kubler-Ross E: *On Death and Dying.* New York, Macmillan Publishing Co, 1970.

Rubin P: *Clinical Oncology,* ed 4. Rochester, New York, American Cancer Society, 1974.

Rubin P: *Current Concepts in Cancer.* Chicago, American Medical Association, 1974.

25

Viral and Bacterial Pneumonias

Lyn Hobson, P.T., R.R.T.

Despite recent advancements in diagnostic techniques and preventive nursing care, the incidence of pneumonia is as high in the United States now as it was prior to the use of antibiotics. Bacterial pneumonia remains the fifth most common cause of death in the United States, occurring more frequently in infants and older people. Pneumonia is the illness of the largest segment of most practitioners' patients, as well as being one of the most common disorders seen in hospitalized patients.

DEFENSE MECHANISMS OF THE LUNG

Pneumonia occurs when the normal defense mechanisms of the respiratory system fail to keep the lower respiratory tract sterile. A brief review of these defense mechanisms will be covered. Therapists desiring further knowledge should review Chapter 1 on anatomy or refer to one of the excellent texts in the references at the end of the chapter.

Air inspired through the nasal passages is cleaned of particulate matter by filtration (cilia sweep it to the nasopharynx); impaction (irregular contour of the chamber causes particles to rain out); swelling of hygroscopic droplet nuclei which then either are filtered or become impacted; and defense factors located in the mucous blanket such as immunoglobulins (IgA), lysozymes, polymorphonuclear leukocytes and specific antibodies. Particles that escape one of these defense mechanisms in the nasopharynx may be prevented from entering the lower

634

airways at the larynx. The mucosa of the larynx is sensitive to chemical irritation or mechanical deformation and responds to this stimuli by producing a cough. The high velocities created by the cough are sufficient to clear several branches of the tracheobronchial tree of particulate matter. The cough reflex is frequently absent or depressed in hosts who are unconscious from drug overdose, epilepsy, alcohol ingestion or head injury. Patients with artificial airways are more susceptible to infection as all the previously mentioned defense mechanisms are bypassed, causing organisms to be deposited directly into the lower airways. In the lower airways the cough mechanism is rendered ineffective as the endotracheal tubes prevent cord approximation and tracheostomy tubes cause air to bypass the cords altogether.

The trachea and the tracheobronchial tree to the level of the respiratory bronchioles are protected by the cough reflex, filtration (again by cilia which transport particles to the pharynx), impaction and chemical factors (IgA). Below the level of the respiratory bronchioles the cough reflex is ineffective, and filtration and transportation of particles by cilia cannot occur as cilia are absent. The alveolar macrophages play an important role in protecting these airways from particulate matter. Macrophages ingest organisms and transport them to the lymphatic system or higher up in the tracheobronchial tree to where cilia can then sweep them to the pharynx. This process of phagocytosis can be slowed or stopped by hypoxia, alcohol ingestion, air pollutants, corticosteroids, immunosuppressant agents, starvation, cigarette smoke, and oxygen. Particulate matter can also be removed from the airways below the level of the respiratory bronchioles by postural drainage.

ROUTES OF INFECTION

A host who has impaired or ineffective defense mechanisms of the respiratory tract becomes susceptible to a variety of organisms. Therapists who become aware of such patients should institute prophylactic bronchial hygiene to prevent respiratory problems. Ineffective organisms are introduced to the respiratory tract by one of four routes—inhalation of airborne organisms, spread of oropharyngeal organisms to the lower respiratory tract, spread by the circulatory system from other septic foci and spread from infected contiguous tissue. The organisms causing a pneumonic focus are usually located near the periphery of the lung and from there are transported to other areas by way of the pores of Kohn and the canals of Lambert.

Airborne Organisms

Most respiratory infections are introduced by airborne organisms that have been expelled from the respiratory tracts of infected individuals. They are expelled by sneezing, coughing, talking and singing. Only the smaller particles are able to penetrate to the lower airways and become sites of infection.

Circulation

Circulatory spread of organisms from other septic foci usually occurs in patients with subacute bacterial endocarditis or drug addicts who frequently inject themselves and develop septicemia. Staphylococci and enteric gram-negative bacilli are the most common organisms that cause respiratory infections by circulatory spread.

Contiguous Infection

Contiguous infections are relatively rare and are usually seen in patients with pancreatitis, cholecystitis, subphrenic abscesses, peritonitis and infections of the bones of the rib cage or soft tissues overlying the rib cage. In these cases the organisms invade the pleural spaces to form emphysemas, or effusions, and from there may spread into the lung tissue itself.

Aspiration

Aspiration into the lower airways usually involves oropharyngeal contents, gastric contents, toxic fluids, nontoxic fluids and solid particles. It usually occurs in a host with an altered level of consciousness and almost always contains pathogenic bacteria and other matter that has toxic effects on the lower respiratory tract. Aspiration into the lower airways is a common, well-tolerated phenomenon that occurs frequently in most individuals, sometimes without their awareness of it. Alterations in the host's defense mechanisms and the nature of the aspirate seem to determine the effect of the aspiration.

The more common aspirated toxic fluids are acids (usually gastric acid), animal fats, mineral oil, alcohol and hydrocarbons. In such cases, patients present with an abrupt onset of acute respiratory distress, with bronchospasm as a characteristic feature. Many of the patients become hypotensive and hypoxemic with normal or low arterial levels of Pco_2, and have a cough producing frothy nonpurulent sputum. Their chest x-rays show mottled densities in the affected lung segments (usually superior or posterior segments of the lower lobes). The area depends on the patient's position when he aspirates. The aspirated contents react like a chemical burn, with inflammation of the bronchial walls, increased production of sputum, peribronchial hemorrhage and exudate, pulmonary edema and areas of necrosis. Some of these patients develop adult respiratory distress syndrome but most recover in 2–5 weeks. Secondary bacterial infections can occur in the debilitated host.

Aspiration of pathogenic bacteria presents with the symptoms of the particular organism; this will be discussed in greater depth in the latter part of this chapter. It usually presents with more insidious symptoms, and the actual episode of aspiration is rarely observed. The more common organisms seen are pneumococci, *Escherichia coli*, *Proteus*, *Pseudomonas*, *Klebsiella pneumoniae* and *Staphylococcus aureus*.

Aspiration of nontoxic fluids (saline solution, water, neutralized gastric contents) generally produces transient respiratory distress with temporary hypoxemia. Large amounts of fluid may cause death by mechanical obstruction and suffocation. Varying degrees of mechanical obstruction also occur with aspirated solid particles. Smaller objects produce a persistent cough, while larger objects may cause obstruction, dyspnea, cyanosis, wheezing, pain, nausea and vomiting. Objects that lodge in the larynx or trachea cause severe respiratory distress, aphonia and possibly death (frequently referred to as "cafe coronaries") if not removed or bypassed with an emergency cricothyroidectomy. Chest PT has been found to be useful in removal of small objects (Raghu and Pierson, 1986). Smaller objects when not removed can cause a variety of lung pathologies, including bacterial pneumonia at the site in 1–2 weeks, bronchiectasis, lung abscesses and empyema.

Classification of Pneumonias

Classification of pneumonias was originally anatomical in origin, but with modern chemotherapy pneumonias have become known by the specific organism involved. Some of the more common anatomical classifications are listed below.

Apical. The pneumonia is limited to the upper lobe of the lung. It is more commonly seen in young children, elderly compromised adults and alcoholics.

Bronchopneumonia. This is a term used to refer to a patchy consolidation of the lungs. It is usually bilateral and frequently associated with interstitial pneumonia and subsequent fibrosis.

Interstitial Pneumonia.   This refers to pneumonias that affect the interstitial spaces and produce fibrosis of the lung tissue. Unlike other pneumonias, the process occurs outside of the alveoli and so sputum production is rare.

Lobar Pneumonia.   This is a term used to refer to a pneumonia that involves an entire lobe of the lung. It frequently is referred to as pneumococcal pneumonia. This type of pneumonia was seen more frequently before the advent of chemotherapy.

Massive Pneumonia.   In this type of pneumonia the alveoli as well as the bronchi are filled with a fibrinous exudate. It is rare and almost always fatal.

Segmental Pneumonia.   This type of pneumonia involves only one or two segments of a lobe.

Traumatic or Contusional Pneumonia.   This type of pneumonia occurs after a traumatic incident (i.e., a car accident) and presents with varying degrees of hemorrhagic lesions. It was frequently fatal when superimposed bacterial infections occurred.

With the advent of chemotherapy, respiratory therapy modalities and aggressive bronchial hygiene, pneumonias have become confined to smaller areas. New terminology has come into existence as x-rays have become more readily available. It includes the classifications below:

Atelectasis.   This refers to a collapse or partial involvement of an area of the lung. The specific area involved is usually mentioned (e.g., atelectasis of the left lower lobe).

Absorption Atelectasis.   Plugging of a larger airway with a mucous plug, tumor or foreign object produces alveolar and airway collapse distal to the obstruction as the gas is absorbed by the bloodstream.

Compression Atelectasis.   This occurs when external forces (tension pneumothorax, pleural effusions, ascites, obesity, pregnancy) apply pressure to the alveoli and airways, causing them to collapse.

Microatelectasis.   This refers to widely spread diffuse areas of alveolar collapse that are too small to be seen by x-ray. The patient usually presents with a fairly normal chest x-ray and acute respiratory distress. The areas of atelectasis and lung involvement usually spread until they are visible on x-ray.

Infiltrates.　These are areas of pneumonia or pneumonitis whose boundaries are ill defined.

Plate-like Atelectasis.　This condition includes thin white lines seen on x-ray and interpreted to be small areas of alveolar collapse. It may or may not be associated with pneumonia and is frequently seen in healthy individuals.

Pneumonitis.　This is an inflammation of lung tissue.

Other methods of classification refer to the causative factor, i.e., chemical, lipid or fat, aspiration, bacterial, viral, hypostatic (seen in compromised, bedridden patients who do not change positions), nosocomial and postoperative pneumonias. Most of the pneumonias can be classified as either viral or bacterial.

VIRAL INFECTIONS

Most respiratory viral infections are contracted by droplets from the respiratory tracts of infected human beings. These viruses are responsible for interstitial pneumonias, tracheobronchitis, bronchiolitis and the common cold. The ciliated cells of the respiratory tract are the most frequent site of infection. They become paralyzed and degenerate with areas of necrosis and desquamation. The mucociliary blanket becomes interrupted as destruction of cilia leaves a thin layer of nonciliated basal replacement cells. Inflammatory responses cause exudation of fluid and erythrocytes in both alveolar septa and airways. Congestion and edema become predominant, with the formation of intra-alveolar hyaline membranes. These changes in the normal mucosal structure and cilia make involved areas of the lung susceptible to superimposed bacterial infections. This is the most common complication seen in viral infections and is usually responsible for the fatalities that occur.

The mechanism by which the host fights the virus infection is still a mystery. Many people feel that antibody production is important in ridding the body of the organism. Others feel antibodies only prevent the spread of the infection. Injection of immunoglobulins may help the host fight the infection, but their role is still questionable. At this time there are no specific antiviral agents available that are effective.

Viral Pneumonia

The patient with viral pneumonia presents with fever, dyspnea, loss of appetite and a persistent nonproductive cough. On auscultation normal breath sounds are heard throughout both lung fields with scattered inspiratory rales. X-ray changes range from minor infiltrates to severe bilateral involvement. Consolidation and pleural effusions rarely occur. Secondary bacterial infections occur frequently, and it is only then that patients develop a productive cough.

Influenza

Influenza includes several acute viral respiratory tract infections characterized by a sudden onset of headache, myalgia and fever. The route of infection is by inhalation of airborne particles from an infected person. The incubation period is 24–72 hours. Patients with pneumonia present with the same clinical picture as in viral pneumonia. The most acutely ill patients are those with pneumonia, which occurs in 1%–5% of the cases. Pulmonary lesions include edema of the respiratory epithelium with necrosis and hemorrhage. At the alveolar level interstitial edema, proliferation of type I cells, hemorrhage and an increased number of macrophages are seen. In patients with pneumonia, secondary bacterial infections are frequent and are the cause of most fatalities. The bacterial organisms causing the infections are *Staphylococcus aureus, Hemophilus influenzae, Diplococcus pneumoniae,* and various gram-negative organisms.

Treatment

Medical treatment of these infections is supportive and preventive. Patients should receive vaccines whenever possible to build up antibodies against specific viruses. Once the patient has contracted the organism, treatment becomes supportive, with bed rest, salicylates and high fluid intake being the main modes of treatment. Patients who become more acutely ill with viral pneumonia should be put on a vigorous preventive program to lessen the possibility of bacterial infection. They must also be closely observed so they can receive mechanical ventilation if any signs of respiratory failure develop.

   Chest physical therapy in these patients should be prophylactic. Patients with viral pneumonias have a persistent nonproductive cough. Therapists who initiate vigorous bronchial hygiene will become very frustrated as they try to mobilize nonexistent secretions. Treatment programs should be directed to the needs of the patient. Patients who are less acutely ill may do well with breathing exercises and positional rotation; more vigorous treatment should be initiated at the first sign of a bacterial infection (i.e., productive cough). At this time, the appropriate respiratory therapy appliances should be ordered. Ultrasonic or medication nebulizers can help liquefy secretions. Percussion and vibration in postural drainage positions should follow the respiratory therapy treatments. Patients should also assume some responsibility for their treatments by performing breathing exercises and positional rotation during the therapist's absence.

BACTERIAL PNEUMONIA

Bacterial pneumonia causes the largest number of deaths per year by an infective agent and is the fifth most common cause of all deaths in the United States today. The patient presents with an abrupt onset of a severe illness characterized by fever, tachypnea, dyspnea, hypoxemia, tachycardia and a cough producing bloody or purulent sputum. The clinical findings depend on the organism involved and the extent of the pneumonia found in the lungs. The infective process may cease with the use of chemotherapeutic agents, respiratory therapy appliances and chest physical therapy, or it may spread to contiguous areas, causing pleural effusions and empyemas.

Bacterial pneumonias can occur as either primary or secondary infections. Primary pneumonias arise in otherwise healthy individuals and are usually pneumococcal in origin. Secondary pneumonias occur when the patient's defense system becomes ineffective. The specific diseases and routes of infection have been discussed earlier in the chapter.

Pneumococcal Pneumonia *(Streptococcus pneumoniae or Deplococcus pneumoniae)*

The pneumococcus, a gram-positive organism, is responsible for the majority of primary and secondary pneumonias. It occurs most frequently in the winter months among adults between 15 and 40 years of age, with a preponderance of males. More than 80 types of pneumococcal organisms have been isolated. Identification of the specific organism causing the infection is unnecessary as all types are treated identically. The patients present clinically with an abrupt onset of illness characterized by fever, cough, purulent or rust-colored sputum and pleuritic chest pain over the affected lung tissue. Physical examination may reveal decreased expansion of the chest over the affected area and muscle splinting. On auscultation there may be bronchial breath sounds (indicating consolidation), decreased or absent breath sounds, wheezes, rales or rhonchi heard over the affected lung. Chest x-rays may show infiltrates, consolidation or atelectasis.

The lung tissue itself goes through four stages—engorgement, red hepatization, gray hepatization and resolution. The *engorgement* stage occurs within the first few days of infection and is characterized by vascular engorgement, serous exudation and evidence of many bacteria. *Red hepatization* occurs within 2–4 days as a result of diapedesis of the red blood cells. The alveoli are full of polymorphonuclear leukocytes, fibrin and red blood cells. The organism continues to multiply within the edematous fluid. Areas of consolidation become evident. *Gray hepatization* occurs within 4–8 days and is characterized by evidence of abundant fibrin, decreased polymorphonuclear leukocytes and dead bacteria. Consolidation continues to be a problem in this stage. *Resolution* occurs after 8 days as the consolidations begin to resolve. There are many macrophages seen and evidence of enzymatic digestion of exudate is present. The affected tissue becomes softer with large amounts of grayish red fluid present within the alveoli. This process continues for 2–3 weeks with the lung gradually assuming a more normal appearance.

Pleural involvement occurs frequently, with the pleural spaces filling with the same type of fluid seen within the alveoli. Resolution is much slower as there are few surfaces available for phagocytosis. Complications that may occur in patients with pneumococcal involvement include empyema, superinfections (occur when large numbers of new organisms invade the lung), abscesses, atelectasis and delayed resolution (defined as taking more than 4 weeks to resolve).

Treatment of pneumococcal pneumonia involves the use of chemotherapeutic agents, with penicillin being the antibiotic of choice. If the patient is allergic to penicillin, erythromycin or lincomycin is used. Thoracentesis is performed when pleural fluid is present. The patient should also receive supplemental oxygen therapy, USN, and aggressive chest physical therapy.

Staphylococcal Pneumonia

Staphylococcal pneumonia is caused by a gram-positive organism. It rarely occurs in the healthy adult but is a frequent cause of pneumonia in children, infants and patients with chronic lung diseases, especially carcinoma, tuberculosis and cystic fibrosis. Clinically the patient presents with the same picture as the patient with pneumococcal pneumonia. There are some differences in the x-ray picture, such as that consolidation occurs infrequently in this pneumonia. Instead one sees on x-ray patchy areas of infiltrates. Pleural effusions, empyema, abscesses, bronchopleural fistulas and pneumatoceles (subpleural cyst-like structures) occur frequently. Treatment is with chemotherapeutic agents, bedrest, increased fluids, USN, or medication nebulizers, and aggressive chest physical therapy.

Streptococcal Pneumonia

Streptococcal pneumonia is caused by a gram-positive organism, *Streptococcus pyogenes* (a member of the A beta-hemolytic streptococci). It occurs most frequently in the very young, the very old or the debilitated patient. The clinical picture is very similar to that of staphylococcal pneumonia. Again consolidation is rare and x-rays usually show one or more areas of patchy infiltrates. Complications are rare, but empyema does occasionally occur. Treatment for this organism is the same as that for pneumococcal pneumonia.

Klebsiella Pneumonia (Friedländer's)

This pneumonia is caused by a gram-negative organism, the *Klebsiella pneumoniae*. It occurs most frequently in older patients (over 50) or in those who have an underlying disease (especially alcoholism, chronic lung disease and diabetes). It occurs most frequently in the upper lobes. The patient presents with the same clinical picture seen in the other bacterial pneumonias. Patients have a cough producing either gelatinous red sputum (rare); thick greenish, purulent sputum streaked with blood (most common); or frankly bloody sputum. On x-ray the bulging of fissures adjacent to the areas of consolidation is distinctive as well as areas of consolidation and atelectasis. Consolidation and atelectasis of more than one lobe occur frequently, with destruction of lung tissue, necrosis and extensive abscess formation occurring early in the disease.

Complications are frequent and include empyema, pneumothorax, chronic pneumonia and spread to contiguous tissues. Treatment must be immediate and very aggressive due to the destructive nature of the disease. Chemotherapeutic drugs used to treat the organism include streptomycin, chloramphenicol, tetracycline and kanamycin. Supplemental oxygen, bronchodilators, USN, and aggressive chest physical therapy are also used to treat the patient.

Hemophilus Influenzae

Hemophilus Influenzae pneumonia is caused by a gram-negative organism and occurs primarily in children (as bronchiolitis) and in adults who have chronic bronchitis or are alcoholics. The clinical picture is the same as for the other bacterial pneumonias, with numerous areas of infiltration evident on x-ray. On auscultation, breath sounds are generally good, with rales heard at the end of inspiration. Treatment of this pneumonia includes chemotherapeutic agents (ampicillin), oxygen, USN, and chest physical therapy.

Miscellaneous

Other gram-negative organisms causing pneumonia are *Escherichia coli*, *Pseudomonas aeruginosa* and *Proteus* species. They are seen most frequently in patients with underlying disease (especially pulmonary) or who are debilitated. They are frequently the cause of superinfections in individuals who have received massive doses of broad-spectrum antibiotics. Clinically these patients present with cough, fever and dyspnea. On auscultation rales, bronchiolar breath sounds and diminished or absent breath sounds are heard. X-ray changes almost always show bibasilar infiltrates, with the amount of involvement being widely variable. As in other bacterial pneumonias, treatment includes chemotherapeutic agents, USN, and chest physical therapy.

TREATMENT

Treatment of a patient with bacterial pneumonia is the same as chest physical therapy in other patients. The initial evaluation, perusal of the chart and chest x-ray will reveal the area of involvement. Assessment of the need for respiratory therapy modalities must be made. Ultrasonic nebulizers are helpful to mobilize secretions. Percussion and vibration to the appropriate area should be done in postural drainage positions when possible. Postional rotation should be done frequently to prevent further areas of involvement and assist drainage of the affected area. The patient's nurse should become involved and assist the patient in positional rotation, breathing exercises and coughing. The patient should play a role in his treatment by performing the breathing exercises, coughing and positional rotation in the therapist's absence.

Lobes that were affected by the pneumonia will remain vulnerable to further infection for some time. Patients who continue to be bedridden, debilitated or have underlying diseases should be put on a pro-phylactic treatment program to prevent further involvement. The patient should be shown positions that will facilitate drainage of his involved lung segments. Usually patients will only be in the hospital up to three days for pneumonia. They will need to follow up with their own home care. The therapist may wish to continue the percussion and vibration in postural drainage positions for a short period of time. Positional rotation should be the most important part of the prophylactic treatment program. Frequent positional changes will prevent secretions from accumulating in dependent positions. The patient should also continue his breathing exercises.

Therapists must remember that their role in the treatment of bacterial pneumonia, while important, is not as essential as the appropriate antibiotics. Once the patient is on the medication, the drug will begin to fight the bacteria and prevent the infection from spreading. Only then can therapy assist the patient in ridding his lung of accumulated secretions and prevent their mechanical transfer to another location.

ACQUIRED IMMUNE DEFICIENCY SYNDROME (AIDS)

Acquired immune deficiency syndrome (AIDS) has reached proportions that must be called epidemic since it was first reported in 1981. The numbers of AIDS victims are increasing and the fatality rate of the disease is remarkable. It is estimated that of patients diagnosed as having AIDS for three years or more, 85% have expired. Social and ethical issues have been brought to light regarding this population of patients. Over 85% of AIDS patients are homosexual men and intravenous drug users (DeVita et al., 1985). Others at risk are parenteral drug users, Haitians, hemophiliacs, recipients of blood or blood products, and female sexual partners of men with AIDS. There is much anxiety on the part of health care workers that deal with these patients. The definition of AIDS "should be reserved for a person with at least one life-threatening opportunistic infection or Kaposi's sarcoma, who has no identifiable reason or profound immunodeficiency."

We see AIDS patients for chest PT; they often have pneumonia and may be ventilated if they go into respiratory failure. We attempt to clear the pneumonia that is reversible. Many AIDS patients develop Pneumocystis carinii pneumonia (60%). *P. carinii* pneumonia often occurs in immunocompromised patients. It is both an alveolar and an interstitial infiltrative pneumonia.

Typical features noted in AIDS patients are low-grade temperatures, often for prolonged periods (i.e., three months), weight loss, lymphadenopathy, fatigue and night sweats. Mucosal *Candida,* herpes simplex, and cytomegalovirus are also common infectious agents seen in the patient with AIDS.

The health care practitioner should take good handwashing precautions and should protect himself while dealing with secretions. If a patient has a very productive cough, he should take care to cover his mouth with a Kleenex. The health care practitioner should avoid standing in front of the patient as he coughs and protect his eyes from droplet infection as the disease is spread through mucous secretions. In our infectious disease precautions, we will use gloves and gown (the same precautions as used with hepatitis B) when treating patients and handling mucous secretions (especially when suctioning patients with very productive coughs, etc.). It is important when these precautions are taken not to have the patient feel "contaminated" and isolated. Psychological support is necessary, as it is for all patients, but especially when isolation procedures are utilized. Each therapist should check the hospital protocol for infectious disease precautions to be utilized. Since this is a relatively new disease, our infectious disease precautions for AIDS patients have changed and may change again as new information is available.

REFERENCES

Periodicals

Bartelett JG, Gorbach SL: The triple threat of pneumonia. *Chest* 1975; 68:4.

Cushing R: Pulmonary infections. *Heart Lung* 1976; 5:4.

Ehrenkranz NJ, et al: Pneumocystitis carinii pneumonia among persons with hemophilia. *MMWR* 1982; 31:365.

Friedman KA, et al: Kaposis sarcoma and pneumocystis pneumonia among homosexual men: New York and California. *MMWR* 1981; 30:305.

Iannini PB, et al: Bacteremic pseudomonas pneumonia. *JAMA* 1974; 230:4.

Lerner AM, Jankauskas K: The classical bacterial pneumonias. *DM,* February 1975.

Raghu G, Pierson DJ: Successful removal of an aspirated tooth by chest physiotherapy. *Respir Care* 1986; 31:1099–1101.

Ziskind MM: The acute bacterial pneumonias in the adult. *Respir Care* 1976; 21:3.

Books

Avers JA, Dale C: AIDS: Reference guide for medical professionals. Center for Interdisciplinary Research in Immunology and Diseases at UCLA, in cooperation with the National Institute of Allergy and Infectious Diseases and the UCLA AIDS Center, 1984.

Baum GL: *Textbook of Pulmonary Diseases* ed 2. Boston, Little, Brown & Co, 1974.

Bendixen HH, et al: *Respiratory Care*. St Louis, CV Mosby Co, 1965.

Brunson JG, Gall EA: *Concepts of Disease*. New York, Macmillan Publishing Co, 1971.

DeVita V, Hellman S, Rosenberg S: *AIDS: Etiology, Diagnosis, Treatment, and Prevention*. Philadelphia, JB Lippincott Co, 1985.

Ebbesen P, et al: AIDS: A Basic Guide for Clinicians. Philadelphia, WB Saunders Co, 1984.

Guenter CA, Welch MH: *Pulmonary Medicine*. Philadelphia, JB Lippincott Co, 1977.

Gupta S: *AIDS-Associated Syndrome*. New York, Plenum Press, 1984.

Hedley-White J, Burgess GE: *Applied Physiology of Respiratory Care*, ed 2. Boston, Little, Brown & Co, 1976.

Mann WN: *Conybeare's Textbook of Medicine*, ed 16. New York, Churchill Livingstone, Inc, 1975.

Scott RB: *Price's Textbook of the Practice of Medicine*, ed 10. London, Oxford University Press, 1966.

Wilson GS, Miles A: *Principles of Bacteriology, Urology and Immunity*, ed 16. Baltimore, Williams & Wilkins Co, 1975.

26

Respiratory Failure

Carol Dickman, P.T., R.R.T.

Judith Ameen Wilchynski, M.S., P.T.

The diagnosis and treatment of respiratory failure has progressed over the last 30 years from the use of the tank or iron lung to mechanical ventilation with intermittent mandatory ventilation (IMV) and positive and expiratory pressure (PEEP). As we continue to learn more about this disease entity, we also learn that our treatment techniques can cause side effects. It was not until 1967 that Nash et al. described the pulmonary morphologic changes that occurred with mechanical ventilation at $F_{I_{O_2}}$ greater than 85%–90%. Today we refer to this as pulmonary oxygen toxicity. Some medical centers have tried extracorporeal membrane oxygenation in an attempt to alter the prognosis of respiratory failure in some patients. This has not altered the course of respiratory failure much and thus is not used frequently.

All health professionals, especially those working with respiratory care patients, should be aware of the incidence and clinical symptoms of respiratory failure.

DEFINITION

Respiratory failure, or insufficiency, occurs when the respiratory system is unable to maintain adequate oxygenation for metabolism, or to eliminate adequate carbon dioxide as a waste product.

As a result tissues are not supplied with adequate oxygen, and alveolar ventilation is not in normal ranges. Clinically this is a pH < 7.30, Pa_{O_2} < 50 mm Hg with or without Pa_{CO_2} > 50 mm Hg along with symptomatic abnormalities. This may require the institution of mechanical ventilation. In severe respiratory failure, the patient may exhibit progressive hypoxemia, hypercarbia, acidemia, and cardiac arrest. Dysfunction in other organ systems concomitantly is also common.

ETIOLOGY

No one factor is responsible for the cause of respiratory failure and the pathologic and physiologic changes produced. Table 26–1 lists some of these factors. When respiratory failure develops as a result of pulmonary disease or injury or with multisystem illness, the mortality rate is high.

Acute respiratory failure may frequently develop in patients who are hypovolemic or in septic shock. Sepsis is very important as an etiologic factor in acute respiratory failure, whose main manifestation may be hypoxemia. As a result of this prolonged ischemia, there is a release of histamine and serotonin and an increase in ADP levels. The effect is an increase in pulmonary capillary permeability, lymphatic flow, and pulmonary extravascular water. The hypoperfusion will injure Type II alveolar cells and result in a decrease of surfactant production. Patients who have acute respiratory failure have low pulmonary capillary wedge pressures (PCWP) and pulmonary edema. The pulmonary capillary injury appears to be primary in acute respiratory failure. Table 26–2 lists some of the disease states that lead to the development of respiratory failure.

TABLE 26–1.
Factors Promoting Respiratory Failure

Preexisting lung disease
Smoking history
Obesity—restriction to breathing
Age—lung volumes decrease with age
Sex—men > women
Pain—decreases deep breathing and may lead
   to atelectasis and infection
Pain medication
Abdominal distention
Anesthesia—decreases ciliary motion and pattern
   of ventilation
Respiratory depressant medications

TABLE 26–2.

Disease Entities Leading to Respiratory Failure

I. Problems in Ventilation
  A. Obstructive defects
    1. Cystic fibrosis, chronic bronchitis, asthma, emphysema
  B. Restrictive defects
    1. Decreased lung expansion—effusion, fibrosis
    2. Decreased thoracic expansion—rib fracture, kyphoscoliosis
    3. Decreased diaphragmatic movement—ascites, abdominal surgery
  C. Neuromuscular defects
    1. Acute—anesthetic agents that block neuromusculature
    2. Chronic—Muscular dystrophy, multiple sclerosis, tetanus, toxic
       agent, Guillain-Barré syndrome, ALS, myasthenia gravis,
       poliomyelitis, cervical spinal cord injury
  D. Central Ventilatory Drive Depression
    1. Narcotics, anesthetics, high flow oxygen therapy uncontrolled,
       drug overdose, stroke, brain trauma, genetic insensitivity to
       elevated Pa_{CO_2} or low Pa_{CO_2}, obesity-related hypoventilation
       (Pickwickian syndrome)
II. Problems With Diffusion and Gas Exchange
  A. Pulmonary fibrosis
  B. Pulmonary edema
  C. Adult respiratory distress syndrome (ARDS)
  D. Obliterative pulmonary vascular diseases
  E. Anatomic loss of functioning lung tissue
  F. Carbon monoxide inhalation
III. Ventilation—Perfusion Abnormalities and Venous Admixture
  A. Upper airway obstruction—tumor, foreign body

ARDS, adult respiratory distress syndrome, is a form of acute respiratory failure as a result of injury to the pulmonary parenchyma (air spaces and pulmonary interstitum). Patients may exhibit normal or low Pa_{CO_2}, have decrease in lung compliance, widespread infiltrates, and rapid deep respirations greater than 40 per minute. Hypoxemia is a result of blood shunting. If treatment is delayed, the hypoxemia worsens and is uncontrollable by FI_{O_2} 1.0. PEEP is often used to increase the functional residual capacity and shunt of blood with resulting improvement in arterial oxygen tension.

Chronic obstructive pulmonary disease, an intrinsic disease, is the most frequent cause of respiratory failure. Others in this category are severe pneumonia, interstitial lung disease, drowning, and toxic substance inhalation. In all of these cases, the lung architecture prevents normal oxygen transport while the chest wall ventilatory drive remains normal. The amount of renal bicarbonate retention will tell if it is of acute or chronic etiology.

Respiratory muscle fatigue plays a role in the development of respiratory failure. There is an increased work of breathing with airway obstruction. Impaired oxygenation and nutrient supply of respiratory muscles leads to dyspnea and respiratory failure associated with pulmonary edema and congestive heart failure.

Sleep disorders may lead to respiratory failure. Sleep apnea syndrome's clinical feature is daytime sleepiness. The symptoms are insidious on onset. Pickwickian syndrome is the syndrome of obesity, cyanosis, and daytime somnolence. These patients exhibit isolated, brief apneic periods at night that increases with age. They rarely exceed 25 and are usually fewer than 10 per night. Systemic and pulmonary arterial hypertension develop with the apneic periods. Sinus bradycardia is also evident. All findings return to normal with respiration. The closing volume is diminished and when lying down is larger than the FRC. Thus, many alveoli close and the patient develops a ventilation-perfusion (V/Q) mismatch. Arterial hypoxemia and hypercapnia develop, and become more severe during the apneic periods.

CLINICAL MANIFESTATIONS

Clinical manifestations are exhibited in a variety of ways in respiratory failure. Table 26–3 shows some of these manifestations. These may occur in conjunction with those of any underlying disease as well. Four major manifestations are hypoxia, hypercapnia, hypotension, and dyspnea. If hypoxia is severe, it may be evident as cyanosis. Tissue hypoxia may result in confusion and restlessness. Hypotension and arrhythmias present with myocardial hypoxia. In order to compensate for this, cardiac output will increase. This results in tachycardia and vasoconstriction. This is evident in an elevated blood pressure. Hypercapnia, an elevated Pa_{CO_2}, will cause general vasodilatation. This may eventually cause cardiovascular failure. Muscle twitching may be evident if the $Pa_{CO_2} > 80$ mm Hg. The third manifestation of hypotension is a result of the previous two manifestations. Hypotension may have an adverse effect on urinary output. Dyspnea, the subjective feeling of shortness of breath, is caused by an increase in the work of breathing and a decrease in functional residual capacity (FRC).

Elderly

As one ages, there are many changes that occur in the pulmonary system. As a result, it may be difficult to differentiate between age-related

TABLE 26–3.
Clinical Manifestations of Respiratory
Failure

Confusion
Restlessness
Tachycardia
Diaphoresis
Headache
Central cyanosis
Hypotension
Tremors, weakness
Poor chest expansion
Depressed respiration
Miosis
Unconsciousness
Hypoxia
Hypercaporia
Dyspnea and cough
Malaise
Difficulty with sleep
Palpitation, arrhythmias
Ascites, edema
Personality change

changes and those of disease. Some of the pulmonary changes related to age are: (1) decrease in PaO_2, (2) decrease in exercise capacity, (3) decrease in vital capacity by age 70 to 75% of that at age 20, (4) decrease in diffusing capacity, (5) decrease in ventilatory response to hypoxia and hypercapnia, (6) decrease in FEV and FEV/VC, (7) prone to infection, (8) ventilation—perfusion mismatching, and (9) deterioration of mucociliary clearance

The elderly are also very susceptible to dehydration, problems with fluid and electrolytes, aspiration, pulmonary emboli, and cardiac arrhythmias. As a result, their clinical manifestations may be less obvious. Clinical signs may include confusion, tachycardia, and restlessness (may often be interpreted as "sundowning" or senility), changes in behavior, mental status, or vital signs. It is extremely important to be judicious in the use of respiratory depressant medication and to supply adequate nutrition.

PATHOPHYSIOLOGY

Gas pressure within the alveoli is formed by the partial pressures of nitrogen (N), oxygen (O_2), carbon dioxide (CO_2) and water (H_2O) vapor. Nitrogen and water vapor are constant, with the oxygen and carbon dioxide varying inversely. Of these, carbon dioxide is highly soluble in liquid and freely diffusible, and oxygen is less soluble and diffusible. As a result, in normal lung, the arterial tension of oxygen is about 10–20 mm Hg less than alveolar tension. The tension of carbon dioxide in alveolar and arterial samples is nearly equal. A main and important cause of high levels of Pa_{CO_2} is alveolar hypoventilation. This may occur in COPD, disorders of the chest wall, neuromuscular deficits, and abnormalities of central ventilatory drive. As the Pco_2 rises, Po_2 will fall unless supplemental oxygen is supplied.

In an abnormal lung, the alveolar-arterial gradient of oxygen may be larger. This is especially true in the presence of COPD. The reasons for an increased gradient and resultant hypoxemia are: (1) increased shunting where blood flow is normal, but there is decreased alveolar ventilation; (2) ventilation-perfusion mismatch (V/Q); (3) impaired diffusion where there is an increased alveolar-capillary distance or presence of interstitial disease; (4) increase in dead space; (5) increased airway resistance resulting in increased work of breathing (asthma, fibrosis, emphysema, pneumonia); and (6) decreased oxygen transport in the blood.

Abnormalities of the central ventilatory drive mechanism occur when chemoreceptor input is inappropriate. PaO_2 sensors are in the carotid body, and Pa_{CO_2} sensors are in the carotid body and brain stem. Normally, a rise in Pa_{CO_2} or drop in PaO_2 would stimulate ventilation. An abnormal response may produce hypoventilation with an increased Pa_{CO_2}. Consequently, the pulmonary artery pressure is increased by constriction of the pulmonary arterioles. If this becomes chronic, right ventricular failure (cor pulmonale) will develop.

A decrease in functional residual capacity and collapse of alveoli contribute to a reduction in lung compliance or increased elastic resistance to lung expansion. The FRC is decreased in patients with severe respiratory failure. If the closing volume is greater than FRC, the number of poorly ventilated alveoli increase and produce atelectasis. The result would be an increase in shunting secondary to normal blood flow, bypassing nonventilated alveoli.

Patients in severe respiratory failure have an increased dead space to tidal volume ratio (VD/VT) which may be precipitated by hypovolemia. Hypercapnia and acidemia may be avoided by increasing ventilation twofold. Most spontaneous breathing patients with severe respiratory failure are unable to achieve this. The increased VD/VT is a result of hypovolemia and reduced cardiac output (Q). Infusion of volume may help to improve the cardiac output and lower the dead space/tidal volume fraction in patients whose hypercapnia resulted from the two factors above.

Acute respiratory failure patients may have an increased CO_2 production secondary to hyperalimentation. This may result in a greater energy expenditure to breathe, and difficulty in weaning.

DIAGNOSIS

The diagnosis of respiratory failure is confirmed through laboratory study of arterial blood gases (ABGs) taken via an arterial puncture. These should be measured immediately if respiratory failure is suspected.

Normal oxygen transport depends on several factors. These include the fraction of inspired oxygen (FI_{O_2}), alveolar ventilation (V_A), the diffusion of gases from alveoli and capillary blood, hemoglobin content, cardiac output (Q), and the relationship of ventilation to pulmonary blood flow distribution. To obtain adequate arterial blood gases, arterial oxygen tension and content, and oxygen transport (cardiac output) to tissues must be sufficient.

Arterial blood gases are measured by analyzing an adequate amount of arterial blood. The arterial blood gas measures partial pressure of oxygen, carbon dioxide, and the pH. Bicarbonate level (HCO_{-3}) is calculated using the values of the other factors. PaO_2 is the measurement of dissolved oxygen in arterial blood. This is related to the oxygen content and oxygen saturation of hemoglobin. The PaO_2 may be altered due to severe pulmonary disease, shunts, hypoventilation and ventilation—perfusion abnormalities. Hypoxemia is a decrease in level of oxygen partial pressure arterial blood. Infants and the elderly (over 60 years old) have different levels of PaO_2. Hypoxemia is one of the earliest manifestations of respiratory failure. An elevated Pa_{CO_2} may not occur until respiratory failure has progressed. Chronic respiratory failure patients retain bicarbonate ions in their kidneys to offset the elevated carbon dioxide level. This occurs in order to return the pH to a normal value.

Pa_{CO_2} refers to the partial pressure exerted by dissolved CO_2 gas in the blood. This level is a measure of the adequacy of alveolar ventilation. The P_{CO_2} is important in determining whether there is normal ventilation, hypoventilation or hyperventilation. Hypoventilation is indicative of an elevated P_{CO_2} or hypercapnia. Hyperventilation would be indicated by a low P_{CO_2} level.

The pH level is the only way to determine if the body is too acidic or too alkaline. A low pH—below 7.35—indicates an acid state. A high pH—above 7.45—indicates an alkaline state. It is a measurement of free hydrogen ion (H+) concentration in arterial blood. If the pH is not normal, the kidneys may or may not retain bicarbonate ions to return it to a normal level. This is dependent on the level of PCO_2. Metabolic imbalances (i.e., diabetes acidosis) will also affect the pH level.

Bicarbonate (HCO_3^-) ions are influenced only by metabolic processes, and regulated by the kidneys. Blood gas values evident in normals and in respiratory failure are shown in Table 26–4.

Other diagnostic measures include radiography, measurement of compliance (tidal volume/peak airway pressure, negative inspiratory pressure (NIF) if on mechanical ventilation), reserved ventilatory effort necessary for deep breathing and coughing, and the arterial-alveolar oxygen difference (Aa_{DO_2}). The Aa_{DO_2} should be measured after 15 to 20 minutes of breathing 100% (FI_{O_2} 1.0) oxygen. Water vapor pressure and CO_2 tension are subtracted to obtain the oxygen difference. A difference greater than 350 mm Hg is indicative of respiratory failure.

The most useful criteria in diagnosing respiratory failure are PaO_2, Pa_{CO_2}, pH, and vital capacity (VC). The lower limit for vital capacity in

TABLE 26–4.

Blood Gas Values

	NORMAL	RESPIRATORY FAILURE
pH	7.35–7.45	<7.30
Pa_{CO_2}	35–45 mm Hg (or torr)	>55 mm Hg
PaO_2	80 mm Hg (or torr)	< 55–60 mm Hg
(on room air)		(without supplemental O_2)
HCO_3^-	22–28 mEq/L	

TABLE 26–5.

Criteria for Diagnosis of Respiratory Failure

PaO_2 (room air)	<60 torr
Pa_{CO_2}	>60 torr
pH	<7.25–7.30
VC	<10 ml/kg
Inspiratory force	< −20 cm H_2O
Vd/Vt (dead space/tidal volume)	>.60
FRC (% of predicted value)	<60
Aa_{DO_2} 1.0	>350 mm Hg
Resting minute volume	>10 L/min
Qs/Qt	>15%–20% (shunt)

order to maintain adequate blood-gas exchange is 10 ml/kg. Most patients require a vital capacity of about 15 ml/kg (three times normal tidal volume) to prevent atelectasis and assist with coughing. It is important in measuring ABGs to record the F_{IO_2}, tidal volume, and respiratory rate to acquire an accurate diagnosis. Table 26–5 lists the criteria necessary to diagnose respiratory failure.

COMPLICATIONS

There are many complications that may occur as a result of respiratory failure and its treatment. Some of these complications are listed in Table 26–6.

NUTRITION

Enteral hyperalimentation is more physiologic for the mechanically ventilated patient. The intubated patient should begin nutritional intake within 24 hours. Starvation and muscle wasting are results of lack of nutritional support. Liquid nourishment may be provided using the nasogastric tube. For long-term use, a smaller pediatric feeding tube is preferred to avoid otitis, increased risk of aspiration, and sinusitis. It is best to avoid nasogastric and nasotracheal use together. In this situa-

TABLE 26–6.
Complications of Respiratory
Failure

Pulmonary
Oxygen toxicity
Infection
Injury
Pneumothorax
Neurologic
Gastrointestinal
Electrolyte and fluid abnormalities
Cardiovascular
Congestive heart failure
Hypotension
Hypertension
Cardiac arrest
Low cardiac output
Arrhythmias
Hepatic and renal

tion, the risk of necrosis of the nasal septum is high. Another source of nourishment is intravenous hyperalimentation.

Nutritional support has become sophisticated and complex. The dietician is a welcome and necessary member of the team caring for the patient on a ventilator.

TREATMENT

There are two priorities in the treatment of acute respiratory failure, which could cause a medical emergency if overlooked. First, it is necessary to provide adequate oxygenation until endotracheal intubation is performed. Second is the reversal of the respiratory acidosis. An increase in alveolar ventilation should correct the CO_2 retention. Initial therapy should provide for an adequate airway, supplemental oxygen and assisted ventilation as required to correct the Pa_{CO_2} and any acid-base abnormality. The most important part of treatment depends on identifying the etiology. If an infection is present that should be treated, chest physical therapy is indicated to remove any obstructing secretions. Oxygen therapy may be indicated to treat hypoxemia or decrease myocardial work due to increased stress on the cardiovascular system secondary to the infection. Medications may be administered as counter-agents to ingested drugs or toxins. In summary, the goal in management of respiratory failure is the correction of the defect in oxygen delivery to tissues, and, the patient's inability to remove CO_2 from the blood.

Endotracheal intubation and mechanical ventilation should be initiated based on clinical evaluation and blood gas abnormalities. If the etiology is massive pneumonia or drug overdose, mechanical ventilation should be initiated immediately. Respiratory failure secondary to COPD is treated first with low flow oxygen therapy, chest physical therapy, bronchodilators, mechanical ventilation as dictated by arterial blood gases, and antibiotics, if necessary.

Oxygen is a drug and can produce toxic effects. All efforts should be made to use an Fi_{O_2} of .70 as an upper limit. ABGs should be taken a half-hour after initiation of ventilation to measure Po_2 and ventilatory effects. The Fi_{O_2} is adjusted according to ABG results.

Endotracheal Tube (ETT)

Mechanical ventilation and the use of an endotracheal tube should be performed in an adequately staffed ICU, with labs available for ABG analysis and physicians skilled in critical care. The position of the endotracheal tube should be checked by radiography, and the end of the tube placed 3–4 cm above the carina. A high compliance cuff should be used to avoid ischemic changes to the cartilaginous rings. The largest diameter tube possible is used to allow for suctioning. A tracheostomy may be necessary for prolonged ventilation and less pressure in the cuff to obtain a sealed airway to deliver ventilation.

General indications for endotracheal intubation and ventilation in the presence of acute respiratory failure are: (1) unconsciousness, inability to protect airway; (2) copious secretions not cleared by coughing (suctioning); and (3) severe hypoxemia or respiratory acidosis not respondent to lesser measures (provide for mechanical ventilation).

Mechanical Ventilation

Mechanical ventilation is the support or control of external respiration. Intermittent positive pressure to the airways requires access via a cuffed endotracheal or tracheostomy tube. Courrand and coworkers were the first to report that intermittent positive pressure breathing in normal subjects decreased cardiac output in direct relation to mean airway pressure elevation. The Type III curve (mean airway pressure 5.7 mm Hg) does not decrease cardiac output and has been the basis for design of mechanical ventilation since 1948.

Intermittent Negative Pressure

The main principle employed here is if the chest wall surface is exposed to a subatmospheric pressure during which time the nose and mouth remain at atmospheric pressure, air will enter the lungs as a result of the pressure gradient that develops. The first type is the tank respirator or iron lung. This type of respirator was in widespread use around 1960, and with poliomyelitis. While the patient lies horizontally in the metal tank, his head projects through a collar. Subatmospheric pressure is cyclically produced within the tank to affect inspiration. Respirations occur without a tracheostomy or endotracheal tube. The disadvantage to the tank is lack of access to the patient for monitoring and care of other body systems. The use today generally is in a patient with thoracic bellow defect who requires ventilation only with sleep. However, there are still postpolio patients who prefer this means of ventilation.

A second type of negative pressure ventilator is the shell or cuirass that has a rubber gasket on the free edge which is fitted to the anterior aspect of the chest. The shell is then connected with a large bore tube to a device that produces intermittent negative pressure, much the same as the tank. This may be used in sitting or in the recumbent position, and allows greater accessibility of the patient. Some irritation to skin surfaces may be evident from the ventilator edge. Leaks develop easily and cause inadequate ventilation. Again, this type of respirator is used in patients with thoracic bellow defect.

Intermittent Positive Pressure

Two classes of ventilators exist in this category. The pressure-cycled ventilator maintains an inspiratory flow until a preset pressure is reached regardless of the volume delivered. It is less expensive than the volume-cycled ventilator, but the volume delivered may diminish if obstruction is present in the tubing or bronchial tree or if there is a decrease in pulmonary compliance.

Volume-cycled ventilation delivers a preset volume. It is limited only by preset airway pressures. The same tidal volume is delivered regardless of peak inspiratory pressure. This system is safer and more versatile. Volume ventilation is preferred in long-term ventilation ($>$ 3 hours) to provide stable Pa_{CO_2} and acid-base balance.

Both systems can be set so the patient initiates ventilation by producing negative airway pressure. This is referred to as the assist mode. Either system may be set to deliver a definite number of respirations per minute, i.e., control mode. Supplemental oxygen is given in concentrations (FI_{O_2}) necessary for maintenance of tissue oxygenation (PaO_2 60–80). All gases should be heated and humdified. An alarm system should be provided on all ventilators to signal any change in pressure in the inspiratory line and if the exhaled tidal volume is low. The delivered volume should be monitored in either system and be maintained at 10–15 ml/kg body weight in patients of normal weight. Respiratory frequency should be such to maintain respiratory acid-base balance (approximately 8–12 breaths per minute). The ventilatory rate should yield the patients normal arterial CO_2 tension.

Intermittent mandatory ventilation (IMV) and positive end-expiratory pressure (PEEP) may be provided on both systems. IMV allows for spontaneous respiratory muscle activity. This also allows for the inspired gas to be preferentially distributed to dependent lung regions. In positive pressure ventilation, distribution of gas favors nondependent regions. The use of IMV allows for a reduced need of sedatives, muscle relaxants, etc.

PEEP is used to open alveoli during expiration and to increase the functional residual capacity. This will aid to decrease the shunt and permit a lower FI_{O_2} to be employed.

Intermittent Expiratory Positive Pressure to the Abdomen

The rocking bed and inflatable abdominal belt (pneumobelt) are the two devices that produce a positive expiratory pressure. In using the rocking bed, the patient has no mobility. It is a motorized bed that alternately produces a controllable degree of head and foot down tilt. Expiration is therefore assisted by the effects of gravity on the abdomen when the head of the bed is down.

The inflatable abdominal belt produces expiration by an increase in intra-abdominal pressure. Inspiration is passive. This may be used with the patient sitting.

Indications

Mechanical ventilation is indicated in respiratory failure as evidenced by: (1) VC< 10 ml/kg; (2) inspiratory force <-20 cm H_2O; (3) minute volume >10 L/min; (4) Aa_{DO_2} 1.0 >350 mm Hg; (5) Qs/Qt > 15%–20% (shunt); (6) Vd/Vt >0.6 (dead space/tidal volume). Arterial blood gases, vital signs, cardiac rhythm, and end organ function should be monitored at all times.

Complications

Some of the complications of mechanical ventilation are: (1) pneumothorax, (2) excessive oxygen and toxicity, (3) stress ulcer, (4) renal complications, (5) infection, (6) air trapping, airway obstruction, (7) starvation, (8) ETT complications—tracheal stenosis, (9) ileus, (10) endobronchial intubation, and (11) inability to wean. A primary complication is nosocomial pneumonia as a result of high-dose antibiotics in the ICU and the patient's condition.

Physiological Effects

Mechanical ventilation may cause an increase in intrathoracic pressure, decreased venous return, intracranial pressure, atelectasis, increased secretions, and alterations in renal blood flow.

Weaning

The main indication for weaning from the ventilator is correction of the underlying etiology, along with increased mechanical and oxygenation capabilities evidenced by: (1) VC >10 ml/kg, (2) IF >-20 cm H_2O, (3) MV < 10 L/min, (4) Aa_{DO_2} 1.0 < 300 mm Hg, (5) Qs/Qt <

10%–15%, (6) Vd/Vt < 0.6, (7) PaO_2 > 60 with F_{IO_2} .4 or less, (8) cardiovascular stability.

Work of breathing is a result of minute ventilation and mechanical characteristics of the chest wall and lung. Minute ventilation is determined by the magnitude of CO_2 production and efficiency of CO_2 elimination. Respiratory work capacity is estimated by clinical observations of strength, endurance, mental status, motivation, reaction to stress, and respiratory muscle coordination. A decrease in FRC with atelectasis is common in mechanical ventilation. During weaning there may be a further reduction.

Before extubation occurs, the patient should be allowed to breathe spontaneously through the endotracheal tube. F_{IO_2} should be the same or slightly more than that with ventilation. Should the Pa_{CO_2} increase or other signs of respiratory failure appear, ventilation should be started again.

Weaning should progress in four stages: (1) from PEEP, (2) from artificial ventilation, (3) from endotracheal tube, (4) from supplementary inspired oxygen. This should take one of two forms. One is abrupt weaning from controlled ventilation to spontaneous breathing via a "T" piece. This is frequently applicable in the recovery room. The second form is gradual reduction of the ventilatory rate for patients provided with intermittent mandatory ventilation. This allows for a more gradual transition. It is often helpful in patients on long-term mechanical ventilation.

Careful note of inspiratory muscle fatigue should be taken in weaning. The respiratory muscle energy requirement increases, and the body may be unable to supply the necessary oxygen and nutrients. As a result, the source of energy may decrease. The patient now either decreases ventilation and becomes hypercapnic or maintains ventilation until the muscles fatigue. A vital capacity equal to three times the tidal volume must be maintained to prevent recurrence of respiratory failure.

PREVENTION

There are several things to watch and correct in order to prevent the development of respiratory failure. In a patient with normal lungs, the oxygen-carrying capacity may be reduced secondary to anemia. The correction of electrolyte and acid-based balance is important. To provide for proper deep breathing and coughing, the patient must maintain an adequate ventilatory effort reserve.

Two important factors in all patients are the presence of abdominal bandages or a cast, and pain. The patient with abnormal lungs may have an elevated CO_2 secondary to retention. Here the work of breathing may be high, and the patient is unable to increase his ventilation in relation to stress. Again the hemoglobin content must be maintained secondary to chronic hypoxemia.

If there is evidence of large amounts of secretions, chest physical therapy, humidification, and possibly bronchodilators should be initiated. In an unconscious patient, careful airway care should be maintained. ABGs should be measured to determine the need for supplemental oxygen or ventilation. The cough reflex may be depressed and the patient prone to an increase in secretions. Aggressive suctioning is indicated.

A surgical patient may benefit from preoperative pulmonary function tests (to determine baseline for patient), and instruction in respiratory care. Postoperatively, chest physical therapy, humidity, position change, and mobilization as soon as possible will help prevent any respiratory problems. If possible, this care should begin immediately postoperatively in the recovery room.

Physical Therapy Role

The role of the physical therapist in treatment of the respiratory failure patient is twofold. First and foremost is the respiratory care of the patient. This should be initiated after mechanical ventilation to prevent atelectasis, infection, and accumulation of secretions. Position change should be encouraged every 1–2 hours. This will also occur with the respiratory treatment, and allows visualization of body parts. Manual techniques should be employed as the therapist sees fit after her evaluation. Because the ventilator delivers constant volume or pressure, the patient is prone to the development of atelectasis. Manual hyperinflations via an ambu bag will help to prevent this, and aid in mobilizing secretions. Aspiration of secretions by *sterile* technique should be done every two hours and whenever necessary. Douglas et al. observed improvement in arterial Po_2 when the prone position was used in patients. If the patient is alert, he should be encouraged to perform relaxation and breathing exercises. If the patient is on mechanical ventilation but strong enough, he may get out of bed or ambulate with a portable oxygen tank and ambu bag.

The second area of physical therapy intervention is in exercise. Passive, active, or active-assistive exercises should be performed to prevent contractures, prevent muscle wasting and increase circulation (Fig 26–1). Resistive exercises should be avoided because of the tendency to

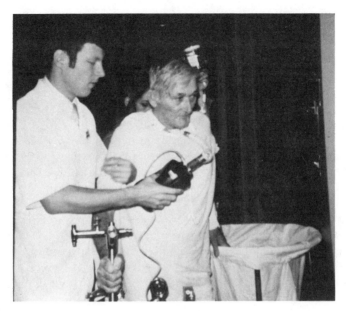

FIG 26–1.
Ambulation of a ventilator patient using self-inflating bag with oxygen. (Note: A laundry cart is used as an improvised support walker.)

perform a Valsalva maneuver which would impede ventilation and blood flow to the heart.

All patients should be encouraged to perform as many activities independently as possible—from rolling, to transferring, to activities of daily living and ambulation. The patient is a "person." Talk *to* the patient, not around him. Ask simple "yes or no" questions or provide a paper and pen or board to write on. The patients have an increased stress and anxiety level, and feel loss of control over their bodies and others. Psychological support is a very important element of treatment. The therapist provides positive impact and facilitates the patient's ability to participate in his progress and recovery.

CHRONIC RESPIRATORY FAILURE

COPD is the main cause of chronic respiratory failure. The work of breathing may be a significant component of total body metabolism because of an inadequate respiratory system. Other causes, to a lesser degree, include neuromuscular disease, dysfunction of central ventilatory drive related to obesity, and interstitial lung disease.

Chronic respiratory failure is defined as alterations of arterial blood gases in respiratory failure existing in a stable clinical state for more than 30 days. The initial response may be (1) decrease in ventilation relative to metabolic demand (i.e., higher Pa_{CO_2}, lower PaO_2), or (2) to shed lean body mass. Both result in a decreased work of breathing. The "blue bloater" tends to compensate by decreasing ventilation, and the "pink puffer" compensates by the latter method. Both compensatory responses may lead to other problems.

The "blue bloater" hypoventilates and exhibits increased hypoxemia and respiratory acidosis. This leads to an increase in pulmonary hypertension and increased onset of cor pulmonale. The cachectic appearance of the "pink puffer" may lead to questioning the presence of a neoplasm.

The use of supplemental oxygen may be hazardous in a patient with an elevated Pa_{CO_2} and chronic respiratory failure. High concentrations of oxygen supplementation may suppress the chemoreceptors to breath and knock out the patient's hypoxemic drive. Nasal oxygen flow of 3 L/min or less may be sufficient to raise the PaO_2 without danger to the patient.

Ventilation in a chronic respiratory failure patient should not be to correct an elevated Pa_{CO_2} if the pH is normal. Renal compensation has been established already, and a rapid decrease in Pa_{CO_2} could lead to severe metabolic alkalosis with hypotension, seizures, and arrhythmias. Here the patient should be ventilated to his previous Pa_{CO_2} for which he has compensated the pH with retention of bicarbonate ions.

A patient with cor pulmonale and chronic respiratory failure can benefit from the continuous use of low-flow (1–2 L/min) nasal oxygen. This may be sufficient to alleviate the pulmonary artery hypertension, correct or prevent congestive right heart failure, and enable the patient to return to a more functional life.

REFERENCES

Periodicals

Bone RC: Treatment of respiratory failure due to advanced chronic obstructive lung disease. *Arch Intern Med* 1980; 140(8):1018–21.

Braun NM, Rochester DF: Muscular weakness and respiratory failure. *Am Rev Respir Dis* 1979; 119(2 Pt 2):123–125.

Brewis RA: Diseases of the respiratory system: Respiratory failure. *Br Med J* 1978; 1(6117):898–900.

Bushnell LS: Management of acute respiratory failure. *Cardiopulmonary Q* 1982; 2:198.

Douglas WW, Kai R, Beynen FM, et al: Improved oxygenation in patients with acute respiratory failure: The prone position. *Am Rev Resp Dis* 1977; 115:559–566.

Hammond GL: Acute respiratory failure. *Surg Clin North Am* 1980; 60(5):1131–1149.

Pontopiidan H, Wilson R, Rie M et al: Respiratory intensive care. *Anesthesiology* 1977; 47:96–116.

Wilson R: The diagnosis and treatment of acute respiratory failure in sepsis. *Heart Lung* 1976; 5:614–620.

Books

Bendixen HH, Egbert LD, Hedley-Whyte J, et al: *Respiratory Care.* St Louis, CV Mosby Co, 1965.

Cherniak R, Cherniak L, Naimark A: *Respiration in Health and Disease,* ed 2. Philadelphia, WB Saunders Co, 1972.

Crews ER, Lapuerto L: *A Manual of Respiratory Failure.* Springfield, Illinois, Charles C Thomas, Publisher, 1972.

Downie PA (ed): *Cash's Textbook of Chest, Heart, and Vascular Disorders for Physiotherapists,* ed 3. Philadelphia, JB Lippincott Co, 1982.

Mitchell RS, Petty TL (eds): *Synopsis of Clinical Pulmonary Disease,* ed 3. St Louis, CV Mosby Co, 1982.

Petty TL: *Intensive and Rehabilitative Respiratory Care,* ed 3. Philadelphia, Lea and Febiger, 1982.

Petty T: *Intensive and Rehabilitative Respiratory Care,* ed 2. Philadelphia, Lea & Febiger, 1974.

Shapiro B, Harrison R, Trout C: *Clinical Application of Respiratory Therapy.* Chicago, Year Book Medical Publishers, 1975.

Shapiro B, Harrison R, Walton J: *Clinical Application of Blood Gases,* ed 2. Chicago, Year Book Medical Publishers, 1977.

Snider GL: *Clinical Pulmonary Medicine.* Boston, Little, Brown & Co, 1981.

Manuals

Patterson CD: Decisions to be Made When Starting Mechanical Ventilation and Weaning from Mechanical Ventilation, Third Annual Critical Care Medicine Course, February 29–March 29, 1976 (Department of Medicine, University of Oklahoma, Oklahoma Heart Assoc, Oklahoma Lung Assoc).

Rogers R, Juers J: Physiologic considerations in the treatment of acute respiratory failure. Basic Respiratory Diseases, 1975.

27

The Neonate and Child

Linda D. Crane, M.M.Sc., P.T.

The application of chest physical therapy to infants and children requires a special understanding of cardiorespiratory, anatomy, physiology, and pathology differences as compared to adults. Infants and children are not merely "miniature adults" but represent a unique population of patients. Chest physical therapy management of this population is both challenging and rewarding. Few areas of health care delivery require creative adaptation and problem solving to the extent that pediatrics does (Fig 27–1).

This chapter reviews the unique cardiorespiratory problems of the neonate and child and discusses chest physical therapy management of this age group. Given the diversity between the premature infant and adolescent and the fact that older children and adolescents can be managed similar to adults (in terms of techniques, not psychosocially), this chapter limits discussion primarily to the neonate and young child.

DIFFERENCES IN STRUCTURE AND FUNCTION

Term Neonate

The full-term neonate is delivered at 38 to 42 weeks gestation. Although the infant's gestational age may be normal, he may be predisposed to respiratory difficulties due to several anatomic and physiologic factors. The factors briefly reviewed below do not normally present problems for a term infant. However, if an infant develops an infection or has pulmonary dysfunction of any etiology, these factors may contribute to respiratory distress and respiratory failure in this age group.

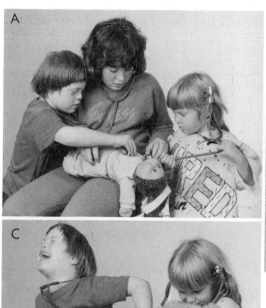
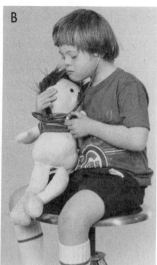
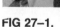

FIG 27–1.
A, B, C, few areas of health care delivery require creative adaptation and problem solving
to the extent that pediatrics does.

Structural differences lead to functional differences. The first difference is airway diameter. An infant's airways are narrower from the nares to the terminal bronchioles. A smaller diameter airway has more resistance to air flow and is more easily obstructed by mucus, edema, and foreign objects.

The second difference is the circular and horizontal position of the lower ribs and concomitant horizontal angle of insertion of the diaphram on the ribs. This, along with the more cartilaginous nature of the rib cage, results in less efficient chest wall mechanics and more distortion of the chest wall leading to an increased work of breathing.

The high laryngeal position of a neonate has long been assumed to result in obligatory nasal breathing (except during crying) for the first 2–3 months of life. Recent literature challenges this theory and has demonstrated initiation of mouth breathing in infants during nasal occlusion.

Structural differences on a submicroscopic level also contribute to altered physiology. First, the diaphragm of a newborn has less Type 1 (high oxidative) muscle fibers (25% compared to 50% in adult). The difference predisposes an infant to earlier diaphragmatic fatigue when stressed. A normal newborn also has less collateral ventilatory channels than an adult. The number of channels are especially reduced in the right middle and upper lobes of neonates, possibly contributing to the relatively higher incidence of atelectasis in these lobes.

In summary, normal term infants have less "functional reserve" to protect them from respiratory compromise. These alterations are even more pronounced and create more problems in the premature infants.

Premature Infant

The infant delivered before 38 weeks gestation is premature and significantly compromised in terms of respiratory structure and function. All of the structural and functional differences previously discussed apply to the premature infant plus several factors unique to the "premie" (Table 27–1).

TABLE 27–1.

Factors Contributing to Pulmonary Dysfunction in the Premature Infant*

ANATOMIC	PHYSIOLOGICAL
Capillary beds not well developed before 26 weeks gestation	Increased pulmonary vascular resistance leading to right-to-left shunting
Type II alveolar cells and surfactant production not mature until 35 weeks gestation; elastic properties of lung not well developed; lung "space" decreased by relative size of the heart and abdominal distention	Decreased lung compliance
Type I, high-oxidative fibers compose only 10% to 20% of diaphragm muscle	Diaphragmatic fatigue: respiratory failure
Highly vascular subependymal germinal matrix not resorbed until 35 weeks gestation, increasing the vulnerability of the infant to hemorrhage	Decreased or absent cough and gag reflexes; apnea
Lack of fatty insulation and high surface area to body-weight ratio	Hypothermia and increased oxygen consumption

*From Irwin S, Tecklin JS (eds): *Cardiopulmonary Physical Therapy*. St. Louis, CV Mosby, 1985. Used by permission.

Child

As the infant grows and develops, most structural and functional disadvantages disappear. One exception is the horizontal position of the rib cage which results in less efficient chest wall motions. This persists until approximately 7 years of age. Another residual structural difference is enlarged lymphatic tissue (especially adenoids), which is a potential cause of upper airway obstruction in infants and children.

One of the disadvantages of developing beyond infancy is loss of passively acquired immunity against disease. Dr. William Waring creatively coined this characteristic of children's pulmonary disease—"immunologic innocence." Another aspect of growth and development that can be protective for an infant and younger child is alveolar multiplication. Alveolar surface area of a full-term infant is approximately 1/20 that of an adult. Alveoli multiply rapidly in the first year of life and continue until approximately 8 or 9 years of age.

COMMON DISORDERS FOR WHICH CHEST PHYSICAL THERAPY IS INDICATED

Hyaline Membrane Disease

The most common respiratory disorder in premature infants is hyaline membrane disease (HMD) or infant respiratory distress syndrome (IRDS). HMD is a direct result of prematurity as it results from lung immaturity. An inadequate level of pulmonary surfactant is the primary etiology of HMD. Surfactant enables the neonate to stabilize terminal air spaces by decreasing alveolar surface tension. The result of surfactant deficiency is alveolar collapse, complicated by a relatively smaller alveolar size in premature infants, right-to-left intrapulmonary shunting of pulmonary blood flow, and increasing metabolic acidosis, resulting in increased pulmonary vascular resistance. Neonates can not use their chest walls to stabilize lung volume because the rib cage is cartilaginous and very compliant.

Clinical signs of respiratory distress occur early in HMD (usually within 1–2 hours) and persist for at least 48–72 hours. The chest x-ray shows a reticulogranular appearance with air bronchograms. Respiratory failure is common in these infants, necessitating oxygen therapy and assisted ventilation.

Chest physical therapy (CPT) is commonly indicated in the management of infants with HMD. There is usually a marked increase in airway secretions in the "recovery" state of the syndrome (after approximately 2–3 days) which is exacerbated by oxygen therapy and endotracheal intubation. To improve airway clearance, bronchial drainage techniques including positioning for postural drainage, chest percussion, vibration, and airway suctioning are judiciously applied. Bronchial drainage is also appropriately continued as a prophylactic measure to prevent pneumonia and atelectasis, especially just prior to and following extubation.

Meconium Aspiration Syndrome

Meconium aspiration syndrome (MAS) is seen less commonly now with improved management. MAS is more common in postmature infants. Meconium is the content of the fetal and newborn bowel which, when passed in utero, is believed to represent fetal compromise. The aspiration of meconium occurs *during* birth with the first breaths. Several studies support the contention that MAS is largely preventable if the upper and lower airways are suctioned immediately after birth. The lower airway especially should be suctioned in babies delivered through thick, particulate ("pea soup") meconium in amniotic material.

Aspiration of meconium can result in serious and devastating pathophysiology. Mortality can be as high as 20%. Meconium obstructs peripheral airways, sometimes creating a ball-valve obstruction which leads to air trapping and ventilation-perfusion mismatch. By 24 to 48 hours, there is usually severe necrotic chemical pneumonitis.

Medical management of MAS is supportive with supplemental oxygenation and mechanical ventilation if necessary. Two common complications of MAS are tension pneumothorax and pulmonary vascular hypertension. Mortality in these babies can be as high as 50%.

Chest physical therapy is an important component of the management of infants with MAS. Bronchial drainage including positioning for postural drainage, chest percussion, vibration, and airway suctioning assist in obtaining airway clearance of residual meconium and secretions produced by the inflammatory response of the airways. CPT is especially advocated during the first eight hours of life but may be necessary for a prolonged period if the infant requires assisted ventilation.

Neonatal Pneumonia

The most common organisms producing pneumonia in neonates are Group B streptococcus and *Hemophilus influenzae*. Neonatal pneumonia mimics HMD in clinical presentation and chest x-ray findings. Compromised neonates are at high risk for developing pneumonia, although true pneumonia is relatively rare in this age group.

Chest physical therapy may or may not be helpful in managing neonatal pneumonia. Bronchial drainage techniques are indicated when secretions are mobilized in the airways, usually during the resolution stage of the disease process. Clinical signs that indicate an airway clearance problem include rales on auscultation, increased volume of secretions, and a change in color and consistency of secretions. Increased apnea and bradycardia in a neonate can also indicate an airway clearance problem.

Bronchopulmonary Dysplasia

As the mortality rates decrease in infants with HMD, the prevalence of chronic lung disease has increased (bronchopulmonary dysplasia—BPD). Although controversial, the etiology of BPD is usually linked with positive pressure ventilation and oxygen therapy. Four pathologic stages of BPD have been identified with the first stage corresponding with HMD progressing to the fourth stage which is consistent with changes seen in chronic lung disease.

Clinically, infants with BPD often present with rales, wheezing, cyanosis, hypoxemia, and an increased incidence of lower respiratory tract infections. Right-sided heart failure (cor pulmonale) is a common finding in the sequelae of this disease, especially in the first few years of life. Medical management for infants with BPD is primarily supportive. Long-term oxygen therapy is often necessary for infants who exhibit persistent severe hypoxemia.

Chest physical therapy is an important component of the management of an infant with BPD. Airway clearance problems are common due to submucosal and peribronchial smooth muscle hyperplasia, increased mucous secretions, oxygen therapy (which drys mucus and slows mucociliary transport), and frequent lower respiratory infections. Infants with BPD also often exhibit poor growth and emotional and behavioral problems. Oral avoidance is not uncommon among these babies who are frequently noxiously stimulated around the mouth and nose and do not have the opportunity to normally develop sucking and swallowing. Therapeutic intervention related to developmental delay and even, in some cases, altered joint range of motion, strength, and endurance is often indicated.

Transient Tachypnea of the Newborn

This is another neonatal problem considered in the differential diagnosis of HMD. Transient tachypnea of the newborn (TTNB) is associated with delayed clearance of amniotic fluid from the lungs, results in early presentation of respiratory distress, and is most common in full-term and postmature neonates (especially if delivered by cesarean). Chest physical therapy is occasionally indicated for infants with this problem, but TTNB is usually self-limited.

Respiratory Problems Secondary to CNS Depression

Central nervous system depression may result from perinatal complications such as asphyxia due to umbilical cord compression, placental insufficiency, or congenital defects like diaphragmatic hernia and trachial web. Infants who sustain significant asphyxia develop shock, hypoxemia, and hypoxia. These infants often have muscular flaccidity and respiratory depression with resulting poor ventilation and decreased airway clearance due to hypoventilation and decreased or absent cough reflexes.

Infants with CNS and respiratory depression are at risk for developing pulmonary atelectasis and infection. Prophylactic CPT is therefore usually indicated.

Genetically Transmitted Disorders/Cystic Fibrosis (CF)

This is a complex disorder transmitted as an autosomal recessive trait which affects the exocrine glands. CF involves almost every organ system and is characterized by increased sweat electrolyte content, chronic obstructive lung disease, and pancreatic insufficiency. Definitive diagnosis of CF includes positive family history; clinical symptoms of poor digestion, growth or recurrent pulmonary infection; and, most importantly, a positive sweat chloride test.

The chronic pulmonary disease in CF is related to increased secretion of abnormally viscous mucus, impaired mucociliary transport resulting in airway obstruction, bronchiectasis, overinflation, and infection. Radiographically, changes are most pronounced in the upper lobes, especially the right upper lobe.

The early institution of prophylactic pulmonary therapy, including chest physical therapy and the judicious use of antibiotics, provides effective measures for controlling or slowing the effects of bronchiolar and bronchial obstruction. Involvement of the patient and his parents in chronic care is particularly important. Understanding the nature of the disease and the purpose of each therapeutic measure promotes successful management of the patient.

A home program of chest physical therapy should be worked out for each individual. The frequency, duration, and appropriate positions for postural drainage must be carefully assessed according to the affected areas of the lungs. There can be no set frequency for treatments since there is no set amount of pulmonary involvement. During an exacerbation, the patient may require postural drainage 2–4 times a day. Patients with mild sputum production may require treatments only once or twice a day. However, in order to prevent the buildup of retained secretions, postural drainage must be a constant feature in the management of the patient.

Breathing exercises are an important part of the home program. Diaphragmatic breathing and basal expansion exercises should be practiced regularly. In order to prevent air trapping, the emphasis in breathing exercises must be on relaxed expiration.

Exercise involving the trunk muscles, such as sit-ups with touching an elbow to the opposite knee, and physical activities such as swimming and jogging, are also encouraged. Physical activity designed to improve exercise tolerance helps patients with CF to mobilize secretions as well as improve body image and cope with stress. Some CF patients with mild disease may be able to use regular exercise in place of bronchial drainage treatments.

The Immotile Cilia Syndrome

It is only recently that immotile cilia syndrome (ICS) has been identified and included in the differential diagnosis of infants and children with chronic recurrent pneumonia, otitis media, and sinusitis. Diagnosis of immotile cilia syndrome is made by electron microscopic (EM) study of nasal or bronchial ciliated mucosa. The older child or adult with ICS often presents with bronchiectasis. This syndrome is closely associated with Kartagener's syndrome, which presents with the triad of situs inversus, bronchiectasis, and sinusitis. Not all patients with ICS, however, have situs inversus; and if diagnosed early, bronchiectasis might not yet have developed.

The ICS is thought to be genetically transferred as an autosomal recessive trait. Incidence is unknown, but it is likely more prevalent than statistics indicate because EM studies of cilia are not routinely available.

Infants and children with ICS are prone to both upper and lower airway infection due to ciliary immotility (due to absence of dyneine arms in the ciliary microstructure). Techniques that assist in airway clearance are generally indicated for these patients. Bronchial drainage treatments including postural drainage, chest percussion, vibration, and cough are recommended once or twice daily. Positions for drainage usually emphasize lower and middle lobe segments prophylactically and should emphasize any segments that are bronchiectatic or frequent sites of recurrent infection. A regular exercise program to assist in airway clearance and general conditioning is also appropriate for patients with ICS.

Neuromuscular Disease

Pediatric neuromuscular diseases often result in hypoventilation, poor cough and chronic aspiration, and respiratory failure. Both inspiration and expiration are involved with many of these diseases as well as swallow and cough. Examples of pediatric neuromuscular diseases transmitted genetically that affect the respiratory system include muscular dystrophy, Werdnig-Hoffman's syndrome, Kugelberg-Welander disease, familia disautonomia (Riley-Day syndrome). Guillian-Barré syndrome and spinal cord injury are not genetically acquired but constitute two major forms of neuromuscular disease that can also affect pulmonary function.

Chest physical therapy for infants and children with these and other related neuromuscular diseases must be individualized based on the stage of the disease and level of impairment. Generally, bronchial drainage techniques are often indicated to assist in removal of secretions, especially in the more severely impaired child. Breathing exercise programs are also extremely appropriate and helpful in improving coordination of breathing patterns, increasing ventilation (therefore, decreasing atelectasis and improving cough), *and* decreasing the work of breathing. Patients with decreased mobility of their chest walls due to weakness or paralysis benefit from manual stretching and mobilization of the rib cage. Diaphragmatic strengthening is another important component of the CPT program of patients with neuromuscular disease, especially those with cervical and high thoracic spinal cord lesions. Diaphragmatic strengthening can be done using abdominal weights, inspiratory resistive breathing, and incentive spirometry in any patient over 4 or 5 years of age (see Chapters 9 and 10).

Bacterial Pneumonia

This is relatively uncommon in infants and children unless they are compromised and therefore more susceptible. Still, pneumonia is a significant cause of pediatric morbidity and mortality, especially in the newborn. In neonates, bacterial pneumonia can be difficult to distinguish from HMD on chest x-ray and by presenting clinical signs. Neonatal bacterial pneumonia can be acquired in utero, during delivery, or postnatally. Group B streptococcal pneumonia is of particular concern due to its association with neonatal septicemia and high mortality.

Medical management of bacterial pneumonia includes specific antibiotic therapy, supportive care to control temperature, maintenance of fluid electrolytes, and close monitoring of ventilatory status and oxygenation.

Chest physical therapy measures, although controversial regarding effectiveness in treating bacterial pneumonia, are warranted. During the resolution stage of the infiltrative process, positioning for postural drainage, chest percussion, vibration, and airway suctioning will help infants and children to clear their smaller diameter airways.

Viral Pneumonia

Viral pneumonia or infant pneumonitis has, until recently, been considered a rare cause of acute respiratory disease in infants less than 3 months of age. With modern viral isolation techniques, the incidence of viral pneumonitis is now believed to be higher. Examples of the more common viruses associated with infant pneumonitis include respiratory syncytial virus (RSV), chlamydia trachomatis, cytomegalovirus (CMV), pneumocystic carinii, and adenovirus.

The clinical presentation of infants with viral pneumonitis generally includes cough, tachypnea, respiratory distress (especially retractions), chest x-ray evidence of bilateral diffuse pulmonary infiltrates with air trapping, and crepitant inspiratory rales. Many of these infants remain afebrile. A few of the previously mentioned viral infections are sensitive to chemotherapy, so a correct and specific diagnosis is important. The possibility of bacterial superinfection can complicate the course and directly affects management of these infants.

Chest physical therapy techniques for bronchial drainage are indicated for these patients only if there are clinical indications of decreased airway clearance. Continuation of therapy requires evidence (after a clinical trial) that the bronchial drainage treatments are affecting airway clearance in these infants (e.g., decreased respiratory distress, infiltrates on x-ray, adventitious sounds and/or productive cough or increased secretions suctioned from the airways). Chest physical therapy techniques are most valuable when a bacterial superinfection is present and if the infant is intubated and receiving assisted ventilation.

Aspiration Pneumonia

This is an unfortunate result of small children's "indiscreet curiosity" in exploring their environment. Aspiration of toxic substances (commonly household cleaning solutions and hydrocarbons such as kerosene and gasoline) and foreign bodies (such as peanuts, popcorn, small toys, etc.) can lead to a host of pulmonary sequelae including pneumonia, bronchiectasis, and severe ventilation/perfusion abnormalities with right to left shunting.

Management of aspiration pneumonia varies according to the specific derangement and clinical course. Bronchial drainage techniques are often indicated as part of the management of infants and children after aspiration to aid to clear the airways and reduce the possibility of bacterial superinfection.

Asthma

Although asthma is discussed in detail in Chapter 4, a discussion of pediatric pulmonary problems would not be complete without some discussion of this common cause of childhood lung disease. Although by definition asthma is a reversible form of obstructive lung disease, it is probably the leading cause of lost time from school. It is estimated that anywhere from 2% to 7% of all children in the United States suffer from asthma at some time. The good news is that approximately half of all children with asthma "outgrow" the disease by their middle teens. Mortality from asthma is rare in children, but morbidity, both physical and emotional, is significant in those children whose disease is not easily controlled.

Childhood asthma can begin at any age and its etiology and clinical course vary from patient to patient. Medical management usually includes avoidance of known precipitants, adrenergic drugs, and corticosteroids (in chronic, severe cases). Chest physical therapy for this disease includes primarily patient/family education in breathing control, relaxation, effective coughing, and occasionally bronchial drainage techniques.

Exercise conditioning is a very important component of the treatment of the asthmatic patient. Although exercise can induce bronchoconstriction in patients with asthma, improved aerobic fitness increases threshold levels of provocation of symptoms. Asthmatic patients who are aerobically trained also seem to cope better during an asthma attack, require less medication, have higher self-esteem and self-confidence, and have decreased absences from school. Swimming has been identified as the aerobic exercise least likely to induce bronchospasm (with running the most likely to cause bronchospasm).

A carefully designed exercise conditioning program (which includes sufficient warm-up and cool-down time) with preexercise aerosol

β_2 agonist or cromolyn sodium administration can result in similar cardiorespiratory improvements for the asthmatic child or adolescent as the nonasthmatic. During the early phase of the training program, interval-type training (which intersperses low-level work, or rest periods, with higher level work) may be necessary to prevent bronchospasm and enable the asthmatic to sustain the activity long enough to achieve a training effect.

Miscellaneous Conditions

Many other diseases and syndromes affect infants and children and cannot be described here due to space limitations. Some of these problems include alpha-1 antitrypsin deficiency, idiopathic pulmonary fibrosis, and allergic bronchopulmonary aspergillosis. All of these problems are relatively rare, but when present, usually indicate or require a concerted team approach including many aspects of CPT management.

Special Respiratory Problems Associated With Intubation/ Tracheostomy of an Infant or Child

Once an infant or child develops respiratory failure, intubation and mechanical ventilation are usually required. The goal of medical management, in these cases, is to treat the cause of the failure as aggressively as possible and wean the patient from the assistive devices as quickly as possible. The presence of an endotracheal tube interferes with mucociliary transport. It is therefore important to augment airway clearance with bronchial drainage including airway suction as a prophylactic measure. Also, it has been dramatically demonstrated that CPT, including postural drainage and vibration emphasizing right upper lobe segments, can significantly decrease the incidence of postextubation atelectasis in infants intubated for more than 24 hours.

If the child's condition necessitates long-term mechanical ventilation or an artificial airway is needed to bypass an upper airway obstruction, a tracheostomy is usually performed. Endotracheal tubes (ETs) and tracheostomy tubes (TTs) that are in place for a prolonged period of time may cause erosion, fibrotic stenosis of the trachea or tracheomalacia, which often means prolonged hospitalization and repeated trials of extubation. Occasionally, an infant will need to remain trached until he grows (and the tracheal diameter increases) sufficiently to permit adequate ventilation.

Infants and children who are intubated and trached for long periods of time require vigorous prophylactic airway management. They also require special attention to the commonly encountered developmental problems which may include but are not limited to oral stimulation interpreted as a noxious stimulus, poor suck and swallow, and delayed speech. These problems are often not considered until later in the hospital course of these patients because the concern is life and death, not normal development. It is important, however, for the health care providers to be aware of the potential consequences of the care and procedures rendered and to begin intervention techniques to minimize the problems as soon as possible.

CHEST PHYSICAL THERAPY FOR INFANTS

The primary goal of chest physical therapy for infants is to improve airway clearance. If techniques of bronchial drainage can increase the diameter of the airways through secretion mobilization, then ventilation may also be improved and the work of breathing reduced. These techniques should be judiciously applied for prophylaxis as well as treatment in infants with documented airway clearance (AWC) problems or who are at risk for developing complications of poor AWC. Applying bronchial drainage techniques including positioning for postural drainage, chest percussion and vibration, cough stimulation and airway suctioning to infants requires modification based on a thorough understanding of each infant's condition.

Positional Rotation

Frequent changing of position can help avoid or treat pooling of secretions by preventing the prolonged dependency of one portion of the lung. Whereas the emphasis of a positional rotation program for adults is often directed toward the lower lobes, it is important that not only the lower lobes but all lung areas be considered when instituting a positional rotation program for infants. The upper lobes and right middle lobe are common sites of airway collapse in infants. Infants often develop atelectasis in the upper lobes and right middle lobe because of a lack of collateral ventilation channels. The right middle lobe bronchus is also surrounded by a collar of lymph nodes and is therefore vulnerable to extrinsic compression by the hilar nodes.

One area of the lung should not be continually emphasized in a positional rotation program. This program is designed to avoid positioning any one segment dependently for any prolonged period of time. Although mobilization of secretions is a primary focus of posi-

TABLE 27–2.

Essentials of a Positional Rotation Program

1. Care should be taken to coordinate any change in the infant's position with other nursing procedures to avoid unnecessary stimulation.
2. Infants should never be left unattended when in a head-down position.
3. Vital signs should be monitored closely by respiration and heart rate monitors. The alarms should be turned on!
4. The infant's chest should be auscultated for bilateral breath sounds after positioning.
5. While the infant is in a drainage position, secretions will be more easily mobilized. The infant's trachea or endotracheal tube should be suctioned as needed.
6. Avoid placing the infant in a head-down position for approximately one hour after eating to avoid aspiration of regurgitated food.
7. Any change in the infant's position should be done slowly in order to minimize stress on the cardiovascular system.
8. Infants with umbilical arterial lines *can* be placed on their abdomens. However, one should always check that the line has not been kinked.
9. Some infants might require modified drainage positions. Infants with severe cardiovascular instability or suspected intracranial bleeding should not be placed in a head-down position.

tional rotation, ventilation is also affected as the chest wall is regionally "freed up" by being placed uppermost at regular intervals. A suggested sequence of positions is found in Figures 27–2 to 27–4. Important considerations and essentials of a positional rotation program for infants are outlined in Table 27–2.

Postural Drainage

Postural drainage (PD) positions to promote gravity-assisted drainage of specific segmental airways can be safely applied to any age or size patient. In the acute care setting, however, many of the head-down positions are modified according to tolerance and adjust for specific precautions and contraindications. The rule for modification of any position for PD is that the position used should be as close as safely possible to the classical (anatomically correct) position for that segment. Examples of the classical PD positions for each bronchopulmonary segment are pictured in Figures 27–5 to 27–17.

Positioning of tiny infants, especially premature infants weighing less than 800 gm, usually requires modifications of the head-down positions to flat or slightly head-up. This modification is due primarily to the high incidence of intraventricular hemorrhage in premature infants. These infants do, however, tolerate and benefit from being positioned prone. Prone positioning in premature infants has been shown

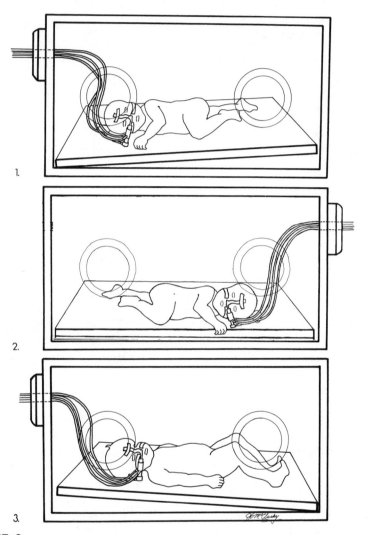

FIG 27–2.

Sequence for positional rotation.

Position 1.—Segments that come off the left lower bronchus posteriorly are drained by positioning the infant on his right side, three-fourths prone with a head-down angle. *Position 2.*—The posterior segment of the right upper lobe is drained by positioning on the left side, three-fourths prone with the bed flat. *Position 3.*—The anterior segments of the upper lobes are drained by positioning supine with the head of the bed elevated or flat. *Position 4.*—Segments that come off the right lower lobe bronchus posteriorly are drained by positioning on the left side, three-fourths prone with a head-down angle. *(Continued.)*

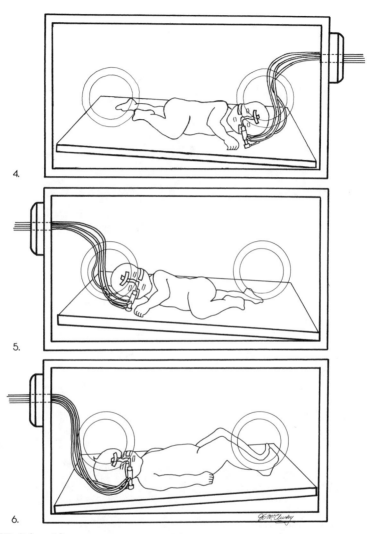

Fig 27–2 (cont.).

Position 5.—The posterior segment of the left upper lobe is drained by positioning on the right side, three-fourths prone with the head of the bed elevated. *Position 6.*—Segments that come off the tracheobronchial tree anteriorly are drained by positioning supine with a head-down angle. *Positions 7 and 8.*—Segments such as the right middle lobe or lingula that come off the tracheobronchial tree anterolaterally will be drained in a three-fourths supine position, slightly head down (see Fig 27–4).

Note: Babies on ventilators may also be positioned prone. This is usually done by the therapist rather than in a *routine* positional rotation (see Fig 27–3).

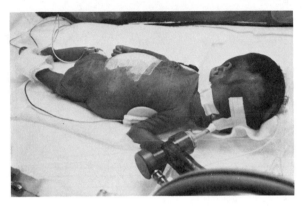

FIG 27–3.
Premies (even those on ventilators with numerous catheters) may be placed prone when care is taken.

to improve oxygenation, tidal volumes, and dynamic lung compliance (see Fig 27–2 and 27–3).

Other precautions for Trendelenburg positioning of infants include but are not limited to abdominal distention, congestive heart failure, arrhythmias, hydrocephalus, frequent episodes of apnea and bradycardia, and acute respiratory distress.

Chest Percussion and Vibration

Percussion and vibration are used in conjunction with postural drainage to augment the effect of gravity in the removal of secretions. There

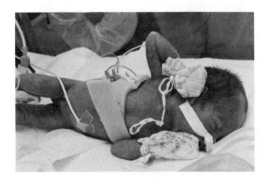

FIG 27–4.
Three-fourths supine position for right middle lobe. Lingula is the same three-fourths supine position with the patient lying on his right side.

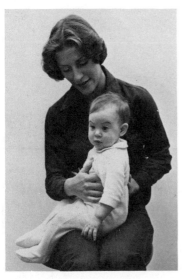

FIG 27–5.
Upper lobes—apical segments.

are several ways of performing percussion on infants. For the larger infant, it is possible to use a cupped hand the same as one would for percussing an adult's chest. For the smaller infant, some modification of this technique is needed. Chest percussion for the smaller infant is accomplished by the use of tenting three fingers (Fig 27–18), four fingers, or using any of the commercially available percussion devices

FIG 27–6.
Left upper lobe—anterior segment.

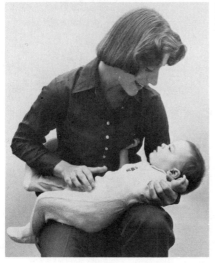

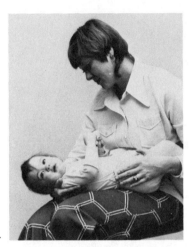

FIG 27–7.
Right upper lobe—anterior segment.

made for the neonates. A small anesthesia mask or "palm cup" can also be used effectively. Some therapists prefer a "contact heel percussion" technique using the thenar-hypothenar eminence of the hand. Precautions for chest percussion in the infant include but are not limited to unstable cardiovascular or oxygenation status (may proceed if continuous transcutaneous monitoring is available), coagulopathy, subcuta-

FIG 27–8.
Lingula.

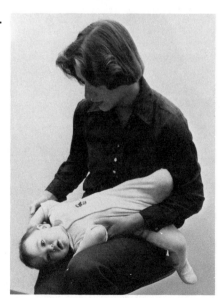

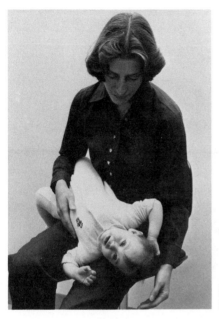

FIG 27–9.
Right middle lobe.

neous emphysema, intraventricular hemorrhage, over a healing thoracotomy incision, and if infant becomes more irritable or displays increased respiratory distress during the treatment.

Vibration is accomplished either by manual vibratory motion transmitted to the infant's chest wall though the therapist's fingers (Fig 27–19) or by mechanical vibrators. An electric toothbrush can be adapted

FIG 27–10.
Right upper lobe—posterior segment.

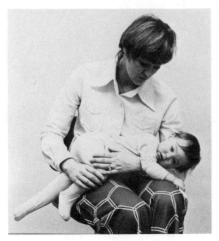

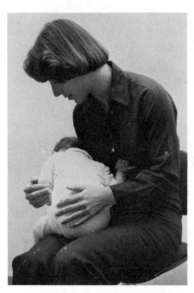

FIG 27–11.
Left upper lobe—posterior segment.

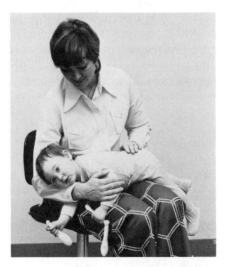

FIG 27–12.
Apical (superior) segments of both lower lobes.

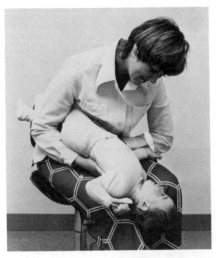

FIG 27–13.
Both lower lobes—anterior basal segments.

by padding the bristle portion of the toothbrush with foam. The most common precaution for vibration is if the infant becomes increasingly irritable and develops bradycardia and increased respiratory distress.

Whether chest percussion and/or vibration are used depends on each infant's condition and how well tolerated if applied in a firm, non-painful, and rhythmic way. Vibration has been observed to occasionally increase irritability and therefore be less well tolerated than percussion

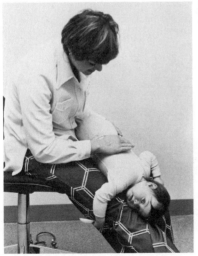

FIG 27–14.
Both lower lobes—posterior basal segments.

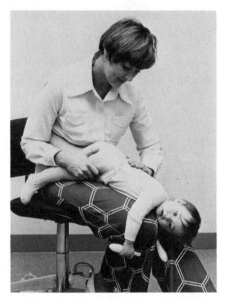

FIG 27–15.
Three-fourths prone modified position for right lower lobe—posterior basal segment.

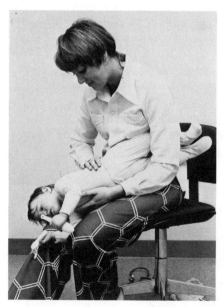

FIG 27–16.
Right lower lobe—lateral basal segment.

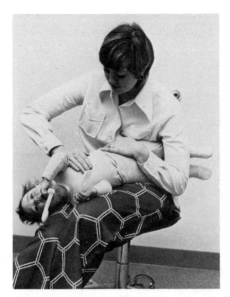

FIG 27–17.
Left lower lobe—lateral basal segment, right lower lobe—cardiac (medial) segment.

in neonates. The time necessary for effective drainage of an area being drained is a minimum of three to five minutes. This time frame may need to be shortened if the position or technique is not well tolerated. Since bronchial drainage is often fatiguing, the areas of greatest involvement should be treated first, followed by the less involved areas.

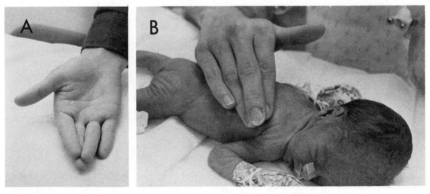

FIG 27–18.
"Tenting" of the finger for percussion of premies or small children.

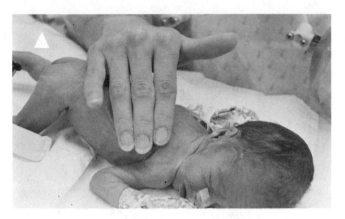

FIG 27–19.
Manual chest wall vibration of a premie.

It may also be necessary to give more frequent treatment sessions to include all involved areas.

Airway Suctioning

Sterile airway suctioning is discussed in detail in Chapter 30. This discussion is meant to highlight some *special considerations* which should be made when suctioning an infant's airway.

1. If possible, suction with a transcutaneous oxygen monitor in place. These monitors give continuous feedback regarding the infant's oxygenation status.

2. Bagging should be done only with a bag attached to a pressure manometer to assure sufficient pressures are being used without exceeding the maximum safe levels (these limits should be similar to the ventilator settings).

3. Suction for no more than five seconds with each catheter withdrawal.

4. Infants should be carefully hyperoxygenated when hyperventilated so as to minimize *hyperoxia* as well as hypoxia. Bagging usually does not need to continue for more than 5–10 seconds to maintain adequate oxygen levels.

CHEST PHYSICAL THERAPY FOR CHILDREN

The goals for chest physical therapy in the child (essentially 2 years of age and up) include more than improving AWC. Children and adolescents are capable of following directions and mimicking a therapist to work on deep breathing, coughing, and active exercise techniques at varying levels. Goals for these patients can include improving ventilation, decreasing work of breathing, increasing strength and endurance of respiratory and other muscles, improving posture, relaxation, breathing control and pacing and improving cardiorespiratory endurance. The application of these techniques often requires patience, understanding, and ingenuity. These patients are of varying ages, emotional makeup, and neuromusculoskeletal development. There are no set ways of accomplishing chest PT goals. Anything goes!

Positional Rotation

The goal of positional rotation and postural drainage is to prevent the accumulation of secretions and to aid in their removal. Any child who is immobile, receiving artificial ventilation, or not expanding his chest adequately should have his position changed at least every two hours. If the child is reluctant to have his position changed, changing the location of the television set may be helpful.

As stated earlier, it may be necessary to be creative in gaining the confidence and cooperation of a youngster. The challenge is to make it seem less like a treatment and more like a game. It is important, however, to be honest in your explanations or you will never be trusted in subsequent sessions. Involving the parents can also be invaluable. In some cases, the parent may do most of the "hands-on" and repeat instructions to the child under the direct guidance of the therapist. This arrangement helps reinforce parent education for home therapy as well.

Breathing Enhancement and Coughing

From the age of 18 months to 3 years, it is usually possible to encourage deep breathing by means of blowing bubbles, tissue paper, paper mobiles, or horns. If one side of the child's chest is expanding poorly, the child can be positioned on each side while doing these exercises. The theory behind sidelying positions is that the downside lung ventilates more effectively (see Chapter 2). However, if the poorly ventilated lung is uppermost, stretch techniques can facilitate deeper breathing (see Chapter 1). Spontaneous coughing at this age often occurs with a change in position or crying. For the child who does not cough spontaneously or whose cough is inadequate to clear secretions, nasopharyngeal suctioning may be necessary.

The preschool child can also be encouraged to take deep breaths by blowing objects. A doll, Happy Birthday Tender Care, may be used as a model to show the child how to use his stomach muscles to blow tissues or party favors. Some children this age can also be successfully taught diaphragmatic breathing, lateral-costal expansion, and coughing.

Older children (not infants) can be stimulated to cough by applying a firm pressure over the trachea in the suprasternal notch. Beware that coughing, whether spontaneous or stimulated, may elicit gagging and vomiting. Be sure to allow at least an hour after oral feedings or meals before treating a child for an AWC problem.

Older children can be instructed in various deep breathing exercises such as diaphragmatic breathing, pursed-lip breathing, and segmental lateral costal breathing. They may also be candidates for using relaxed deep breathing for relaxation, control, and pacing of activity. Older children and adolescents may use an incentive spirometer or an inspiratory resistive breathing device for specific inspiratory muscle endurance training.

Preoperative and Postoperative Care

Postoperative pulmonary complications may not be as prevalent in the pediatric age group as adults, but they still occur. The most common complications are atelectasis, infection secondary to pooling of secretions, and airway obstruction. Infants and children who represent the following situations are at higher risk for developing postoperative pulmonary complications: (1) preexisting lung disease; (2) incision in thorax or upper abdomen; (3) if long bed rest or restricted mobility postoperatively; (4) coexisitng neuromuscular problem affecting ability to cough, deep breathe, and be generally mobile.

The effectiveness of preoperative and postoperative CPT has been well documented. The appropriate application of preoperative assessment, instruction, and treatment by therapists has been associated with decreased incidence of postoperative complications.

Prevention is the key, particularly in a high-risk patient.

Preoperative teaching is extremely important for the child and the parent. Parents can often be more anxious than the child and transfer that apprehension to the child. The level of preoperative training depends on a child's age.

If the client is an infant or very young child (i.e., less than 2 years), the therapist will meet with the parents and explain and demonstrate the following: Purpose of bronchial drainage treatments, potential airway clearance problems, and complications. Stress *preventive* nature of these treatments. Demonstrate various procedures that might be done to the infant following surgery: (1) positioning; (2) percussion (chest); (3) vibration; (4) airway suctioning. Ask parents for questions and answer them as best you can (refer all specific medical questions to the physicians involved).

If the client is able to understand simple concepts and will cooperate some with the therapist (approximately 2–7 years), the above orientation with the parents should be done. Also, try to talk to the child and explain the same concepts in very simple terms. Additional instruction might include: (1) various breathing games, (2) instruction in using the incentive spirometer, (3) coughing practice, (4) upper and lower extremity exercises.

In older or more mature children (i.e., 8 years or older), the following procedures will be explained and demonstrated when appropriate (the parents may be present but the child is the one who should be spoken to primarily). (1) Reason why deep breathing, coughing and bronchial hygiene are important. (2) Demonstration of log-rolling, sitting, chest percussion, vibration, etc. (3) Teach the child deep breathing exercises (diaphragmatic and pursed-lip with inspiratory-hold maneuver). Teach the child the use of the incentive spirometer if appropriate. (4) Teach leg and arm exercises (active, through full range of motion). (5) Teach effective cough; show how the incision can be splinted; discuss the *importance* of the cough. (Do not say it won't hurt; be honest.)

Postoperative treatments generally focus on improving ventilation, coughing to maintain clear airways, and gradually increasing activity. Specific bronchial drainage is used only if the child is unable to clear his airways or is at risk due to chronic lung disease.

Following high abdominal or thoracic surgery, there may be a tendency for the child to splint on the side of his incision. Arm, shoulder, and trunk movement should be encouraged to prevent any postoperative complications. For the younger child, chest mobility can be encouraged by clapping the hands over the head or by dramatizing songs such as "The Itsy Bitsy Spider." More conventional exercises may be taught to the older child. Incentive spirometry can be extremely helpful in encouraging a sustained maximal inspiration and preventing atelectasis.

Children tend to mobilize very quickly (unless they are prevented due to disease or specific procedure). Once a child is out of bed and moving about, essentially afebrile, lungs clear to auscultation, and coughing effectively, postoperative CPT treatments can generally be discontinued.

Pulmonary Rehabilitation

Rehabilitation programs for pediatric patients with chronic lung disease include the same components and have essentially the same goals as those of an adult (see Chapter 13). The major difference between comprehensive rehabilitation programs for adults versus children and adolescents is related to the diagnoses most prevalent in the two age groups. Asthma and cystic fibrosis (CF) are the most common diagnoses of children and adolescents who are candidates for pulmonary rehabilitation. The most common diagnosis in the adult population are chronic bronchitis and emphysema.

Conditioning exercise for the asthmatic patient was discussed earlier in this chapter. The asthmatic patient's response to exercise conditioning is similar to that of an individual without chronic pulmonary disease. Children and adults with asthma can improve cardiovascular fitness as well as the many disease-specific benefits mentioned earlier.

The effects of exercise conditioning on patients with cystic fibrosis are similar to those of adults with chronic obstructive lung disease (other than asthma). The major physiologic benefit of conditioning appears to be improving the endurance of the respiratory muscles.

A comprehensive pulmonary rehabilitation program for the older child and adolescent with CF ideally includes the following components:

1. Continuing patient and parent education regarding adapting to changing life-style to the disease (i.e., sports and physical education, independent bronchial drainage, college or vocational training, marriage, and family). The adolescent and young adult with CF need special counseling and sensitivity to the fears and decisions they are facing as they make the transition to adulthood.

2. Bronchial hygiene.

3. Prevention program for postural deformities.

4. Breathing retraining and relaxation.

5. Exercise training program.

It is vital to carefully assess aspects of the neuromuscular, skeletal, and cardiorespiratory systems of these patients in preparation for developing an appropriate program. Evaluation should include but not be limited to:

1. Range of motion, strength, posture.

2. Exercise tolerance (ideally this test should be done with EKG, BP and O_2 saturation monitored.

3. Evaluation of ADL tolerance/limitation.

4. Complete chest evaluation.

5. Inspiratory muscle strength (maximal inspiratory negative pressure at the mouth) and endurance testing (can be done with an inspiratory muscle training device by having the patient breathe for a predetermined length of time at progressively increased resistances until tolerance is reached).

The adolescent with chronic lung disease has a special need for increased independence and an improved body image. The health care team must recognize these needs and plan evaluation treatment and education programs prophylactically as well as in response to identified problems.

REFERENCES

Periodicals

Bacsik RD: Meconium aspiration syndrome. *Pediatr Clin North Am* 1977; 24(3):463–479.

Barnes CA, Asonye VO, Vidyasagar D: The effects of bronchopulmonary hygiene on $P_{Tc}O_2$ valves in critically ill neonates. *Crit Care Med* 1981; 9(12):819–822.

Cerny FJ, Pullano TP, Cropp GJA: Cardiorespiratory adaptations to exercise in cystic fibrosis. *Am Rev Respir Dis* 1982; 126:217–220.

Chawla H, Finnegan L: Acute pneumonia in the newborn: Changing picture. *Pediatr Ann* 1977; 6(7):18–31.

Crane LD: Physical therapy for neonates with respiratory dysfunction. *Phys Ther* 1981; 61(12):1764–1773.

Demers RD, Saklad M: The etiology, pathophysiology, and treatment of atelectasis. *Respir Care* 1976; 21(3):234–239.

Dunn D, Lewis AT: Some important aspects of neonatal nursing related to pulmonary disease and family involvement. *Pediatr Clin North Am* 1973; 20(2):491–498.

Finer NN, Boyd J: Chest physiotherapy in the neonate: A controlled study. *Pediatrics* 1978; 61:202–285.

Finer NN, Mariarty RR, Boyd J, et al: Postextubation atelectasis: A retrospective review and a prospective controlled study. *Pediatrics* 1979; 94(1):110–113.

Fitch RD: Comparative aspects of available exercise systems. *Pediatrics* 1975; 56(suppl):904–907.

Gregory GA, et al: Meconium aspiration in infants: A prospective study. *J Pediatr* 1974; 85:848.

Holsclaw DS: Pediatric pulmonary disease: An overview. *Pediatr Ann* 1977; 6(7):10–17.

Kaneko K, Milie-Emili J, Dolowich MB: Regional distribution of ventilation and perfusion as a function of body position. *J Appl Physiol* 1966; 21(3):767–777.

Keens TG: Exercise training programs for pediatric patients with chronic lung disease. *Pediatr Clin North Am* 1979; 26(3):517–524.

Krastins IRB, Corey ML, McLead A, et al: An evaluation of incentive spirometry in the management of pulmonary complications after cardiac surgery in a pediatric population. *Crit Care Med* 1982; 10(8):525–528.

Laitman JT, Crelin ES: Developmental change in the upper respiratory system of human infants. *Perinatal Neonatal* 1980; 4:15.

Lew CD, Ramos AD, Plaztzker ACG: Respiratory distress syndrome. *Clin Chest Med* 1980; 1(3):297–309.

Martin RJ, Herrell N, Rubin D, et al: Effect of supine and prone positions on arterial oxygen tension in the preterm infant. *Pediatrics* 1979; 63(4):528–531.

McFadden R: Decreasing respiratory compromise during infant suctioning. *Am J Nurs* 1981; 12:2158–2161.

Mellins RB, et al: Committee report: Respiratory care in infants and children. *Am Rev Respir Dis* 1972; 125:461–483.

Morton AF, Fitch KD, Hahn AG: Physical activity and the asthmatic. *Physician Sports Med* 1981; 9(3):51–64.

Muller NL, Bryan AC: Chest wall mechanics & respiratory muscles in infants. *Pediatr Clin North Am* 1979; 26:503.

Rockwell GM, Campbell SK: Physical therapy program for the pediatric cardiac surgical patient. *Phys Ther* 1976; 56(6):670–675.

Rodenstein DO, Perlmutter N, Stanesw DC: Infants are not obligatory nasal breathers. *Am Rev Respir Dis* 1985; 131(3):343–347.

Rooklin AR, McGeady SJ, Mikaelian DO, et al: The immotile cilia syndrome cause of recurrent pulmonary disease in children. *Pediatrics* 1980; 66(4):526–531.

Seligman T, Randel HO, Stevens JJ: Conditioning program for children with asthma. *Phys Ther* 1970; 50(5):641–650.

Stagno S, Brasfield DM, Brow MB, et al: Infant pneumonitis associated with Cytomegalovirus, Chalamydia, Pneumocystic and Ureaplasma: A prospective study. *Pediatrics* 1981; 68(3):322–329.

Thurlbeck WM: Postnatal growth and development of the lung. *Am Rev Respir Dis* 1975; 111:803.

Tudehope DI, Bagley C: Techniques of physiotherapy in intubated babies with respiratory distress syndrome. *Aust Pediatr J* 1980; 16:226–228.

Voyles JB: Pulmonary problems in infants and children: Bronchopulmonary dysplasia. *Am J Nurs* 1981; 81:510.

Wagoman MJ, Shutack JG, Moomjian AS: Improved oxygenation and lung compliance with prone positioning of neonates. *J Pediatr* 1979; 99(5):787–791.

Waring WW: Respiratory diseases in children: An overview. *Respir Care* 1975; 20:1138–1145.

Wood RD: Cystic fibrosis: Diagnosis, treatment, and prognosis. *South Med J* 1979; 72(2):189–202.

Wood RD, Boat RF, Doershuk CF: Cystic fibrosis: State of the art. *Am Rev Respir Dis* 1976; 113:883–877.

Zach M, Oberuwaldner B, Hausler F: Cystic fibrosis physical exercise versus chest physiotherapy. *Arch Dis Child* 1982; 57:587–589.

Books

Crane L, Physical therapy for the neonate with respiratory disease, in Irwin S, Tecklin JS (eds): *Cardiopulmonary Physical Therapy*. St. Louis, CV Mosby Co, 1985.

Johnson TR, Moore WM, Jeffries JE (eds): *Children Are Different: Developmental Physiology*, ed 2, Columbus, Ohio, Ross Laboratories, 1978.

Scarpelli EM, Auld PAM, Goldman HS (eds): *Pulmonary Disease of the Fetus, Newborn and Child*. Philadelphia, Lea & Febiger, 1978.

Tausig LM, Lemen RJ: *Chronic Obstructive Lung Disease*. Chicago, Year Book Medical Publishers, 1979.

Wetzel J, Lunstord BR, Peterson MJ, et al: Respiratory rehabilitation of the patient with spinal cord injury, in Irwin S, Tecklin J (eds): *Cardiopulmonary Physical Therapy*. St Louis, CV Mosby Co, 1985.

Miscellaneous

Evans HE: What happens when a child has asthma. American Lung Association Publication 7.84.

PART FOUR

Related Aspects of Respiratory Care

28

Body Mechanics—The Art of Moving and Positioning Patients

Donna Frownfelter, P.T., R.R.T.

Body mechanics may be defined as the efficient use of one's body as a machine and a locomotive entity. It is extremely important that therapists and nurses (especially those working with critically ill, *dependent* patients) understand and utilize proper body mechanics. This is necessary to reduce stress and trauma for both the patient and the nurse/therapist. Positioning and moving dependent patients is an art quite different than working with a patient who can move independently and assume any given position with ease. In this chapter, we will discuss the principles of body mechanics and suggest guidelines for their practical applications.

LIFTING

There has been a change from earlier concepts and principles of lifting. As was discussed, the body has been thought of as a machine. It was believed that improper mechanics of lifting would result in tremendous loads on the discs. The key components of lifting were to "keep it close," bend knees, "lift with the legs." Later the spinal posture was the center of attention during lifting.

During observation, it was seen that lifting seemed to be "naturally" done from slightly bent knees and then during the raise to left butt-end first, rearing backwards at the start as he started to extend his knees prior to lifting. The predominance of injuries seems to occur with the back in flexion. There is a rationale for strengthening abdominal muscles to promote safer lifting. The abdominal strength is necessary to support a pelvic tilt during lifting.

Another current school of thought advocates lifting with the lordotic lumbar curve intact. This is the technique utilized by weight lifters. When these individuals are questioned about any backaches, they usually deny any problems.

The lifting technique may be modified by other factors: limited space (i.e., small hospital rooms), clothing, degenerative knee joints.

The first consideration in body mechanics is the need for maintenance of proper posture and balance (body stability). Consideration should be paid to the relationship between gravity, posture and body stability (Fig 28–1). It is commonly known that gravitational force is always exerted in a vertical direction toward the center of the earth. In addition, that point in a patient or object at which all of its mass is centered is the *center of gravity* (the point at which the patient's maximum weight is concentrated). In the standing position, the human body's center of gravity is approximately 55% of the body's total height, in the pelvic cavity, slightly anterior to the upper part of the sacrum. The lower the center of gravity, the greater the body stability. Consequently, when the human body is used as a machine to lift an object, muscular effort great enough to maintain stability as well as to lift against the force of gravity is necessary, especially when the patient's center of gravity is further removed from your own. *Therefore,* one way to conserve energy and maintain stability is to carry the weight of the patient (or object) as close to one's own center of gravity as possible. This allows maximum concentration of one's own energy toward movement of the patient, with minimal stress or injury to oneself. To help accomplish this, the bed should be adjusted so the therapist/nurse can reach the patient comfortably. Usually adjusting the bed to one's hip level is adequate. This makes the patient close to the therapist's center of gravity.

All lifting should be done with the legs (knees) and not by straining to lift with the arms and back (Fig 28–2). Whenever there is a question about one's ability to lift a patient alone, generally it should not be done, and assistance should be obtained.

Another point to consider is the base of support while lifting. The base of support is defined as the area between the feet that provides the body's stability. It is easily appreciated that the wider the base of support, the greater the body's stability. To enlarge on this concept, one needs to define also the *line of gravity* and its relationship to body stability. The line of gravity is an imaginary line passing through the

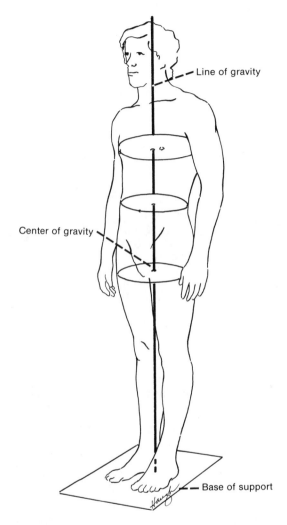

FIG 28–1.
The line of gravity passes through the center of gravity and the base of support to maintain body stability.

center of gravity of an object and perpendicular to the surface on which the object (body) rests (see Fig 28–1). The closer the line of gravity passes to the *center* of the *base of support,* the greater is the body's (object's) stability. Increased muscular effort needs to be exerted in proportion to the distance the line of gravity shifts away from the base of support.

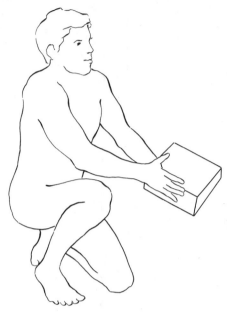

FIG 28–2.
Reach work level by bending the knees and hips rather than the back. Lift with the legs!
This can also be done with a full double knee squat similar to techniques by weightlifters.

To summarize and apply these concepts, one can list the following guidelines:

1. The lower the center of gravity, the wider the base of support, and the nearer the line of gravity falls to the center of the base of support, the *greater the body's (object's) stability*. When lifting, stand with feet well apart, knees slightly flexed and one foot forward. Keep head and trunk in proper alignment.

2. When our bodies are used as machines, the external weight upon which we are working displaces the center of gravity in the direction of the weight being lifted. To conserve energy and maintain stability, carry the weight as close to your own center of gravity as possible. Lower your hips to the level of the surface supporting the weight you plan to lift by flexing your hips and knees. Adjust the bed up as high or down as low as you need for comfortable and efficient work.

3. The effort to perform a given activity depends upon the weight of the object to be lifted. Know your limits. Don't attempt to lift alone

if you have any doubts about your ability to do so. Don't be a hero in a back brace! Obtain assistance for the sake of both the patient and yourself.

4. Other general tips for lifting are as follows:

Lift with your legs. Keep legs in a position that permits them to supply most of the force for shifting your trunk.

Do not attempt to lift with your arms and back.

When lifting, avoid rotation of the spine. Shift feet into position for weight shift when moving or lifting patient.

Stabilize your body against a stationary object whenever possible.

For best efficiency, coordinate the move by a verbal expression understood by therapists and patient, such as "1–2–3 lift," to synchronize the effort.

As we now come to the actual mechanics of how to lift and position patients, one additional consideration must be noted—moving against the resistance of friction. *Friction* is defined as a force that opposes the movement of one object over the surface of another. Friction is reduced as the amount of surface area contact between two objects is reduced.

When moving a patient side to side or up and down in bed, the therapist/nurse attempts to reduce the contact of the patient's body surface with the bed. This can be accomplished by several maneuvers: use a turning sheet (placed just above the patient's shoulders to just below the patient's hips), cross the patient's arms over his chest or abdomen, flex the patient's knees and hips, and ask the patient to flex his neck and raise his head as he is lifted (if the patient is unable to do this, the therapist/nurse will assist) (Fig 28–3).

MOVING DEPENDENT PATIENTS

I. Moving the patient up or down.
   A. Using a turning sheet (Figs 28–4 to 28–6).
      1. Sheet should cover from shoulders to hips.
      2. Gather material as *close* to the patient's body as possible.
      3. Hold at shoulders and hips, with a flexion pattern (see Fig 28–5).
      4. Cross patient's arms over chest, flex knees and hips.
      5. Ask patient to raise head if possible.
      6. Synchronize action by counting "1–2–3 lift."

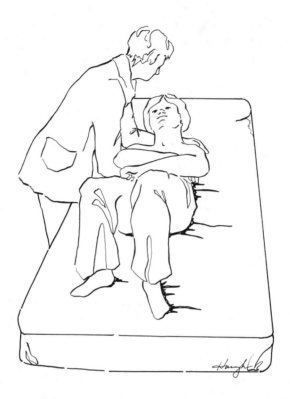

FIG 28–3.
The patient should be prepared for a position change: knees bent, arms crossed over chest and head lifted up to reduce friction between the patient's body and the bed.

       7. Shift weight from one leg to the other rather than lifting up and pulling on back.
   B. Without turning sheet (up or down), two people.
       1. Follow basic procedure—cross arms, lift head, flex knees and hips.
       2. The therapist places his hands and forearms under the patient's shoulders and hips.
       3. If patient is extremely heavy or tall, another person can bend knees and assist.
 II. Moving the patient to the side of the bed.
   A. With turning sheet.
       1. Cross arms, etc., toward the side to which the patient is to be moved.
       2. Therapist's hands at patient's hips and shoulder on material close to patient's body.

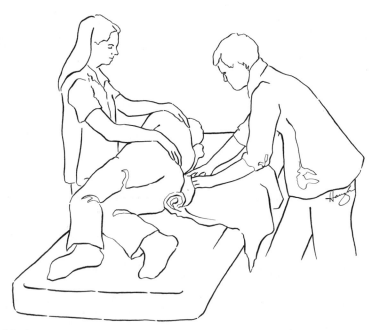

FIG 28–4.
To insert the drawsheet, the patient is turned to his side and the half-rolled drawsheet is tucked under him (from just above the shoulders to just below the hips). He rolls over the drawsheet and it is pulled out behind him.

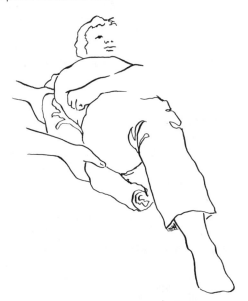

FIG 28–5.
The drawsheet should be rolled close to the patient's body. A flexion hand grip at the patient's shoulders and hip is most efficient.

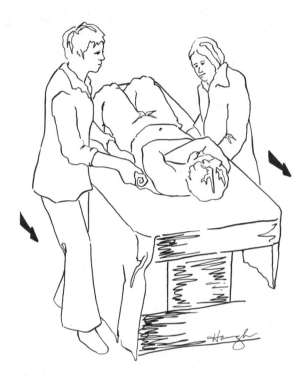

FIG 28–6.
Moving the patient toward the head of the bed. The patient is prepared. The therapist is positioned to move toward the head of the bed in order to shift his body weight to move the patient.

       3. One therapist pushes, the other pulls.
   B. Without turning sheet.
      1. *Both persons* stand on the desired side.
      2. One therapist's forearms under patient's shoulder, the others under patient's hips.
      3. Synchronize action by counting "1–2–3 pull."
 III. Turning the patient to his side.
   A. With turning sheet (to right side) (Figs 28–7 and 28–8).
      1. Move patient supine to *opposite* side of turn (e.g., if turning to right side, move patient to left side of bed).
      2. Bring right arm to the side at a 90-degree angle up and away from body.
      3. Place left arm across chest.
      4. Place left leg over right leg.
      5. Pull sheet at patient's back to turn.

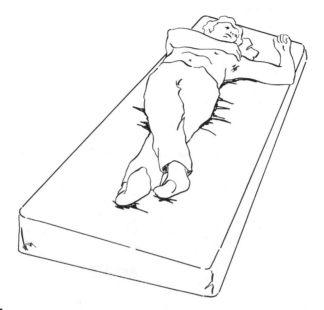

FIG 28–7.
Preparation for the patient to turn to his left side: move patient to the right side of the bed, position his left arm up to the side at a 90-degree angle, cross the right leg and arm over his body and turn the patient's head to the left.

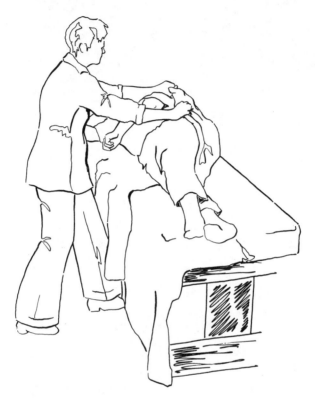

FIG 28–8.
A one-person turn to the right side using a drawsheet. The patient's body position is the same as for the turn to the side. The therapist is positioned with one foot forward, the other back. He pulls the sheet with his hands positioned at the hips and shoulders of the patient.

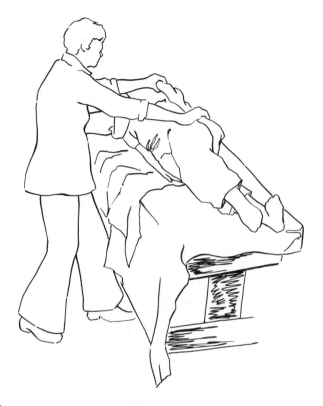

FIG 28–9.
Positioning patient prone (example: Rolling to the right side). The patient's right arm is tucked in at his side with the left arm and leg crossed over.

    B. Without turning sheet (to right side).
        1. Move to opposite side (therapist's hands and forearms under patient's shoulders and hips).
        2. Same steps as 2, 3, and 4 above.
        3. Roll to right side using left shoulder and left hip to push or pull.
  IV. Turning the patient prone (e.g., roll to right side) (Fig 28–9).
    A. With or without turning sheet.
        1. Move patient to opposite side of bed from side toward which he is turning.
        2. Cross left arm and left leg over body.
        3. Right hand and arm *at body side* tucked in as close as possible.
        4. Use hips and shoulders to turn.

5. Free both arms, do not allow patient to lie on arm or hand.
6. May want pillow under hips and lower legs to bend knee and relieve back strain at lumbar spine.

To summarize, we find patient movement is a necessary and integral function of chest physical therapy. It is so often taken for granted and performed with little thought or planning. Therapists and nurses need to analyze beforehand their physical activity in relation to the principles of efficient movement and the proper application of body mechanics. The practical application of body mechanics will not only conserve energy and preserve muscles and joints but will also allow the patient to be moved with a minimum amount of pain and discomfort.

REFERENCES

Periodicals
Neil C: Body management in nursing. *Nurs Times* 1959; 55:163.

Books
Fuerst, E., and Wolff, L: *Fundamentals of Nursing* (4th ed; Philadelphia: JB Lippincott Co, 1969).
Lewis L: *Fundamental Skills in Patient Care.* Philadelphia, JB Lippincott Co, 1976.
Rantz M, Courtial D: *Lifting, Moving and Transferring Patients: A Manual.* St Louis, CV Mosby Co, 1977.
Rauch B: *Kinesiology and Applied Anatomy.* Philadelphia, Lea & Febiger, 1971.
Roper N: *Principles of Nursing,* ed 2. New York, Churchill Livingstone, Inc, 1973.
Wells K: *Kinesiology.* Philadelphia, WB Saunders Co, 1971.

Miscellaneous
Is there a right way to lift? *Physical Therapy Forum* 1985; 4:23.

29

Respiratory Therapy Review for Nurses and Physical Therapists

Cassandra Jahntz Pecaro, R.R.T.

Donna L. Frownfelter, P.T., R.R.T.

This chapter is a generalized summary of respiratory therapy principles and equipment. It is geared to the physical therapist and nurse. As one works in the field of respiratory care, it becomes evident that all personnel involved need to understand the principles and equipment in order to effectively deal with the patient. We will discuss oxygen therapy, aerosol therapy, IPPB and medications generally used in treatments. A brief discussion of ventilators used in continuous modes will also be included. (This was discussed in Chapter 26 on respiratory failure.)

OXYGEN THERAPY

Oxygen is the single most important life-sustaining element required by humans. Its vital role in modern medicine has caused it to be recognized as a drug and to be administered as such.

Oxygen therapy modalities are used to increase alveolar oxygen tension, decrease the work of breathing and decrease myocardial work.

The fraction of inspired oxygen F_{IO_2} is a term used to indicate a particular percentage of oxygen present at any given time. For example, ambient air is composed of 20.95% oxygen, 78.08% nitrogen and various other trace gases. Oxygen is only a portion of the entire atmosphere; however, it functions independently of the other constituent parts and renders its fraction of the whole F_{IO_2} at 21%.

Guidelines have been established regarding individual oxygen appliances, suggested liter flows and the approximate F_{IO_2} values delivered. However, a precise response to a given dose of oxygen cannot be predicted. Therefore, the effectiveness is determined by arterial blood gases which reflect the partial pressure of oxygen in the arterial blood (PaO_2) and the clinical observation of the patient.

Oxygen therapy can be administered by one of two methods—low-flow and high-flow systems.

Low-Flow System

A low-flow system is one in which the total flow is not adequate to meet the inspiratory requirements of the patient. Therefore, a portion of the inspired gas is composed of ambient air. The resultant F_{IO_2} is a balance between the inspired gas obtained from these two sources. Variance in respiratory rate and/or depth alters these proportions, which in turn alter the F_{IO_2}. A low-flow oxygen system is effective only for: 1) patients with an intact upper airway, 2) a stable ventilatory pattern, 3) stable respiratory rate and minute volume in order to approximate the desired F_{IO_2}.

Low-Flow Oxygen Devices

Cannula—Nasal Prongs (Fig 29–1)

The nasal cannula is a two-prong device placed within the nares, extended behind the ears and secured under the chin of the patient. This appliance allows the patient to eat and talk without removing the device. The approximate liter flow and resultant F_{IO_2} values are as follows:

FLOW (L/MIN)	F_{IO_2} (%)
1	24
2	28
3	32
4	36
5	40
6	44

Providing the patient meets the requirements previously listed for the use of the low-flow system, the F_{IO_2} values rendered will remain

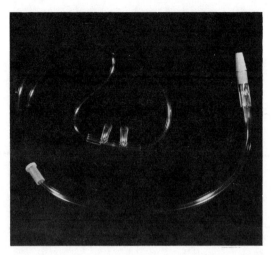

FIG 29–1.
Oxygen cannula.

fairly consistent. A variability in $F_{I_{O_2}}$ will occur with changes in rate and depth of respiration. Liter flows in excess of 6 L/min should not be used with the nasal cannula due to extreme irritation of the nasal mucosa, drying of the mucous blanket and crusting of the airway which in turn cause increased resistance to breathing.

Nasal Catheter (Fig 29–2)
The nasal catheter is inserted through one nare and should rest approximately one-fourth inch above the uvula between the oropharynx and the nasopharynx. The nasal catheter must be secured to the nare when in place and reinserted in the opposite nare every eight hours, due to nasal irritation. If functioning properly, the catheter will deliver approximately the same $F_{I_{O_2}}$ values as the nasal cannula; that is, 1–6 L/min render an $F_{I_{O_2}}$ of 24%–44% O_2.

The $F_{I_{O_2}}$ delivered is dependent on respiratory rate and depth as with the cannula. The nasal catheter is used very little in modern hospitals due to irritation and the need for frequent reinsertions.

Mask (Fig 29–3)
The simple mask creates a reservoir through which oxygen is introduced and room air is entrained via side ports to provide the inspired atmosphere. Higher concentrations of oxygen can be delivered with the mask. However, consistency of $F_{I_{O_2}}$ is dependent, once again, on

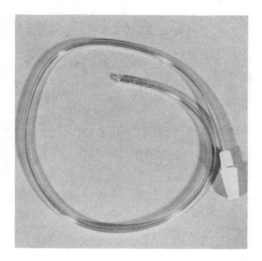

FIG 29–2.
Oxygen catheter.

the stability of the patient's rate and volume intake, as well as on good mask fit. The approximate liter flow and F_{IO_2} are as follows:

FLOW (L/MIN)	F_{IO_2} (%)
5–6	40
6–7	50
7–8	60
8–9	70
9–10	80

The oxygen mask restricts the patient from eating while the appliance is in use and is generally cumbersome while talking and sleeping. Many patients also complain of feeling claustrophobic.

Partial Rebreathing Mask (Fig 29–3)

The partial rebreathing device is composed of a mask with a reservoir bag. The inspired volume consists of source oxygen and anatomic dead space from the previous exhalation. Anatomic dead space is that portion of the exhaled volume, approximately the first one-third, that does not participate in gas exchange and is therefore rich in oxygen. Source oxygen and anatomic dead space mix together in the reservoir bag and are rebreathed, while the remaining two thirds of the exhaled volume is vented out the side ports of the mask. If this

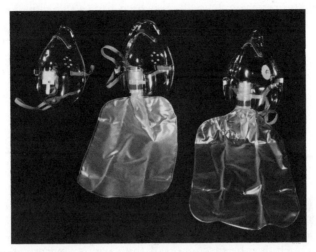

FIG 29–3.
Left to *right,* mask without bag, partial rebreathing bag, nonrebreathing bag (note the valves on the mask and at the junction between the mask and bag).

appliance is used properly, the amount of CO_2 that is rebreathed is negligible. Approximate flows and F_{IO_2} values are:

FLOW (L/MIN)	F_{IO_2} (%)
6–7	60
7–8	70
8–9	80
9–10	90

High oxygen concentrations are delivered with the partial rebreathing mask. *Providing* the flow is sufficient to meet the inspiratory requirements of the patient, the F_{IO_2} values will remain consistent.

Nonrebreathing Mask (Fig 29–3)

The principle of the nonrebreather is to create a one-way system which is made possible by the valve separating the mask from the reservoir bag. The reservoir bag is filled with source oxygen. On inspiration, the one-way valve rises and allows oxygen from the reservoir bag to be emitted to the patient. The flutter flaps covering the side ports of the mask close on inspiration, preventing a large amount of ambient air from entering the mask and in turn being introduced as a portion of the inspired volume. On exhalation, the one-way valve between the mask and the reservoir bag closes, which forces the *entire* exhaled volume through the side ports and out to the ambient room air. Consequently, rebreathing does not occur. Approximate flows and F_{O_2} values are:

FLOW (L/MIN)	F_{O_2} (%)
6	60
7	70
8	80
9	90
10	99+

Under *stable* conditions, only a small amount of ambient air is drawn into the system via the side ports; however, tachypnea and hyperpnea will alter the F_{O_2} values.

This concludes the discussion of the various devices categorized as low-flow systems. As one can see, *low flow does not necessarily refer to the administration of low concentrations of oxygen.* The major point to bear in mind is that the F_{O_2} values delivered by a cannula, catheter, mask, partial rebreather or nonrebreather are subject to change if the inspiratory requirements of the patient are not satisfied.

High Flow System

A high-flow system is the second means by which oxygen therapy is delivered. This method is based on two principles of physics—Bernoulli's law and Venturi's principle. Bernoulli's law states that lateral pressure exerted by a flow of gas in a conducting tube varies inversely with the velocity. The Venturi principle elaborates on the Bernoulli law as applied to oxygen and states that at the point of restricted orifice the lateral pressure becomes negative, causing a secondary source gas to be entrained into the main source gas. *Therefore, 100% of the inspired atmosphere in a high-flow system is delivered via the device, and the total flow in liters per minute is sufficient to compensate for all inspiratory demands. The F_{O_2} will remain constant.*

High-Flow Oxygen Devices

Venturi Mask (Fig 29–4)
At the point of restriction, the secondary source gas (ambient air) is entrained into the main source gas (oxygen). Inspired gases from

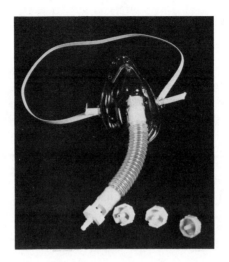

FIG 29–4.
Venturi mask.

both sources combine and provide the total atmosphere required by the patient as seen below.

TOTAL FLOW (L/min)	ENTRAINMENT (L/min)	O_2 (L/min)	LITER FLOW (L/min)	$F_{I_{O_2}}$ (%)
84	20	1	(4)	24
44	10	1	(4)	28
48	5	1	(8)	35
32	3	1	(8)	40

The total flow in liters per minute exceeds the patient's inspiratory flow rate. Therefore, the $F_{I_{O_2}}$ is precise. Changes in respiratory rate and/or depth will *not* alter the $F_{I_{O_2}}$ value.

A high-flow system does not necessarily indicate administration of high concentrations of oxygen. Devices using the Venturi principle render $F_{I_{O_2}}$ values ranging from 24% to 100% oxygen. The orifice size and the entrainment ratio (amount of ambient air drawn into the system) will vary with every appliance within that range.

HUMIDITY AND AEROSOL THERAPY

Humidity Therapy

During the inspiratory cycle, ambient air is 100% saturated with water vapor proximal to the carina. Humidification of the inspired air is important to mucus production, ciliary activity and a healthy respiratory tract. When normal function is interfered with, other methods of adding moisture to the respiratory system must be undertaken.

Adequate humidification is an absolute necessity in preventing respiratory complications and is indicated: (1) whenever a dry gas is administered, (2) in the presence of thick tenacious secretions and (3) when an artificial airway, endotracheal or tracheostomy tube is in place.

A humidifier is the device designed to deliver a maximum amount of water vapor to the respiratory tract.

Aerosol Therapy

The use of aerosol therapy in acute and/or chronic periods of bronchopulmonary disease has become an integral part of the total respiratory care regime.

An aerosol is defined as actual particulate matter (water particles) suspended in a gas. This particulate water introduced into the respiratory tract plays an important role in liquefying and mobilizing the tenacious pulmonary secretions that so often occur in short-term as well as long-term disease processes.

The sizes of the aerosol particles determine their entry or nonentry into the respiratory tract. Particles larger than 5 μ (1 μ equal 1/25,000 in.) will be trapped in the nose and not allowed entry. Particles 2–4 μ in size will deposit somewhere proximal to the alveoli; particles 1–2 μ in size can enter the alveoli; and particles 0.15–0.25 μ account for the greatest alveolar deposition.

The device that produces an aerosol is a nebulizer. Nebulizers are classified by the power source that enables them to function, either pneumatic or electric. A pneumatic nebulizer is one in which the power is derived from a 50 psi compressor or cylinder source, such as the oxygen piping system in every hospital. An electrically driven nebulizer utilizes a standard household electric current.

Pneumatic jet nebulizers classically consist of a water reservoir and a capillary tube submerged in the water (Fig 29–5). A high-velocity gas flow is introduced into the system, which causes the water from the reservoir to advance upward through the tube (Bernoulli's principle) to create a fine mist of particles which are in turn subjected to a baffle.

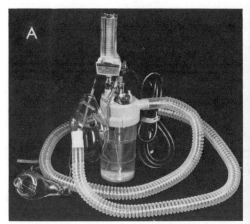
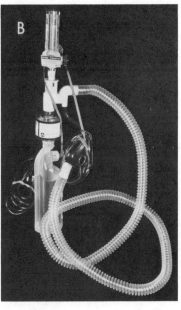

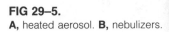

FIG 29–5.
A, heated aerosol. **B,** nebulizers.

A baffle is a device situated in the direct path of the gas carrying the particulate water. The aerosol particles hit the baffle, become fragmented, and smaller particles are created. Therefore, a baffle assures uniform particle size.

A Venturi device provides the total flow of gas—entrained ambient air plus source oxygen: This makes a readily available oxygen dilution system for combining controlled oxygen therapy with aerosol therapy.

Pneumatic jet nebulizers produce uniform particles in the range of 3–5 μ in size, and approximately 55% of these aerosol particles are within effective range.

The electrically driven aerosol unit is the *ultrasonic nebulizer* (Fig 29–6). Electrical energy is converted by virtue of the piezoelectric transducer to mechanical vibrational energy with an ultrahigh frequency of 1.35 megacycles/second. The piezoelectric crystal disk transmits ultrasound vibration to the couplant, which is a water reservoir. Slightly submerged in the couplant is the nebulizer cup, which also receives the vibrational energy, and an aerosol geyser effect is created. The nebulus is then transmitted to the patient by a compressor blower which provides the carrier gas.

The total aerosol output of the ultrasonic nebulizer ranges from 1 to 6 ml/min as compared to the total ouput of the pneumatic nebulizer at 1–2½ ml/min. The particle size of the ultrasonic aerosol is 0.5–3 μ

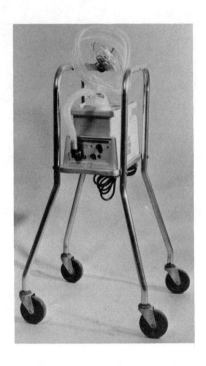

FIG 29–6.
Ultrasonic nebulizer.

and approximately 90% of these particles are within the effective range for deposition in the alveoli.

Proper instruction as to the use of aerosol therapy is *essential*. For optimal benefit, it is suggested that a sitting position be assumed for gravity to facilitate deposition of the aerosol. The patient is then instructed to breathe slowly and deeply through the mouth, pausing slightly after each inspiration. Nose breathing may filter out particles of optimal size. Diaphragmatic exercises will aid even aerosol distribution, and cough instruction is of primary importance.

There are potential hazards associated with the administration of aerosol therapy which will be mentioned as a precautionary note to the therapist.

Bronchospasm.   Involuntary contraction of the bronchial smooth muscle due to entry of foreign bodies and aerosol particles.

Swelling of Secretions.   The addition of water to dry retained secretions may cause them to swell and occlude small or large airways, causing extreme shortness of breath and respiratory distress. The therapist should be present and the aerosol advanced only as tolerated. USN should not be given to patients who cannot cough and mobilize secretions without the therapist or nurse present.

Cross Contamination. Proper sterilization techniques and frequent changing of equipment are of the utmost importance due to the fact that aerosol devices harbor microorganisms which may be transmitted to the patient.

IPPB

Intermittent positive pressure breathing (IPPB) is a mode of therapy that, when used with discretion and administered by a knowledgeable and skilled therapist, may offer beneficial results to patients with long-term chronic disease as well as with a short-term acute episode.

IPPB therapy is a form of mechanical ventilation used on an intermittent basis and is defined as a mechanical device that augments respiratory gas flow. Machines most commonly used for this purpose are pressure-preset ventilators (Fig 29–7).

Pressure-preset ventilators are designed to inflate the patient's lungs until a fixed pressure is reached, at which time inspiration ends and expiration begins.

This form of assisted ventilation is used for patients who have spontaneous respiration but inadequate vital capacity, i.e., below 1000 cc TV.

Indications for IPPB

Intermittent positive pressure breathing is used to improve effective alveolar and total ventilation, prevent or remove microatelectasis and deliver aerosolized medication. Studies have shown the metered dose inhalers and oral bronchodilators deliver the same benefits of medication so the last reason is not enough alone to order IPPB.

MECHANICAL VENTILATION

As discussed in Chapter 26, mechanical assistance of ventilation may be required for supportive respiratory care in many disease states. The two principles of operation of a mechanical ventilator are negative

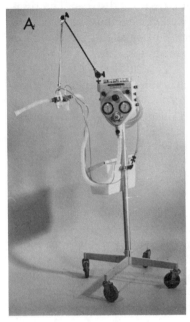

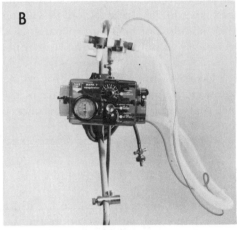

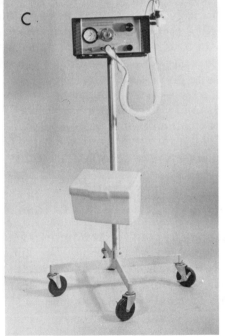

FIG 29–7.
A, IPPB (Bennett PR-2). **B,** IPPB (Bird).
C, IPPB (AP-4) electrically operated.

pressure, as in the classic "iron lung," and positive pressure, as in the majority of ventilators presently used. Positive pressure ventilators are further subclassified by describing the mechanism of ending or limiting inspiration and beginning expiration of the ventilatory cycle: (1) preset pressure level limits inspiration in machines such as the Bird Mark series; (2) a preset flow limit ends inspiration in the Bennett PR series and (3) a preset time and/or volume limits the inspiration in most other ventilators.

MECHANICAL VENTILATION

Controlled Ventilation

The ventilator completely controls the patient's ventilation. The patient is either too weak to initiate the inspiratory cycle to trigger an assisted ventilation or may have been given medication such as Pavulon or morphine and valium to allow the ventilator to control the patient.

Intermittent Mandatory Ventilation (IMV)

IMV allows the patient to breathe spontaneously from a resevoir in addition to a preset number of positive pressure breaths from the ventilator at adjustable levels of volume and time intervals. It is usually used for weaning from the ventilator.

One problem that arises is if the positive pressure breath is out of synchrony from the patient. The Siemens-Elema Servo Ventilator provides for this with an SIMV (synchronus intermittent mandatory ventilation). This may also be called intermittent demand ventilation (IDV). This produces *patient*-triggered "sighs" rather than just time-edged sighs.

PEEP, CPAP

Positive end expiratory pressure and continuous positive airway pressure may be used to prevent alveolar collapse by maintaining positive airway pressure all during the respiratory cycle. Benefits seen are a higher FRC and improved ventilation/perfusion ratios.

The Siemens-Elema Servo Ventilator 900C (Fig 29–8) will be used in this discussion as an example of a positive pressure, pneumatically and electronically controlled time-cycled ventilator. It is used commonly in medical center settings for mechanical ventilation. It may be used as a controlled mechanical ventilator (CMV), assist, synchronized intermittent mandatory ventilation (SIMV), or spontaneous mode. The ventilator is capable of many varying respiratory flows and breathing patterns. PEEP and CPAP are available. If a patient-initiated or controlled breath doesn't occur for more than 15 seconds, visual and audible alarms activate.

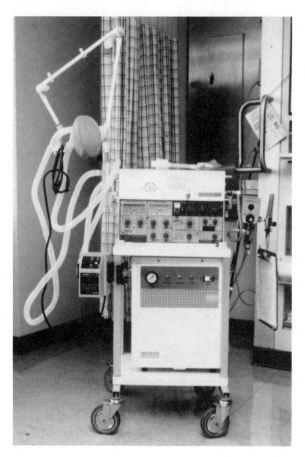

FIG 29–8.
The Siemens-Elema Servo Ventilator 900C.

All health care practitioners should become familiar with the types of ventilators utilized in their facilities. Alarms should not be turned off and should be valued as excellent sources of information rather than a nuisance. Often when a pressure alarm responds, there are secretions in the patient's airway indicating a need for suctioning. Disconnected or low reservoir pressure alarms warn of lack of ventilation. As health care practitioners get more comfortable with treating patients on ventilators alarms are more appreciated.

REFERENCES

Periodicals

Anthonisen NR: Long-term oxygen therapy. *Ann Intern Med* 1983; 99(4):519–527.

Ashutosh K, Mead G, Dunsky M: Early effects of oxygen administration and prognosis in chronic obstructive pulmonary disease and cor pulmonale. *Am Rev Respir Dis* 1983; 127(4):399–404.

Baxter WD, Levine RS: An evaluation of IPPB in the prevention of postoperative pulmonary complications. *Arch Surg* 1969; 98:795.

Braun SR, Smith FR, McCarthy TM, et al: Evaluating the changing role of respiratory therapy services at two hospitals. *JAMA* 1981; 245(2):2033–2037.

Curran FJ: Night ventilation by body respirators for patients in chronic respiratory failure due to late stage Duchenne muscular dystrophy. *Arch Phys Med Rehabil* 1981; 62(6):270–274.

Curtis JK, et al: IPPB therapy in chronic obstructive pulmonary disease. *JAMA* 1968; 206:1037.

Dehaven CB, Jr, Hurst JM, Branson RD: Postextubation hypoxemia treated with a continuous positive pressure mask. *Crit Care Med* 1985; 13(1):46–48.

Egan DF: Humidity and water aerosol therapy. *Conn Med* 1967; 31:353.

Hedley-Whyte J, Winter PM: Oxygen therapy. *Clin Pharmacol Ther* 1967; 8:696.

Minscher M, Vincent JL, Ros AM, et al: Influence of incentive spirometry on pulmonary volumes after laparotomy. *Acta Anaesthesiol Belg* 1982; 33(3):203–209.

Morrison DR, Powers WE, Boocks RD: A proposal for the more rational use of IPPB. *Respir Care* 1976; 21:318.

Ros AM, Vincent JL, Kahn RJ: Incentive spirometry: Prevention of pulmonary complications after abdominal surgery. *Acta Anaesthesiol Belg* 1981; 32(2):167–174.

Sheldon GP, Pressure breathing in chronic obstructive lung disease. *Medicine* 1963; 42:197.

Stock MC, Downs JB, Cooper RB, et al: Comparison of continuous positive airway pressure after cardiac operations. *Crit Care Med* 1984; 12(11):969–972.

Stock MC, Downs JB, Gauer PK, et al: Prevention of postoperative pulmonary complications with CPAP, incentive spirometry and conservative therapy. *Chest* 1985; 87(2):151–157.

Timms RM, Khaja FR, Williams GW: *Ann Intern Med* 1985; 102(1):29–36.

Van De Water JM: Preoperative and postoperative techniques in the prevention of pulmonary complications. *Surg Clin North Am* 1980; 60(6):1339–1348.

Weaver TE: New life for lungs. . . .through incentive spirometers. *Nursing (Horsham)* 1981; 11(2):54–58.

Woodcock AA, Musca A, Violi F, et al: Oxygen relieves breathlessness in "pink puffers." *Lancet* 1981; 25:1(8226):907–909.

Wright JL, Lawson L, Parie PD, et al: The structure and function of the pulmonary vasculature in mild chronic obstructive pulmonary disease: The effect of oxygen and exercise. *Am Rev Respir Dis* 1983; 128(4):702–707.

Books

Asperheim MK, Eisenhauer LA: *The Pharmacologic Basis of Patient Care.* Philadelphia, WB Saunders Co, 1973.

Cash JE: *Chest, Heart and Vascular Disorders for Physiotherapists.* London, Faber and Faber, 1975.

Cherniak RM, Cherniak L: *Respiration in Health and Disease.* Philadelphia, WB Saunders Co, 1962.

Crews ER, Lapuerta L: *A Manual of Respiratory Failure.* Springfield Illinois, Charles C Thomas, Publisher, 1972.

Egan DF: *Fundamentals of Respiratory Therapy.* St Louis, CV Mosby Co, 1973.

Hatch TF, Gross P: *Pulmonary Deposition and Retention of Inhaled Aerosols.* New York, Academic Press, 1964.

Mitchell RS: *Synopsis of Clinical Pulmonary Disease.* St Louis, CV Mosby Co, 1974.

Modell W, Schied HO, Wilson A: *Applied pharmacology.* Philadelphia, WB Saunders Co, 1976.

Shapiro B, Harrison R, Trout C: *Clinical Application of Respiratory Care.* Chicago, Year Book Medical Publishers, 1975.

Wade JF: *Respiratory Nursing Care.* St Louis, CV Mosby Co, 1973

30

Care of the Patient
With an Artificial Airway

Lisa Sigg Mendelson, M.S.N., R.N.

An artificial airway is a tube inserted in the trachea either through the mouth or nose, or by a surgical incision. Artificial airways have been known to medical science for 2,000 years, and they have become a highly specialized technique in patient care. In today's clinical practice, artificial airways have four basic purposes: (1) to bypass upper airway obstruction, (2) to assist or control respirations over prolonged periods, (3) to facilitate the care of chronic respiratory trace infections and (4) to prevent aspiration of oral/gastric secretions. There are multiple disease processes and traumatic problems that can require an artificial airway (Table 30–1) but each situation, simple or complex, can fit into one or several of these categories.

INDICATIONS OF NEED—OBSERVATIONS

The respiratory care team can play a vital role in recognizing patient need for a tracheostomy from physiologic changes that indicate respiratory distress. Cardinal signs of dangerous airway obstruction are stridor and chest wall retractions. Early clinical signs may include restlessness, agitation, tachycardia, confusion and motor dysfunction. These signs may be accompanied by headache, flapping tremor and diaphoresis. Cyanosis from impaired oxygenation of the blood is a late, ominous sign.

TABLE 30–1.

Disease Processes That Could Require an Artificial Airway Due to Respiratory Insufficiency*

1. Primary lung disease—e.g., emphysema, chronic bronchitis, pulmonary fibrosis, cystic fibrosis, severe pneumonia, burned lung and toxic inhalation.
2. Systemic disease with secondary lung involvement—e.g., cardiac failure, renal failure (fluid overload) and adult respiratory distress syndrome (shock lung).
3. Neuromuscular disease—e.g., polio, Guillain-Barré syndrome, myasthenia gravis, use of muscle relaxants and tetanus.
4. Central nervous system depression—e.g., drugs, postanesthesia, metabolic coma, cerebrovascular accident, meningitis and central nervous system tumors.
5. Trauma—e.g., head/neck/chest surgery or injuries.
6. Diseases complicated by extremes of age—e.g., premature infant or elderly.
7. Mechanical obstruction—e.g., upper airway infection, laryngeal paralysis, tumor, edema, bleeding, foreign body and thyroid malignancy.
8. Recurrent aspiration—e.g., glottic incompetence, occlusive diseases of the esophagus and swallowing disorders of various causes.

*From Selecky PA: Tracheostomy—a review of present day indications, complications and care. *Heart Lung* 1974; 3:272–283. Used by permission.

In children, restlessness must be due to lack of oxygen unless another factor (for instance, thirst), is clearly evident. Extreme fatigue and an inability to sleep indicate impending danger. Apprehension, restlessness and mental confusion at any age may be taken as early signs of oxygen deficiency.

The selection of the appropriate airway is made by several factors: (1) What is the best means of accomplishing the goal? (2) Is it an emergency or a controlled, determined situation? (3) Will the airway be needed for long-term care? In general, oral endotracheal tubes are inserted in emergencies. They are the quickest and easiest tubes to insert, even for relatively untrained personnel. A nasotracheal tube will generally replace the oral endotracheal tube for a long-term intubation. The nasal tube is more efficient in that it is better secured, the patient may eat, it is easier to suction and it is generally more comfortable for the patient.

There are certain complications with endotracheal tubes. Among these are sinus blockage and pain, vocal cord damage or pressure necrosis to the cartilaginous structure of the nose. To reduce these complications, the airway should be evaluated daily. The tube should be removed as quickly as possible when the indication for intubation is reversed. However, if there appears to be a need for a more long-term airway, a tracheostomy should be considered. The procedure should not be taken lightly as many additional complications may occur.

Complications of tracheostomy can be surgical, postoperative or physiologic. Complications that occur at the time of the operation are more frequently direct results of the surgical procedure itself. Delayed complications may result directly or indirectly from surgery, from postoperative care and from the abrupt physiologic changes resulting from tracheostomy. Nursing objectives in caring for the patient after a tracheostomy are to maintain patency of the tube, cleanliness of the wound site, good aeration and to observe any changes in the patient's vital signs.

In patients with artificial airways, the normal physiologic mechanism for adding moisture to the air via the nasal mucosa obviously is bypassed. Therefore, supplemental humidification is *extremely* important to protect the mucosa from drying and crusting, with resulting obstruction.

The dressing under the tracheostomy tube should be changed when it becomes soiled because dried blood and other secretions near the incision can encourage bacterial growth. The incision should be checked frequently for bleeding. The skin may be cleaned with hydrogen peroxide and sterile saline when a new dressing is applied. The dressing should be folded into place—never cut. This eliminates the possibility of lint or frayed threads from being aspirated. Commercially prepared dressings best meet these criteria.

When changing the tapes that hold the tube in place, it is best to have one nurse hold the tube in place while another replaces the old tapes. An angle is cut at the end of the tape to facilitate its placement through the flange of one side of the tube. It is then threaded through the back of the tracheostomy tube and through the other flanged opening and tied securely with a *square knot* placed on one side of the patient's neck.

Immediate Surgical Complications of Tracheostomy

A rather uncommon immediate complication is hemorrhage, since there are few, if any, major blood vessels in the midline of the neck. However, some blood may leak into the trachea around the cannula and the aspirated blood may plug the smaller or even the larger bronchi with clots that could lead to atelectasis. If not removed by suction or coughing, the clots become an excellent culture medium for bacterial growth.

Pneumothorax can occur immediately due to laceration of the mediastinal pleura at the time of surgery or within 24 hours (can arise often in children and in patients with chronic obstructive lung disease). Other problems include air embolism, aspiration and subcutaneous and mediastinal emphysema. Recurrent laryngeal nerve damage or posterior tracheal penetration may occur but is uncommon.

Postoperative Physiologic Complications

Attentive nursing care is the single most essential factor in postoperative management. A ratio of one nurse for each patient is the ideal; however, since this is not often possible, increased vigilance by the entire respiratory care team is of vital importance.

A patient with an artificial airway is understandably apprehensive and has special communication needs. He should also be reminded that his inability to phonate is only temporary. He must be reassured that he will be attended to constantly and will be able to trust and depend fully upon the nursing staff to attend to his needs. If alert, he must be equipped with a signal light or bell, paper and pencil or magic slate so he can communicate.

Airway obstruction is the foremost complication that exists for the postoperative tracheostomy patient. Tracheal secretions are the major source of obstruction, particularly if they are excessive or viscous. When using a cuffed tube, acute obstruction might occur from overinflating the cuff, allowing it to balloon over the end of the tube. Other causes of obstruction are dislodgment of the tube into a false tract anterior to the true tracheal opening, occlusion by an overinflated cuff and kinking of a softened plastic cannula.

Tracheobronchitis is a complication resulting primarily from irritation due to incorrect suctioning technique.

Crusting is a common and complex problem that emphasizes the need for adequate humidification of inspired air or may be due to dehydration. In many instances, ulceration of the tracheal mucosa results from irritation by the airway or incorrect suctioning. This ulcerated area becomes infected with various organisms and is virtually covered by a crust. Further suctioning removes the crust, causing discharge of serum and even bleeding. The discharge produces a wet eschar which is covered with mucus. Because of the drying effect of air passing over this mass, a hard crust can form. This process can compound the difficulty as the development of this crust in the trachea might eventually produce a mass large enough to completely plug the tracheal cannula and almost completely obstruct the trachea. Cases have been cited where an entire cast of the tracheobronchial tree has been removed.

Other physiologic complications may be related to (1) *hypoxia* developing prior to or during the procedure and resulting in an uncontrollable patient, cardiac arrest and increased myocardial sensitivity to adrenalin; (2) *alkalosis* developing from rapid CO_2 wash-out following establishment of the airway and resulting in myocardial fibrillation and apnea; and (3) *cardiac failure* resulting in profuse bronchorrhea from pulmonary edema and shock.

Postoperative Mechanical Complications

Dislocation of the tube might result from unsatisfactory nursing care, poor attention to the airway during positioning or ventilator tubing pulling on the airway. If the tracheostomy tube tapes are not kept tight and tied with a square knot, or if they become loose as a result of cervical emphysema or edema, the tube may be coughed out of the trachea and become lodged in the tissues of the neck and obstruct the airway.

Stay sutures are useful in tracheostomy patients when there is the possibility of tube displacement. These sutures are valuable during recannulization of the tube if it becomes dislodged before a tract has been well established. These sutures will prevent entry into a false tract. Advantages of this technique include: (1) blocked or displaced tubes can be rapidly replaced; (2) exposure of the trachea at surgical intervention is improved; (3) firm anchoring of the trachea at the moment of incision; (4) decreased trauma associated with entubation; and (5) uniform tracheostomy technique for all ages.

Dislodgment of the outer cannula or required removal before a tract has been well established (usually 4–7 days) again requires diligence and quick action by the nurse. No attempt at reinsertion should be made without adequate light, satisfactory tissue retraction, tracheal hook and Trousseau's dilator. A Trousseau dilator, tracheal hook and spare tracheostomy tube of the correct size should be kept at the patient's bedside at all times. Then, should the tube be coughed out, the nurse uses the Trousseau dilator to hold the wound apart while summoning the physician. Tragedies have occurred from inserting the tube into the soft tissues of the neck or mediastinum due to a dislodged cannula and the frantic efforts to replace it. Once the tracheostomy tract has been firmly established, the tube can be replaced by the nurse upon written order of the physician.

TRACHEOSTOMY TUBES

Metal Tubes

Tracheostomy tubes are of two basic types: metal and disposable plastic. Metal tubes can be made of either stainless steel or sterling silver and are composed of three parts: (1) an outer cannula which fits into the tracheal incision, (2) an inner cannula which fits into the outer cannula and (3) an obturator. Before the outer cannula is inserted into the tracheal incision, the obturator is placed inside. The lower end of the obturator protrudes from the end of the outer cannula and facilitates its insertion into the trachea. This is the only purpose of the obturator. The protruding end of the obturator obstructs the lumen of the outer cannula. When the obturator is removed, immediately replace it with the inner cannula. When dealing with metal tubes, the parts of each set are not interchangeable and fit only one particular set. If one part is lost or damaged, the entire set is useless. Therefore, each part, including obturator, is carefully accounted for. Plastic tubes generally have interchangeable parts.

Care should be exercised in handling sterling silver tubes as silver is very soft and will dent easily.

Mucus that has dried inside the inner cannula cannot be cleaned by merely rinsing in water. The cannula should be soaked in hydrogen peroxide, then rinsed with saline. Scrub with a tracheostomy brush and rinse with saline to be sure all secretions have been removed. If the silver inner cannula is discolored, it may be cleaned with silver polish.

The inner cannula should always be inspected to be sure it is clean and clear of secretions before it is reinserted. Be sure to lock the inner cannula in position after reinsertion.

Plastic Disposable Tubes

The development of plastic tracheostomy tubes came about for three important reasons: (1) application of silicone to the inner surface of the plastic tube minimizes crusting and adherence of secretions; (2) there is greater ease in placing a safe, dependable, permanent inflatable cuff to the plastic tube which cannot slip off to occlude tracheal opening; and (3) lower costs allow the tube to be disposable.

The cuffed tracheostomy tube (Fig 30–1) is primarily used in conjunction with a positive pressure ventilator to form a closed system. It is also used to reduce the possibillity of aspiration due to absent, protective laryngeal and pharyngeal reflexes. The inflatable cuff is located

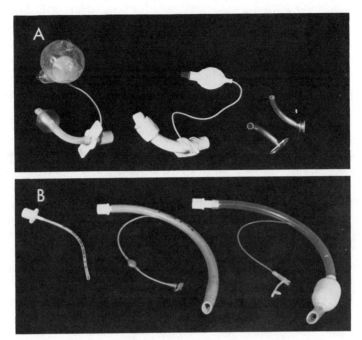

FIG 30–1.
A, cuffed adult tracheostomy tubes, uncuffed pediatric tracheostomy tube *(far left).* **B,** cuffed adult endotracheal tubes, uncuffed pediatric endotracheal tube *(far left).*

around the lower portion of the tube and, when inflated, seals the trachea from most airflow except through the tube itself. The cuff, usually made of pliable plastic, is inflated by injecting air into the fine-bore tubing. A small pilot balloon is located proximally in the tubing and, when inflated, indicates that the cuff is inflated. The nurse *must* check the inflation end of the cuff and the balloon prior to insertion of the tube into the trachea to be certain that there are no leaks. The ends of some inflation tubings may be self-sealing, whereas other tubings require the use of a hemostat to seal the end to maintain the pressure.

Once the cuff is inflated, the only route for air exchange is through the patient's tracheostomy tube; therefore careful observation of the patient by the nurse is essential. If the patient is on mechanical ventilation, observation is essential if there is ventilator failure, as asphyxiation may occur. Some means of resuscitation, such as a manual resuscitating bag with mask, should also be available at the bedside to ventilate the patient in the event the tracheostomy tube comes out or is dislodged.

Inspired air must be continuously and adequately humidified by means of nebulizing equipment to prevent the formation of crusts. The equipment used for this purpose can be a possible source of infection. Therefore, the nebulizer and tubing should be changed ideally every 8 hours, but at least once in 24 hours.

Considerable emphasis has been given to the incidence of tracheal ischemia and resulting stenosis from the use of a cuffed tube. This ischemia results from the pressure of the cuffed tube against the tracheal wall which heals with scar formation, resulting in subsequent stenosis. This complication can be reduced or eliminated by the following procedure: Inflate the cuff until there is no air leak between the wall of the trachea and the cuff, and then release a small amount of air to allow only a slight air leak between the walls of the trachea and the cuff. This reduces the pressure of the cuff, still allows the ventilator to function properly and reduces the likelihood of tracheal ischemia. In the past, it has been the practice to deflate the cuff for five minutes every hour to reduce the possibility of tracheal ischemia. The need for this practice has been eliminated by the above technique.

If the tracheostomized patient is conscious, he may attempt to speak. If the cuff is properly inflated, he will be aphonic since no air can pass over the vocal cords. If he needs to speak, the cuff can be deflated and the patient may be given a sterile dressing to hold over the tube. This will allow him to speak and also simulate a cough by rapid exhalation to clear secretions.

The Communitrache I is a new tracheostomy tube that permits the removal of secretions above the infected cuff without nasotracheal suctioning. The other plus factor to this new tracheostomy tube is the patient's ability to communicate, especially while on a ventilator. When the patient is weaned from the ventilator, a fenestrated trache tube may be used. Fenestrated comes from the French word *fenestre,* meaning window. There is a window (fenestration) in the outer cannula. When the tube is used for speaking, the cuff is down, the inner cannula removed, and an external "plug" is inserted to "cap" the tracheostomy tube to allow the patient to speak. The cuff must be deflated when the cap is in place. If the cuff was inflated the patient would be unable to breathe air into the lungs. The patient exhibits immediate distress if this mistake is made.

The Olympic trache button is used as an interim airway following tracheostomy tube removal. This method is another example of weaning a patient from tracheostomy tube but still maintain the stoma should a tracheostomy be again needed. The patient that benefitted most from the procedure was the COPD patient. This was one method used to facilitate secretion removal posthospitalization when it became necessary due to their disease process. The Olympic trache button allowed the tracheostomy patient the opportunity to reestablish an unobstructed airway and at the same time allowed the patient to speak.

The management of major airway obstruction by tracheal tumor, external compression, or tracheal disease below the thoracic inlet still present difficult problems. The Montgomery T-tube is a bifurcated silicone rubber stent designed to preserve patency of the airways in a patient with injury to the trachea or main bronchi. When the T-tube is in place, the patient breathes normally through nose and mouth and can speak. The T-tube is a method in which secretions can be removed if necessary and is helpful in long-term therapy to alleviate obstruction or during reconstructive surgery. This device does not cause any adverse tissue reaction on a long-term basis. Any difficulty in properly inflating the cuffed tracheostomy tube should be immediately reported to the physician.

Airway Care

Normally the mucociliary escalator and the cough reflex provide airway clearance. When these mechanisms fail, suctioning of the airways is indicated. Suctioning does have potential hazards, but with proper guidance and care should be a safe procedure.

Suctioning

Proper explanation of the suctioning technique to the patient helps allay apprehension and enhance his cooperation. Always maintain a calm and reassuring manner.

Maintain aseptic technique throughout the entire procedure. Use sterile gloves and a sterile disposable catheter for each suctioning.

Position the patient properly unless contraindicated. Nasotracheal and/or pharyngeal suctioning should be done with the patient in the Fowler or semi-Fowler position with the neck hyperextended (Fig 30–2). The supine position is best for the patient with tracheostomy or endotracheal tubes (Fig 30–3).

Pharyngeal suctioning may be necessary prior to deflating the cuffed tracheostomy tube. The nurse should not suction the pharynx and then the trachea with the same catheter, but the trachea may be suctioned first and then the pharynx with the same catheter.

Duration of suctioning is of extreme importance. Each suctioning procedure should last no longer than 5–10 seconds to avoid hypoxia.

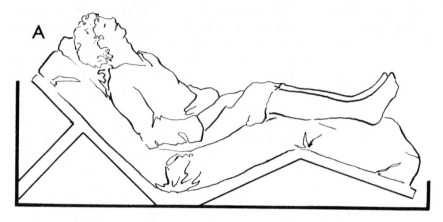

Fowler 60-70 degrees

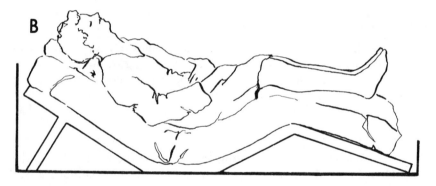

Semi-Fowler 10-12"

FIG 30–2.
Fowler's and semi-Fowler's positions.

Prolonged suctioning may result in precipitating an arrhythmia or cardiac arrest. A good way to judge the elapsed time is to hold one's own breath and be guided by the development of discomfort. This is most important for the patient who is dependent on ventilatory assistance.

The *lowest possible vacuum* settings are best. The higher the setting is raised, the greater the risk of trauma to the tracheal mucosa. Caution should be exercised to avoid kinking the suction tubing or catheter. When negative pressure is excessive and released suddenly, inadvertent removal of portions of tracheal mucosa may occur.

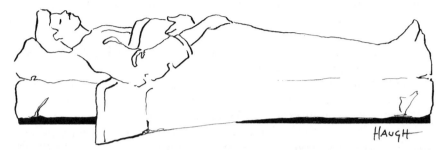

FIG 30–3.
Supine position.

Insertion of the suction catheter should be done gently. The catheter should first be moistened in sterile saline or with a water-soluble gel. Suction is not applied while the catheter is passed down into the trachea. Proper insertion of the catheter will stimulate coughing when it contacts the carina (Fig 30–4). It is then immediately withdrawn 1 cm

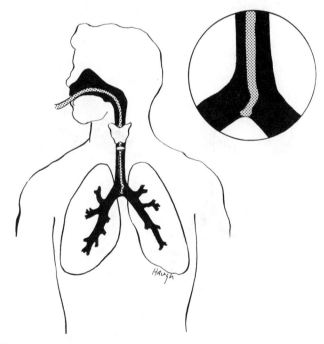

FIG 30–4.
The catheter will stimulate coughing when it contacts the carina (in a patient with intact cough reflex).

before suction is applied (Fig 30–5). Do not force the catheter up and down while suctioning. Suction is applied only while the catheter is being withdrawn. Rotating the catheter during withdrawal results in suctioning a larger area and increases the surface contact of the trachea and tracheostomy tube (Fig 30–6).

Left main-stem bronchus aspiration is more difficult because of the anatomical arrangement of the bronchus. It was formerly thought that left bronchial aspiration was facilitated by turning the patient's head to the right. Recent studies indicate, however, that this is not true and that left bronchial aspiration is best accomplished by using a Coudé tip catheter. After its insertion into the trachea, the curved tip should be positioned to point toward the left main-stem bronchus. Even so, insertion is difficult and auscultation by stethoscope is necessary to thoroughly access the suctioning.

Right main-stem bronchus aspiration is the usual case because of the more direct alignment of this bronchus with the trachea. This can be carried out almost always with a straight tracheal catheter.

Excessive suctioning can be harmful. Use judgment to determine just how often a patient requires suctioning. Auscultation by stetho-

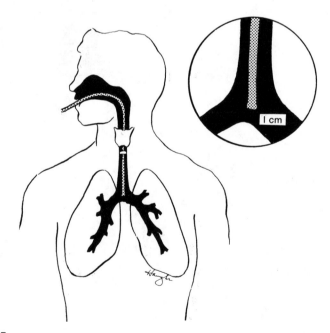

FIG 30–5.
The catheter is withdrawn 1 cm after it reaches the carina, before applying suction.

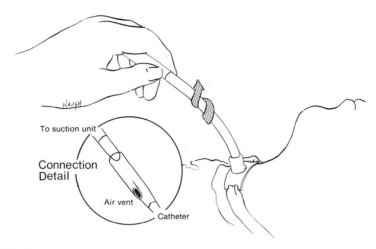

FIG 30–6.
The catheter is rotated during withdrawal in order to suction a larger surface area.

scope should be used to determine the thoroughness of suctioning. Allow the patient to rest and breathe between each insertion of the suction catheter and, if necessary, ventilate him for a few minutes before further suctioning. Remember each suctioning attempt removes air as well as secretions. Preoxygenation has been suggested with better results and fewer complications.

Nasotracheal Suctioning Procedure

1. Check equipment.

2. Check monitors.

3. Inform patient of the procedure.

4. Preoxygenate patient.

5. Place patient's neck in extension.

6. Lubricate catheter with water soluble gel.

7. Pass catheter (without suction) upward and backward with short increments. Continue until an obstruction (the carina) is reached.

8. When the carina is stimulated, the patient will generally cough reflexly unless his/her reflexes are obtunded.

9. The catheter should be pulled back slightly, then suction applied as catheter is withdrawn.

10. The aspiration time should be within 10–15 seconds total (a good guideline is for the therapist to hold his or her breath during suctioning as the patient is also not breathing and it gives the therapist a better sensitivity for what the patient experiences).

11. The patient should be allowed to rest for several seconds and again be preoxygenated.

12. The procedure should be repeated if necessary to remove more secretions.

Nasopharyngeal Airways

When frequent, aggressive nasopharyngeal suctioning is indicated in a semicomatose patient, a nasopharyngeal airway (NPA) will lessen the trauma of frequent passage of the catheter. The NPA is a soft latex material that provides easy access to the trachea for nasopharyngeal suctioning. The nasal and pharyngeal mucosa are protected and the procedure thus becomes more comfortable to the patient. In addition, a fiberoptic bronchoscope may be passed through the airway if the procedure is indicated:

Endotracheal or Tracheostomy Suctioning

The procedures are the same, except sterile technique is followed and no lubrication is usually necessary, although it may be used if there is difficulty passing the catheter.

Sterile Suctioning

The technique for correct sterile suctioning of artificial airways is perhaps the most important and vital segment of care for the patient because it removes secretions that would otherwise obstruct the airway. If suctioning is not performed properly, it can cause physiologic or psychological trauma to the patient.

The equipment necessary for proper sterile suctioning includes proper mechanical apparatus, connecting tubing, sterile gloves, sterile saline, suction catheters and dressings. While suctioning the patient, it should be remembered that the patient's only air passage is being partially occluded. Thus, the suction catheter should never be larger than one-half the diameter of the tube opening; if it is larger, it may completely occlude the patient's air passage.

One method of determining the size of the catheter used for suctioning is to double the size of the trache tube in place and add two. Example: if the patient has a #6 tube, the calculation would be as follows: $6 + 6 = 12 + 2 = 14$; therefore, a 14fr catheter would be used for suctioning. The catheter used for *pharyngeal* suctioning should never be used for subsequent suctioning of the artificial airway, but the reverse of using an artificial airway suction catheter for pharyngeal suction is acceptable. Aseptic technique is absolutely necessary to minimize the risk of infection and, ideally, only disposable catheters should be used.

Suctioning may be necessary every few minutes when the patient initially returns from surgery because there is an increase in secretions which usually results from irritation of the endotracheal tube plus a reflex mechanism initiated by the surgical trauma. Usually by paying attention to the patient's color and respiration, the nurse or therapist can determine the amount of secretions present. Excessive mucus in the trachea or large bronchi is usually indicated by coarse rattling sounds. Fine bubbling sounds usually suggest fluid located more peripherally, i.e., in the alveolar spaces. If accumulated secretions are not cleared, they can cause respiratory and cardiac rates to increase; effective O_2 and CO_2 transfer is impaired, causing cyanosis to appear and low-grade fever to develop.

Extubation

Extubation or decannulation is the removal of the artificial airway. The patient is helped to gradually relearn normal breathing through his upper respiratory tract before the tube is removed. This can be a time of considerable fear and anxiety for patients because they have learned they can breathe safely through their tracheostomy but may become apprehensive when asked to breathe in a normal manner. The relearning process can be accomplished under the physician's direction by reducing the lumen of the tube for a day or two or by partially obstructing the tube's outer opening for increasing lengths of time. Eventually, the patient is able to tolerate the complete occlusion of his tracheostomy opening. This is sometimes difficult and similar to breathing through a straw with very *small* tubes.

Note: When occluding the tracheostomy opening with a cuffed tube, the cuff must be deflated first. Failure to do this will result in total obstruction of the patient's airway as you occlude the tube opening.

Fenestrated tubes have also been excellent for weaning the patient from the tracheostomy tube. Actually, they do not increase the airway resistance as in the above method and are probably more effective. They also allow the patient to talk and attempt to cough to mobilize secretions.

Close supervision should continue after extubation. After a tracheostomy tube is removed, the skin edges are usually taped together with butterfly strips for a few days until the wound heals. While healing, air will escape through the wound and reduce the effectiveness of the patient's cough. The patient should be instructed that the noise from the partially closed trachea is normal and small secretions should be removed from this area. The patient should be taught to hold a sterile dressing firmly over the incision when coughing until it is healed.

REFERENCES

Periodicals
Burke A: The advantages of stay sutures with tracheostomy. *Ann R Coll Surg Engl* 1981; 63:426–428.
Ching N, Nealon T: Clinical experience with new low-pressure high-volume tracheostomy cuffs. *NY State J Med* 1974; 74:2379.
Connor GH, et al: Tracheostomy. *Am J Nurs* 1972; 72:68.
Grielo H, et al: A low pressure cuff for tracheostomy tubes to minimize tracheal injury. *J Thorac Cardiovasc Surg* 1971; 62:898.
Kirimli B, King J, Pfaeffle H: Evaluation of tracheobronchial suction techniques. *J Thorac Cardiovasc Surg* 1970; 59:340.
Long J, West G: The Olympic trache button as an interim airway following tracheostomy tube removal. *Respiratory Care* 1981; 26:1269–1272.
Meade J: Tracheostomy—its complications and their management. *N Engl J Med* 1961; 265:519.
Pratt L: Complications of tracheotomy. *Eye Ear Nose Throat Mon* 1969; 48:119.
Seleckly P: Tracheostomy—a review of present day indications, complications and care. *Heart Lung* 1974; 3:272.
Trout C: Artificial airways: Tubes and tracheas. *Respir Care* 1976; 21:513.
Wanner A: Nasopharyngeal airway: A facilitated access to the trachea. *Ann Intern Med* 1971; 75:593–595.
Westaby S, Jackson JW, Pearson FG: A bifurcated silicone rubber stent for relief of tracheobronchial obstruction. *J Thorac Cardiovasc Surg* 1982; 83:414–417.
Yanagisawa E, Kirchner J: The cuffed tracheotomy tube: Its uses and its dangers. *Arch Otolaryngol* 1964; 79:80.
Books
Bendixen H, et al: *Respiratory Care*. St Louis, CV Mosby Co, 1965.

Goldin M: *Intensive Care of the Surgical Patient.* Chicago, Year Book Medical Publishers, 1971.

Airway Care

Burke A: The advantages of stay sutures with tracheostomy. *Ann R Coll Surg Engl* 1981; 63:426–428.

Gal TJ: Effects of endotracheal intubation on normal cough performance. *Anesthesiology* 1980; 52:324–329.

Orringer MB: Endotracheal intubation and tracheostomy: Indication, techniques, and complications. *Surg Clin North Am* 1980; 60:1447–1464.

Selecky PA: Tracheostomy: A review of present day indications, complications, and care. *Heart Lung* 1974; 3(2):272–283.

Selecky PA: Tracheal damage and prolonged intubation with a cuffed endotracheal or tracheostomy tube. *Heart Lung* 1976; 5(5):733.

Stauffer J, Silvestri R: Complications of endotracheal intubation, tracheostomy, and artificial airways. *Respiratory Care* 1982; 27(4):417–434.

Wanner A, Zighelboim A, Sackner M: Nasopharyngeal airway: A facilitated access to the tracheal. *Ann Intern Med* 1971; 75:4.

Wen-Hsien W, Il-Taik L, et al: Pressure dynamics of endotracheal and tracheostomy cuffs. *Crit Care Med* 1973; 1:4.

31

Respiratory and Cardiovascular Drug Actions

Arthur Prancan, Ph.D.

The respiratory and cardiovascular systems have many built-in mechanisms for controlling their function during health and disease. In healthy individuals, both systems act quickly and positively to maintain proper function under the most complicated conditions. Even during trauma or disease, these systems often overcome distress and regain normal function. The physiology of respiration or circulation is sometimes altered by a disease so that the homeostatic mechanisms are no longer effective. In such a case, a drug with the appropriate action becomes necessary to restore normal physiologic function.

Before a drug can be used effectively, the system it is to modify must be understood. Furthermore, how the mechanism of the drug action relates to the biologic system must be clear before an effect can be predicted.

This chapter describes much of the basic respiratory and cardiovascular physiology that underlies the action of the drugs presented. Hopefully, the relationship between basic physiology and the drug mechanism of action will also be evident.

All pharmacologic interventions for the respiratory and cardiovascular systems have not been covered. Certainly no attempt has been made to describe the pharmacology of other systems or disease states. For further study, I highly recommend any of the books listed in the reference section at the end of the chapter.

AUTONOMIC PHARMACOLOGY

This section introduces the basic aspects of drug action related to both components of the autonomic nervous system—the sympathetic and parasympathetic nervous systems. For both systems, synthesis, storage, and release of the chemical transmitter will be described to emphasize the places in that metabolic scheme where drugs can intervene. The sites of action for the adrenergic (sympathetic) and cholinergic (primarily parasympathetic) transmitters and blockers will also be described.

The autonomic nervous system controls all the bodily functions over which you have no voluntary control, and perhaps which you might not control so well if you had the opportunity. The functions include regulation of respiratory airway diameter, respiratory secretions, blood vessel diameter, heart rate, intestinal motility, pupil size, and many others. It is easy to see that it might take more than the talents of a well-trained expert to keep an active person functioning day and night.

The sympathetic nervous system is the half of the autonomic system that takes a dominant role in the cardiovascular and respiratory systems when some sort of bodily activity is necessary. This includes actions such as increasing ventilation capacity, elevating blood pressure, and shunting blood flow to the skeletal muscles. Classically, the sympathetic component of the autonomic nervous system has been called the "fight or flight" system. The other half of the autonomic system is called the parasympathetic nervous system. It is most important in maintaining the less exciting functions of the body like digestion, salivation, and urination. In some organs, the two systems work against each other to provide very fast and very fine control. For example, the size of the pupil responds quickly to an increase in light intensity. The parasympathetic system actively functions to decrease the size of the opening while the sympathetic system relaxes, thereby causing a quick decrease in pupil size. If the light is turned down, the opposite occurs just as fast. This is a good example of the antagonistic action of the two components of the autonomic nervous system.

Some organs, however, have only one innervation. Much of the arterial blood vessel network is controlled only by sympathetic nerves. Also, gastric secretion and gastric motility are primarily regulated by one system—the parasympathetic.

SYMPATHETIC NEUROTRANSMISSION

Sympathetic nerves transport impulses from the vasomotor center in the medulla of the brain through the spinal cord and out to the smooth muscle, heart muscle, and secretory cells. These tissues have receptor sites that will accept the norepinephrine released from the nerve ending. Norepinephrine, also called noradrenalin, is synthesized in the nerve ending only in the sympathetic neurons. It is stored in the terminal until an electric impulse reaches the terminal, then it is released into the synapse.

The norepinephrine molecule attaches to a receptor molecule on a cell surface in the immediate vicinity of its release. This drug-receptor combination causes a biologic change, such as stimulation of the pacemaker cells in the heart to fire more frequently (increased heart rate). The effect is terminated when the norepinephrine is reabsorbed into the nerve terminal. About 90% of the released norepinephrine is taken back into the neuron. There, it is either restored into granules for future release or it is destroyed by the enzyme monoamine oxidase (MAO).

There are two types of sympathetic receptors—alpha and beta. The alpha receptor is found in the arterioles, and the beta receptor is found in the arterioles, heart, and bronchioles. Stimulation of the alpha receptor in the arteriole causes vasoconstriction which results in increased blood pressure. The beta receptor in the arterioles causes vasodilation and a lowered blood pressure. Some drugs stimulate both receptors, and in those cases the effect will be determined by the degree of alpha or beta activity of the drug. An example is norepinephrine: it has 90% alpha activity and 10% beta activity, and it always causes vasoconstriction. Epinephrine is 50% alpha and 50% beta and may cause a rise or drop in blood pressure.

Stimulation of the beta receptor in the heart results in increased heart rate (beats per minute) and increased stroke volume (number of milliliters of blood the left ventricle pumps out into the aorta every time it contracts). Incidentally, the combination of these two changes (heart rate [HR] × stroke volume [SV]) is another way of saying cardiac output (CO) (milliliters of blood pumped per minute):

$$\text{beats/min(HR)} \times \text{ml/beat(SV)} = \text{ml/min(CO)}$$

This expression, cardiac output, is a common one and it constitutes half of the blood pressure regulation equation: $CO \times TPR = BP$, where CO is cardiac output, TPR is total peripheral resistance, and BP is blood pressure. Total peripheral resistance is determined by vasoconstriction or vasodilation in the arterioles. Vasoconstriction increases resistance so TPR goes up and BP goes up.

Stimulation of smooth muscle beta receptors will relax these tissues wherever they are found. Respiratory airway smooth muscle will decrease tension when the beta receptor is activated by beta-acting drugs like epinephrine or isoproterenol. The functional result will be an increase in air flow due to a larger airway diameter. Likewise, blood vessels respond to beta-acting drugs by increasing in diameter, allowing a greater rate of flow. In this case, TPR has decreased and blood pressure will drop.

Adrenergic Drugs

Norepinephrine, Levarterenol (Levophed)

As mentioned above, this is a mixed activity drug (90% alpha, 10% beta). It stimulates beta receptors in the heart, which results in an increase of heart rate and stroke volume (increased cardiac output). In the arterioles, norepinephrine causes vasoconstriction via the alpha receptor, resulting in increased total peripheral resistance. The total effect, of course, is an increase in blood pressure. Norepinephrine has little effect on the bronchioles. This drug is given only intravenously, and it can be used clinically to raise blood pressure. The natural sympathetic compounds are known as *catecholamines*.

Epinephrine (Adrenalin)

This is also a mixed activity drug (50% alpha, 50% beta). It is naturally produced in the adrenal medulla and can be released during sympathetic nervous system activation. When this occurs, it acts as a circulating hormone, stimulating both alpha and beta receptors. This drug will increase heart rate and stroke volume and may slightly increase or decrease total peripheral resistance at the arterioles. In any case, cardiac output always goes up; blood pressure may go up or down slightly.

In the bronchioles, epinephrine exerts a dramatic dilating effect which is mediated by the beta receptor. Epinephrine can be administered by inhalant aerosol to reverse a bronchoconstrictive episode. It is also administered intramuscularly and subcutaneously to treat asthma, anaphylactic reactions to an allergic response, low blood pressure, cardiogenic shock, and as a mild vasoconstrictor to keep local anesthetics at the injection site.

Isoproterenol (Isuprel)

This is a synthetic compound that has 100% beta activity. This means that it can increase heart rate and stroke volume to produce a great rise in cardiac output, while it stimulates the beta receptor on the arterioles to effect a profound vasodilation. The final result can be a high cardiac output with low blood pressure. This drug improves blood circulation in shock patients by increasing local blood flow (vasodilation) and elevating cardiac output. Isoproterenol is considered very useful for treating acute asthmatic conditions because of its bronchodilating action.

Phenylephrine (Isophrin, Neo-Synephrine) and Metaraminol

Both of these drugs are powerful and prolonged stimulators of alpha receptors. The action is directly on the receptor site itself. The response to the administration of either of these drugs is a rise in blood pressure due to vasoconstriction accompanied by a reflex bradycardia, which causes a decrease in cardiac output. Reflex alterations of cardiovascular function are explained later in this chapter. The primary usefulness of these drugs is in various hypotensive states. Phenylephrine is used as a nasal decongestant and a mydriatic and for the relief of paroxysmal atrial tachycardia. Phenylephrine affords relief from the tachycardia because it increases blood pressure and evokes the cardiovascular reflex which is marked by high vagal tone and bradycardia.

Ephedrine

Ephedrine has both alpha and beta activity as direct effects and it also causes release of epinephrine and norepinephrine. Its pharmacologic actions are similar to epinephrine, with the main exception that duration of action of ephedrine is longer. Ephedrine increases cardiac output and vascular resistance, resulting in increased blood pressure. Ephedrine also causes bronchial muscle relaxation which is less potent than that of epinephrine but has a longer duration. This drug is useful in controlling milder cases of bronchoconstriction that require long-term drug therapy.

Amphetamine (Benzedrine)

This drug has pharmacologic properties related to the catecholamines because it causes release of norepinephrine from the nerve terminal. Amphetamine has both alpha and beta receptor activity, although indirectly, through its release of norepinephrine. The usual cardiovascular response is an increase in blood pressure often accompanied by a reflex bradycardia. Amphetamine also has potent central nervous system (CNS) activity. It is a stimulant of the medullary respiratory center, and it can antagonize drug-related central nervous system depression. Respiratory depression often accompanies overdoses of CNS depressant drugs, and this effect may be overcome by amphetamine. This drug is usually used for its central nervous system effects and not for peripheral cardiovascular or respiratory effects.

β₂Receptor Stimulants

There are several drugs that act primarily at the β₂ smooth muscle receptor site, causing selective actions in the bronchioles and arterioles, but not in the heart. These drugs will produce a bronchodilation without increasing cardiac output. This particular lack of cardiovascular effect makes them safer and more useful than isoproterenol or epinephrine in treatment of bronchial asthma. The drugs are metaproterenol (Alupent, Metaprel), terbutaline (Brethaire, Brethine, Bricanyl), albuterol (Proventil, Ventolin), ritodrine and isoetharine (Bronkosol, Bronkometer).

Alpha-Adrenergic Blocking Drugs

Phentolamine (Regitine)

This is a competitive alpha receptor blocker. Its action is reversible. This drug prevents the hypertensive effect of norepinephrine, and it reverses the blood pressure elevating effect of epinephrine ("epinephrine reversal"). Epinephrine reversal looks like an isoproterenol effect with high cardiac output and low blood pressure. Phentolamine may be used clinically as a vasodilator. It is also useful as a clinical diagnostic agent in evaluating hypertensive patients who may have pheochromocytoma, which is a tumor that grows in the gastrointestinal chromaffin tissue. The tumor produces epinephrine and norepinephrine, and may be responsible for one aspect of a clinical hypertension.

Phenoxybenzamine (Dibenzyline)

This drug is also an alpha adrenergic blocking agent. It has effects similar to phentolamine in the cardiovascular system, but it is less reversible. This drug is gaining some usefulness in the treatment of shock syndromes characterized by high vascular tone.

Beta-Adrenergic Blocking Drugs

Propranolol (Inderal)

Propranolol is a beta-adrenergic blocker. This drug occupies the beta receptor sites of the heart, the blood vessels, and the bronchioles. It prevents the beta-adrenergic effect usually seen with drugs like epinephrine, norepinephrine, and isoproterenol. In the arterioles, when epinephrine is given following propranolol, the usual mixed alpha and beta effect is eliminated, leaving only an alpha-adrenergic action. This causes profound vasoconstriction, allowing greater increase in blood pressure than is normally seen with epinephrine alone. In the heart, the beta receptors are blocked, and since there are no alpha-adrenergic receptors in this organ, all effects of catecholamine drugs on the heart are effectively eliminated, allowing the vagal influence on the heart to predominate. Propranolol decreases the heart's requirement for oxygen because it blocks the cardiac stimulant action of norepinephrine. In the respiratory system, the administration of propranolol results in bronchoconstriction. This effect is increased dramatically in patients who are susceptible to asthma. The main use for propranolol is in conditions related to hypertension and tachycardia, where a decrease in cardiac output is beneficial.

Norepinephrine-Depleting Drugs

Reserpine

Reserpine is an alkaloid of *Rauwolfia serpentina,* also known as the Indian snake root plant. There are many commercial preparations of this compound, but it is widely sold as the simple plant extract. This compound depletes norepinephrine from the nerve endings in the various tissues of the body that produce and store norepinephrine, including the brain. The depletion takes several days to accomplish, and it may take several weeks to restore catecholamine levels to normal after therapy is discontinued. During this time, there is a decrease in catecholamine response to sympathetic stimulation. Blood pressure in humans does not drop dramatically with therapeutic doses of reserpine, but when reserpine is used in combination with diuretics or other antihypertensive agents, a significant hypertensive effect is obtained. Reserpine is used in this way to treat essential hypertension. One serious side effect related to reserpine use is the behavioral modification that can result in severe depression and suicide.

Guanethidine (Ismelin)

This is an adrenergic neuron-blocking agent that works by replacing norepinephrine in the nerve terminal. Norepinephrine is usually taken up by the nerve terminal after its discharge and is reused to maintain granule concentrations. Guanethidine takes the place of norepinephrine in the granules and prevents the reuptake of norepinephrine, thereby causing its metabolism outside of the neuron and its eventual depletion. The result on the cardiovascular system of this action is postural hypotension. The patient is unable to control blood pressure by sympathetic activity. This drug is used in treatment of severe hypertension, usually after diuretics and reserpine are shown to be ineffective.

Methyldopa (Aldomet)

This drug is also used in the treatment of hypertension. It enters the norepinephrine synthetic pathway and replaces dopa in that scheme. It goes through the metabolic scheme to produce methylnorepinephrine instead of norepinephrine. The methylnorepinephrine is a false transmitter and is released as norepinephrine would be, following a sympathetic stimulus, but it is ineffective in producing the biologic response required. This drug also causes postural hypotension because the sympathetic terminals are functionally ineffective. Methyldopa is used with diuretics to treat a hypertensive state. An additional action of this drug is to decrease the activity of the sympathetic nervous system at its control center in the brain. The consequence is a total decrease in sympathetic activity in the heart and blood vessels leading to a reduction in blood pressure.

Parasympathetic Neurotransmission

The center for parasympathetic control is the vagal nucleus in the medulla. The vagus nerves pass through the spinal cord and out to the heart, the smooth muscle and exocrine glands (salivary glands and pancreas). In all of these tissues, acetylcholine is released from the nerve terminals and combines with receptor sites to cause an effect such as bradycardia (slowing of the heart) or an increase in gastric motility. Acetylcholine is found in many parts of the central and peripheral nervous system. Acetylcholine is the only transmitter used in the parasympathetic system. It is used to transmit impulses from the nerve that comes out of the spinal cord to the nerve that finally reaches the cells in the organ being affected. This connection is called a *ganglion* and exists in both sympathetic and parasympathetic systems. Acetylcholine is also the neurotransmitter that makes the connection between the voluntary (somatic) nerves and the skeletal muscle.

There are two types of receptors in these systems. Acetylcholine affects both, but some drugs affect only one and not the other. The two types of receptors are called nicotinic and muscarinic, and they are named after the drugs that selectively stimulate them. Nicotine stimulates only those receptors in the ganglia and at the neuromuscular junction. The muscarinic receptor site is found everywhere a parasympathetic nerve terminal synapses at a tissue. The biologic effects usually attributed to the parasympathetic nervous system, such as bradycardia, salivation, and bronchoconstriction, for example, are produced when the muscarinic receptors are stimulated. Of course, it is also possible to stimulate muscarinic receptors indirectly with a nicotinic drug by activating the parasympathetic ganglia. In fact, in a similar way, it is possible to stimulate the entire sympathetic nervous system. The neurotransmitter at the sympathetic ganglia is acetylcholine and it affects nicotinic receptor sites there. One of the toxic effects of acetylcholine and drugs that act like it is hypertension with tachycardia, due to stimulation of the sympathetic postganglionic fibers.

To better understand the action of acetylcholine and related drugs, let us consider the synthesis, release, and inactivation of this transmitter. Acetylcholine is synthesized inside the nerve terminal from acetyl-CoA and choline. The acetylcholine is then stored in granules and is released out into the synapse when an action potential reaches the terminal. The acetylcholine molecule attaches to a receptor site, muscarinic or nicotinic, or to the enzyme that breaks it apart. Combination with the receptor site results in biologic action, and coupling with the enzyme ends in destruction. The enzyme, acetylcholinesterase, is found at all cholinergic synaptic sites. A nonspecific variety of the enzyme is also prevalent in many other tissues. It too will break down acetylcholine. The final action of either enzyme is the production of acetic acid and choline. The acetic acid is washed away for further metabolism, and the choline is reabsorbed into the nerve terminal for resynthesis to acetylcholine.

Cholinergic Drugs

Acetylcholine

This is the endogenous cholinergic transmitter that accounts for nicotinic and muscarinic actions within the autonomic nervous system.

It is rapidly hydrolyzed by acetylcholinesterase and the nonspecific cholinesterases, and therefore has a short duration of action if administered parenterally. This makes acetylcholine (ACh) a poor drug. Nicotinic effects of acetylcholine are (1) stimulation of parasympathetic ganglia causing occurrence of all muscarinic effects, (2) stimulation of sympathetic ganglia causing increase in vascular resistance and cardiac output to produce hypertension, and (3) stimulation of the neuromuscular junction (NMJ) at the skeletal muscle (muscle contraction and movement). Muscarinic effects of acetylcholine are bradycardia, salivation, pinpoint pupils, bronchial constriction, gastric and intestinal hypermotility, increased gastric acid and mucous secretion and facilitated urination. Toxic effects of cholinergic stimulation include diarrhea, urinary incontinence, bradycardia, bronchoconstriction, excessive salivation, CNS excitement, and respiratory collapse. In all of these toxic effects, atropine, a competitive muscarinic blocker, is the antidote of choice.

Bethanecol (Urecholine)

This drug is a synthetic choline ester that is not destroyed as easily as acetylcholine by cholinesterase enzymes. It is useful in treating patients with urinary retention and paralytic ileus, and it is administered orally or subcutaneously. The side effects and toxicities for this drug are exactly those for ACh. However, since the drug is not given intravenously, cardiac and respiratory effects are minimized.

Carbachol (Carcholin)

Carbachol is a mixed nicotinic and muscarinic drug because it releases acetylcholine from the nerve ending, producing the expected cholinergic effects at all receptor sites. The drug is useful for treatment of glaucoma (applied topically), paralytic ileus, and urinary retention (orally, subcutaneously).

Pilocarpine

This is a cholinomimetic that is useful in ophthalmology as an antiglaucoma agent. Cholinergic compounds decrease intraocular pressure by relieving the obstruction to the canal of Schlemm, a drainage circuit for the eye. Miosis (pinpoint pupils) is one feature of cholinergic therapy and may be beneficial to glaucoma treatment because the muscular base of the relaxed iris may contribute to the drainage block. Another use of pilocarpine is to promote salivary flow in patients with a ganglionic blockade.

Anticholinesterases

Before proceeding to specific anticholinesterase drugs, it is important to understand the basic mechanism of action for these compounds. Acetylcholinesterase is the enzyme responsible for destroying acetylcholine at the various nerve junctions where it is released. The class of drugs that interfere with this function is called anticholinesterases. These drugs attach to the enzyme and thereby block the enzymatic hydrolysis of ACh, causing ACh to accumulate outside of the nerve ending. This results in a greater response than normal to any cholinergic nerve stimulation. Some of these anticholinesterases are relatively short-acting compounds and are therapeutically important, while others are extremely long-lasting and potent compounds that are important only as poisons. The long-acting compounds have been used as insecticides and as nerve gases in chemical warfare. The therapeutically useful anticholinesterases are beneficial in problems related to the eye, intestine, and the skeletal neuromuscular junction (NMJ). In these applications, these drugs increase the amount of ACh available for activity, an effect that is especially important in cases where the synthesis or release of acetylcholine is lower than normal, as in myasthenia gravis.

There is also great medical interest in the toxicology of the anticholinesterases, especially the extremely potent irreversible anticholinesterases. Toxicity due to these compounds is not uncommon and is often severe. When a toxic irreversible anticholinesterase such as diisopropylfluorophosphate (DFP) or sarin is ingested, inhaled, or absorbed across the skin, a great variety of toxic cholinergic effects are seen. The first effects seen after exposure to an anticholinesterase are often ocular and respiratory effects. In the eyes, marked miosis is produced quickly. In the respiratory system, bronchoconstriction and bronchial secretions combine to produce tightness in the chest and wheezing. Gastrointestinal symptoms include nausea, vomiting, cramps, and diarrhea. Other muscarinic effects are severe salivation, involuntary defecation and urination, sweating, lacrimation, bradycardia, and hypotension.

Further effects are related to nicotinic functions of acetylcholine. These include skeletal muscle twitching, weakness, and paralysis. CNS effects include depression of the respiratory and cardiovascular control centers, leading to respiratory collapse. At the time of death, respiratory paralysis is evident and it is due to a combination of bronchoconstriction, bronchosecretions, respiratory muscle paralysis from overstimulation, and CNS and control depression. The treatment of this toxicity is closely related to preserving respiratory function. Administration of atropine, a muscarinic blocker, will effectively decrease bronchoconstriction and secretion. Another drug, pralidoxime (Protopam), is used to reactivate the acetylcholinesterase. It is most effective shortly after exposure to the toxic agent as it breaks down the anticholinesterase so it can be removed from the enzyme site. Additional measures are related to physiologic support of the patient. Maintenance of any airway, artificial respiration, and oxygen administration are important therapeutic applications for these patients.

Physostigmine (Eserine)

This drug is useful in glaucoma and in selected therapeutic measures where a cholinergic effect is beneficial. It functions as an indirect cholinomimetic by blocking the acetylcholinesterase.

Neostigmine (Prostigmine)

Neostigmine is useful in patients with nonobstructive paralytic ileus to increase tone and motility of the small and large intestines. It is also useful for stimulating the skeletal NMJ. Neostigmine is used for treating myasthenia gravis because it indirectly increases acetylcholine at the NMJ and it acts directly at the nicotinic receptor site itself. The disease is marked by subnormal response to acetylcholine, resulting in skeletal muscle weakness. Neostigmine temporarily restores muscle strength.

Edrophonium (Tensilon)

This is a very short-acting anticholinesterase. It is primarily useful as a diagnostic agent in myasthenia gravis to reveal, for a few minutes, if the dose of neostigmine is appropriate. A longer-acting drug would risk a serious cholinergic toxicity if the neostigmine dose was already at the therapeutic limit.

Cholinergic Blocking Drugs

Cholinergic antagonists block the various receptor sites where acetylcholine is a transmitter. There are specific blocking drugs for each type of acetylcholine receptor. Atropine blocks all cholinergic action right at the muscarinic receptor site on smooth muscle, exocrine glands, and myocardium. Another cholinergic antagonist, curare, works only at the neuromuscular junction to block the nicotinic effect of acetylcholine, resulting in paralysis of skeletal muscle. Still another type of nicotinic blocker is the ganglionic blocker, hexamethonium, which blocks both sympathetic and parasympathetic ganglia by occupying the acetylcholine receptor there. These drugs are useful wherever sympathetic or parasympathetic tone needs to be decreased. It is possible to selectively inhibit cholinergic effects in the body in order to produce a desired effect or to eliminate an undesirable effect. Because of this selectiveness, cholinergic antagonists have widespread use in many areas of medicine.

Atropine

Atropine is an extract from the plant *Atropa belladonna,* also known as the deadly nightshade. Another plant extract, scopolamine, has action similar to atropine. Atropine works by establishing a competitive blockade at the muscarinic receptor site, which is the effector at all tissues innervated by the parasympathetic nervous system. This blockade is selective for the tissue effect of the parasympathetic system and does not counteract the nicotinic ganglionic effects or the nicotinic effects at the NMJ.

Because heart rate is controlled by both sympathetic and parasympathetic tone, atropine will eliminate the parasympathetic effect on the heart, allowing the sympathetic system to increase heart rate and stroke volume to cause an increase in cardiac output. In fact, tachycardia may occur following atropine administration. In cases where bradycardia exists due to high vagal tone, atropine can be used to reverse this depression.

In the respiratory tract, atropine is a bronchodilator. It is also possible to delay respiratory depression associated with anesthetic, tranquilizing and anticholinesterase drugs by using atropine, either as a pretreatment agent or as an antidote during overdose.

Atropine is used widely as preanesthetic medication to prevent bronchiolar secretions and laryngeal spasm, as well as bradycardia. A more general medical use for atropine exists as an emergency tool. It is the antidote of choice for all cholinergic toxicities.

One of the most important clinical uses for atropine is the gastrointestinal tract as a antiulcer and antispasmodic agent. This drug acts to decrease motility in the GI tract so that other antiulcer agents can remain in contact with the GI mucosa longer, and it is possible that it also decreases acid secretion. Other problems related to hypermotility of the GI tract are treated with atropine, mainly to decrease gastric muscle activity during treatment of conditions such as cramping and diarrhea.

In ophthalmology, atropine is useful for producing mydriasis, which is pupillary dilation. It is contraindicated in glaucoma patients because it may precipitate an acute attack.

Atropine itself is also capable of producing toxic effects. These are mydriasis, tachycardia, dry mouth, constipation, and urinary retention.

Effects related to the central nervous system are also apparent, and these include sedation initially, followed by delirium and hallucinations, which lead to a coma. In severe toxicities, the patient convulses and experiences severe respiratory depression which may be the final course. Anticholinesterase drugs such as physostigmine and neostigmine are effective antidotes for atropine because they increase the amount of acetylcholine which will compete with atropine for the receptor site.

Homatropine (Novatrin) and Cyclopentolate (Cyclogyl)

These are anticholinergic drugs related in action to atropine. They are useful in ophthalmology to produce mydriasis.

Dicyclomine (Bentyl)

This drug is considered very useful in the gastrointestinal tract to decrease secretions and motility. It is sometimes called a chemical vagotomy.

Trihexyphenidyl HCL (Artane) and Benztropine Mesylate (Cogentin)

These are antiParkinson drugs that enter the CNS to reverse the imbalance between the cholinergic and dopaminergic systems in this disease. They have some of the same side effects as atropine.

Pentolinium (Ansolysen) and Hexamethonium (Methium)

These are nicotinic antagonists. They block the acetylcholine receptor site in the ganglia in both the sympathetic and parasympathetic nervous systems. They are used to control hypertension, which is due to a high sympathetic tone. Because of their blocking action at the sympathetic ganglion, these drugs will produce a postural hypotension. They will also decrease cholinergic effects at the parasympathetic effector sites because they block the ganglia for the entire parasympathetic nervous system as well. This means that a patient may experience blurred vision, dryness of mouth, and tachycardia, as well as other atropine-like peripheral effects.

The Cardiovascular Reflex

The cardiovascular reflex involves many of the components of the autonomic nervous system to maintain a normal blood pressure. This mechanism is important for maintaining blood pressure within certain limits during all phases of physical activity. Even the simple act of standing from a sitting position requires prompt compensation by this reflex system. If in some way this reflex is interrupted, a condition known as *orthostatic* hypotension will exist. A common manifestation of this condition is fainting upon standing due to inadequate blood flow to the brain. This section is devoted to the functional aspects of the reflex following a change in blood pressure.

The Carotid Baroreceptors

Neuronal elements, known as *baroreceptors,* exist in the sinus of the carotid arteries supplying the brain. These are stretch receptors that fire electrical impulses at a rate directly related to the blood pressure. As the pressure in the artery increases, the vessel wall (and baroreceptor) stretches, causing an increase in the receptor firing rate. Conversely, a decrease in blood pressure results in a decrease in stretch receptor firing rate. This firing rate signal is sent directly to the brain, where the vasomotor center and vagal nucleus respond to it.

The Functional Reflex

To create an example for demonstrating this reflex, let us assume we have just experienced a loss of blood pressure. The carotid baroreceptors shorten and slow their firing. This message is then delivered to the brain, and the vasomotor center responds by increasing sympathetic nerve activity. This control always responds to information regarding blood pressure in the carotid artery by doing the opposite of the baroreceptors. If the pressure had risen, the baroreceptors would have increased their firing rate and the vasomotor center would have responded by slowing the sympathetic nerve firing rate. Since the blood pressure in this example is low, the vasomotor center increases sympathetic nerve firing, resulting in increased release of norepinephrine from the nerves that reach the heart and arterioles. Norepinephrine increases the heart rate and stroke volume, thereby producing an increase in cardiac output. In the arterioles, norepinephrine stimulates the alpha receptors, producing vasoconstriction, which results in increased resistance to blood flow. Elevation of cardiac output and vascular resistance result in raised blood pressure. A third component of the sympathetic nervous system can be involved during sympathetic activation. Epinephrine released from the adrenal medulla will also increase cardiac output.

Meanwhile, the vagal nucleus is responding to the decreased baroreceptor firing by decreasing its own activity. The vagus nerve to the heart will release less acetylcholine, allowing the sympathetic effect to predominate. The total effect becomes an increase in blood pressure, which is the response required to return the systemic pressure to normal. If the original pressure alteration had been an increase above normal, the opposite reflexive actions would have occurred to return pressure to a normal range. In this case, the predominant effect would have been an increase in vagal nerve tone, releasing high amounts of acetylcholine at the heart, causing a dramatic slowing of heart rate, accompanied by a decrease in stroke volume. This combination produces a decrease in cardiac output. The sympathetic system would have responded to the increased baroreceptor firing by decreasing firing in all sympathetic nerves, thereby decreasing norepinephrine and epinephrine release. All of these factors combine to decrease blood pressure to normal.

Drugs Used in Airway Obstructive Disease

Patients suffering from asthma, emphysema, and chronic bronchitis may have an obstructed airway for several reasons. Acute asthmatic obstruction and some chronic airway obstruction are due to bronchial smooth muscle contraction, resulting in a smaller diameter airway. Inflamed passageways, which are swollen due to edema, may also constitute an airway obstruction. A further complication seen in many respiratory diseases is the thickening and collection of secretions that cannot be eliminated from the respiratory tree and subsequently block the airway. In this section, the various drugs that can reverse smooth muscle contraction, inflammatory edema, and collection of secretions will be presented.

A variety of therapeutic mechanisms are useful against this collection of obstructive conditions. The single most effective mechanism for relief of smooth muscle spasm is the β_2 activity that is available in some of the adrenergic agents. Other useful mechanisms aim at potentiating the beta activity of adrenergic agents, decongesting the inflamed airway, decreasing release of histamine, and in a broader approach, the general stabilization of cells that can release mediators of the disease, thereby lowering the severity of the disease.

Sympathomimetic Drugs

Isoproterenol (Isuprel) and Epinephrine (Adrenalin)

The muscle relaxant bronchodilator effect attributed to the beta-adrenergic sympathomimetic compounds is most commonly required for asthmatic or allergic emergencies. Isoproterenol is often self-administered by inhalation to reverse mild to moderate obstructive episodes. However, during a severe acute obstruction, the airway is unable to pass the drug to the alveoli, and the intramuscular or subcutaneous routes for epinephrine and isoproterenol are used. Isoproterenol is a purely beta compound. Epinephrine has 50% beta-adrenergic activity and also exerts a great bronchodilating effect. Both of these agents are useful when given parenterally or by inhalation. The most common side effects of isoproterenol are flushing of the skin, headache, palpitation, and tachycardia. Epinephrine may cause an anxiety reaction in a patient along with headache, palpitations, and respiratory difficulty. Both drugs can cause serious cardiac reactions (arrhythmias), which have resulted in death.

Metaproterenol (Alupent) and Isoetharine (With Phenylephrine, Bronkosol-2)

These are isoproterenol analogs that exert most of their action on respiratory or vascular smooth muscle but have little effect on the heart. They are useful compounds for selectively relaxing bronchial smooth muscles without directly affecting the heart. The major advantage of these drugs is that their action on the heart is approximately one-tenth that of isoproterenol or epinephrine, and their potential for inducing cardiac toxicities is correspondingly reduced. However, because vascular smooth muscle responds much like respiratory smooth muscle to these drugs, arterial resistance will be decreased, leading to a drop in blood pressure and a reflexive tachycardia. The β agonists are often given by inhalation.

Ephedrine

Ephedrine is a sympathomimetic that acts by liberating norepinephrine and epinephrine from storage sites in addition to having a possible direct effect on adrenergic receptors. Its usefulness and side effects are similar to those of epinephrine. One beneficial factor in ephedrine use is that it can be administered orally for convenient long-term therapy.

Phenylephrine (Neo-Synephrine)

This drug is useful for its alpha-adrenergic effects when treating airway obstruction due to edematous swelling. It may be used in conjunction with isoproterenol because it can exert a decongestant action in the respiratory tract that reduces edema or swelling of those tissues. Using an alpha-adrenergic agonist with isoproterenol has been shown to be more effective than using isoproterenol alone. The side effects of phenylephrine include an increase in systemic blood pressure (because of its alpha-adrenergic vasoconstricting activity) with a reflex decrease in the heart rate. This reflex bradycardia moderates the usual increase in heart rate associated with using isoproterenol alone. The reflex bradycardia can also be used to advantage when the drug is combined with the β_2 drugs. Phenylephrine would not be combined with epinephrine because one-half of epinephrine action is an α_1 component.

Xanthines

These drugs have effects similar to the catecholamines in the respiratory and cardiovascular systems. This similarity in effect may be due to the elevation of cyclic AMP. Both the catecholamines and xanthines are known to produce elevated cyclic AMP levels in the tissues they stimulate. The catecholamines activate adenyl cyclase, the enzyme that converts ATP to cyclic AMP. The newly formed cyclic AMP exerts its effects on the local tisssue (e.g., bronchial muscle relaxation) and is inactivated by the enzyme phosphodiesterase. The xanthines inhibit phosphodiesterase, conserving cyclic AMP and thereby promoting its effects. An additional action of xanthines may be a direct smooth muscle relaxation that could increase airway diameter.

Theophylline and Aminophylline

Drugs in this class are structurally very similar to caffeine. They are used to control asthma when given orally or intravenously. Theophylline is often used orally for long-term maintenance of mild to moderate disease. One of the most common uses for aminophylline is the treatment of acute asthmatic airway obstruction, especially in cases that do not respond to epinephrine alone. Intravenous administration of this drug increases the opportunity for serious side effects, which are hypotension and cardiac arrhythmias.

Corticosteroids

The anti-inflammatory steroids are related to the naturally occurring glucocorticoid, cortisol (Prednisone, Methylprednisolone, Beclomethasone). Many compounds have been synthetically derived to produce a variety of anti-inflammatory potencies. The usefulness of corticosteroids in treating respiratory diseases depends upon the ability of these drugs to depress the symptoms of inflamed tissue. The mechanism of action for the drugs, however, has not clearly been defined. Some specific effects of corticosteroids that relate to the anti-inflammatory action are decreased capillary dilation and permeability, and stabilization of lysosomal membranes in white blood cells. In addition, these compounds decrease the synthesis of compounds that can promote broncho-obstructive disease: prostaglandins and leukotrienes. The long-term use of the corticosteroids is recommended only after other measures fail. The reason for this caution is that they produce serious side effects and permanent changes if used for two weeks or longer. After one week of corticosteroid therapy, behavioral changes and acute peptic ulcers may be observed. However, when longer therapy is instituted and adrenal suppression occurs, the patient requires supplemental corticosteroid therapy until normal adrenal cortex function is restored. This state of insufficiency may last for as long as several months after suppression. Most patients who receive corticosteroids for long-term therapy develop a condition called Cushing's syndrome. It is characterized by wasting of muscles due to the breakdown of protein and by redistribution of fat from the extremities to the face and the trunk. Eventually these patients develop osteoporosis and diabetes. Other serious complications are peptic ulcers, psychosis, glaucoma, intercranial hypertension, and growth retardation.

Antihistamine

Sodium Cromoglycate (Intal)
Cromolyn has a limited usefulness compared to the other drugs presented here—it can only prevent an asthmatic episode. The mechanism of action is probably the stabilization of the mast cell which synthesizes, stores, and releases histamine. Since histamine can precipitate broncho-obstructive reactions, this drug is useful in preventing its release. Cromolyn is administered by inhalation.

Mucolytics and Expectorants

Acetylcysteine (Mucomyst) and Pancreatic Dornase (Dornavac)
These drugs act by breaking the chemical bonds that hold together the large protein structure that contributes to the viscosity of mucus. Mucolytics are inhaled to liquify mucus so that it can be moved out of the bronchial tract to prevent airway obstruction. Side effects associated with these drugs are bronchospasm, nausea, and vomiting. Acetylcysteine also inactivates the penicillin antibiotics and is contraindicated in their presence.

Trypsin (Tryptar)
This proteolytic enzyme may also be useful for liquifying respiratory secretions. It can be administered by inhalation although it can

cause irritation to the eyes, nose, and throat. An additional problem with this drug is a possible anaphylactic reaction in sensitized patients. There is a variety of other enzymes with specific actions on protein that may be useful in liquifying secretions.

Sodium Iodide and Potassium Iodide

These expectorants act by increasing the amount of respiratory secretion so that it is relatively less viscous and can be more easily removed. The iodide salts are often used in late bronchitis, bronchiectasis, and asthma, and they break up especially tough bronchial secretions by attracting fluid to the respiratory tract. Characteristic side effects with these compounds are gastric irritation, nausea, and vomiting. More serious complications occasionally involve the respiratory tract. These patients wheeze and experience bronchial spasm. Other expectorants that are usually used in mixtures or administered as cough syrups are ammonium chloride, syrup of ipecac, and glyceryl guaiacolate. These are useful for patients who cannot tolerate the iodide salts.

REFERENCES

Gilman A, Goodman L, Rall T, et al (eds): *The Pharmacological Basis of Therapeutics,* ed 7. New York, Macmillan Publishing Co, 1985.

Goth A: *Medical Pharmacology: Principles and Concepts,* ed 11. St Louis, CV Mosby Co, 1984.

Gurwitz D, Levisonit J, Mindorff C, et al: Assessment of a new device (aerochamber) for use with aerosol drugs for asthmatic children. *Ann Allergy* 1983; 50(3):166–170.

Lee HS: Proper aerosol inhalation techniques for delivery of asthma medications. *Clin Pediatr (Phila)* 1983; 22(6):440–443.

Melmon KL, (ed): *Clinical Pharmacology: Basic Principles in Therapeutics,* ed 2. New York, Macmillan Publishing Co, 1978.

Milner AD: Steroids and asthma. *Pharmacol Ther* 1982; 17(2):229–238.

Pederson S: Aerosol treatment of bronchoconstriction in children with or without a tube spacer. *N Engl J Med* 1983; 2:308(22):1328–1330.

Weiner P, Greif J, Fireman E, et al: Bronchodilating effect of cromolyn sodium in asthmatic patients at rest and following exercise. *Ann Allergy* 1984; 53(2):186–188.

32

Principles of Chest X-ray Interpretation

Thomas Johnson, M.D.

There are three general categories of radiographic studies of the chest—fixed-position studies, suspended motion studies, and motion studies. The routine posteroanterior (PA) and lateral chest film is a fixed-position, suspended motion study. The patient is positioned with his chest against the x-ray film holder and is asked to hold his breath in deep inspiration.

The radiograph is named from the source of the x-rays to the film. Thus, a PA chest film is positioned so that the source of the x-rays is behind the patient and the film is in front. An anteroposterior (AP) chest film is the reverse, with the back of the patient against the film. During interpretation, the conventional position of the film on the view box is as if you were facing the patient.

One of the first things to check before interpreting the film is the quality of the film. An optimal PA chest film is one in which you see the dim outline of the vertebral bodies through the mediastinum. Films may be overpenetrated (of increased density) or underpenetrated (of decreased density) and still be adequate for interpretation. Suboptimal films may also hide pathology and cause misinterpretation.

The purpose of a radiograph (x-ray) is to see inside the otherwise opaque body by shifting the spectrum of light to above the high ranges of the visible spectrum, thus converting the body structures into densities rather than colors. The densities recorded on the x-ray film are shades of gray to black depending on the amount of x-ray energy the structures of the body absorb as the x-ray passes through them.

There are five basic densities, varying from very radiolucent to very radiopaque. The darkest or most radiolucent density is gas or air. Fat is moderately radiolucent. An intermediate or water density is seen reflecting the connective tissues, blood, muscle, skin and other structures. Bone and deposited calcium are moderately radiopaque. Metal is the most opaque (white or clear). The structures of the body absorb most of the x-rays as they pass through the body, and the remainder of the rays expose the film.

During the process of radiography, familiar fruits or objects are converted into a two-dimensional reproduction of densities (Fig 32–1). Three-dimensional structures are reduced to two dimensions and only the edges or structures tangential to the beam of the x-rays are recorded. Thus, two views, taken at 90 degrees from each other (PA and lateral), are required for a mental reconstruction of the third dimension, which we use to interpret the internal problems of a patient.

The routine examination of the chest should include a PA and lat-

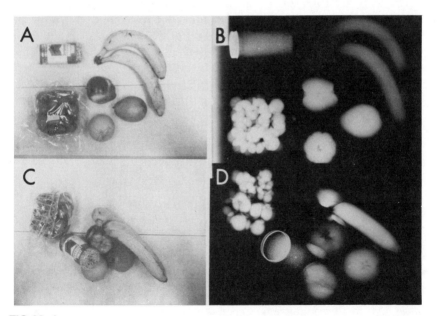

FIG 32–1.
Familiar fruits such as an apple, orange, pear and banana **(A and C)** transform into two-dimensional objects when x-rayed **(B and D).** The pictures **(A and C)** also show a box of cherry tomatoes and a jar of bird seed (millet seed) and their x-rays. **B** is the radiograph of **A,** and **D** is the radiograph of **C.** Changes in position of the same objects from **A** to **C** illustrate the changes of shape in the corresponding x-rays, **B** to **D,** and emphasize the need for PA and lateral x-rays for evaluating three-dimensional structures.

eral chest film at least for the first examination. Without the lateral film, disease processes behind the heart and posterior in the thorax may be missed. Very ill patients who cannot be transported to the radiology department must often be evaluated from a single PA or AP view (taken with the portable x-ray unit). The size of the patient introduces mechanical limitations to the performance of a lateral chest film. Portable x-ray units are not as powerful as the stationary departmental machines.

Additional radiographic views may be ordered to verify or elucidate findings. These include (1) oblique views; (2) apical lordotic views; (3) decubitus views; (4) laminograms; (5) inspiration and expiration films; (6) special studies requiring contrast materials; and (7) physiologic motion evaluation with the fluoroscope.

Film interpretation requires a solid knowledge of gross anatomy and gross pathology. You are literally looking at the internal structures of the body without an autopsy or surgical operations. The structures of the body are thus converted into the densities of air, fat, water, calcium and metal. Look at the entire film, not just one area—don't get "tunnel vision." Once an abnormality is found, continue to evaluate the remainder of the film; do not stop at that point since other pathologies may be present. Remember to look at all the anatomical structures on the film, including the soft tissues, bony thorax, mediastinal structures, hilar areas, lung fields and the corners of the film (Fig 32–2).

The tools of radiographic interpretation include:

1. The principle of bilateral symmetry (when structures are paired, then in general one should look like the other).

2. The presence or absence of air fluid levels (there are almost no straight lines in the chest). If a line appears to be straight then it must be explained.

3. The silhouette sign. When densities are next to each other, they obliterate the margins and show no separation. When densities or structures are in front or in back of other densities or structures, then a margin is seen.

4. An air bronchogram is seen when the air around a bronchus is pathologically filled with fluid or other material.

5. Lobar and segmental collapse follows the anatomy of the lung.

6. Pleural changes may be manifested by gas in a pneumothorax, fluid in a pleural effusion or calcium. A hydropneumothorax demonstrates an air fluid level. Pleural reaction is residual fibrosis.

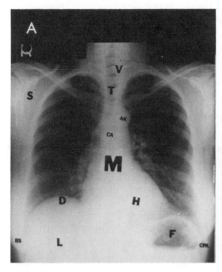 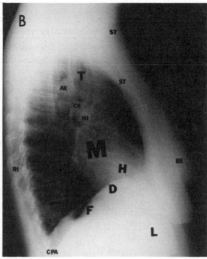

FIG 32–2.
These PA **(A)** and lateral **(B)** x-rays anatomically localize the basic structures that must be reviewed during chest x-ray evaluation. Some of the structures are seen in both views and others are seen in only one view. During evaluation, one should identify and see the following basic anatomical structures.

Soft tissues and *extrathoracic structures:* soft tissues *(ST)*, breast shadows *(BS)*, diaphragm *(D)*, liver *(L)*, and fundus of stomach *(F)*.

Bony thorax: ribs *(RI)*, vertebrae *(V)*, scapulae (*S*, seen best on PA), clavicles (*CL*, seen best on PA) and sternum (*ST*, seen best on lateral).

Mediastinal structures: mediastinum *(M)*, trachea *(T)*, carina *(CA)*, aortic knob *(AK)*, heart *(H)*, anterior clear space *(ACS*, seen on lateral) and hilus of lungs *(HI)*.

Lung fields: hilus of lungs *(HI)*, pulmonary vessels (arise from hilus and branch outward), costophrenic angles *(CPA)* and lung apices (*LA*, seen best on PA).

There are many other structures that must be evaluated in addition to these basic ones, and pathologies must be identified.

7. The presence or absence of mass formation as in tumors, nodular changes or miliary changes. The conventional terminology depends on the size of the abnormality.

The key to what happens in the lung fields is an evaluation of the vascularity. Bronchi are not usually seen unless they are surrounded by fluid or have a disease causing thickening of the walls. The vascular pattern may be distorted, blurred, increased or decreased by pulmonary disease.

Air space or alveolar disease is manifested by opacification (white appearance) of air-filled structures of the lung in a logical progression from the periphery to the center. Thus, pneumonia may appear as patchy coalescent areas of acini, or segmental and/or lobar consolidation. An air bronchogram is seen when the air-filled lung tissue about the bronchus is filled with fluid or other material and the bronchus is filled with air. There is usually a moderately rapid change of findings in air space or alveolar disease, with changes occurring in approximately 24 hours or less (Fig 32–3).

Interstitial pulmonary disease is manifested by distortion or loss of the vascularity. The normal tissues are affected and scarring may be the end result. A loss of alveolar walls with enlargement of the air-containing spaces is characteristic of emphysema. Enlargement of the bronchi may result in bronchiectasis. End-stage fibrosis may result from many causes and is irreversible (Fig 32–4).

Translated from the original language *pneumonia* means inflammation of the lung. Pneumonias are identified by their anatomical characteristics and causative agents. A lobar pneumonia is one that involves the entire lobe, and a segmental pneumonia involves the anatomical segment of a lobe. Generalized pneumonic processes occur with aspiration or vascular spread of an infectious agent (Fig 32–5).

Pulmonary abscesses and cavities may occur secondary to pneumonia or atelectasis or both. An abscess occurs when there is a break-

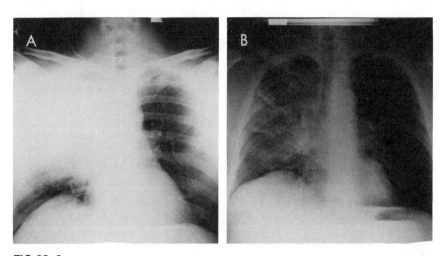

FIG 32–3.
A, there is total pneumonic consolidation of right upper lobe with complete alveolar and bronchial filling. **B,** approximately 24–36 hours later, the consolidation has cleared markedly with patchy coalescent residual. A few air bronchograms are seen in the perihilar region.

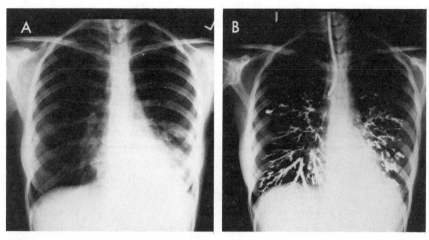

FIG 32–4.
A, fibrosis and saccular bronchiectatic changes are present in the left lower lobe. A few cystic "circular" changes are present in the right upper lobe but are best seen on the bronchogram. **B,** the bronchogram demonstrates the dilated abnormal bronchi of cystic and saccular bronchiectasis in the left lower lobe with fibrosis around them. The right upper lobe reveals a few cystic changes.

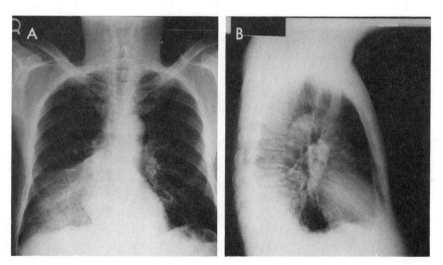

FIG 32–5.
A, the PA chest film demonstrates the water density of a pneumonic consolidation in the right lower lobe. The diaphragm is blurred. **B,** the lateral film shows obliteration of the posterior right diaphragm and the costophrenic angle by the pneumonic consolidation.

down of the tissues of the lung, with the area replaced by infectious materials. When the infectious materials empty into the bronchus, a cavity develops in that area of the lung. Since lung abscesses often result from aspiration, they are frequently found in the areas dependent at the time of the aspiration. Thus, abscesses occur in the area that is downward by gravity, depending on the upright or lying position of the individual (Fig 32–6). If the pleura is penetrated by the abscess, then a pneumothorax develops with a bronchopleural fistula.

A pneumothorax or gas in the pleural space develops when the pleural space communicates with the air around us through either a defect in the chest wall or a defect in the pleural surface of the lung because the normal pleural pressure is less than the atmospheric pressure (Fig 32–7). Chronic interstitial disease and emphysema are often complicated by a spontaneous pneumothorax. Traumatic causes, such as automobile accidents or insertion of central venous pressure catheters, may result in a traumatic pneumothorax. The appearance is fairly characteristic and there may be an associated air fluid level with a hydropneumothorax.

Atelectasis is the term used for incomplete expansion of a portion or all of the lung. There is a loss of air in the alveoli in the atelectatic

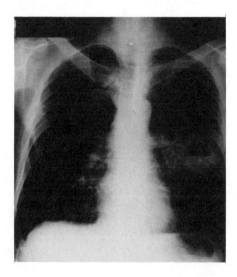

FIG 32–6.
A 5-cm cavitary abscess is seen on the left with an air fluid level and a relatively smooth wall. This patient was probably recumbent and lying slightly on his left side to aspirate materials to this area, which was first a pneumonic process in the superior segment of the left lower lobe and progressed to an abscess cavity.

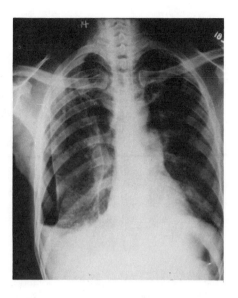

FIG 32–7.
The chest x-ray reveals separation of the visceral from the parietal pleural line and absence of vessels laterally. A "straight line" is seen at the right base, indicating a gas fluid level in a hydropneumothorax. Fibrotic and irregular pulmonary changes in the lungs indicate underlying interstitial disease, which was a pneumoconiosis (silicosis).

area. Atelectasis is a sign of disease since it is always secondary to another lesion, such as: (1) obstruction of a bronchus; (2) decreased motion secondary to paralysis or pleural disease; or (3) loss of ability for pulmonary expansion due to pleural disease, diaphragmatic disease and masses in the thorax.

Atelectasis is a loss of volume in the area involved and results in a decrease in size or a change in position of the surrounding structures (Fig 32–8).

Congestive failure, uremia and pulmonary edema may be manifested by a "butterfly" pattern on the chest film. Fluid is seen opacifying the central area of the lungs with sparing of the periphery (Fig 32–9). From congestive failure to pulmonary edema is a logical progression in most patients. The first manifestation is an increase in the antigravity vasculature of the lungs. In the upright patient this would be in the upper lung fields. The next stage is interstitial edema which is manifested by a loss of the distinct margins of the vessels and blurring of the margins. Pulmonary edema is present when the fluid seeps from the interstitium and opacifies the alveoli. At that time, pulmonary edema is indistinguishable from pneumonia. Congestive failure usually

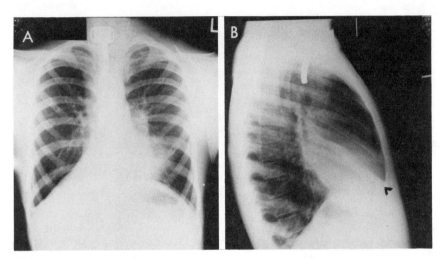

FIG 32–8.
A, the PA film demonstrates loss of the right heart border and the downward shift of the minor fissure, with atelectasis of the right middle lobe secondary to a radiolucent foreign body in the right middle lobe bronchus. No air remains in the middle lobe, thus it is dense. **B,** the *arrow* on the lateral view points to the residual tissue density of the right middle lobe, which is atelectatic.

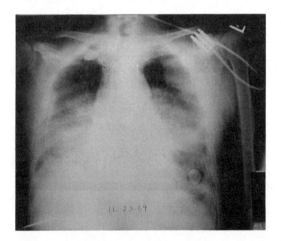

FIG 32–9.
The central lung fields reveal increased density and there is sparing of the peripheral areas in "butterfly" pulmonary edema. The patient has had a thoracotomy and chest tubes are in place.

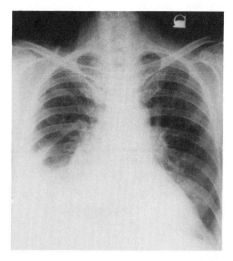

FIG 32–10.
The chest film reveals cardiomegaly (enlargement of the cardiopericardial silhouette) and bilateral pleural effusions are more marked on the right than on the left. Vascular structures are blurred with interstitial edema.

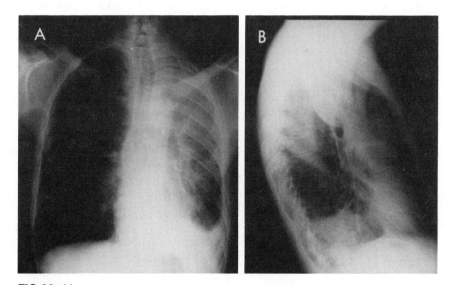

FIG 32–11.
A, a mass is present in the left hilar area obstructing the left upper lobe bronchus. There is atelectasis of the left upper lobe and lingula secondary to the malignancy. **B,** the lateral view reveals an S-shaped curve of tumor mass and atelectasis.

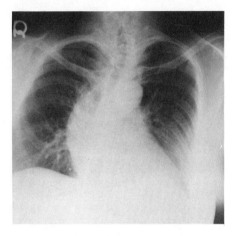

FIG 32–12.
This chest x-ray of a kyphoscoliotic patient reveals a markedly abnormal, reverse S-shaped curve of the thoracic spine deforming the mediastinal structures and ribs. This patient is breathing primarily with her diaphragms.

is associated with cardiomegaly (enlargement of cardiac silhouette) and may be associated with pleural effusions and/or pericardial effusions (Fig 32–10).

Pulmonary malignancies may be both primary and metastatic. Mass formation is characteristic and there may be atelectasis when the mass obstructs a bronchus (Fig 32–11). Secondary findings such as widening of the mediastinum, rib metastasis, pleural masses and/or pleural fluid, and encasement of vasculature with hyperlucency beyond may be seen. Alveolar cell carcinoma may appear like a pneumonia. Involvement of the phrenic nerve may result in paralysis of the diaphragm with elevation.

Thoracic deformities such as kyphoscoliosis may severely impair the respiration of an individual (Fig 32–12). The abnormal shape and direction of the spine interfere with the leverage necessary for movement of the ribs with respiration. Severe impairment of respiration may occur when there is fusion of the articulating facets in rheumatoid arthritis of the spine. A very fat individual (medically termed a *Pickwickian*) may have severe difficulty with respiration not only due to the excess fat and weight on the thorax but also because of the increased load on the cardiovasculature system which may result in congestive failure.

REFERENCES

Periodicals

Johnson TH, Gajaraj A, Feist JH: Vascular key to diagnosis of pulmonary interstitial disease. *Am J Roentgenol Radium Ther Nucl Med* 1971; 113:518.

Books

Felson B: *Fundamentals of Chest Roentgenology* ed 2. Philadelphia, WB Saunders Co, 1973.

Fraser RG, Pare JA: *Diagnosis of Diseases of the Chest.* Philadelphia, WB Saunders Co, 1970.

Meschan I: *An Atlas of Normal Radiographic Anatomy.* Philadelphia, WB Saunders Co, 1965.

Meschan I: *Synopsis of Analysis of Roentgen Signs in General Radiology.* Philadelphia, WB Saunders Co, 1976.

Paul LW, Juhl JH: *The Essentials of Roentgen Interpretation,* ed 3. New York, Paul B Hober Inc, 1972.

33

Case Studies: Clinical Application of Chest Physical Therapy

Ludi Isaac, B.S.N., R.N.

Mary Mathews, B.S., R.N., C.C.R.N., R.R.T.

In the previous chapters, patient assessment and treatment techniques were described. Each patient must be seen as an individual with an individually tailored treatment program planned to meet his or her needs.

The following case studies are meant to help in the clinical application of chest PT. There are a variety of patient cases from surgical, medical, pediatric, and geriatric units. First, a schematic will be demonstrated as a guide for treatment planning. Then, in each case, specific considerations and precautions will be discussed. Finally, a treatment plan will be presented. Obviously, the treatment plan will not be limited to only the therapy suggested. It is meant as a guideline or minimum treatment plan. For example, in a surgical patient with atelectasis, bronchial hygiene and positional rotation are done predominantly to clear the atelectasis. However, later, ambulation, breathing exercise, and chest mobilization may be indicated. If the patient is prone to chronic increased mucus secretion and frequently has pneumonia or atelectasis, a home program will be given.

PROBLEM-SOLVING MODEL (From Maureen Fogel Perlstein)

There are six steps involved in a problem-solving model: (1) evaluation, (2) defining the problem, (3) determining the goals, (4) identifying appropriate techniques, (5) application of techniques, and (6) reevaluation.

Step 1: Evaluation

This is the process of gathering both objective and subjective information. Objective information may be obtained from the patient's chart, including history, physical exam, x-ray reports, lab data, and progress notes. Additional objective data are collected during the therapist's examination of the patient. These data include respiratory rate, pattern of breathing, exercise tolerance, chest auscultation, cough evaluation, and sputum examination.

During the initial session, the therapist is also able to obtain subjective information from an alert, cooperative patient. He should ask questions such as: Is it difficult for you to breathe? Are you able to cough? Do you cough up any mucus? Almost all patients complain of increased incisional pain with coughing. So, rather than asking, "Does your incision hurt when you cough?," the therapist may ask, "Does your pain medication make it easier for you to cough?" or "Can you cough better after you take your pain pill (shot)?" An occupational and smoking history may also be obtained at this time if such information is lacking from the history taken on admission (see Chapter 6 on evaluation).

Step 2: Defining the Problem

From the above information, a specific problem or problems are defined that answer the question: How is the patient's illness affecting his pulmonary status? The physician's prescription should answer this question in a broad sense. For example, a patient's diagnosis may be right lower lobe atelectasis following coronary artery bypass surgery. It is within the therapist's area of expertise to define more specific problems such as decreased right basal expansion, poor cough, interruption of the mucociliary escalator due to inadequate humidification, retained secretions, and immobility due to muscular weakness.

Step 3: Determining Goals

As with peanuts, so also with questions; one always leads to another. The next question to be answered is: With the skills of chest physical therapy and respiratory therapy, what goals can you help the patient to achieve? Logically, the answer should be to treat the problems defined in Step 2. Consider, for example, the following goals for the patient with right lower lobe atelectasis: (1) improve right lateral basal expansion; (2) improve cough effectiveness; (3) improve humidification to restore the mucous blanket to promote expectoration; (4) mobilize secretions; and (5) prevent venous stasis.

Step 4: Identifying Appropriate Techniques

Determine which techniques are appropriate to achieve the goals set in Step 3. Techniques should be specific to goals.

1. Breathing exercises to improve right lateral basal expansion.

2. Postural drainage, percussion and vibration to mobilize secretions.

3. Cough instruction and/or stimulating a cough to improve cough effectiveness.

4. The use of ultrasonic nebulizer or heated aerosol to restore the mucous blanket.

5. Range of motion exercises to prevent venous stasis.

6. Discussion and suggestions to the nursing staff on appropriate positional rotations and simple exercises that can be done with the patient. This would provide continuity of care and prevent the accumulation of secretions. In many hospitals, the therapist's suggestions may be incorporated into the nursing care plans or cardex.

Step 5: Application of Techniques

Only after obtaining and processing the above information should chest physical therapy techniques be applied to the patient. During the treatment session, the therapist must monitor the patient carefully for changes in vital signs, color of mucous membranes, complaints of dyspnea, nausea, dizziness, or intolerance due to pain. Specific techniques will be discussed later in this chapter.

Step 6: Reevaluation

The therapist should continually reevaluate the patient's progress. This process includes writing initial and additional notes whenever there is a significant change in the patient's condition, or at least once a week. As the patient's condition changes, goals will also change and techniques will be updated. For example, two days after initiating treatment, the patient's right lower lobe atelectasis is resolving as determined by chest auscultation, x-ray, temperature, and amount and color of sputum. The goal now is to upgrade the patient's exercise tolerance through simple strengthening exercises and gradual ambulation.

SURGICAL CASES

Case 1. Mr. Jones is a 65-year-old white male with a right upper lobe adenocarcinoma. He underwent a right upper lobectomy. He has 35-packs per year history of smoking and hypertension.
Preoperative blood work count normal; ABG showed hypoxemia corrected by O_2 at 2 L/min; bone scan normal; chest x-ray, right upper lobe mass.

Two days postop, right upper lobectomy, the patient's temperature was 102° F, auscultation revealed diminished bibasilar breath sounds. Chest tubes were in place on the right, functioning without a leak, no subcutaneous emphysema. Chest tube drainage is small amount serous fluid. Patient tends to splint and lean toward his incision. Cough effort is poor and nonproductive. It is at this time chest PT is ordered.

USING THE PROBLEM-SOLVING MODEL

Step 1: Evaluation

Special consideration preop was baseline hypoxemia. If the patient was already on oxygen preop, his postop course may be more difficult. He may retain secretions that could cause increased shunting and consequently decreases the Po_2. He will be at higher risk for postop problems and will be a priority patient.

We did not receive an order preop, so we can not compare our assessments. Postop, he has decreased breath sounds and is febrile to 102° F. We know most postop temperatures are due to respiratory problems. He is splinting toward his incision. His cough is poor and unproductive. His cough effort is weak, but contributing factors are pain and dehydration of the respiratory mucosa (preop fluids are held from 12 midnight the night before surgery). Fluids are carefully replaced postoperatively, but patient's respiratory mucosa tends to be dehydrated. The patient may not be drinking much water and secretions are thick. Pain seems to be a limiting factor.

Step 2: Defining the Problem

The patient is febrile, postop he coughs poorly and is unproductive; breath sounds decreased at bases, splinting from pain, will not want to lie on right side due to incision and right chest tube; consequently, left lung problems with retained secretions.

Step 3: Determining Goals

To reduce temperature by mobilizing secretions, improve cough effectiveness, improve breathing mechanics.

Step 4: Identify Appropriate Techniques

Mobilize secretions. Postural drainage both lower lobes with percussion and vibration.

Improve posture. Promote symmetry, encourage proper positioning.

Pain. Coordinate pain medication prior to chest PT treatment.

Decreased chest mobility. Breathing exercise—segmental lateral costal breathing exercise. Incentive spirometry, in sitting and sidelying positions. Range of motion exercise to right shoulder. Poor cough—encourage allowable fluid intake, wet mouth, teach incisional support, cough techniques.

Step 5: Application of Technique

Step 6: Reevaluation

Follow patient's clinical course when the patient is afebrile, able to be responsible for positioning self, and performing deep breathing exercises independently; chest x-ray has cleared, and breath sounds have improved; he may be discontinued from bronchial hygiene treatment. Active exercise encouraged gradually increasing ambulation; chest mobilization by active upper extremity exercises postdischarge.

Case 2. Mr. Ynot is a 55-year-old male patient with admitting diagnosis of descending abdominal aortic aneurysm. He has a history of hypertension. S/P ABG one year prior to admission. During that hospitalization he developed infiltrates postoperatively. Chest PT order received preoperatively. Breath sounds clear, fair chest wall mobility, patient anxious as he had difficulty postop previous admission; 48 hours postop—poor cough effort; decreased chest wall mobility; febrile temperature 101.6°F; decreased inspiratory effort; breath sounds upper airway transmitted noise, rales left lower lobe area; complaining of pain.

Step 1: Evaluation

Patient seen preop, breath sounds normal; anxious, previously had respiratory distress postoperatively. S/p aneurysm repair, febrile, decreased inspiratory effort and cough. Fair physical condition, does not exercise at home, fair exercise tolerance.

Step 2: Defining the Problem

High-risk surgical patient with history of pulmonary problems postop. CV status needs monitoring due to history of hypertension. Aggressive bronchial hygiene and breathing exercise, early mobilization.

Step 3: Determining Goals

Treat following pain medication; need breathing exercises to improve chest mobility; encourage support of incision; early mobilization; hydration; make sure patient doesn't Valsalva (breathhold).

Step 4: Identify Appropriate Techniques

Pain medication prior to treatment; postural drainage both lower lobes in modified flat bed position secondary to hypertension, percussion, and vibration; lateral costal breathing exercise; general exercise upper extremities done gently and bilaterally; posture correction; ambulation.

Step 5: Reevaluation

When patient is afebrile, chest x-ray and breath sounds clear, and patient is ambulating, acute treatment may be discontinued. Recommend joining cardiac rehab group postdischarge.

MEDICAL CASES

Case 1. Patient is a 55-year-old male admitted to MICU, s/p anterior wall myocardial infarction (AWMI), having atrial and ventricular arrhythmias. He has a 120-pack year smoking history. Three days post-MI the patient developed an episode of low blood pressure and increased shortness of breath. Chest x-ray suggestive of congestive heart failure (CHF) and pulmonary edema. Subsequently patient developed respiratory failure and was placed on a ventilator. The endotracheal tube was suctioned frequently, and a large amount of frothy white secretions was obtained. After 48 hours on the ventilator the patient's temperature spiked to 102° F. The chest x-ray revealed a left lower lobe infiltrate. Copious yellow thick secretions were suctioned. Breath sounds demonstrated rales/ronchi in left lower lobe area.

Step 1: Evaluation

Unstable patient with recent MI developed respiratory failure, ventilated, now developed a left lower lobe infiltrate.

Step 2: Defining the Problem

Cardiovascular status is a special consideration in patient with recent MI with atrial and ventricular arrhythmias. Copious secretions will be primary consideration.

Step 3: Determining Goals

Mobilize secretions; when lungs clear, facilitate weaning; promote exercise as patient becomes stable to prevent deconditioning.

Step 4: Select Appropriate Techniques

Postural drainage with emphasis to left lower lobe—modified bed flat (as arrhythmias improve and the infarction resolves, use Trendelenburg) with percussion and vibration; frequent suctioning to promote airway clearance; graded exercise to tolerance; refer to cardiac rehab program.

Step 5: Applying Techniques

Step 6: Reevaluation

Become more aggressive with therapy as patient's condition stabilizes. Encourage exercise to tolerance as cardiopulmonary status improves.

Case 2. Patient is a 69-year-old woman with COPD. She complains of increased shortness of breath and loose, nonproductive cough. Afebrile on auscultation, bilateral rales, rhonchi, and expiratory wheezing. Patient is on bronchodilators and chronic low-dose steroids.

Step 1: Evaluation

Patient with COPD experiencing increased SOB; assessment reveals airway secretions.

Step 2: Defining the Problem

SOB probably secondary to increased secretions in woman with COPD. Would be helpful to do chest PT after bronchodilators. Percussion can trigger bronchospasm in patients with asthma. In patient that is SOB, would benefit to have maximum bronchodilation prior to treatment.

Step 3: Determining Goals

Promote airway clearance; encourage relaxation and breathing exercise; encourage exercise to promote airway clearance.

Step 4: Identifying Appropriate Techniques

Postural drainage, modify initially until less SOB; then Trendelenberg with percussion and vibration, gently due to long-term steroids therapy. Emphasis on both lower lobes as no specific area of pathology. Patient will tend to sit up due to SOB so lower lobes will be involved.

Relaxation exercises for upper chest and neck, abdominal areas; teach home postural drainage; good candidate for pulmonary rehabilitation; should have exercise test; evaluate O_2 saturation with exercise—patient may need O_2.

Step 5: Apply Techniques

Step 6: Reevaluation

Will wait until secretions are mobilized and patient is breathing more effectively and relaxed before starting exercise program. Progress slowly as patient is deconditioned. Encourage patient to remain active to prevent loss of therapy gains.

NEONATE

Case 1. Patient is a 28-week premature infant. Birth weight was 1,040 gm. Patient is intubated and on ventilator for respiratory distress in isolette. Chest x-ray shows RUL atelectasis. Ultrasound shows intracranial bleeding.

Step 1: Evaluation

Unstable premature baby on ventilator with intracranial bleeding has RUL atelectasis.

Step 2: Defining the Problem

Ventilated baby needs CPT to clear RUL atelectasis. Do not put babies with intracranial bleeding in Trendelenburg. Other special considerations: all areas treated in neonates; no percussion due to low birth weight.

Step 3: Goals of Treatment

Reexpand RUL atelectasis; treat all areas; watch for bleeding with handling or suctioning; suction airways, oxygenate before, during, and after; watch for cyanosis (not an early sign of hypoxia) and bradycardia.

Step 4: Select Appropriate Treatment

Postural drainage to all lobes with emphasis on right upper lobe; modify to flat bed secondary to ICB, no percussion secondary low birth weight; vibrations 20 times in each position; may instill very small amounts of normal saline solution to thin secretions and suction to keep tiny ET tubes clear using 0.2–0.3 cc.

Step 5: Apply Techniques

Step 6: Reevaluation

Follow chest x-rays for improvement; as weight increases above 1,200 gm, can consider also using percussion; home program shown to family consisting of bronchial hygiene and infant stimulation programs.

CYSTIC FIBROSIS

Case 1. The patient is a 10-year-old female admitted with a diagnosis of cystic fibrosis. On admission, the child was SOB, febrile to 101° F and produced large amounts of thick green mucus. The PFTs revealed severe obstructive and restrictive lung disease. On auscultation, there was decrease in air entry with rales and rhonchi present in all lung fields.

Step 1: Defining the Problem

Chronic patient being admitted acutely with increased SOB and secretions, febrile, probably has pulmonary infection. Need to consider treating initially; before patient goes home, patient should assume responsibility for bronchial hygiene treatments and be involved in an exercise regime.

Step 2: Determining Goals

Mobilization of secretions; relaxation and breathing exercises (pursed lip breathing as well); chest mobilization; home program by patient; exercise program.

Step 3: Select Appropriate Technique

Postural drainage with percussion and vibration; breathing exercise—diaphragmatic and active chest mobilization; cough facilitation; walking, bicycling; inspiratory resistance exercise.

Step 4: Apply Techniques

Step 5: Reevaluation

Ten-year-old who has been ill may need assistance from mother in CPT treatment (child can learn to do percussion and vibration on all chest surface areas except the posterior chest); need to reinforce child's responsibility for self-treatment; may skip some bronchial hygiene treatments if engaging in heavy exercise, especially with upper extremities and chest wall movement, i.e., jumping jacks, volleyball, basketball, jogging, and swimming; if volume of sputum raised with heavy exercise, similar or larger than with postural drainage.

SUMMARY

The basic treatment techniques can be utilized in a variety of ways. It is important that the outcome goals for the patient be kept in mind as the treatment plan is formulated. As the goals change, the treatment will also vary. Patient education accompanies the treatment, and the patient should be as involved in and participative as possible. In patient with chronic problems, the goal of self-treatment is primary. There should be a smooth transition from therapist treating and teaching the patient to overseeing the patient perform the treatment to being available for questions or consultation.

Index